Lecture Notes in Computer Science 9520

Commenced Publication in 1973
Founding and Former Series Editors:
Gerhard Goos, Juris Hartmanis, and Jan van Leeuwen

More information about this series at http://www.springer.com/series/7407

Roberto Moreno-Díaz · Franz Pichler
Alexis Quesada-Arencibia (Eds.)

Computer Aided Systems Theory – EUROCAST 2015

15th International Conference
Las Palmas de Gran Canaria, Spain, February 8–13, 2015
Revised Selected Papers

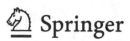 Springer

Editors
Roberto Moreno-Díaz
Universidad de las Palmas de Gran Canaria
Las Palmas de Gran Canaria
Spain

Alexis Quesada-Arencibia
Universidad de las Palmas de Gran Canaria
Las Palmas de Gran Canaria
Spain

Franz Pichler
Johannes Kepler University Linz
Linz
Austria

ISSN 0302-9743   ISSN 1611-3349 (electronic)
Lecture Notes in Computer Science
ISBN 978-3-319-27339-6   ISBN 978-3-319-27340-2   (eBook)
DOI 10.1007/978-3-319-27340-2

Library of Congress Control Number: 2015956351

LNCS Sublibrary: SL1 – Theoretical Computer Science and General Issues

Printed on acid-free paper

This Springer imprint is published by SpringerNature
The registered company is Springer International Publishing AG Switzerland

Preface

The concept of CAST as computer-aided systems theory was introduced by Franz Pichler in the late 1980s to refer to computer theoretical and practical development as tools for solving problems in system science. It was thought of as the third component (the other two being CAD and CAM) required to complete the path from computer and systems sciences to practical developments in science and engineering.

Franz Pichler, of the University of Linz, organized the first CAST workshop in April 1988, which demonstrated the acceptance of the concepts by the scientific and technical community. Next, the University of Las Palmas de Gran Canaria joined the University of Linz to organize the first international meeting on CAST (Las Palmas, February 1989) under the name EUROCAST 89. This proved to be a very successful gathering of systems theorists, computer scientists, and engineers from most European countries, North America, and Japan.

It was agreed that EUROCAST international conferences would be organized every two years, alternating between Las Palmas de Gran Canaria and a continental European location. From 2001 the conference has been held exclusively in Las Palmas. Thus, successive EUROCAST meetings took place in Krems (1991), Las Palmas (1993), Innsbruck (1995), Las Palmas (1997), Vienna (1999), Las Palmas (2001), Las Palmas (2003), Las Palmas (2005), Las Palmas (2007), Las Palmas (2009), Las Palmas (2011) and Las Palmas (2013), in addition to an extra-European CAST conference in Ottawa in 1994. Selected papers from these meetings were published as Springer's *Lecture Notes in Computer Science* volumes 410, 585, 763, 1030, 1333, 1798, 2178, 2809, 3643, 4739, 5717, 6927, 6928, 8111, and 8112 and in several special issues of *Cybernetics and Systems: An International Journal*. EUROCAST and CAST meetings are definitely consolidated, as has been shown by the number and quality of the contributions over the years.

EUROCAST 2015 took place in the Elder Museum of Science and Technology of Las Palmas, February 8–13, and it continued with the approach tested at previous conferences as an international computer-related conference with a true interdisciplinary character. There were different specialized workshops, which, on this occasion, were devoted to the following topics:

1. Systems Theory and Applications, chaired by Pichler (Linz) and Moreno-Díaz (Las Palmas)
2. Modelling Biological Systems, chaired by Nobile and Di Crescenzo (Salerno)
3. Intelligent Information Processing, chaired by Freire and Castro-Souto (A Coruña)
4. Theory and Applications of Metaheuristic Algorithms, chaired by Affenzeller and Jacak (Hagenberg) and Raidl (Vienna)
5. Computer-Based Methods and Virtual Reality for Clinical and Academic Medicine, chaired by Rozenblit (Tucson), Klempous (Wroclaw), and Suárez-Araujo (Las Palmas)

6. Mobile and Autonomous Transportation Systems, chaired by González, Godoy, and Villagrá (Madrid)
7. Signals and Systems in Electronics, chaired by Huemer (Linz), Lunglmayr (Klagenfurt), and Jungwirth (Wels)
8. Traffic Behavior, Modelling and Optimization, chaired by Avineri (Tel Aviv), Paz (Las Vegas), Rossetti (Porto), Rubio-Royo and Sánchez-Medina (Las Palmas)
9. Computer Vision, Sensing, Image and Medical Images Processing and Visualization; Image Processing, chaired by Penedo (A Coruña) and Llorca (Madrid)
10. Model-Based System Design, Verification and Simulation, chaired by Ceska (Brno) and Nikodem (Wroclaw)
11. Digital Signal Processing Methods and Applications, chaired by Astola (Tampere), Moraga (Dortmund), and Stankovic (Nis)
12. Modelling and Control of Robots, chaired by Müller and Gattringer (Linz)
13. Mobile Computing Platforms and Technologies, chaired by Mayrhofer and Holzmann (Austria)
14. Process Modelling and Simulation, chaired by Grossmann and Rinderle Ma (Vienna)
15. Cloud and Other Computing Systems, chaired by Schwartzel (Munich)
16. Marine Sensors and Manipulators, chaired by Khatib (Stanford), Kruusmaa (Tallinn), Silva (Porto), and Sosa (Las Palmas)

In this conference, as in previous ones, most of the credit for the success is due to the chairs of the workshops. They and the sessions chairs, with the counseling of the International Advisory Committee, selected from 161 initially presented papers, after oral presentations and subsequent corrections, the 107 revised papers included in this volume.

The event and this volume were possible thanks to the efforts of the chairs of the workshops in the selection and organization of all the material. The editors would like to express their acknowledgement to all contributors and participants and to the invited speakers, Milan Ceska from Brno, Teresa de Pedro from Madrid, and Harmut Bremer from Linz, for their readiness to collaborate. We would also like to thank the director of the Elder Museum of Science and Technology, D. José Miranda, and the members of the museum. Special thanks are due to the staff of Springer in Heidelberg for their valuable support.

September 2015

Roberto Moreno-Díaz
Franz Pichler
Alexis Quesada-Arencibia

Organization

Organized by

Instituto Universitario de Ciencias y Tecnologías Cibernéticas
Universidad de Las Palmas de Gran Canaria, Spain

Johannes Kepler University Linz,
Linz, Austria

Museo Elder de la Ciencia y la Tecnología
Las Palmas de Gran Canaria, Spain

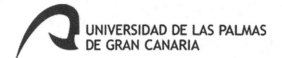

Conference Chair

Roberto Moreno-Díaz, Las Palmas

Program Chair

Franz Pichler, Linz

Honorary Chair

Werner Schimanovich, Austrian Society for Automation and Robotics

Organizing Committee Chair

Alexis Quesada Arencibia
Instituto Universitario de Ciencias y Tecnologías Cibernéticas
Universidad de Las Palmas de Gran Canaria
Campus de Tafira
35017 Las Palmas de Gran Canaria, Spain
Phone: +34-928-457108
Fax: +34-928-457099
e-mail: aquesada@dis.ulpgc.es

Contents

Modelling Biological Systems

Intelligent Information Processing

Theory and Applications of Metaheuristic Algorithms

**Computer Methods, Virtual Reality and Image Processing
for Clinical and Academic Medicine**

Signals and Systems in Electronics

Model-Based System Design, Verification and Simulation

Digital Signal Processing Methods and Applications

Modelling and Control of Robots

Mobile Platforms, Autonomous and Computing Traffic Systems

Cloud and Other Computation Systems

Marine Sensors and Manipulators

Systems Theory and Applications

Which State Feedback Control Laws will not Alter the System's Transfer Function?

Vladimír Kučera$^{(\boxtimes)}$

Institute of Informatics, Robotics and Cybernetics,
Czech Technical University in Prague, Zikova 4, 166 36 Prague, Czech Republic
kucera@ciirc.cvut.cz

Abstract. A parameterization of all state feedback control laws that do not alter the system's transfer function matrix is presented. The problem is recognized as a special case of another problem, the model matching by state feedback. The parameterization is thus obtained by parameterizing a qualified solution set of a linear matrix polynomial equation.

Keywords: Linear systems · State feedback · Transfer function · Model matching

1 Problem Formulation

Given a linear, time-invariant, differential system (A, B, C, D) described by the equations

$$\dot{x}(t) = Ax(t) + Bu(t), \quad y(t) = Cx(t) + Du(t),$$

where $x \in R^n$ is the state, $u \in R^m$ is the input, and $y \in R^p$ is the output of the system. The system gives rise to the $p \times m$ proper rational transfer function matrix

$$T(s) = C(sI - A)^{-1}B + D.$$

We seek to determine any and all state feedback control laws (F, G), with G square and nonsingular, of the form

$$u(t) = Fx(t) + Gv(t),$$

where $v \in R^m$ is an external input, such that the compensated closed-loop system transfer function matrix

$$T_{F,G}(s) := (C + DF)(sI - A - BF)^{-1}BG + DG$$

equals $T(s)$.

This work was supported by the Technology Agency of the Czech Republic under the project TE01020197 Centre for Applied Cybernetics 3.

R. Moreno-Díaz et al. (Eds.): EUROCAST 2015, LNCS 9520, pp. 3–9, 2015.
DOI: 10.1007/978-3-319-27340-2_1

This is a problem of interest in systems and control theory. In applications, such a problem arises when feedback compensation is desirable to improve system's performance without altering its transfer function.

The solution of the problem amounts to determining all pairs (F, G) such that $(A+BF, BG, C+DF, DG)$ is equivalent to (A, B, C, D), that is to say,

$$A + BF = PAP^{-1}, \quad BG = PB, \quad C + DF = CP^{-1}, \quad DG = D$$

holds for some nonsingular matrix P.

This is a difficult problem related to similarity [1] and feedback equivalence [2, 3]. To address the problem from a different point of view, the problem is recognized as a particular case of model matching by regular state feedback in which the model transfer function matrix equals $T(s)$.

2 Model Matching by State Feedback

Model matching is a problem of compensating a given system so as to achieve a specified transfer function matrix.

Given a linear, time-invariant, differential system (A, B, C, D) described by the equations

$$\dot{x}(t) = Ax(t) + Bu(t), \quad y(t) = Cx(t) + Du(t),$$

where $x \in R^n, u \in R^m$, and $y \in R^p$. The system gives rise to the $p \times m$ proper rational transfer function matrix

$$T(s) = C(sI - A)^{-1}B + D.$$

Also given is a proper rational matrix $T_m(s)$, the target model transfer function matrix, of size $p \times r$.

The problem of model matching by state feedback is to determine a control law (F, G) of the form

$$u(t) = Fx(t) + Gv(t),$$

with $v \in R^r$, such that the transfer function matrix of the compensated closed-loop system

$$T_{F,G}(s) := (C+DF)(sI - A - BF)^{-1}BG + DG$$

equals $T_m(s)$.

For our purposes, we shall restrict our attention to the case of regular state feedback, for which $r = m$ and G is square and nonsingular.

Necessary and sufficient conditions for a matching feedback law to exist are well known [4]. Let $N_1(s)$, $D(s)$ be right coprime polynomial matrices such that

$$(sI - A)^{-1}B = N_1(s)D^{-1}(s). \tag{1}$$

Denote

$$N(s) := CN_1(s) + DD(s), \tag{2}$$

so that $T(s) = N(s)D^{-1}(s)$ and suppose that $D(s)$ is column reduced with column degrees $d_1, d_2, \ldots, d_m$. Note that the polynomial matrices $N(s)$, $D(s)$ may not be right coprime. Let $N_m(s)$, $D_m(s)$ be right coprime polynomial matrices such that

$$T_m(s) = N_m(s)D_m^{-1}(s). \tag{3}$$

Then the exact model matching problem is solvable if and only if for some non-singular polynomial matrix $V(s)$ the following conditions hold
(i)

$$N(s) = N_m(s)V(s) \tag{4}$$

(ii) $D_m(s)V(s)$ is column reduced with column degrees $d_1, d_2, \ldots, d_m$.
The matching state feedback law (F, G) that corresponds to a particular matrix $V(s)$ is obtained by solving the polynomial equations (5, 6),

$$XD(s) + YN_1(s) = D_m(s)V(s) \tag{5}$$

for constant matrices X, Y such that X is nonsingular and putting

$$F = -X^{-1}Y, \ G = X^{-1}. \tag{6}$$

Any and all solutions to the exact model matching problem are described [6] by any and all polynomial matrix solutions $V(s)$ to the equation

$$N_m(s)V(s) = N(s)$$

such that the matrix $D_m(s)V(s)$ is nonsingular and column reduced with column degrees equal to those of $D(s)$. The solution matrices are given by

$$V(s) = V_0(s) + K(s)L(s) \tag{7}$$

where $V_0(s)$ is a particular solution, the columns of $K(s)$ form a minimal polynomial basis for the kernel of $N_m(s)$, and $L(s)$ is an arbitrary polynomial matrix.

3 Parameterization of State Feedback Control Laws

The problem under consideration, namely the determination of all feedback control laws that will not alter the system's transfer function matrix, is clearly a particular case of model matching via regular state feedback with the target model transfer function matrix $T_m(s)$ equal to $T(s)$.

Clearly, then, the conditions (i) and (ii) are satisfied. In fact, a particular solution $V_0(s)$ of (4) is provided by a greatest common right divisor of $N(s)$ and $D(s)$. Such a solution will result in the trivial feedback control law $F = 0$, $G = I$. The set of all solutions $V(s)$ parameterized in (7) is then used to parameterize all feedback pairs (F, G) that do not alter $T(s)$.

It is also of interest to solve the model matching problem with the further constraint that the resulting system be stable. Under the proviso that (A, B, C, D) is a stabilizable system and the poles of $T(s)$ are all in the domain $\mathrm{Re}\,s < 0$, the matching state feedback law (F, G) that corresponds to a solution matrix $V(s)$ will stabilize the closed-loop compensated system [6] if and only if $\det V(s)$ is a Hurwitz polynomial, i.e. all of its roots lie within $\mathrm{Re}\,s < 0$.

The stability result may be useful when solving a stable exact model matching problem. Once a match has been found, for example by constructing a cascade compensator, then the system can be stabilized by state feedback without affecting the match.

4 Example

Consider a simple illustrative example.

Given a system (A, B, C, D) described by

$$A = \begin{bmatrix} 1 & 0 \\ 0 & -1 \end{bmatrix}, \quad B = \begin{bmatrix} 0 & 1 & 0 \\ 0 & 0 & 1 \end{bmatrix},$$

$$C = \begin{bmatrix} 0 & 0 \\ 0 & 1 \end{bmatrix}, \quad D = \begin{bmatrix} 1 & 0 & 0 \\ 0 & 1 & 0 \end{bmatrix},$$

which gives rise to the transfer function matrix

$$T(s) = \begin{bmatrix} 1 & 0 & 0 \\ 0 & 1 & \frac{1}{s+1} \end{bmatrix}.$$

We wish to determine in parametric form all state control feedback laws (F, G) with G nonsingular that will not change $T(s)$.

We have the input-to-state transfer function matrix

$$(sI - A)^{-1}B = \begin{bmatrix} 0 & \frac{1}{s-1} & 0 \\ 0 & 0 & \frac{1}{s+1} \end{bmatrix}$$

and calculate the right coprime factors in (1) to be

$$N_1(s) = \begin{bmatrix} 0 & 1 & 0 \\ 0 & 0 & 1 \end{bmatrix}, \quad D(s) = \begin{bmatrix} 1 & 0 & 0 \\ 0 & s-1 & 0 \\ 0 & 0 & s+1 \end{bmatrix}.$$

We obtain the numerator matrix (2) as

$$N(s) = \begin{bmatrix} 1 & 0 & 0 \\ 0 & s-1 & 1 \end{bmatrix}.$$

We further determine a right coprime factorization (3) for $T_m(s)$: $= T(s)$ to be

$$N_m(s) = \begin{bmatrix} 1 & 0 & 0 \\ 0 & 1 & 1 \end{bmatrix}, \quad D_m(s) = \begin{bmatrix} 1 & 0 & 0 \\ 0 & 1 & 0 \\ 0 & 0 & s+1 \end{bmatrix}.$$

The polynomial matrix Eq. (4) admits a particular solution

$$V_0(s) = \begin{bmatrix} 1 & 0 & 0 \\ 0 & s-1 & 0 \\ 0 & 0 & 1 \end{bmatrix}.$$

As a minimal polynomial basis for the kernel of $N_m(s)$ is

$$K = \begin{bmatrix} 0 \\ 1 \\ -1 \end{bmatrix},$$

all solutions (7) to Eq. (4) are of the form

$$V(s) = V_0(s) + \begin{bmatrix} 0 \\ 1 \\ -1 \end{bmatrix} [\alpha(s) \quad \beta(s) \quad \gamma(s)] = \begin{bmatrix} 1 & 0 & 0 \\ \alpha(s) & s-1+\beta(s) & \gamma(s) \\ -\alpha(s) & -\beta(s) & 1-\gamma(s) \end{bmatrix},$$

where $\alpha(s), \beta(s)$, and $\gamma(s)$ are polynomial parameters. Calculate

$$\det V(s) = (1 - \gamma(s))(s - 1) + \beta(s) \tag{8}$$

to see that $V(s)$ will be nonsingular if and only if (8) is a nonzero polynomial. Now

$$D_m(s)V(s) = \begin{bmatrix} 1 & 0 & 0 \\ \alpha(s) & s-1+\beta(s) & \gamma(s) \\ -\alpha(s)(s+1) & -\beta(s)(s+1) & (1-\gamma(s))(s+1) \end{bmatrix}$$

will have column degrees equal to those of $D(s)$, namely 0, 1, 1, if and only if $\alpha(s) = 0$, $\beta(s)$ is an arbitrary constant, and $1 - \gamma(s)$ is a nonzero constant. Note that the resulting matrix

$$D_m(s)V(s) = \begin{bmatrix} 1 & 0 & 0 \\ 0 & s-1+\beta & \gamma \\ 0 & -\beta(s+1) & (1-\gamma)(s+1) \end{bmatrix}$$

is column reduced. Solving (5) for constant matrices X and Y such that X is nonsingular, one obtains

$$X = \begin{bmatrix} 1 & 0 & 0 \\ 0 & 1 & 0 \\ 0 & -\beta & 1-\gamma \end{bmatrix}, \quad Y = \begin{bmatrix} 0 & 0 \\ \beta & \gamma \\ -2\beta & 0 \end{bmatrix}.$$

Then any and all feedback gains that do not alter $T(s)$ are given by (6) as

$$F = \begin{bmatrix} 0 & 0 \\ -\beta & -\gamma \\ -\beta\frac{\beta-2}{1-\gamma} & -\frac{\beta\gamma}{1-\gamma} \end{bmatrix}, \quad G = \begin{bmatrix} 1 & 0 & 0 \\ 0 & 1 & 0 \\ 0 & \frac{\beta}{1-\gamma} & \frac{1}{1-\gamma} \end{bmatrix}.$$

In case we wish to impose the constraint of stability on the compensated system, we note from (8) that

$$\det V(s) = (1-\gamma)s + (\beta+\gamma-1)$$

will be Hurwitz if and only if

$$(1-\gamma)(\beta+\gamma-1) > 0.$$

The compensated closed-loop system will have the eigenvalues -1 and $-\frac{\beta+\gamma-1}{1-\gamma}$.

5   Conclusions

We have parameterized all state feedback control laws that do not alter the system's transfer function matrix by means of parameterizing all solutions of a particular model matching problem. Within this class of control laws, we have identified all stabilizing control laws.

It is clear from (1) that the polynomial matrix $D(s)$ represents the controllable dynamics of the given system and it follows from Eq. (5) that the polynomial matrix $D_m(s)V(s)$ represents the controllable dynamics of the compensated system. The matrix $D_m(s)$ captures the controllable-and-observable dynamics and $V(s)$ describes the controllable-but-unobservable dynamics. While $D_m(s)$ is fixed for all feedback control laws that do not alter $T(s)$, the matrix $V(s)$ describes the degrees of freedom in the compensated system that are cancelled when forming $T(s)$. That is why $V(s)$ plays the key role in the parameterization result and in the ability and/or inability to achieve stable compensated systems.

References

1. Antsaklis, P.J., Michel, A.N.: Linear Systems. Birkhäuser, Boston (2006)
2. Fuhrmann, P.A.: Linear Systems and Operators in Hilbert Space. McGraw-Hill, New York (1981)
3. O'Halloran, J.: Feedback equivalence of constant linear systems. Syst. Control Lett. **8**, 241–246 (1987)
4. Wolovich, W.A.: The use of state feedback for exact model matching. SIAM J. Control **10**, 512–523 (1972)
5. Kučera, V., Zagalak, P.: Constant solutions of polynomial equations. Int. J. Control **53**, 495–502 (1991)
6. Kučera, V., Castañeda Toledo, E.: A review of stable exact model matching by state feedback. In: Proceedings of 22nd Mediterranean Conference on Control and Automation, pp. 85–90, Palermo, Italy (2014)

A Simple Linearisation
of the Self-shrinking Generator

Sara D. Cardell[1]([✉]) and Amparo Fúster-Sabater[2]

[1] Departamento de Estadística e Investigación Operativa,
Universidad de Alicante, Ap. Correos 99, E-03080 Alicante, Spain
s.diaz@ua.es
[2] Instituto de Tecnologías Físicas y de la Información (CSIC),
144, Serrano, 28006 Madrid, Spain
amparo@iec.csic.es

Abstract. Nowadays stream ciphers are the fastest among the encryption procedures, thus they are performed in many practical applications. Irregularly decimated generators are very simple sequence generators to be used as keystream generators in stream ciphers. In this paper, a linearisation method for the self-shrinking generator has been developed. The proposal defines linear structures based on cellular automata (rules 102 or 60) able to generate the self-shrunken sequence. The obtained cellular automata are simple, easy to be implemented and can be extended to other sequence generators in a range of cryptographic interest.

Keywords: Self-shrinking generator · Self-shrunken sequence · Cellular automata · Rule 102 · Rule 60 · Stream cipher · Cryptography

1 Introduction

Symmetric key ciphers are usually split into two large classes: stream and block ciphers depending on whether the encryption function is applied either to each individual bit or to a block of bits, respectively.

At the present moment, stream ciphers are the fastest among the encryption procedures so they are implemented in many technological applications e.g. the encryption algorithm RC4 [1] used in Wired Equivalent Privacy (WEP) as a part of the IEEE 802.11 standards, the encryption function E0 in Bluetooth specifications [2] or the recent proposals HC-128 or Rabbit from the eSTREAM Project [3] that are included in the latest release versions of CyaSSL [4] (open source implementation of the SSL/TLS protocol). In fact, from a short secret key (known only by the two interested parties) and a public algorithm (the sequence generator), stream cipher procedures consist in generating a long sequence, the so-called keystream sequence, of seemingly random bits. For encryption, the sender performs the bit-wise XOR operation among the bits of the plaintext and the keystream sequence. The result is the ciphertext to be sent to the receiver. For decryption, the receiver generates the same keystream, performs the same bit-wise XOR operation between the received ciphertext and the keystream sequence and recovers the original plaintext.

© Springer International Publishing Switzerland 2015
R. Moreno-Díaz et al. (Eds.): EUROCAST 2015, LNCS 9520, pp. 10–17, 2015.
DOI: 10.1007/978-3-319-27340-2_2

Most keystream generators are based on maximal-length Linear Feedback Shift Registers (LFSRs) [5], that is linear structures characterized by their length (the number of memory cells), their characteristic polynomial (the feedback function) and their initial state (the seed or key of the cryptosystem). Their output sequences, the so-called PN-sequences, are combined in a nonlinear way to break their inherent linearity as well as to produce new pseudorandom sequences of cryptographic application. Combinational generators, nonlinear filters, clock-controlled generators, LFSRs with dynamic feedback or irregularly decimated generators are just some of the most popular keystream sequence generators found in the literature [6,7].

Irregularly decimated generators produce good cryptographic sequences [8] characterized by long periods, good self-correlation, excellent run distribution, balancedness, simplicity of implementation, etc. The underlying idea of this kind of generators is the irregular decimation of a PN-sequence according to the bits of another one. The result of this decimation is a binary sequence that will be used as keystream sequence in the cryptographic procedure. A well known design in the class of irregularly decimated generators is the self-shrinking generator proposed by Meier and Staffelbach [9] that includes only one LFSR. A natural extension of this sequence generator is the generalized self-shrinking generator [10] that generates a whole family of cryptographic sequences.

It is a well known fact that some one-dimensional linear cellular automata [11] generate exactly the same PN-sequences as those generated by LFSRs. Therefore, a cellular automata can be considered as an alternative generator to the maximum length LFSRs [12]. Moreover, some keystream generators can be modeled in terms of linear cellular automata. In [13], the authors modeled the self-shrinking generator by using rules 150 and 90. In this work, we model the same generator by using rules 102 and 60. A comparison between both modelings is also provided.

The main contribution of this work is to define one-dimensional linear CA able to generate the self-shrunken sequence. The generation of such a sequence from a linear model simplifies the cryptanalysis of the self-shrinking generator.

2   Fundamentals and Basic Notation

First of all, different features and properties of the two basic structures (self-shrinking generator and linear binary CA) considered in this paper are introduced.

2.1   The Self-shrinking Generator

The **self-shrinking generator** was designed by Meier and Staffelbach [9] for potential use in stream cipher applications. This generator consists of a maximal-length Linear Feedback Shift Register (LFSR) [5] of L stages whose output sequence the PN-sequence $\{a_i\}$ is self-decimated giving rise to the self-shrunken sequence $\{s_j\}$ or output sequence of the self-shrinking generator. This sequence generator is attractive by its simplicity and easy implementation as it involves a unique LFSR. The decimation rule is very simple; let (a_{2i}, a_{2i+1}), with $i = 0, 1, 2, \ldots$, be pairs of consecutive bits of the PN-sequence, then the self-shrunken sequence $\{s_j\}$ is given by:

$$\begin{cases} \text{if } a_{2i} = 1 \text{ then } s_j = a_{2i+1} \\ \text{if } a_{2i} = 0 \text{ then } a_{2i+1} \text{ is discarded} \end{cases}$$

The key of this generator is the initial state of the LFSR. Period, linear complexity and statistical properties of the self-shrunken sequence [9] are very adequate for their application in stream cipher. In brief, the self-shrinking generator is a simplified version of the shrinking generator, suggested by Coppersmith et al. [14], which satisfies the same decimation rule but includes two maximal-length LFSRs.

2.2   Cellular Automata

A one-dimensional **Cellular Automata** (CA) is a device composed by memory cells whose content (binary in this work) is updated according to a state transition rule that determines the new state of each cell in terms of the current state of the cell and the states of the cells in its neighbourhood [11]. In fact, the value of the cell in position i at time $\tau + 1$, notated $x_i^{\tau+1}$, depends on the value of the k neighbour cells at time τ.

The cellular automata considered in this work are **linear** (only XOR operations are used), **regular** (every cell follows the same rule) and **null** (cells with null content are adjacent to extreme cells). In this work, our attention is focused on one-dimensional linear CA with binary contents whose time evolution is determined by two simple linear transition rules: rule 102 and rule 60.

Rule 102: $x_i^{\tau+1} = x_i^{\tau} + x_{i+1}^{\tau}$

111	110	101	100	011	010	001	000
0	1	1	0	0	1	1	0

Rule 60: $x_i^{\tau+1} = x_{i-1}^{\tau} + x_i^{\tau}$

111	110	101	100	011	010	001	000
0	0	1	1	1	1	0	0

Recall that both rules are linear and that just involve the addition of two bits. The numbers 01100110 and 00111100 are the binary representations of 102 and 60, respectively. That is the reason why they are called rule 102 and rule 60.

In Fig. 1, we can see these rules using the notation introduced by S. Wolfram [15], where 1 is represented by a black square and 0 is represented by a white square.

Rule 102   Rule 60

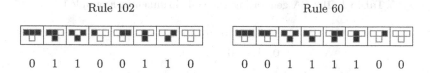

0   1   1   0   0   1   1   0   0   0   1   1   1   1   0   0

Fig. 1. Rules 102 and 60 depicted in Wolfram's notation

3   The Self-shrinking Generator in Terms of Linear CA

In this section, we propose a family of uniform, null, linear CA that generate the self-shrunken sequence. The following facts characterize the linearisation of the shrunken sequence in terms of CA with rules 102 or 60.

Fact 1. Given a positive integer t, the polynomial $p_t(x)$ is defined $p_t(x) = (1+x)^t$ where $p_t(x) = (1+x)\, p_{t-1}(x)$.

Fact 2. The characteristic polynomial of the shrunken sequence generated by a maximal-length LFSR of length L is [16]:

$$p_n(x) = (1+x)^n, \quad 2^{L-2} < n \le 2^{L-1} - (L-2).$$

Fact 3. If the characteristic polynomial of a binary sequence $\{s_i\}$ is $p_n(x)$, then the characteristic polynomial of the sequence $\{u_i\} = \{s_i + s_{i+1}\}$ is $p_{n-1}(x)$.

Fact 4. According to the previous fact, if the first column of a linear CA with rule 102 and length n is the shrunken sequence, then the successive columns of CA will be sequences with characteristic polynomials $p_{n-1}(x), p_{n-2}(x)$, $\ldots, p_2(x)$, $p_1(x)$, respectively, where $p_1(x)$ corresponds to the identically 1 sequence.

Fact 5. A uniform, null, linear CA of length n whose first column is the shrunken sequence defined in fact 2 will generate:

- $n - 2^{L-2}$ sequences of period 2^{L-1},
- 2^{i-1} sequences of period 2^i, for $1 \le i \le L - 2$,
- one sequence of period 1 (the identically 1 sequence).

It is worth noticing that the previous facts also hold for uniform, null, linear CA with rule 60. In this case, the CA provides the same sequences but they are obtained in reverse order. The previous results are illustrated in the following example.

Example 1. Given an LFSR with characteristic polynomial $p(x) = 1+x^3+x^4$ and initial state 1001, the self-shrunken sequence obtained is 01001011, with period 2^3. The characteristic polynomial of this sequence is $p_5(x) = (1+x)^5$. In Table 1, a one-dimensional, uniform, null, linear CA with rule 102 and length 5 is given. Starting at initial state 01011, this CA generates the self-shrunken sequence, in bold, at the first column. It is easy to check that the characteristic polynomials of the remaining sequences are $p_4(x), p_3(x), p_2(x)$ and $p_1(x)$, respectively.

If we consider the same CA of length 5 with rule 60 starting at the symmetric initial state 11010, then the output sequences are the same but they appear in reverse order. See Table 2.

Table 1. 102 CA generating the self-shrunken in Example 1

102	102	102	102	102
0	1	0	1	1
1	1	1	0	1
0	0	1	1	1
0	1	0	0	1
1	1	0	1	1
0	1	1	0	1
1	0	1	1	1
1	1	0	0	1

Table 2. 60 CA generating the self-shrunken in Example 1

60	60	60	60	60
1	1	0	1	**0**
1	0	1	1	**1**
1	1	1	0	**0**
1	0	0	1	**0**
1	1	0	1	**1**
1	0	1	1	**0**
1	1	1	0	**1**
1	0	0	1	**1**

4   90/150 CA Versus 102/60 CA

Now, we compare the linearisation of the self-shrunken sequence in terms of 102/60 CA with that of [13] carried out in terms of 90/150 CA. In [13], the authors proposed CA based on rules 90/150 that generate the self-shrunken sequence. In fact, the rules 90 and 150 can be defined as follows:

$$\textbf{Rule 90: } x_i^{\tau+1} = x_{i-1}^{\tau} + x_{i+1}^{\tau}$$

111	110	101	100	011	010	001	000
0	1	0	1	1	0	1	0

$$\textbf{Rule 150: } x_i^{\tau+1} = x_{i-1}^{\tau} + x_i^{\tau} + x_{i+1}^{\tau}$$

111	110	101	100	011	010	001	000
1	0	0	1	0	1	1	0

As before, the numbers 01011010 and 10010110 are the binary representations of 90 and 150, respectively.

90/150 CA generating the self-shrunken sequence had a defined structure: rule 90 in extreme cells and rule 150 in the intermediate cells. The length of this CA equals the period of the self-shrunken sequence, 2^{L-1}. In Table 3, the same self-shrunken sequence as that of Example 1, in bold at the first column, is generated by means of these rules. See references [17,18] for a more detailed description.

Table 3. 90/150 CA generating the self-shrunken in Example 1

90	150	150	150	150	150	150	90
0	1	1	1	0	0	0	1
1	0	1	0	1	0	1	0
0	0	1	0	1	0	1	1
0	1	1	0	1	0	0	1
1	0	0	0	1	1	1	0
0	1	0	1	0	1	0	1
1	1	0	1	0	1	0	0
1	0	0	1	0	1	1	0

In this work, 102/60 CA generating the self-shrunken sequence have a well defined structure too. At the last column the sequence of 1s appears. Besides, there is always a sequence of period 2 (0101... or 1010...). Next, there are 2 sequences of period 4, 4 sequences of period 8 and so on, until we find 2^{L-3} sequences with period 2^{L-2}. The remaining sequences (the length of the CA minus 2^{L-2}) have period 2^{L-1}, including the self-shrunken sequence.

On the other hand, we know that the linear complexity n of the self-shrunken sequence satisfies $2^{L-2} < n \leq 2^{L-1} - (L - 2)$. Hence the length of these CA, n, is less than 2^{L-1}, the length of the CA proposed in [13]. For example, in order to model the self-shrunken sequence in Example 1, we need CA of length 5 (see Tables 1 and 2). If we use the CA proposed in [13], then we need CA of length 8. This difference is more remarkable as far as the length L of the maximal-length LFSR increases.

5   Application of the CA to the Self-shrinking Generators Cryptanalysis

Assume that n is the linear complexity of the self-shrunken sequence. Given $2n$ intercepted bits, it is possible to recover the characteristic polynomial of the maximal-length LFSR that generates the sequence by means of the Berlekamp-Massey algorithm [19].

In our case, we know that there exist CA that generate the self-shunken sequence as well as that the last sequence for rule 102 is the identically 1 sequence (the first sequence for rule 60 is the identically 1 sequence). Therefore, it is enough to know $n - 1$ bits of the self-shrunken sequence to recover the initial state of the CA and thus, to recover the whole sequence. Notice that this amount is half the needed bits to apply the Berlekamp-Massey algorithm so that the required amount of intercepted bits is reduced by a factor 2.

In Example 1, the self-shrunken sequence had period 8 and linear complexity 5. In Table 4, we can see that intercepting 4 bits of the self-shrunken sequence, we can determine the initial state of the CA and, consequently, the whole self-shrunken sequence.

Table 4. Necessary bits to recover the initial state

102	102	102	102	102
0	1	0	1	1
1	1	1		1
0	0			1
0				1
				1
				1
				1
				1

6 Conclusions

In this work, it is shown that the sequences generated by self-shrinking generators are output sequences of one-dimensional, linear, regular and null cellular automata based on rules 102 and 60. In fact, the linearisation procedure to convert a given self-shrinking generator into the linear cellular model here proposed is quite immediate. It must be noticed that, although the self-shrunken sequences come from PN-sequences irregularly decimated, in practice they can be modeled by means of linear structures. This fact establishes a subtle link between irregular decimation and linearity that as it is shown can be conveniently exploited in cryptanalysis.

A natural extension of this work is the generalization of this procedure to many other cryptographic sequences: (a) The sequences generated by the shrinking generator and the generalized self-shrinking generator as more simple examples of decimation-based keystream generators. (b) The so-called interleaved sequences, as they present very similar structural properties to those of the sequences obtained from irregular decimation generators.

Acknowledgments. The work of the first author was partially supported by Generalitat Valenciana (Spain) with reference APOSTD/2013/081 and by FAPESP with number of process 2015/07246-0. The work of the second author was supported by Ministerio de Ciencia e Innovación (Spain) under Project TIN2014-55325C2-1-R and by Comunidad de Madrid (Spain) under Project CIBERDINE, S2013/ICE3095-CM.

References

1. Paul, G., Maitra, S.: RC4 Stream Cipher and Its Variants. Discrete Mathematics and Its Applications. CRC Press, Taylor & Francis Group, Boca Raton (2012)
2. Bluetooth, Specifications of the Bluetooth system, Version 1.1. http://www.bluetooth.com/
3. eSTREAM, the ECRYPT Stream Cipher Project, Call for Primitives. http://www.ecrypt.eu.org/stream/
4. Yet Another SSL (YASSL). http://www.yassl.com
5. Golomb, S.W.: Shift Register-Sequences. Aegean Park Press, Laguna Hill (1982)
6. Menezes, A.J., et al.: Handbook of Applied Cryptography. CRC Press, Boca Raton (1997)
7. Peinado, A., Fúster-Sabater, A.: Generation of pseudorandom binary sequences by means of LFSRs with dynamic feedback. Math. Comput. Model. **57**(11–12), 2596–2604 (2013)
8. Fúster-Sabater, A.: Linear solutions for irregularly decimated generators of cryptographic sequences. Int. J. Nonlinear Sci. Numer. Simul. **15**(6), 377–385 (2014)
9. Meier, W., Staffelbach, O.: The self-shrinking generator. In: De Santis, A. (ed.) EUROCRYPT 1994. LNCS, vol. 950, pp. 205–214. Springer, Heidelberg (1995)
10. Hu, Y., Xiao, G.: Generalized self-shrinking generator. IEEE Trans. Inf. Theory **50**(4), 714–719 (2004)
11. Das, A.K., Ganguly, A., Dasgupta, A., Bhawmik, S., Chaudhuri, P.P.: Efficient characterisation of cellular automata. IEE Proc. E: Comput. Digit. Tech. **137**(1), 81–87 (1990)
12. Fúster-Sabater, A., Caballero-Gil, P.: Linear solutions for cryptographic nonlinear sequence generators. Phys. Lett. A **369**, 432–437 (2007)
13. Fúster-Sabater, A., Pazo-Robles, M.E., Caballero-Gil, P.: A simple linearization of the self-shrinking generator by means of cellular automata. Neural Netw. **23**(3), 461–464 (2010)
14. Coppersmith, D., Krawczyk, H., Mansour, Y.: The shrinking generator. In: Stinson, D.R. (ed.) CRYPTO 1993. LNCS, vol. 773, pp. 22–39. Springer, Heidelberg (1994)
15. Wolfram, S.: Cellular automata as simple self-organizing system. Caltrech preprint CALT 68–938 (1982)
16. Blackburn, S.R.: The linear complexity of the self-shrinking generator. IEEE Trans. Inf. Theory **45**(6), 2073–2077 (1999)
17. Fúster-Sabater, A., Caballero-Gil, P.: Strategic attack on the shrinking generator. Theoret. Comput. Sci. **409**(3), 530–536 (2008)
18. Caballero-Gil, P., Fúster-Sabater, A., Pazo-Robles, M.E.: Using linear equations to model nonlinear cryptographic sequences. Int. J. nonlinear Sci. Numer. Simul. **11**(3), 165–172 (2010)
19. Massey, J.L.: Shift-register synthesis and BCH decoding. IEEE Trans. Inf. Theory **15**(1), 122–127 (1969)

Systems Theory and Model of Diversification in Building of Information Systems

Cestmir Halbich[1]([⊠]), Vaclav Vostrovsky[2], and Jan Tyrychtr[1]

[1] Faculty of Economics and Management,
Department of Information Technologies,
Czech University of Life Sciences at Prague, Prague, Czech Republic
halbich@pef.czu.cz

[2] Faculty of Economics and Management,
Department of Information Engineering,
Czech University of Life Sciences at Prague, Prague, Czech Republic

Abstract. First the paper characterizes the current situation in the field of building of information systems (IS). It discusses a model based on systems theory which describes some possibilities in diversification of risk in developing of IS. To minimize risk in the process of building information systems it is recommended to use components produced by worldly recognized manufacturers of the highest quality. The main subject of investigation by the present model is to quantify risk and to find the minimum. Finally, the paper mentions the direction for further research of the model described by use of correlations and covariances.

Keywords: Model of diversification in information system · Building of information systems · Minimization of risk

1 Introduction

Information systems appear as critical components in every business and organization, and managers have a fundamental role in the initiation, design and implementation of a new information system. The main goal is to ensure organizational efficiency, effectiveness and profitability. The considered model helps managers to decide how to improve abilities of their information systems. The correct selection of information technology in wide sense plays a key role in modern business information systems. On the other hand human knowledge is based on historical experience. The year 2015 marks the 350th anniversary of the introduction of Philosophical Transactions - the world's first journal dedicated to science. Philosophical Transactions originated the concepts of scientific priority and peer review which, together with archiving and dissemination, provide the model for over 40,000 scientific and technical journals today.

2 Current Situation in Building of Information Systems

At first, we describe the basis of model building. In the real world there are objective laws of physics, for example. Hook's law. The law is named after 17th century British physicist Robert Hooke. He first stated the law in 1660 as a Latin anagram *ceiiinosssttuv*

© Springer International Publishing Switzerland 2015
R. Moreno-Díaz et al. (Eds.): EUROCAST 2015, LNCS 9520, pp. 18–24, 2015.
DOI: 10.1007/978-3-319-27340-2_3

[1]. In the first phase the law verbalized later expressed mathematically in vector form. The generalized form is used using tensor notation. The existence of this law is reflected e.g. to ISO standards describing screws or other fasteners. From the common sense we can say, that the chain is only as strong as its weakest link. This we can consider as an extension of Hook's law. On the other hand, standards dealing with e.g. in the field of information systems security otherwise known as the Information Security Management System (ISMS) family of standards (ISO/IEC 27000 family) [2] are more subjective. They started from common sense and led to so called best practices in field of information systems security. From common sense about chain properties we can derive so called information security chain model, see Finne [3]. Finne created own model as a chain with 12 modules and 80 submodules (lines). He defined his model as a conceptual only. One element of information systems are also people therefore we can also find such analogies systems as in Fig. 1 where the chain model is presented in more visible form. The forces Fmax are limits before breakage of weakest link. This value is exceeding of values from Hook's law. More subjective are models based at the law. In Czech Republic for example the Act no. 181/2014 Coll. on the Cyber Security and on the Amendments of the Related Acts (Cyber Security Law) has been published in the Collection of Laws on August 29, 2014.

It was effective as of January 1, 2015. The model described by these documents are more subjective and react at political requirements. In the paper presented mathematical model is designed in the best possible way. The presented mathematical model is better one than none.

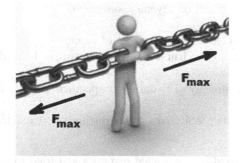

Fig. 1. Visualization of chain model with forces F_{max} (Source: own processing)

3 Proposed Model in Building of Information Systems

When we compare two models, i.e. first traditional model of diversification of investments where this model shows to investors how to combine securities to minimize risk, versus model of diversification of building of information systems, we can say that both models are similar. Many authors consider the desirability of diversification. For example Daniel Bernoulli (1738) in his well-known article about the St. Petersburg Paradox, argues by example that risk averse investors will want to diversify: "… it is advisable to divide goods which are exposed to some small danger into several portions rather than to risk them all together." The following Shakespeare's quote is yet an earlier. In The Merchant of Venice, Act I, Scene I, William Shakespeare has Antonio say:

"…I thank my fortune for it,
My ventures are not in one bottom trusted,
Nor to one place; nor is my whole estate
Upon the fortune of this present year…"

Although this turns out to be a mistaken security in the Shakespeare's comedy, Antonio rests easy at the beginning of the play because he is diversified across ships, places and time.

The fundamental problem of traditional model of diversification investment lies in the fact that for the estimation of future data we use data from the past (it certainly can work, but it does not have to). That was why, in the history of investment theory to many attempts to alleviate this deficiency - e.g. by help of newer theories of risk diversification for example the so called post-modern portfolio theory [4], etc. Markowitz [4] created his model on the basis of historical monitoring data specific securities and therefore interpret real data. The compilation of the portfolio consists of two parts. First, you need to get the data (and the various observations) and use them to express expectations of future developments, and consequently it is necessary to select a suitable portfolio. Markowitz theory deals only with the selection of the portfolio and anticipates that expectations obtained in the first step are correct and can be taken as a given value.

Markowitz model is based on several assumptions:

- Investor has frontloaded a certain amount of capital,
- a predetermined time period in which the investment is made (considering one period model)
- passive investment strategy (i.e. during a specified period, the structure of the portfolio unchanged)
- the investor pursues two objectives - maximizing the (expected) return and minimize portfolio risk.

If an investor followed only expected revenues and tried to maximize this model would not lead to diversification, because the investor would always invested all the funds into assets with the highest expected return. Similarly, if the investor is trying simply to minimize risk by investing any funds to assets with the lowest risk.

While watching both goals (maximizing revenues and minimizing risk) has been mostly a portfolio diversification. For the calculations, it is important the last of assumptions:

$$r_\mathrm{p} \to \max \quad \sigma_\mathrm{p} \to \min$$

where r_p is the asset return and σ_p is the risk of changes in the profitability of the asset return.

These two objectives are contradictory to one solution and it is necessary to express the investor's attitude to risk. This problem can be formulated in various ways.

The basic idea of the Markowitz's model lay in the fact that by help of the central limit theorem it can be proved (the proof is trivial and general) that risk can be minimized when we invest into securities. Markowitz defined a number of risks, unfortunately some of these risks cannot be minimized. The model best minimizes the risk if the purchased securities are independent, it means that their coefficient covariance, correlation is zero. This fact is known at the time of purchase of securities and the entire history of the data we have on the stock market, but may not apply in the future. Securities will become addicted possibly longer time after the purchase. The reasons are numerous, for example companies go through fusion, some sectors suffer crisis, a perfect substitute of key product of the company emerges, the crisis of the entire economy etc. There are plenty of possible events and adverse scenarios. On the other hand the proposed model was created by analogy from the Markowitz's model.

The proposed model is focused on future investments in the area of building of information systems generally and on future investments in the area of information systems security specifically. Historical data are usually mostly known (in many cases there are time series longer than ten years, which is often in the field of information technologies close to eternity due the rapid development of these technologies.) The Markowitz's model was focused at only one risk - future income of purchased securities and the only one functionality - profit from the transactions. In proposed model, we have essentially infinite number of risks fortunately with different importance, so that a wide range of minor risks can be neglected.

Consider N risky assets with random return vector R_{i+1} and a risk-free asset with known return R_i. Define the excess returns $r_{i+1} = R_{i+1} - R_i$ and denote their conditional means (or risk premium) and covariance matrix by μ_i and $\sum_i$ respectively. Assume, for now, that the excess returns are i. i. d. with constant moments.

Suppose our investor can only allocate wealth to the N risky security measures to improve security of his information system. Of course each proposed measure improves security of his information system in different way with different investments. In the absence of a risk-free asset, the mean–variance problem is to choose the vector of portfolio weights x, which represent the investor's relative allocations of wealth to each of the N risky measures, to minimize the variance of the resulting portfolio return $R_{p,\ i+1} = x'R_{i+1}$ for a predetermined target expected return of the portfolio $R_i + \mu$.

Consider a project of building an IS with n different assets where asset number i will give the return R_i. Let μ_i and σ_i^2 be the corresponding mean and variance and let $\sigma_{i,j}$ be the covariance between R_i and R_j. Suppose the relative weighting coefficients of the value of the portfolio invested in asset i is x_i. If R is the return of the whole project then proposed model is described by next equations (Table 1 and Fig. 2).

$$\mu = \mathrm{E}[R] = \sum_{i=1}^{n} \mu_i x_i$$

$$\sigma^2 = \mathbf{Var}[R] = \sum_{i=1}^{n} \sum_{j=1}^{n} \sigma_{i,j} x_i x_j$$

$$\sum_{i=1}^{n} x_i = 1$$

$$x_i \geq 0, \quad i = 1, 2, \ldots n$$

Table 1. Example for investments to two security measures (Source: own computation)

Investment into security measure	A	B
Started price	1.00	1.00
1. month	1.05	1.16
2. month	1.08	1.12
3. month	1.04	1.08
4. month	1.09	1.00
5. month	1.01	1.06
6. month	1.11	1.00
7. month	1.00	1.16
8. month	1.10	0.90
The ratio of investments	0.50	0.50

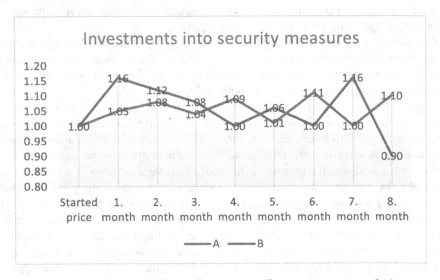

Fig. 2. Investments into security measures (Source: own computation)

From a simple view is seen that the selected investments are in their development to a large extent contradictory. This means that when one decreases, the second growing. To demonstrate the proposed model, this contradiction is necessary. If we examine the values obtained as shown in Table 2, we find that the correlation between examined investments is −0.67 which indicates a strong negative relationship. An important fact

Table 2. Indikators of risk and portfolio performance (Source: own computation)

Covariance	−21.75
Portfolio risks	5.09
Risk A	3.87
Risk B	8.43
(Risk A + Risk B)/2	6.15
Correlation	−0.67
Average return	0.06
Return A	6.0 %
Return B	6.0 %
Total return	6.0 %

is that both generate the same income investments. Proceeds individual investments as well as the portfolio is therefore the same. This is of course in reality difficult to reach, but here for illustration appropriate. The risk of individual investments to security measures are 3.87 and 8.43 (measured by standard deviation). At any given representation as shown in Table 2, we achieved risk 5.09, which is better than the average of individual risk 6.15 (at the same rate of return of the portfolio).

The proposed model allows two possible risky solutions select risk with less correlation to the whole system. Any other solution is less optimal. In the model we consider e.g. the risk of information system performance, safety (for example - time to repair security holes, frequency and severity of errors in the past (does not apply in the future)), price risk - whether the so-called freeware or closed software total cost of ownership (TCO) and return on investment (ROI). In the model, the partial risks modified used weights. The weighting coefficients mentioned above, we find by Saaty's method using the weights of criteria. The importance of the characteristics or sub-characteristics of quality defined by the ISO 9126 standard depends on a certain IS in proposed model. We wrote that Finne created own model as a chain with 12 modules and 80 submodules (lines). This describes complexity of the observed domain. On the other hand Thomas [6] writes that in a portfolio the unique risk normally diminishes strongly with the first 15–20 stocks included.

Then, the model is described in more details here [7]. In terms of risk diversification model very nicely often comes the so-called Open Source Software (OSS) because it reduces their risk through diversification. If you buy one mighty powerful but closed information system, the risk is not diversified at all. TCO and ROI of the past may be optimal, but in the future may discover new requirements that the system will not be able to meet (and it need not meet it even in distant future or only in the new version, the purchase of substantially worsen TCO and ROI). When I need to change one particular procedure - for closed software it is impossible. On the other hand, in the OSS it is possible. In other example the supplier goes bankrupt or will be imposed an embargo on the export of this product in certain countries where we export our products assembled like. There are other future risks. In both the above cases, the choice of OSS and this way of risk diversification is beneficial. In good example to use instead of a whole range of complex software less complex or in the limiting case of single purpose, which data among themselves gradually transmit and receive at the output IS exactly what data we need. In this case if the above mentioned risks, the candidate method for risk diversification software development minimizes these risks. If there are new requirements to run the IS, it is just added to a dedicated software or we write new software that complements the functionality needed.

4 Conclusion

The proposed model helps decrease general risks in field of building of information systems generally and in field of information systems specifically. The model is based on diversification of risks in this problem domain by means of diversification of objects and subjects in built information systems. The model allows two possible risky solutions to select risk with less correlation to the whole system. Any other solution is less optimal. In further studies weighting coefficients and values of correlations and covariances will be searched which can better describe the model.

Acknowledgments. This work was supported by a grant of the Czech University of agriculture at Prague, Faculty of economics and management, project number: IGA PEF 20141040

References

1. Petroski, H.: Invention by Design: How Engineers Get from Thought to Thing, p. 11. Harvard University Press, Cambridge (1996). ISBN 0674463684
2. ISO 27000: 2014 Information technology — security techniques — information security management systems - overview and vocabulary
3. Finne, T.: The information security chain in a company. Comput. Secur. 15(4), 297–316 (1996)
4. Markowitz, H.M.: Portfolio Selection: Efficient Diversification of Investments. Wiley, New York (1959). (reprinted by Yale University Press, 1970)
5. Rom, B.M., Ferguson, K.: A software developer's view: using post-modern portfolio theory to improve investment performance measurement. Managing Downside Risk in Financial Markets: Theory, Practice and Implementation. Butterworth-Heinemann Finance, Oxford (2001)
6. Thomas, L.C.: Financial risk management models. In: Ansell, J., Wharton, F. (eds.) Risk Analysis, Assessment and Management. Wiley, Chichester (1992)
7. Halbich, C.: Patent application PV 2014 involvement to increase the reliability of systems – in Czech language. Industrial Property Office Prague (2014)

Time Sub-Optimal Control of Triple Integrator Applied to Real Three-Tank Hydraulic System

Pavol Bisták[(⊠)]

Slovak University of Technology in Bratislava,
Ilkovičova 3, 812 19 Bratislava, Slovakia
Pavol.Bistak@stuba.sk
http://uamt.fei.stuba.sk

Abstract. Control of nonlinear systems with input constraints is an interesting topic of control theory that must be solve adequately because of the presence of constraints in almost each real system. There are many authors and several techniques trying to solve this problem (anti-windup structures, positive invariant sets, variable structure systems, global, semi-global and local stabilization of systems with constraints, optimization problems solved by linear matrix inequalities).

This paper shows a different approach that originates in the time optimal control and is improved by decreasing the sensitivity to uncertain model parameters that is balanced by sub-optimality. The design of constrained controller is carried out on the triple integrator system and this is later applied to the nonlinear three-tank hydraulic system after its exact linearization.

Keywords: Input constraints · Time sub-optimal control · Nonlinear systems · Exact linearization · Computer algebra system

1 Introduction

The optimal control belongs to the basic study field of the control engineering. Its serious development started in 50-ties of the previous century and in 60-ties it was further worked out by many famous scientists (see [1] and references therein). The aim of the optimal control is to minimize or maximize given criteria under existing constraints. For instance, the time optimal control minimizes the time necessary to reach a desired state when the control value or the states values are limited. Using Pontryagin's Maximum Principle [8] many optimality problems have been theoretically solved. The disadvantage of the optimal control is given by its high sensitivity to model uncertainties, parametric variations, disturbances and noise always presented in real systems. This was also the reason why later the optimal control has been suppressed by pole assignment control.

The idea of the pole assignment control consists in the introduction of a desired dynamics into control circuits. The choice of poles can slow responses and so the sensitivity can be decreased to the level acceptable also in real systems. The problem of the pole assignment control in real applications is determined

© Springer International Publishing Switzerland 2015
R. Moreno-Díaz et al. (Eds.): EUROCAST 2015, LNCS 9520, pp. 25–32, 2015.
DOI: 10.1007/978-3-319-27340-2_4

by the linear character of this method that has been not designed to respect nonlinear elements in a control circuit such as constraints of inputs or states. In order to keep the stability and quality of control the resulting responses are often over-damped.

There exist several methods that are able to cope with input and state constraints. A practical solution is to extend the linear control circuit by an anti-windup structure that will keep the circuit in desired states. Another possibility is to construct positive invariant sets where the states and control are within the specified interval [4]. Also variable structure systems represent the method that is able to respect constraints. Other methods solve global, semi-global and local stabilization of systems with constraints and many optimization problems can be solved by linear matrix inequalities [2,5].

This paper combines the qualities of the time optimal control with the decreased sensitivity of the "slow" pole assignment control that results in the design of a time sub-optimal controller that is fast enough but it respects given constraints. Similar design methods have been developed for lower order systems in [6]. In [9] the sub-optimal controller has been applied to the triple integrator and in [3] a simplified version of it has been applied to the simulated hydraulic system. The main contribution of this paper consists in application of the previously designed sub-optimal controller to the real system that shows the sophisticated theory can be successfully applied in practice.

The paper is organized in six chapters. After introduction the problem is stated in the second chapter. The third chapter offers analysis in the phase space after applying nonlinear decomposition. The fourth chapter shows possible explicit solutions for the time sub-optimal control algorithm. Its application to the three-level hydraulic system can be found in the fifth chapter and the paper is finished by short conclusions.

2   Problem Statement

Consider a linear system of the third order representing the triple integrator

$$\dot{\mathbf{x}} = \mathbf{A}\mathbf{x} + \mathbf{b}u$$
$$y = \mathbf{c}^t\mathbf{x} \tag{1}$$

where

$$\mathbf{A} = \begin{pmatrix} 0 & 1 & 0 \\ 0 & 0 & 1 \\ 0 & 0 & 0 \end{pmatrix}, \ \mathbf{b} = \begin{pmatrix} 0 \\ 0 \\ 1 \end{pmatrix}, \ \mathbf{c}^t = (1 \ 0 \ 0) \tag{2}$$

Further take into account that the control signal u is constrained

$$U_1 \leq u \leq U_2 \tag{3}$$

Then the aim is to design such a time sub-optimal controller that will bring the system from an initial state $\mathbf{x} = (x \ y \ z)^t$ to the desired state $\mathbf{x}_w$ in the minimum time t_{min} under an additional condition that limits the changes between two opposite values U_1, U_2 of the control signal u (3). It is required that these changes will correspond to an exponential behavior that could be expressed by the exponential decrease of the distance between the current state $\mathbf{x}$ and a corresponding part of a switching plane in the phase space. If the distance will be expressed by a scalar function $\rho_i : \mathbf{R}^3 \to \mathrm{R}$, the condition of the exponential decrease can be mathematically formulated by the differential equation

$$\frac{\mathrm{d}\rho_i}{\mathrm{d}t} = \alpha_i \rho_i, \ \alpha_i \in \mathrm{R}^-, \ i = 1, 2, 3 \tag{4}$$

From this equation the value of the time sub-optimal controller can be calculated. To simplify the problem it is possible to set the desired state $\mathbf{x}_w$ to be equal to the origin of the phase space due to a suitable coordinate transformation. Further simplifications will be necessary in order to derive an explicit solution for the control value.

After evaluating the sub-optimal controller for the triple integrator it is our goal to apply it for the real hydraulic system. In order to use the control law originally derived for the linear system (triple integrator) a linearization technique must be applied first. This will influence also control limits U_1, U_2 that should be transformed. Exact linearization method uses Lie algebra formalism to convert a nonlinear system to a linear one [7].

3 Nonlinear Decomposition

The design of the time-suboptimal control is based on a nonlinear dynamics decomposition [3]. This is done in the phase space and it enables to express the state of the system $\mathbf{x}$ as a sum of subsystem states $\mathbf{x}_i, i = 1, ..., n$

$$\mathbf{x} = \sum_{i=1}^{n} \mathbf{x}_i(q_i, t_i), \ \mathbf{x}_i(q_i, t_i) = e^{-\mathbf{A}t_i} \mathbf{v}_i q_i + \int_0^{-t_i} e^{\mathbf{A}^\tau} \mathbf{b} \mathrm{d}\tau q_i \tag{5}$$

where $\mathbf{A}$ is the system matrix corresponding to the triple integrator (2), $\mathbf{b}$ is the input vector (2), $\mathbf{v}_i = (1/\alpha_i^n, ..., 1/\alpha_i)^t$ represent eigenvectors (with different eigenvalues α_i), $U_j, j = 1, 2$ are control limits (3), q_i and t_i are parameters of the decomposition that have to be solved from this system of nonlinear algebraic equations under following conditions

$$\text{if } q_i \in \left[U_1 - \sum_{k=1}^{i-1} q_k, \ U_2 - \sum_{k=1}^{i-1} q_k \right] \text{ then } t_i = 0$$
$$\text{else } q_i = U_j - \sum_{k=1}^{i-1} q_k \text{ and } 0 < t_i \leq t_{i-1} \tag{6}$$

for $i = 1, \ldots, n$, $j = 1, 2$, $t_0 = \infty$. Then the control law can be computed as

$$u = \sum_{i=1}^{n} q_i \tag{7}$$

The nonlinear decomposition (5) fulfills the aim of the control expressed by the condition (4) when the current state vector is decomposed to the individual subsystem state vectors and each of them is either time optimally controlled by one of the limit values of q_i or it decreases the distance ρ_i from the phase space origin.

In the case of the triple integrator it is valid $n = 3$. Suppose we have three different eigenvalues with ordering $\alpha_3 < \alpha_2 < \alpha_1 < 0$. After substitution of (2) into (5) one gets the system of three algebraic equations (8) that is necessary to be solved under the condition (6) in order to evaluate the parameters q_1, q_2 and q_3 that according to (7) determine the resulting control law u.

$$\mathbf{x} = \begin{pmatrix} \sum_{i=1}^{3} \left(q_i \left(\frac{1}{\alpha_i^3} - \frac{t_i}{\alpha_i^2} + \frac{1}{2}\frac{t_i^2}{\alpha_i} \right) - \frac{1}{6}q_i t_i^3 \right) \\ \sum_{i=1}^{3} \left(q_i \left(\frac{1}{\alpha_i^2} - \frac{t_i}{\alpha_i} \right) + \frac{1}{2}q_i t_i^2 \right) \\ \sum_{i=1}^{3} \left(\frac{q_i}{\alpha_i} - q_i t_i \right) \end{pmatrix} \tag{8}$$

Generally, it is not possible to solve this system analytically because of the resulting polynomial of the sixth order. Therefore it is helpful to use graphical interpretation in the phase space. (8) spans the whole phase space but if we consider $t_3 = 0$ then only a part of the phase space is given by it. This part defines the set of states corresponding to the proportional control called proportional band (PB) (Fig. 1). If we were able to localize the actual state within PB the control action u could be easily calculated on the proportional base. This has been used in [9] where the localization has been made with the help of the computer algebra system Maple.

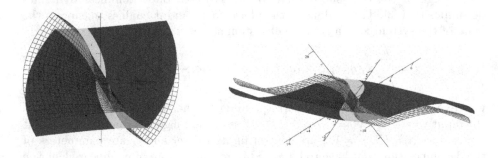

Fig. 1. Proportional band of control

4   Time Sub-Optimal Solution

In order to get an analytical solution it is necessary to accept some simplifications in the nonlinear decomposition. For this reason we will change the third subsystem of the decomposition (5) to be $\mathbf{x}_3 = (1\ 0\ 0)^t q_3$. This will enable a projection along the axis x and a reduction of the order of equations by one.

By application of another limit condition, i.e. $q_3 = 0$, the above mentioned PB reduces to a two dimensional object in the phase space called reference braking surface RBS. According to values of the parameters q_1, q_2, t_1 and t_2, the RBS consists of several regions depicted in the Fig. 2. If the region of RBS corresponding to the actual state is known the control law u can be evaluated by application of (4) to the distance between the actual state and the RBS region. This procedure has been used in [3] where the RBS has been projected along the axis x into the plane y, z. Then the actual state could be localized into the corresponding RBS region by solving quadratic equations. This has enabled to solve the designed time sub-optimal algorithm analytically.

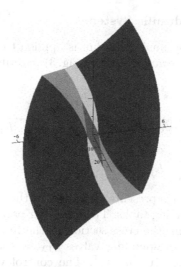

Fig. 2. Reference braking surface splitted to segments (Color figure online)

As an example we describe a procedure of computation of the time sub-optimal control value for one of the regions of RBS denoted by TQ. Consider the parameters of RBS are $q_1 = U_j$, $q_2 \in [0, U_{3-j} - U_j]$, $t_1 > 0$ and $t_2 = 0$. The region of RBS corresponding to these parameters is depicted in the Fig. 2 by green color. After substitution of these parameters into (8) we can determine the unknown parameters q_2 and t_1 from the subsystem of (8) for coordinates y and z by solving a system with one quadratic equation and one linear equation

$$\begin{pmatrix} y \\ z \end{pmatrix} = \begin{pmatrix} U_j \left(\frac{1}{\alpha_1^2} - \frac{t_1}{\alpha_1} \right) + \frac{1}{2} U_j t_1^2 + \frac{q_2}{\alpha_2^2} \\ \frac{U_j}{\alpha_1} - U_j t_1 + \frac{q_2}{\alpha_2} \end{pmatrix} \tag{9}$$

After substitution of the calculated parameters q_2 and t_1 into the (8) (when $q_3 = 0$) we can get from the subsystem of (8) for the coordinate x the equation representing the region TQ of RBS in the form $x = f(y, z)$; $f(y, z) : \mathbf{R}^2 \to \mathrm{R}$. Then the distance between the actual state (with the coordinate x) and the corresponding segment of RBS measured along the axis x can be expressed as $\rho_3 = x - f(y, z)$. Finally, the resulting control value u can be evaluated from (4) when $i = 3$.

A similar procedure is possible to derive for each segment of RBS. The localization of the actual state $\mathbf{x}$ to the corresponding region of RBS is performed in the y, z-plane where for the triple integrator only the equations of second order are necessary to be solved. The complete description of the time sub-optimal controller design can be found in [3].

5   Application to the Real Three-Tank Hydraulic System

5.1   Model of the Hydraulic System

The simplified time sub-optimal algorithm is applied to the control of the level in the third tank of the hydraulic system (Fig. 3) described by

$$
\begin{aligned}
\dot{h}_1 &= \frac{1}{A_1} q_1 - c_{12}\sqrt{h_1 - h_2} \\
\dot{h}_2 &= c_{12}\sqrt{h_1 - h_2} - c_{23}\sqrt{h_2 - h_3} \\
\dot{h}_3 &= c_{23}\sqrt{h_2 - h_3} - c_3\sqrt{h_3} \\
y &= h_3
\end{aligned}
\tag{10}
$$

where the control action q_1 represents the inflow in the first tank and h_1, h_2, h_3 are the levels in corresponding tanks. The following parameters have been identified from the real system: the cross-section of the first tank $A_1 = 1 \cdot 10^{-3} m^2$ and the coefficients of corresponding valves $c_{12} = 1.48 \cdot 10^{-2} m^{\frac{1}{2}} s^{-1}$, $c_{23} = 1.52 \cdot 10^{-2} m^{\frac{1}{2}} s^{-1}$, $c_3 = 6 \cdot 10^{-3} m^{\frac{1}{2}} s^{-1}$. The control value q_1 is constrained: $Q_{min} = 0 \, m^3 s^{-1}$ and $Q_{max} = 1.562 \cdot 10^{-5} m^3 s^{-1}$. The aim is to control the height of the level in the third tank.

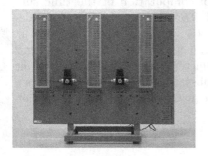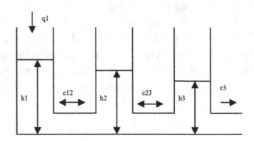

Fig. 3. Three-tank laboratory system

5.2   Exact Linearization Method

Using the exact linearization method [7] the nonlinear system (10) can be expressed in the form of a triple integrator and previously derived control can be applied after taken into account the change of control limits caused by linearization feedback. After denoting the Lie derivative of a scalar function y along a vector field $\mathbf{f}$ by $L_f y$ the desired exact linearization feedback can be expressed as

$$q_1 = \frac{u - L_f^3 y}{L_g L_f^2 y}, \quad \mathbf{f} = \begin{pmatrix} -c_{12}\sqrt{h_1 - h_2} \\ c_{12}\sqrt{h_1 - h_2} - c_{23}\sqrt{h_2 - h_3} \\ c_{23}\sqrt{h_2 - h_3} - c_3\sqrt{h_3} \end{pmatrix}, \quad \mathbf{g} = \begin{pmatrix} \frac{1}{A_1} \\ 0 \\ 0 \end{pmatrix} \quad (11)$$

and new control constraints are

$$U_1 = L_g L_f^2 y \, Q_{min} + L_f^3 y$$
$$U_2 = L_g L_f^2 y \, Q_{max} + L_f^3 y \quad (12)$$

5.3 Control of the Real System

The real three-tank system has been controlled using the designed time suboptimal controller and the exact linearization method. The desired height of the third level has been $0.07\,m$ and the controller parameters have been $\alpha_1 = -0.1$, $\alpha_2 = -0.15$, $\alpha_3 = -0.1$. The output and control responses are shown in the Fig. 4. From the control response one can notice that it does not include the third pulse as it could be expected according to the time optimal control theory. It has been caused by non-modeled dynamics and resulting over-damped suboptimal control law. Moreover, there is a small overshoot. In practice, to avoid model mismatch, noisy measurements and disturbances it is necessary to extend

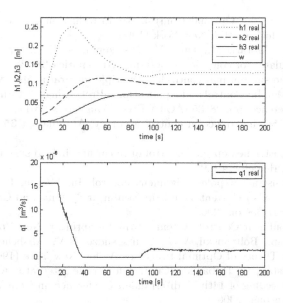

Fig. 4. Three-tank hydraulic system control: output and control transients

the whole control structure by the nonlinear disturbance observer that will also influence the transformation of the original control limits.

The designed controller is focused to improve the dynamics of time responses and this has been successfully carried out. Even derived for the triple integrator the sub-optimal controller works well also for nonlinear systems. It respects the constraints of the control signal as it can be seen from the control responses and switching to the opposite control limit is smooth.

6   Conclusions

This paper summarizes the design of the time sub-optimal controller based on the nonlinear decomposition and its application to the real hydraulic system. Although the resulting expressions for the control law are sophisticated using todays computer technology it has been no problem to implement the developed control strategies to the real system. Here the simplified nonlinear decomposition has played an important role as it allowed to derive the analytical solution. Using the exact linearization method has been also significant. Due to it the time suboptimal controller originally designed for the triple integrator system could have been used also for the nonlinear hydraulic system.

Acknowledgments. This work has been partially supported by the grants VEGA 1/0937/14 and APVV-0343-12.

References

1. Athans, M., Falb, P.: Optimal Control: An Introduction to the Theory and its Applications. McGraw-Hill, New York (1996)
2. Bemporad, A., Morari, M., Dua, V., Pistikopoulos, E.N.: The explicit linear quadratic regulator for constrained systems. Automatica **38**, 3–20 (2002)
3. Bisták, P.: The sub-optimal controller for triple integrator applied to three-level hydraulic system. In: Control and Applications: Proceedings of 13th IASTED International Conference, pp. 28–35. ACTA Press, Vancouver (2011)
4. Blanchini, F.: Set invariance in control a survey. Automatica **35**(11), 1747–1767 (1999)
5. Borelli, F.: Constrained optimal control of linear and hybrid systems. LNCIS, vol. 290. Springer, Heidelberg (2003)
6. Huba, M.: Constrained pole assignment control. In: Menini, L., Zaccarian, L., Chaouki, T.A. (eds.) Current Trends in Nonlinear Systems and Control, pp. 163–183. Birkhäuser, Boston (2006)
7. Isidori, A.: Nonlinear Control Systems, 3rd edn. Springer, New York (1995)
8. Pontryagin, L.S., Boltyanskii, V.G., Gamkrelidze, R.V., Mishchenko, E.F.: The Mathematical Theory of Optimal Processes. Wiley, New York (1962)
9. Tapák, P., Bisták, P., Huba, M.: Control for triple integrator with constrained input. In: Proceeding of 14th Mediterranean Conference on Control and Automation. IEEE, Ancona (2006)

Use of the Automatic Identification System in Academic Research

Miluše Tichavska[1], Francisco Cabrera[2(✉)], Beatriz Tovar[1],
and Víctor Araña[2]

[1] Departamento de Análisis Económico Aplicado, Universidad de Las Palmas
de Gran Canaria (ULPGC), Campus Universitario de Tafira, Edificio
Departamental de CC.EE y EE. Módulo D, 35017 Las Palmas de G.C., Spain
mtichavska@acciones.ulpgc.es, btovar@daea.ulpgc.es
[2] Departamento de Señales y Comunicaciones (DSC),
Instituto para el Desarrollo Tecnológico y la Innovación
en las Comunicaciones (IDeTIC), Universidad de Las Palmas
de Gran Canaria (ULPGC), Las Palmas de G.C., Spain
{francisco.cabrera, victor.arana}@ulpgc.es

Abstract. The Automatic Identification System (AIS) is a Very High Frequency
(VHF) radio broadcasting system frequencies (161.975 MHz and 162.025 MHz)
that transfers packets of data over the data link (HDLC) [1, 2] and enables
AIS-equipment vessels and shore-based stations to send and receive identification information that can be displayed on a computer. It was originally conceived
as a navigational aid for ship monitoring and collision avoidance at sea that over
time, has evolved into a system with a multitude of additional applications,
including experimental systems in academic and research environments.

1 Introduction

The Automatic Identification System is a Very High Frequency (VHF) radio broadcasting system frequencies (161.975 MHz and 162.025 MHz) that transfers packets of
data over the data link (HDLC) [1, 2] and enables AIS-equipment vessels and
shore-based stations to send and receive identification information that can be displayed on a computer. It was originally conceived as a navigational aid for ship
monitoring and collision avoidance at sea that over time, has evolved into a system
with a multitude of additional applications, including experimental systems in educational environments.

Nowadays, the AIS is one of the most widely used marine systems around the
world. It has proven to be an essential tool for professionals in the maritime sector, ship
enthusiasts and a large community of researchers around the globe. According to the
International Maritime Organization (IMO) regulation 19.2 of Safety Of Life at Seas
(SOLAS) Convention [3], an AIS transceiver shall be equipped in every sea-going ship
larger than 300 gross tons and every passenger vessel irrespective of size. Its system
transmits static and voyage-related information every 6 min in addition to dynamic
information with a frequency related to the vessel's speed underway (2–10 s) and
navigational status (3 min when anchored). In a global context and a managing network

© Springer International Publishing Switzerland 2015
R. Moreno-Díaz et al. (Eds.): EUROCAST 2015, LNCS 9520, pp. 33–40, 2015.
DOI: 10.1007/978-3-319-27340-2_5

of over 1,800 coastal AIS stations [4], this could result in over 90,000 vessels visible at any time, 120,000 vessels reporting daily and information of over 200,000 vessels and BigData access through actionable information with millions of positions recorded daily and billions of positions archived.

The present study aims to present the value of the use of the AIS as a data resource for education, academic research and public interests (policy implications and improvements) when related to the operation and performance of vessels. The paper is structured as follows. In Sect. 2 we provide a brief but comprehensive AIS functional overview. In Sect. 3 we enumerate research areas where academic institutions could benefit from the use of AIS. Section 4 presents an overview of the MarineTraffic Academic AIS Network. Section 5 describes empirical research applications based on terrestrial AIS data gathered by BMT-IDeTIC station covering Las Palmas Port. Section 6 concludes.

2   The AIS Functional Overview

The AIS system is capable of handling over 2250 reports per minute and updates as often as every second. It uses a Self-Organising Time Division Multiple Access (SOTDMA) scheme to meet this high broadcast rate and to ensure reliable ship-to-ship operation. Each SOTDMA is designed to cope with path delays not longer than 12 bits, which translates into a maximum range of about 200 nautical miles, but typically the radio frequency coverage is limited to about 40 nautical miles. The AIS uses 9.6 kbps FM/GMSK modulation over 25 or 12.5 kHz channels for transmissions. The AIS uses High Level Data Link Control (HDLC) packet protocols. The AIS stations are divided into mobile AIS and Fixed AIS stations (Table 1).

The AIS receiver should be capable of operating on 25 kHz. Bandwidth adapted frequency modulated Gaussian-filtered minimum shift keying (GMSK/FM) is used in the AIS physical layer. A non-return to zero inverted (NRZI) waveform is used for data encoding. The NRZI encoded data are then GMSK encoded before frequency modulating the carrier.

Table 1. Summary of the AIS protocol parameters

Operational frequency bands	VHF (161.975 MHz and 162.025 MHz)
Transmission power	12.5 W (Class A only)
Modulation	FM/GMSK
Symbol rate	9.6 Kbps
Number slots in TDMA frame	2250
Multiple access method	Self-organised TDMA (SOTDMA)
TDMA frame length	60 s
Burst structure	Training sequence: 24 bits Start flag: 8 bits Data: up to 168 bits FCS: 16 bits End flag: 8 bits

3 AIS Research Environments

The use of the AIS over academic and research institutions covers a wide range of areas and interests. Among others, these are:

- *Radio propagation channel techniques.*

The radio propagation environment uses a VHF channel and it can be modeled using the data of the vessels with the historical data [5, 6]. Explore ship detection capabilities of the AIS and surface wave HF radars [7].

- *Interactive information systems design.*

The interactive information systems may satisfy the requirements of a variety of application areas including engineering, environmental economics, tourism and others. For instance, interactive information systems that address the modelling of oil spills and its visualization through geospatial techniques that support the management and processing of this information. These customized systems commonly allows remote users to run and retrieve oil spill models outputs (GIS resources) and multimedia response information [8].

- *Real-time statistical processing of traffic information.*

The design of databases and the creation of statistics from real-time vessel traffic information (Fig. 1) can be of use to a variety of purposes including operational research and public policy [9].

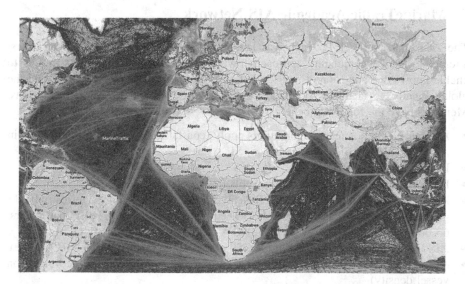

Fig. 1. Vessel traffic information based on the AIS and data globally collected by MarineTraffic

- *Ship traffic management*

Ship traffic management is used for safety assessment and commonly as part of risk management program. Additionally, this is also applied to ship security assessment in areas of piracy risk as the Indian Ocean or in the Horn of Africa [10]. Moreover, this is also of use within governance structures that manage shipping sectors in areas as the Arctic Canada and provide a critical evaluation of its effectiveness considering recent and rapid growth [11].

- *Green and effective operations at port*

Vessel operations share positive effects and economic benefits in ports and cities. Nevertheless, negative impacts, including air pollution are also implied and vary according to operative type (hotelling, manoeuvring, cruising), time, and engine load variations while at port [12, 13]. In this sense, emission inventories based on the AIS can be effectively used to identify operative and polluting profiles at port. This guarantees location, speed and route are always acknowledged, providing the additional possibility to model high-resolution maps with the geographical characterisation of results. This includes among others, the emissions released at source and its dispersion in the atmosphere in areas, which affect port-city areas.

- *Sustainable transport solutions*

The comparative analysis of gas, crude oil and oil gaseous and liquid derivative transportation in terms of quality, efficiency and safety criteria. Historical and statistical data is provided using an AIS system [14].

4   MarineTraffic Academic AIS Network

The Academic Network Program was launched by MarineTraffic in 2013 as a first attempt to start a community approach towards MT Academic users. Its aim is to enable knowledge and support non-funded, non-profit Academic Research around the globe. Finally, to facilitate AIS data access to Academic and Research Institutions. Members have the following benefits:

- AIS receiver and antenna – conditions apply (coastal regions of high interest: Latin America, W&E Africa, Indian Ocean, SE Asia).
- Installation assistance.
- Participation in the AIS Academy events.
- Access to the MarineTraffic.com Research Plan, which includes terrestrial AIS global coverage, a fleet of 50 vessels, 300 email alerts per month, vessel particulars, 60 days voyage history, export of 3,000 records per month.
- AIS historical data: on request, up to 250,000 position records per year (CSV file).
- AIS current data: NMEA or API data feed for your region (area defined based on vessel density).

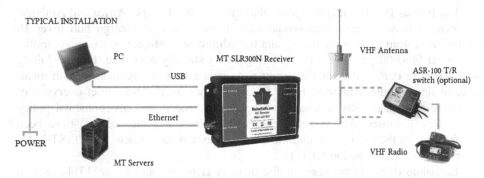

Fig. 2. BMT-IDeTIC node

BMT-IDeTIC is a node of the MarineTraffic Network [15] since April 2013. This node is situated in of the ULPGC *Science and Technology Park* (28.08°N/15.46°W). This location was considered ideal due to its proximity to Las Palmas port. This node has an Antenna with an effective height of 375 m, an AIS Receiver (MT SLR300N) and Ethernet Connection. The SLR300N enables AIS data to be viewed directly, or shared on a local network. The unit can also be mounted at a remote location and AIS data sent via the Internet to a fixed IP address for use on a dedicated server. Figure 2 shows the BMT-IDeTIC Node.

5 Some Empirical Applications Related to Las Palmas Port

AIS range of coverage varies according to weather conditions (so far, from 82.73 to 685.52 nautical miles) and receives data from an average of 100 vessels. In order to demonstrate the coverage of the system, Fig. 3 presents the variation of coverage under different conditions and its extension from the port of Las Palmas to the south of Portugal and to the southward to the Gulf of Guinea.

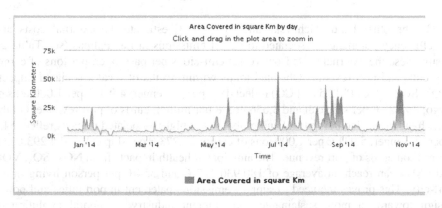

Fig. 3. BMT-IDeTIC radio coverage

Las Palmas Port is a major logistic platform between Europe, Africa and America. Its location between main commercial trade routes makes it a cargo hub (over 19 million tons from loading, unloading and transshipments). Moreover, passenger traffic, with over 908,000 passengers in 2011 is growing steadily over time. Finally, jointly with Tenerife Port, is the main transport node connecting the archipelago with mainland Spain and other countries. In the following lines we present a brief overview of recent research and local case-studies for vessel emission and environmental policy assessment purposes, AIS vessel tracks (with at least a 2 min update) have been combined with the full bottom-up Ship Traffic Emission Assessment Model (STEAM) over a twelve-month period (2011).

Emissions derived from vessel traffic share in Tichavska and Tovar [13] have been grouped by categories as transmitted by the AIS (see Fig. 3). In summary it can be observed from results that the, passenger, container and tanker vessel categories have contributed with the highest share of emissions related to local detriments on air quality (NOx, SOx, PM2.5, CO) and global GHG effects caused by exhausts (CO_2). When compared to the others (Fig. 4) it is noticeable that these sectors are the ones that release the largest share of emissions by spending less time at port.

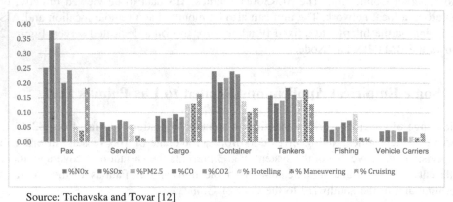

Source: Tichavska and Tovar [12]

Fig. 4. Share of emissions and operative time by shipping sector in Las Palmas Port (2011).

On the other hand, Tichavska and Tovar [13] estimate the external costs and eco-efficiency parameters associated to vessel emissions in Las Palmas (see Table 2). Results describe external costs from vessel emissions per passenger, per tons of cargo, ship calls and port revenue. Obtained totals within results of local associated impacts (NOx, SO2, VOC, PM2.5 and CO) reflect 48 € per passenger; 4,960 € per 1,000 tons of cargo; 19,822 € per ship call and 3,656,463 € per million euros of port revenue. On the other hand, totals including local and global (CO2 high) associated impacts reflect 54.2 € per passenger; 5,931 € per 1,000 tons of cargo; 23,273 € per ship call and 4,293,063 € per million euros of port revenue. The anticipated health impacts from NOx, SO_x, VOC and $PM_{2.5}$ can reach an average of 180,930,427 € and 554 € per person living in the port-city. This proves the need to support emission abatement in port cities and policy design towards a more sustainable and efficient industry. Temporal evolution of

Table 2. Port external cost and eco-efficiency performance

Exhaust emissions	Total external costs	Eco-efficiency performance			
		Emission external cost per passenger (€/ pax)	Emission external cost per tons of cargo (€/ 1,000 tons)	Emission external cost per ship call (€/call)	Emission external cost per port revenue (€/ million euros)
NOx	47,744,771	9.8	1,453	5,231	964,875
SO$_2$	62,661,360	19.1	1,597	6,865	1,266,324
VOC	146,191	0.029	4	16	2,954
PM$_{2.5}$	70,378,105	19.2	1,905	7,710	1,422,272
CO	1,877	0.0003	0.06	0.206	38
CO$_2$ High	31,500,803	6.2	971	3,451	636,600
Total (local only)	212,433,107	48	4,960	19,822	3,656,463
Total (local and global)	212,433,107	54.2	5,931	23,273	4,293,063

Source: Tichavska and Tovar [13]

external costs reflects a largest share of costs from NOx and PM$_{2.5}$ and, noticeable peaks can be seen over January, March and November.

6   Conclusions

The present study brings notice to the value of the use of the AIS for academic research and public interests such as policy implications and improvements when related to the operation and performance of vessels. The data received by the AIS receiving stations may serve among others, for studies such as the simulation of vessel movements, radio propagation channel techniques, interactive information systems design, real-time statistical processing of traffic information, ship traffic management, green and effective operations at port and sustainable transport solutions.

References

1. ITU-R M.1371-5 Technical characteristics for a universal shipborne automatic identification system using time division multiple access in the VHF maritime mobile band
2. ISO/IEC 3309:1993: Information technology – Telecommunications and Information Exchange Between Systems – High-Level Data Link Control (HDLC) Procedures-Frame Structure (1993)

3. International Maritime Organization: International Convention on the Safety of the Life at Sea (SOLAS) (1974)
4. IMO (International Maritime Organization). www.imo.org
5. Report ITU-R M.2123: Long range detection of automatic identification system (AIS) messages under various tropospheric propagation conditions
6. Green, D., Fowler, C., Power, D.: VHF Propagation Study, C-Core (2011)
7. Vesecky, J.F., Laws, K.E., Paduan, J.D.: Using HF surface wave radar and the ship automatic identification system (AIS) to monitor coastal vessels. In: 2009 IEEE International Symposium on Geoscience and Remote Sensing, IGARSS 2009, vol. 3. IEEE (2009)
8. Howlett, E., Mulanaphy, N., Menton, A., Sontag, S.: Web based oil spill response system. In: The International Oil Spill Conference Proceedings. American Petroleum Institute (2014)
9. Boubeta-Puig, J., Medina-Bulo, I., Ortiz, G., Fuentes-Landi, G.: Complex event processing applied to early maritime threat detection. In: The Proceedings of the 2nd International Workshop on Adaptive Services for the Future Internet and 6th International Workshop on Web APIs and Service Mashups. ACM (2012)
10. Sullivan, A.K.: Piracy in the horn of Africa and its effects on the global supply chain. J. Transp. Secur. 3(4), 231–243 (2010)
11. Dawson, J., Johnston, M.E., Stewart, E.J.: Governance of Arctic expedition cruise ships in a time of rapid environmental and economic change. Ocean Coast. Manage. 89, 88–99 (2014)
12. Tichavska, M., Tovar, B.: Port-city exhaust emission model: an application to cruise and ferry operations in Las Palmas Port. Transp. Res. Part A: Policy Pract. 78, 347–360 (2015)
13. Tichavska, M., Tovar, B.: Environmental cost and eco-efficiency from vessel emissions in Las Palmas Port. Transp. Res. Part E: Logist. Transp. Rev. 83, 126–140 (2015)
14. Tudorica, D.: A comparative analysis of various methods of gas, crude oil and oil derivatives transportation. Int. J. Sustain. Econ. Manage. 3(1), 16–25 (2014)
15. MarineTraffic, http://www.marinetraffic.com

Application of Multi-valued Decision Diagrams in Computing the Direct Partial Logic Derivatives

Jozef Kostolny[1]([✉]), Elena Zaitseva[1], Suzana Stojković[2],
and Radomir Stanković[2]

[1] Department of Informatics, University of Zilina, Zilina, Slovakia
{jozef.kostolny,elena.zaitseva}@fri.uniza.sk
[2] Faculty of Electronic Engineering, University of Niš, Niš, Serbia
suzana.stojkovic@elfak.ni.ac.rs, Radomir.Stankovic@gmail.com

Abstract. Multi-State Systems (MSSs) are mathematical models often used in reliability engineering since allow a rather detailed evaluation of system reliability. These models represent the system reliability/availability behavior from the perfect functioning to the fault, but allow to distinguish several intermediate states. The calculation of related reliability measures can be performed in terms of Direct Partial Logic Derivatives (DPLDs). A drawback of this approach is high dimensionality of MSSs. To overcome this problem, we propose to use Multi-valued Decision Diagrams (MDDs) as a data structure to represent multi-state systems and perform computations of reliability measures in terms of DPLDs.

Keywords: Multi-valued decision diagram · Direct partial logic derivative · Reliability analysis · Multi-state systems

1 Introduction

In reliability engineering, usually two mathematical models are used for representation and analysis of systems to be investigated. The first model is the Binary-state system (BSS), which allows to distinguish two states of a system, the correct or faulty functioning. The second model is the Multi-state system (MSS) that permits to observe more than two states of a system, permitting therefore a more detailed evaluation of its reliability. Due to this, there are engineering applications where the usage of MSS is more preferable. Examples of such applications are analysis of power systems, transport systems, oil transmission systems, etc., [3,9]. Several mathematical approaches to the analysis and estimation of MSSs have been proposed in reliability engineering. One of these approaches is based on the description of a given MSS by the so-called structure function that defines the correlation between the states of the system components and the system performance level [3]. This approaches imposes no particular requirements on the systems to be represented and, therefore, can be used to define and represent arbitrary systems.

© Springer International Publishing Switzerland 2015
R. Moreno-Díaz et al. (Eds.): EUROCAST 2015, LNCS 9520, pp. 41–48, 2015.
DOI: 10.1007/978-3-319-27340-2_6

In [7], the relationship between the MSS structure functions and the Multiple-Valued Logic (MVL) functions is pointed out, which allows borrowing mathematical methods used in MVL for the estimation of MSS reliability [9]. In particular, it is possible to use Multi-valued Decision Diagrams (MDDs) to represent the structure functions and perform computation of reliability measures. In this way, the restriction related to the high dimensionality of structure functions is relaxed since MDDs are data structures purposely defined to represent large functions [5].

For a system, different reliability measures can be computed from its structure function in terms of the Direct Partial Logic Derivatives (DPLDs). Therefore, efficient computation of DPLDs is an important task in related practical applications. In this paper, we propose an algorithm for computing DPLDs over MDDs and discuss the application of the algorithm to computing reliability measures.

2 Background Theory

Consider a system consisting of n components x_i, each of which can be in m_i states, and having M performance levels. The structure function of such a system is defined as a mapping

$$f(x) : \{0, \ldots, m_1 - 1\} \times \ldots \times \{0, \ldots, m_n - 1\} \to \{0, \ldots, M - 1\}. \qquad (1)$$

where x_i is the i-th component of the state and $x = (x_1, \ldots, x_n)$ is the vector of component states.

The Direct Partial Logic Derivative (DPLD) is a particular concept in the Logic Differential Calculus which can be used for analysis of dynamic properties of MVL functions including MSS structure functions as particular examples.

For a given MSS structure function (1), the DPLD with respect to the variable x_i permits to analyze the system performance level change from j to $j - 1$ when the i-th component state changes from s to $s - 1$ [8].

Definition 1. *For a structure function $f(x)$, the co-factors with respect to a variable x_i are defined as $f(x_i = s) = f(x_1, \ldots, x_{i-1}, s, x_{i+1}, \ldots, x_n)$, and $f(x_i = s - 1)(x_1, \ldots, x_{i-1}, s - 1, x_{i+1}, \ldots, x_n)$, with $s, s - 1 \in \{0, 1, \ldots, m_i - 1\}$, $j \in \{0, 1, \ldots, M - 1\}$. The direct partial logic derivative (DPLD) is defined as*

$$DPLD_i^{(j,s)} = \frac{\partial f(j \to j - 1)}{\partial x_i(s \to s - 1)} \qquad (2)$$

$$= \begin{cases} 1, \text{ if } f(x = s_i) = j \text{ and } f(x = (s - 1)_i) = j - 1, \\ 0, \text{ otherwise.} \end{cases}$$

3 Representation of Structure Functions by MDDs

Multi-Valued Diagrams (MDD) are a classical approach in MVL for representation and analysis of large MVL functions [4,5]. The representation MSS structure function by MDDs is discussed in [8,9].

It is clear from (1) that a structure function $f(x)$ is a multiple-valued function in multiple-valued variables. Since the number of states can be large, $f(x)$ is a function of many variables and its compact representation is of an essential importance for further manipulation and computations with it. A possible way could be to represent $f(x)$ by a Multiple-valued Decision Diagram (MDD) [5].

Example 1. *Consider a system that consists of three components. First two components have two states, while the third component has four states. The performance of the system has three levels. Therefore, in this case, $n = 3$, $x_1, x_2 = \{0,1\}$, $x_3 \in \{0,1,2,3\}$, and $M \in \{0,1,2\}$. Thus, the structure function of this system is a mapping*

$$f(x_1, x_2, x_3) : \{0,1\} \times \{0,1\} \times \{0,1,2,3\} \rightarrow \{0,1,2\},$$

defined as $f(x) = (x_1 \vee x_2) \wedge x_3$, where $\vee$ and $\wedge$ are operations MIN and MAX corresponding to the logic operations AND and OR in the binary case. The MDD for $f(x)$ shown in Fig. 1, has three levels with nonterminal nodes corresponding to variables x_1, x_2, and x_3. Therefore, nodes for the first two variables have two outgoing edges, while the node for x_3 has four outgoing edges. Three constant nodes show three levels of performances 0, 1, and 2. Attributes at the edges are probabilities $p_{i,j}$ that component x_i will be in the state j. For simplicity, in further considerations in this paper, these probabilities will not be shown in the corresponding figures.

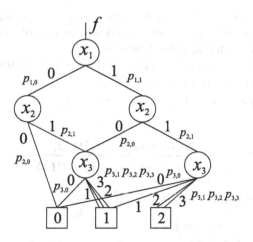

Fig. 1. MDD for $f(x)$ in Example 1.

The structure function is a very useful tool in computing different MSS measures. As an example of MSS measures, in this paper, we will use the structural importance (I) since it takes into account the topology of the system.

Definition 2. *If $\rho_i^{s,j}$ is the number of states that change from s to $s-1$, and m_i is the number of states, then the structural importance is defined as*

$$I_i^{(j,s)} = \frac{\rho_i^{s,j}}{m_1 \cdots m_{i-1} m_{i+1} \cdots m_n}. \tag{3}$$

4 Direct Partial Logic Derivative and MSS Measures

By Definition 1, the DPLD of $f(x)$ of a MSS is a binary-valued function of multiple-valued variables and, therefore, can be represented by a binary-valued vector $\mathbf{DPLD}_i^{(j,s)}$, or alternatively by a MDD. Therefore, in computing over MDDs, the MDD for $f(x)$ is converted into the MDD for $DPLD_i^{(j,s)}$ by processing the nodes and cross points in the MDD for $f(x)$. Recall that in a decision tree, the nodes are connected by paths between successive levels in the tree. Thus, in a decision tree, all paths are of the length 1. After reduction of a decision tree into a decision diagram, there can be paths longer than 1, i.e., connecting nodes at non-successive levels. Cross points are imaginary points where a path longer than 1 crosses a line connecting nodes to which the same variable is assigned [6].

Since $f(x)$ is a multiple-valued function, and $DPLD_i^{(j,s)}$ is a binary-valued function, we define the characteristic function $f_i(x)$ as

$$f_i(x) = \begin{cases} 1, \text{ if } f(x) = i, \\ 0, \text{ otherwise.} \end{cases} \tag{4}$$

DPLDs are purposely defined to compute various MSS reliability measures. The size of instances that can be considered is considerably increased if MDDs are used as the corresponding data structures. In this section, we illustrate how to compute the MSS measures in terms of DPLDs over MDDs by the example of computing the structural importance $I_i^{(j,s)}$.

The key idea in computing $I_i^{(j,s)}$ over MDDs in terms of $DPLD_i^{(j,s)}$ is the observation that

$$I_i^{(j,s)} = \frac{\text{Number of 1 in } \mathbf{DPLD}_i^{(j,s)}}{\text{Number of elements in } \mathbf{DPLD}_i^{(j,s)}}. \tag{5}$$

Algorithm 1. *Algorithm(Computing $I_i^{(j,s)}$)*

1. *Construct MDD for a given $f(x)$,*
2. *Construct MDDs for characteristic functions f_j and f_{j-1},*
3. *Construct MDD for co-factors $f_j(x_i = s)$ and $f_{j-1}(x_i = s-1)$,*
4. *Construct MDD for $\mathbf{DPLD}_i^{(j,s)}$ as $f_j(x_i = s) \wedge f_{j-1}(x_i = s-1)$,*
5. *Compute $I_i^{(j,s)}$ by (5),*
6. *Repeat steps 3, 4, and 5 for each x_i, $i = 1, 2, \ldots, m$.*

Example 2. *For the system in Example 1, the structure function is defined by the function vector* $\mathbf{F} = [0,0,0,0,0,1,1,1,0,1,1,1,0,1,2,2]^T$. *For the illustration, we will compute the structural importance* $I^{(1,1)}$ *by using the Algorithm 1. Figure 2 shows the MDDs for* f *and its characteristic functions* f_1 *and* f_0, $MDD(f)$, $MDD(f_1(x_1 = 1))$, $MDD(f_0(x_1 = 0))$. *This corresponds to steps 1 and 2 of the Algorithm 1. Then, we determine the MDD for* $\mathbf{DPLD}_1(1,1)$ *as the MDD for the function* $f_1(x_1 = 1) \wedge f_0(x_1 = 1)$ *by performing the logic operation AND over the corresponding subdiagrams of* $MDD(f_1(x_1 = 1))$, *and* $MDD(f_0(x_1 = 0))$ *as shown in Fig. 3. In this figure, the* $MDD(DPLD_1^{(1,1)})$ *represents a vector* $DPLD_1^{(1,1)} = [0,1,1,1,0,0,0,0]^T$, *which has 8 elements, three of which are equal to 1. Thus,* $I_1^{(1,1)} = 3/8 = 0,375$. *We repeat the steps 3,4, and*

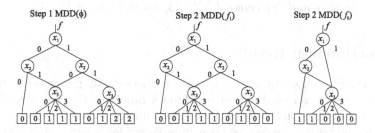

Fig. 2. MDD for $f(x)$ in Example 1.

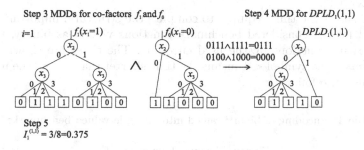

Fig. 3. Computing $I_1^{(1,1)}$.

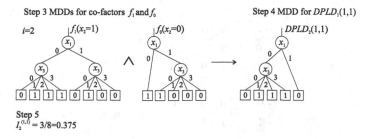

Fig. 4. Computing $I_2^{(1,1)}$.

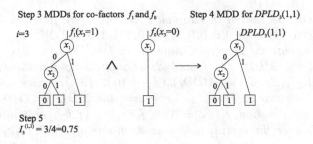

Step 3 MDDs for co-factors f_1 and f_0 Step 4 MDD for $DPLD_3(1,1)$

Step 5
$I_3^{(1,1)} = 3/4 = 0.75$

Fig. 5. Computing $I_3^{(1,1)}$.

5, for $i = 2$ as shown in Fig. 4 and determine that $I_2^{(1,1)} = 3/8 = 0,375$. We do the same procedure and determine $I_3^{(1,1)} = 3/4 = 0,75$ as in Fig. 5.

5   Experimental Results

To examine efficiency of computing DPLD over decision diagrams, we performed experiments over a set of standard benchmark functions that are usually used in evaluation of algorithms where the decision diagrams are the data structure to perform computing. Since these benchmarks are for binary valued functions, we performed encoding of inputs and outputs as shown in Table 1 by following the usual way of converting binary-valued benchmarks into multiple-valued benchmarks [1,2].

Table 2 shows the time required to compute the structural importance functions $I^{(1,1)}$ for the considered benchmark functions viewed as binary, ternary, and quaternary functions by the used encoding. The times are shown in milliseconds [ms]. The symbol < 1 means the time shorter than 1 ms. The notation in this able is the following

Table 1. Encoding of binary-valued into multiple-valued benchmarks.

Binary	Ternary		Quaternary
	In	Out	In/Out
0 0	0	0	0
0 1	1	1	1
0 -	0	0	0
1 0	2	2	2
1 1	*	0	3
1 -	2	2	2
- 0	0	0	0
- 1	1	1	1
- -	-	-	-

Table 2. Times to compute values of $I^{(1,1)}$ for binary-valued and multiple-valued benchmarks.

f	In/Out	$p = 2$				$p = 3$				$p = 4$			
		Size	T_c	T_{is}	T_{is1}	Size	T_c	T_{is}	T_{is1}	Size	T_c	T_{is}	T_{is1}
9sym	9/1	33	< 1	15	1.67	26	< 1	< 1	< 1	46	< 1	< 1	< 1
Alu4	14/8	1352	452	172	1.54	519	125	16	0.57	1177	468	84	3.36
Apex4	9/19	1021	172	78	0.46	198	16	15	0.30	524	156	16	0.32
B12	15/9	91	46	15	0.11	65	31	< 1	< 1	77	46	15	0.38
Checker	10/1	39	< 1	< 1	< 1	12	< 1	< 1	< 1	20	< 1	< 1	< 1
Clip	9/5	254	15	16	0.36	78	15	< 1	< 1	114	16	< 1	< 1
Con1	7/2	18	< 1	< 1	< 1	7	< 1	< 1	< 1	7	< 1	< 1	< 1
Cu	14/11	65	< 1	< 1	< 1	21	< 1	< 1	< 1	32	< 1	< 1	< 1
Ex5	8/63	311	31	47	0.09	177	15	< 1	< 1	403	31	16	0.12
Ex1010	10/10	1079	265	94	0.94	190	31	< 1	< 1	523	234	16	0.64
F51m	8/8	70	< 1	< 1	< 1	18	< 1	< 1	< 1	31	< 1	< 1	< 1
Inc	7/8	89	< 1	< 1	< 1	49	< 1	< 1	< 1	59	< 1	< 1	< 1
Misex1	8/7	47	< 1	< 1	< 1	21	< 1	< 1	< 1	21	< 1	< 1	< 1
Misex3	14/14	1301	561	358	1.83	325	125	15	0.31	658	436	78	1.60
Pdc	16/40	696	47	125	0.20	253	16	15	0.09	364	47	31	0.19
Rd53	5/3	23	< 1	< 1	< 1	10	< 1	< 1	< 1	14	< 1	< 1	< 1
Rd73	7/3	43	16	< 1	< 1	14	< 1	< 1	< 1	24	< 1	< 1	< 1
Rd84	8/4	59	16	15	0.47	12	< 1	< 1	< 1	24	15	< 1	< 1
Sao2	10/4	154	15	16	0.40	29	< 1	< 1	< 1	58	< 1	< 1	< 1
Spla	16/46	625	93	109	0.15	211	15	16	0.09	346	78	31	0.17
Sqrt8	8/4	42	< 1	16	0.5	12	< 1	< 1	< 1	16	< 1	< 1	< 1
T481	16/1	32	47	31	1.94	16	31	16	2	19	31	15	1.88
Table3	14/14	941	63	171	0.87	107	< 1	< 1	< 1	492	47	31	0.63
Table5	17/15	873	62	203	0.80	318	16	15	0.21	594	62	77	0.65

1. In/Out - the number of inputs and outputs. In the case of ternary and quaternary functions, the number of inputs and outputs are determined as $\lceil In/2 \rceil$, and $\lceil Out/2 \rceil$, where In and Out are the number of inputs and outputs in considered binary functions.
2. Size - the number of non-terminal nodes in the MDD,
3. T_c - time to cerate the MDD,
4. T_{is1} - time to compute a single value of $I^{(1,1)}$.
5. T_{is} - time to compute all values of $I^{(1,1)}$.

6   Concluding Remarks

The structure functions used in Multi-State Systems (MSSs) can be compactly represented by Multiple Decision Diagrams (MDDs) which can be used as a data structure to perform computing of various reliability measures in terms of Direct Partial Logic Derivatives (DPLDs). Experimental results show that representation and analysis of relatively large structure functions of MSSs and computing of related reliability measures can be performed very efficiently.

References

1. Fu, C., Falkowski, B.J.: Ternary fixed polarity linear Kronecker transforms and their comparison with ternary Reed-Muller transform. J. Circ., Syst., Comput. **14**(4), 721–733 (2005)
2. Lozano, C.C., Falkowski, B.J., Łuba, T.: Two classes of Fixed polarity linearly independent arithmetic transforms for quaternary functions. In: Proceedings of 17th European Signal Processing Conference, pp. 421–425 (2009)
3. Lisnianski, A., Levitin, G.: Multi-State System Reliability: Assessment, Optimization and Applications. World Scientific, Singapore (2003)
4. Miller, M., Drechsler, R.: On the construction of multiple-valued decision diagrams. In: Proceedings of the IEEE International Symposium on Multiple-Valued Logic, pp. 264–269 (2002)
5. Sasao, T., Fujita, M. (eds.): Representations of Discrete Functions. Kluwer Academic Publishers, Boston (1996)
6. Stanković, R.S., Sasao, T., Moraga, C.: Spectral transform decision diagrams. In: [5], pp. 55–92
7. Zaitseva, E., Levashenko, V.: Dynamic reliability indices for parallel, series and k-out-of-n multi-state system. In: Proceedings of the IEEE 52nd Annual Reliability and Maintainability Symposium (RAMS), vol. 94(2), pp. 253–259 (2006)
8. Zaitseva, E., Levashenko, V., Kostolny, J., Kvassay, M.: A multi-valued decision diagram for estimation of multi-state system. In: EuroCon 2013, pp. 645–650 (2013)
9. Zio, E.: Reliability engineering: old problems and new challenges. Reliab. Eng. Syst. Saf. **94**(2), 125–141 (2009)

Identification of First Order Plants by Relay Feedback with Non-symmetrical Oscillations

Peter Ťapák[✉] and Mikuláš Huba

Slovak University of Technology in Bratislava,
Ilkovičova 3, 812 19 Bratislava, Slovakia
{peter.tapak,mikulas.huba}@stuba.sk

Abstract. The paper deals with the approximation of the systems with dominant first order dynamics by the Integrator Plus Dead Time (IPDT) model. They are attractive especially in control of unstable plants, where an open-loop identification may not be applied. This paper updates a previously published contribution based on analysis of the non-symmetrical oscillations with possible offset arising typically under relay control that has been improved to prevent computational errors in the case of a negligible disturbances, when the relay on and off times are nearly equal over one control period. The analytical results are followed by the experiments with several laboratory plant models. The obtained model parameters are used to tune disturbance observer based controllers to illustrate the performance of the proposed method in real applications.

Keywords: Closed loop identification · Relay control · First order model

1 Introduction

Relay feedback test has been very popular in several commercial autotuners for decades. The research in this area was deeply analyzed in [9–11]. This paper updates an earlier contribution [7] in which the algorithm failed in situations when the disturbances were negligible and the relay on and off times were almost equal over one control period. The results of the previous paper [7] can be summarized in the following way: the proposed method can be used for plants with unknown load disturbances without additional controller (see e.g. [14]). There is not necessary to bias the relay reference value to compensate the static disturbance, which does not have to be known in advance (see e.g. [2,12,13]). This paper starts with a method derivation, then the disturbance observer based PI controller is presented followed by a demonstration of the results of the identification and control using a laboratory model of a real plant.

1.1 Method Derivation

The main advantage of constraining the plant approximation to the IPDT model is that both the experiment setup and the corresponding analytical formulas

© Springer International Publishing Switzerland 2015
R. Moreno-Díaz et al. (Eds.): EUROCAST 2015, LNCS 9520, pp. 49–56, 2015.
DOI: 10.1007/978-3-319-27340-2_7

remain relatively simple and robust against measurement noise.

$$S(s) = \frac{K_s}{s}e^{-T_d s} \tag{1}$$

Let us consider the control loop with a relay with the output $u_r = \pm M$ and a piecewise constant input disturbance $v = const$. Then, the actual plant input will be given as a piecewise constant signal $u_A = \pm M + v$. Possible transients are shown in Fig. 2. Let us assume relay switching from the positive relay output $u = M$ to the negative value $u = -M$ (point 1) at the time t_{21i-1}, the influence of the positive plant input $U_2 = (v + M)K_s$ will remain over interval with the length equal to the dead time value T_d. Then, after reaching output value y_{21} at the time moment τ_{21i-1} (point 2) due to the effective plant input $U_1 = (v-M)K_s$ the output starts to decrease. After the time interval t_1 it reaches the reference value w (point 3). At this moment the relay switches to the positive value $u = M$, however the plant output keeps decreasing for the time T_d and reaches the value y_{12} (point 4). The duration of the interval with negative relay output will be denoted as t^-. While the output of the relay is positive the plant output starts to increase and reaches the reference value after the time t_2 (point 5). Let us

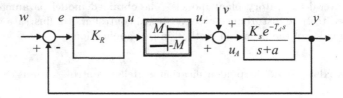

Fig. 1. Relay identification with nonsymmetrical plant input

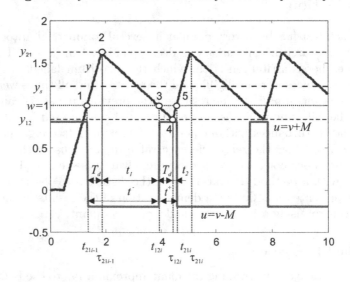

Fig. 2. Transients of basic variables of the loop in the Fig. 1

denote the total duration of the positive relay output as

$$t^+ = t_2 + T_d \tag{2}$$

As a result of the time delay, the plant output turnover time instants τ_{21i} are shifted with respect to the relay reversal moments t_{21i} by T_d. Similar time shift exists among time instants τ_{12i} and t_{12i}, i.e.

$$\tau_{21i} = t_{21i} + T_d \tag{3}$$

$$\tau_{12i} = t_{12i} + T_d \tag{4}$$

For a single integrator one can formulate relations

$$y_{21} - w = U_2 T_d; t_1 = (w - y_{21})/U_1$$
$$y_{12} - w = U_1 T_d; t_2 = (w - y_{12})/U_2 \tag{5}$$

Let us denote the period of one cycle as

$$P_u = t^+ + t^- = 2T_d + t_1 + t_2 = \frac{4T_d M^2}{M^2 - v^2} \tag{6}$$

For a known value of the relay amplitude M and a known ratio of the positive and negative relay output duration over one cycle

$$\epsilon = \frac{t^+}{t^-} = \frac{t_2 + T_d}{t_1 + T_d} = -\frac{v - M}{v + M} \tag{7}$$

it is possible to express the identified disturbance as

$$v = u_0 + v_n \tag{8}$$

This may consist of a known and intentionally set offset at the relay output and of an unknown external disturbance v_n that may be calculated as

$$v = M \frac{1 - \epsilon}{1 + \epsilon} \tag{9}$$

Then from (6) it follows

$$T_d = \frac{P_u}{4} \left[1 - \left(\frac{v}{M} \right)^2 \right] = P_u \frac{\epsilon}{(1 + \epsilon)^2} \tag{10}$$

Since the identification of the plant gain K_s proposed in [7] and based on an average output value over a limit cycle does not work well for negligible disturbances and a symmetrical relay output, one may either introduce a relay offset to make the cycle assymetrical, or to derive K_s by identifying the cycle limits. From (5) one gets

$$y_{21} - y_{12} = U_2 T_d + w - U_1 T_d - w \tag{11}$$

Substituting $U_1 = (v - M)K_s$ and $U_2 = (v + M)K_s$ into (11) yields

$$K_s = \frac{y_{21} - y_{12}}{2T_d M} \tag{12}$$

Substituting (10) into (12) finally yields formula for the plant gain

$$K_s = \frac{1}{2} \frac{(y_{21} - y_{12})(1 + \epsilon)^2}{M P_u \epsilon} \tag{13}$$

2   PI$_1$ - Controller

The PI$_1$ - controller (sometime denoted as DO-PI controller) employs disturbance observer (DO) as the I-action. The controller structure consisting of P-action and DO is presented in Fig. 3. Index "1" used in its title has to be related to one saturated pulse of the control variable that can occur in accomplishing large reference signal steps. In this way it should be distinguished from the PI$_0$ - controller reacting to a reference step by monotonic transient of the manipulated variable. To achieve fastest possible transients without overshooting in a closed loop with an integrator and a dead time, the closed loop pole corresponding to the fastest monotonic output transients using simple P-controller is [3]

$$\alpha_e = -1/(T_d e) \tag{14}$$

When using the P-controller together with the DO based I-action, some "slower" closed loop pole should be used

$$\alpha_{eI} = \alpha_e/c = 1/(T_d ec); c = [1.3, 1.5] \tag{15}$$

The gain of P-controller corresponding to the closed loop pole (15) is then

$$K_p = -\alpha_{eI}/K_s \tag{16}$$

For the time constant of the filter used in the DO one gets

$$T_f = -1/\alpha_{eI} \tag{17}$$

A preciser controller tuning may be derived by using the performance portrait method [6], or the dead-time may also be included into the DO [4].

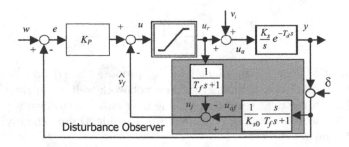

Fig. 3. PI$_1$ - controller

3   Real Experiment - Fan RPM

In this section, several experiments will be reported carried out by using the laboratory thermo-optical plant [8].

3.1   Identification

The input of the plant is the fan power, values from 0 to 100 % can be used in the Simulink model. The system output is the fan rpm filtered by the first order low pass filter with time constant set to one second. Several closed loop experiments have been made to cover a large operational range. Table 1 shows the plant is non-linear, the process gain varies from 21.34 to 30.82. The parameters for each working point in Table 1 were obtained in the following way: The system started from a steady state, the relay control was applied until at least 10 oscillations were measures. The first three relay cycles were omitted, then for the each one left the identification algorithm has been applied separately. The average value of these parameters were put into Table 1. The model and the real data are compared in Fig. 4. The corresponding parameters from Table 1 have been used, the real plant and the model use the same input.

Table 1. System parameters - fan rpm

Setpoint	1000	1500	2000	2500	3000	3500	4000	4500	5000	5500	6000
K_s	21.34	30.81	29.03	28.06	27.29	25.73	20.75	21.26	21.68	21.77	21.82
T_d	0.49	0.29	0.36	0.42	0.48	0.50	0.47	0.48	0.49	0.49	0.49
v	-17.26	28.38	24.38	21.23	18.03	14.98	11.32	6.29	0.91	-4.74	-10.66

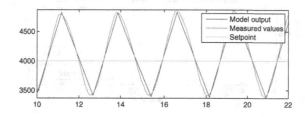

Fig. 4. Real system identification results - fan rpm, model vs real data

3.2   Control

The highest values of the process gain and of the time delay from Table 1 have been used in the experiment for controller tuning. Figure 5 shows the control results for one setpoint step change from a steady state. The system output reaches monotonically the new setpoint. Due to the plant nonlinearity and long dead time, the control signal remains without an extreme point typical for the PI_1 control.

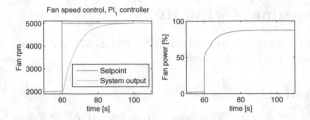

Fig. 5. Fan closed loop control performance of the controller based on the obtained model

4   Real Experiment - Temperature

4.1   Identification

A linear plant approximation corresponds to a plant with fast and slow channels [1], where the fast channel is represented by the heat radiation and the slow one corresponds to the heat conduction via body of the plant. One can expect that with the closed loop relay control, the fast channel would be dominant. Table 2 shows the identification results for various operating points. The model and the real data are compared in Fig. 6. Again the plant is non-linear, process gain varies from 0.0022 to 0.0068 and the time delay ranges from 0.3312 to 1.0533. The system parameters vary from one period to another. Since the simulation in the Fig. 6 was made using the average values of the system parameters calculated for each cycle and using the same input as the real system, one can see a difference in the amplitude of the real system and a model in Fig. 6.

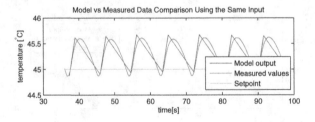

Fig. 6. Real system identification results - temperature, model vs real data

Table 2. System parameters - temperature channel

Setpoint	40	45	50	55	60	65	70
K_s	0.0068	0.0056	0.0048	0.0041	0.0034	0.0026	0.0022
T_d	0.7263	0.9113	1.0305	1.0533	0.9805	0.7325	0.3312
v	39.1122	31.8356	24.2042	16.3182	8.1374	-1.6944	-11.4774

4.2   Control

The highest value of the process gain and time delay from Table 2 have been used in the experiment to tune the controller. Figure 7 shows the control results for setpoint step changes from a steady state. The system output transients are close to the desired monotonic ones. Due to the system nonlinearity and two dynamic modes, the control signal transients show more than one pulse. Nevertheless, when considering the simplicity of the used model, the control performance is satisfactory.

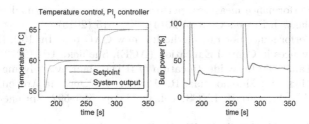

Fig. 7. Temperature closed loop control performance of the controller based on the obtained model

5   Conclusion

The carried out experiments show that the developed identification approach yields results applicable in control of a broad range of linear and nonlinear plants with a dynamics that is considerably more complex than the approximation used. Together with new performance portrait method for the controller tuning [5] and new DO based filtered PI control [4] it considerably simplifies control of the simple plants with significantly increasing reliability of the controller tuning and achievable performance.

Furthermore, when evaluating the dependency of the identified disturbances on the setpoint (or, more precisely, on the average output value), the method may be easily extended also to identification of static plants with a linear, or a nonlinear internal feedback and thus also to precise the subsequent controller tuning, which may bring significant improvements especially in control of static systems with a longer dead time.

Acknowledgment. This work has been partially supported by the grants APVV-0343-12 Computer aided robust nonlinear control design and VEGA 1/0937/14 Advanced methods for nonlinear modeling and control of mechatronic systems.

References

1. Astrom, K., Panagopoulos, H., Hagglund, T.: Design of PI controllers based on non-convex optimization. Automatica **34**(5), 585–601 (1998)
2. Hang, C., Astrom, K., Ho, W.: Relay auto-tuning in the presence of static load disturbance. Automatica **29**(2), 563–564 (1993)
3. Huba, M.: Constrained pole assignment control. In: Menini, L., Zaccarian, L., Abdallah, C.T. (eds.) Current Trends in Nonlinear Systems and Control, pp. 163–183. Birkhäuser, Boston (2006)
4. Huba, M.: Comparing 2DOF PI and predictive disturbance observer based filtered PI control. J. Process Control **23**(10), 1379–1400 (2013)
5. Huba, M.: Performance measures, performance limits and optimal PI control for the IPDT plant. J. Process Control **23**(4), 500–515 (2013)
6. Huba, M.: Performance portrait method: a new CAD tool. In: 10th IFAC Symposium on Advances in Control Education (ACE), Sheffield, UK (2013)
7. Huba, M., Ťapák, P.: Relay identification of IPDT plant by analyzing nonsymmetrical oscillations. In: Moreno-Díaz, R., Pichler, F., Quesada-Arencibia, A. (eds.) EUROCAST 2011, Part II. LNCS, vol. 6928, pp. 585–592. Springer, Heidelberg (2012)
8. Huba, T., Huba, M., Ťapák, P., Bisták, P.: New thermo-optical plants for laboratory experiments. In: IFAC World Congress, Cape Town, South Africa (2014)
9. Liu, T., Gao, F.: Industrial Process Identification and Control Design: Step-test and Relay-experiment-based Methods. Advances in Industrial Control. Springer, London (2011)
10. Liu, T., Gao, F.: A generalized relay identification method for time delay and non-minimum phase processes. Automatica **45**(4), 1072–1079 (2009)
11. Liu, T., Wang, Q.G., Huang, H.P.: A tutorial review on process identification from step or relay feedback test. J. Process Control **23**(10), 1597–1623 (2013)
12. Park, J.H., Sung, S.W., Lee, I.B.: Improved relay auto-tuning with static load disturbance. Automatica **33**(4), 711–715 (1997)
13. Shen, S.H., Wu, J.S., Yu, C.C.: Autotune identification under load disturbance. Ind. Eng. Chem. Res. **35**(5), 1642–1651 (1996)
14. Sung, S.W., Lee, J.: Relay feedback method under large static disturbances. Automatica **42**(2), 353–356 (2006)

Managing Certificate Revocation in VANETs Using Hash Trees and Query Frequencies

F. Martín-Fernández$^{(\boxtimes)}$, P. Caballero-Gil$^{(\boxtimes)}$, and C. Caballero-Gil

Department of Computer Engineering, University of La Laguna,
Santa Cruz de Tenerife, Spain
{francisco.martin.07,pcaballe,ccabgil}@ull.edu.es

Abstract. Due to the proliferation of technology in different areas of daily life, many new types of communication networks are emerging. Among the most interesting wireless networks, Vehicular Ad-hoc Networks are remarkable because road safety and traffic efficiency are two advances that any developed society should undertake. Therefore, research on such networks should evolve to take the final step and move from theory to reality. However, first, it is necessary to improve many aspects related to security. In particular, identification and management of malicious users within the network are major research issues. The traditional method using revocation lists to manage these users becomes very inefficient when the network grows. This paper proposes an alternative method to efficiently manage malicious users, which uses hash trees and query frequencies in order to fit better with the needs of Vehicular Ad-hoc Networks.

1 Introduction

Security is a crucial requirement in any communication network. In particular, the identification of misbehaving nodes and their consequent exclusion from the network are absolutely necessary to guarantee trustworthiness of network services. One of the basic solutions to accomplish these tasks in networks where communications are based on a Public-Key Infrastructure (PKI) is certificate revocation. Thus, a critical part in such networks is the management of revoked certificates. Related to this issue, in the bibliography we can find two different types of solutions. On the one hand, decentralized proposals enable revocation without the intervention of any centralized infrastructure, based on trusting the criteria of network nodes. On the other hand, a centralized approach is based on the existence of a central Certificate Authority (CA), which is the entity responsible for deciding on the validity of each node certificate, and all nodes trust it. This second approach usually requires the distribution of the so-called Certificate Revocation Lists (CRLs), which can be seen as blacklists of revoked certificates.

Research supported by TIN2011-25452, BES-2012-051817, IPT-2012-0585-370000 and RTC-2014-1648-8.

R. Moreno-Díaz et al. (Eds.): EUROCAST 2015, LNCS 9520, pp. 57–63, 2015.
DOI: 10.1007/978-3-319-27340-2_8

Vehicular Ad-hoc NETworks (VANETs) are self-organizing networks built up from moving vehicles that communicate with each other mainly to prevent adverse circumstances on the roads, but also to achieve a more efficient traffic management. VANETs can be seen as an extension of Mobile Ad-hoc NETworks (MANETs) where there are not only mobile nodes, there called On-Board Units (OBUs), but also static nodes, which are the so-called Road-Side Units (RSUs). Once VANETs are implemented in practice on a large scale, their size will grow and the use of multiple temporary certificates will become necessary to protect the privacy of the users. Thus, it is foreseeable that CRLs will grow up to become very large. Moreover, in this context it is also expected a phenomenon known as implosion request, consisting of several nodes who synchronously want to download the CRL at the time of its updating, producing serious congestion and overload of the network, what could ultimately lead to a longer latency in the process of validating a certificate.

The proposal described here uses a Huffman [6] k-ary hash tree as an Authenticated Data Structure (ADS), for the management of certificate revocation in VANETs. By using this ADS, the process of query on the validity of certificates will be more efficient because OBUs will send queries to RSUs, who will answer them on behalf of the CA. In this way, at the same time, the CA will no longer be a bottleneck and OBUs will not have to download the entire CRL. In particular, the used Huffman k-ary hash trees are based on the application of a duplex construction [1] of the Secure Hash Algorithm SHA-3 [2] that was recently chosen as standard, because the combination of both structures allows improving efficiency of updating and querying of revoked certificates.

This paper is organized as follows. Section 2 addresses the general problem of the use of certificate revocation lists in VANETs, and provides a succinct revision of related works. Then, Sect. 3 introduces the main ideas of the proposal for managing certificate revocation. Afterwards, Sect. 4 includes full details of the operations to build the tree. Finally, Sect. 5 discusses some conclusions and possible future research lines.

2 Related Work

Many proposals for the revocation of fraudulent users on computer networks have been published in recent years. Among them, the two main technologies to check the revocation status of a particular certificate are: Online Certificate Status Protocol (OCSP) and Certificate Revocation List (CRL). The OCSP provides revocation information about an individual certificate from an issuing CA, whereas a CRL provides a list of revoked certificates and may be received by users less frequently.

The CRL was the first system proposed to solve the problem, and actually nowadays it is the most popular method, so it can be considered the practical standard to provide information about revoked certificates. Regarding research on VANETs, both possibilities of revocation have been evaluated [11]. [10], and the first one has been adapted to the scheme referred to as ADOPT (Ad-hoc

Distributed OcsP for Trust). In particular, ADOPT is based on a distributed version of the OCSP, which uses caches of OCSP responses to examine certificates validity. These OCSP caches are distributed, updated dynamically, and stored on intermediate nodes, avoiding the exchange of extended certificate status lists. Each node has to use an on-demand protocol to find the closest OCSP cache that is able to provide the status of the requested peer's certificate.

Since almost one thousand million cars exist in the world [8], considering the use of certificates, a direct conclusion is that the number of revoked certificates might reach soon that quantity, one thousand million. Assuming that each certificate takes at least 224 bits, the CRL size would be 224 Gbits, what means that its management following the traditional approach would not be efficient. Even though regional CAs were used and the CRLs could be reduced to 1 Gbit, by using the 802.11a protocol to communicate with RSUs in range, the maximum download speed of OBUs would be between 6 and 54 Mbit/s depending on vehicle speed and road congestion, so on average an OBU would need more than 30 s to download a regional CRL from an RSU. A straight consequence of this problem is that new CRLs cannot be issued very often, what would affect the freshness of revocation data. Besides, if a known technique for large data transfers were used for CRL distribution as solution for the size problem, this would result in higher latencies, what would also impact in the revocation data validity.

In order to overcome some of the aforementioned issues, delta CRLs (d-CRLs) have been proposed. In such a solution, the CA initially signs a base CRL, and later, short CRLs are issued to announce only the certificates that have been revoked after the issuance of the base CRL. Several authors have proposed other methods based on CRLs to avoid different problems such as demand bottlenecks or size overheads. These methods are, for example, segmented CRLs [3], or sliding window d-CRLs [4].

Other authors have tried to improve efficiency of communication and computation in the management of revocations in VANETs by proposing the use of different Authentication Data Structures such as Merkle trees [5], Huffman Merkle trees [9] and skip lists [7]. However, to the best of our knowledge, no previous work has described in detail the use of Huffman k-ary trees as hash trees for revoked certificates management.

3   Managing Certificate Revocation

This work proposes the use of a combinatorial structure known as k-ary tree, which is a rooted tree in which each node has no more than k children, and each internal node is obtained by hashing the concatenation of all the digests contained in its children. Specifically, we propose the use of a Huffman k-ary tree in which leaf nodes are ordered from left to right, based on which revoked certificates the most queried. Thus, we propose the introduction of the combination of both concepts of Huffman coding and k-ary trees applied to trees based revocation. The generated tree structure can be seen in Fig. 1.

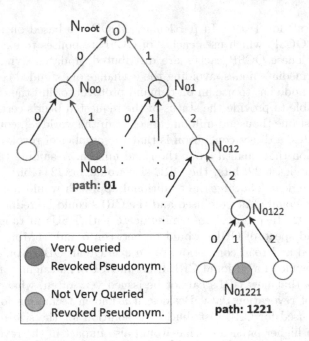

Fig. 1. Query frequencies used in a 3-ary hash tree.

The tree-based model proposed here is based on the notation shown in Table 1.

Regarding the cryptographic hash function h used in the hash tree, this proposal is based on the use of a new version of the Secure Hash Algorithm SHA-3. In SHA-3, the basic cryptographic hash function called Keccak contains 24 rounds of a basic transformation and its input is represented by a 5×5 matrix of 64-bit lanes.

Table 1. Proposal notation

Notation	Meaning
$h(...)$	hash function used to define the revocation tree
$h(A_0\|A_1\|...)$	Digest obtained with the hash function h applied on the concatenation of the inputs $A_i, i = 0, 1, ...$
$D(\geq 1)$	Depth of the hash tree, which indicates the number of different types of vehicles used in the scheme
$d_x(< D)$	Depth of a node x in the tree
t	total number of revoked certificate
$RC_j(j = 1, 2, ..., t)$	$j - th$ Revoked Certificate
$N_{ij}(i = D - d_{N_{ij}}, j = 0, 1, ...)$	Node of the hash tree
k	Maximum number of children for each internal node

In contrast, our proposal is based on 32-bit lanes. Another proposed variation of SHA-3 is the use of a duplex version of the sponge structure of SHA-3. On the one hand, like the sponge construction of SHA-3, the proposal based on a duplex construction also uses Keccak as fixed-length transformation, the same padding rule and data bit rate. On the other hand, unlike a sponge function, the duplex construction output corresponding to an input string might be obtained through the concatenation of the outputs resulting from successive input blocks.

The authenticity of the used hash tree structure is guaranteed thanks to the CA signature of the root node. When an RSU answers to an OBU about a query on a certificate, it proceeds in the following way. If it finds the digest of the certificate among the leaf nodes of the tree, which means that it is a revoked certificate, the RSU sends to the OBU the route between the root and the corresponding leaf node, along with all the siblings of the nodes on this path. After checking all the digests corresponding to the received path, and the CA signature of the root, the OBU gets convinced of the validity of the received evidence on the revoked certificate. Conceptually, thanks to the proposal of using a Huffman tree, queries regarding the most usually queried certificates involve less data transmission and computation.

4   Building the Tree

In the presented proposal, every new revoked node is inserted in the hash tree, if possible, as a new sibling to the right. In such a case, if insertion is possible at the corresponding level, all internal nodes of the path to the root must be updated. Otherwise, if the corresponding level is complete, a new insertion requires the deletion of expired revocations, and afterwards, if necessary, a novel solution that can be based either on the insertion of a new sub-tree, redefinition of neighboring categories, or creation of a new level, depending on the case.

Furthermore, the proposal makes use of the idea under Huffman codes to divide the tree into different levels depending on the frequency of queries about vehicles and/or the time each vehicle spends on the road. Thus, leaf nodes placed in positions closer to the root node correspond to revoked vehicles that spend more time on the road and/or for which more queries about them exist.

This proposal fits real world because vehicles can be ranged into different categories depending on the time they spend on the road: taxis, public transport buses, private transport buses, trucks, emergency vehicles, delivery vehicles, private vehicles, etc., and this classification can be used to assume that those vehicles that spend more time on the road are the vehicles for which more queries exist.

In this proposal, the CA, which is responsible for generating the tree, builds a Huffman tree structure that is prepared to contain all foreseeable revoked nodes. As soon as a certificate of a vehicle is revoked, all certificates of such a vehicle must be inserted in this structure.

During the initialization of the tree, in order to estimate its size, the CA uses actual data of vehicles. Thus, it asks the competent authority that owns the data in order to know the number of vehicles of each type so that it can estimate the number of levels (according to Huffman Codes) and the k parameter of the k-ary tree. The size of the certificate is assumed to be 228 bits, according to the typical size of a classic CRL in VANET.

The procedure applied to calculate the initial parameters of the tree is shown in Algorithm 1.

Algorithm 1. Initial Parameters, k Calculation

---

1 Select *firstK* as the minimum numbers of vehicles of a certain type;
2 Assign *firstK* to *newK*;
3 //*depth* is numbers of vehicle types
4 **for** *i* ← *depth* **to** 1 **do**
5 ⎸   Calculate the number of internal nodes needed in the $(i-1)$ level to accommodate nodes of i level
6 ⎿   with $k = newK$;

7 *maxK* is last calculation of previous loop;
8 **for** *iterateK between (firstK, maxK]* **do**
9 ⎸   Assign *iterateK* to *newK*;
10 ⎸   **if** *newK changed* **then**
11 ⎸   ⎸   **for** *i* ← *depth* **to** 1 **do**
12 ⎸   ⎸   ⎿   Calculate the number of internal nodes needed in the $(i-1)$ level to accommodate nodes of i level with $k = newK$;
13 ⎸   ⎸   Assign last calculation of previous loop to *newK*;
14 ⎸   **else**
15 ⎿   ⎿   Break Loop;

16 Assign *newK* to *optimalK*;
17 **return** *optimalK*;

---

5   Conclusions

Road safety is one of the major concerns of modern society. Therefore, Vehicular Ad-hoc Networks are generating special interest in the most relevant research in recent years. Various innovation fields are appearing in such networks. Besides, every aspect related to computer security in these networks is a fundamental aspect needed to make of VANETs a popular tool. This paper proposes a new management scheme to detect fraudulent users and to prevent communications with illegitimate users. Traditional methods use classical certificate revocation lists, which are inefficient if the number of users of the network increases. The method defined in this paper proposes replacing the traditional method by another one based on a new structure. Such a new structure is an ADS based on hash trees that are k-ary trees. This choice provides many benefits, especially when inserting new revoked certificates. Query frequencies are also used to optimize and prioritize the position of a revoked certificate in the hash tree. Thus, the method of query about a revoked certificate becomes much quicker and efficient because it is achieved by prioritizing those certificates that are more likely to be queried. Early tests show that this approach is more efficient than other classical proposals both regarding the insertion of new revoked nodes and during the query process. This work is part of a work in progress, so the next phases involve the implementation and comparison of the proposed scheme with other schemes.

References

1. Bertoni, G., Daemen, J., Peeters, M., Van Assche, G.: Duplexing the sponge: single-pass authenticated encryption and other applications. In: Miri, A., Vaudenay, S. (eds.) SAC 2011. LNCS, vol. 7118, pp. 320–337. Springer, Heidelberg (2012)
2. Bertoni, G., Daemen, J., Peeters, M., Van Assche, G.: Keccak sponge function family main document version 2.1, Updated submission to NIST (Round 2) (2010)
3. Cooper, D.A.: A model of certificate revocation. In: Proceedings of the 15th Annual Computer Security Applications Conference (1999)
4. Cooper, D.A.: A more efficient use of delta CRLs. In: Proceedings of the IEEE Symposium on Security and Privacy (2000)
5. Gañán, C., Muñoz, J.L., Esparza, O., Mata-Díaz, J., Alins, J.: Toward revocation data handling efficiency in VANETs. In: Vinel, A., Mehmood, R., Berbineau, M., Garcia, C.R., Huang, C.-M., Chilamkurti, N. (eds.) Nets4Trains 2012 and Nets4Cars 2012. LNCS, vol. 7266, pp. 80–90. Springer, Heidelberg (2012)
6. Huffman, D.: A method for the construction of minimum-redundancy codes. Proc. IRE **40**(9), 1098–1101 (1952)
7. Jakobsson, M., Wetzel, S.: Efficient attribute authentication with applications to Ad Hoc networks. In: ACM Workshop on Vehicular Ad Hoc Networks, pp. 38–46 (2004)
8. McMichael, A.J.: The urban environment and health in a world of increasing globalization: issues for developing countries. Bull. World Health Organ. **78**(9), 1117–1126 (2000)
9. Muñoz, J.L., Forné, J., Esparza, O., Rey, M.: Efficient certificate revocation system implementation: huffman merkle hash tree (HuffMHT). In: Katsikas, S.K., López, J., Pernul, G. (eds.) TrustBus 2005. LNCS, vol. 3592, pp. 119–127. Springer, Heidelberg (2005)
10. Papapanagiotou, K., Marias, G.F., Georgiadis, P.: A certificate validation protocol for VANETs. In: Globecom Workshops IEEE, pp. 1–9 (2007)
11. Serna Olvera, J., Casola, V., Rak, M., Luna, J., Medina, M., Mazzocca, N.: Performance analysis of an OCSP-Based authentication protocol for VANETs. Int. J. Adapt. Resilient and Auton. Syst. (IJARAS) **3**(1), 19–45 (2012)

Constrained Pole Assignment Control for a 2nd Order Oscillatory System

Mikuláš Huba$^{(\boxtimes)}$ and Tomáš Huba

Slovak University of Technology in Bratislava, Ilkovičova 3,
812 19 Bratislava, Slovakia
{mikulas.huba,tomas.huba}@stuba.sk
http://uamt.fei.stuba.sk

Abstract. The paper brings phase plane design of a constrained Proportional Derivative (PD) controller for undamped second order oscillatory plants. The approach is focused on achieving the possibly best tracking dynamics considering the control signal saturation. The linear pole assignment control and relay minimum time control are included as its limit solutions. The paper shows that such a task has infinitely many solutions. The existing degree of freedom follows from a free choice of a distance definition in evaluating deviation of the operating point from the considered invariant set specified by the required reference braking trajectory. It may be used to choose the simplest controller equations, or to modify the loop performance in the case of an unmodeled dynamics.

Keywords: Constrained control · Pole-assignment control

1 Introduction

Control saturation represents nonlinearity present practically in all applications. For a double integrator, one of possible solutions including the relay minimum time control and the linear pole assignment control as limit situations has been proposed in [1,2]. Approximations of the plant dynamics by undamped oscillatory models ($a_0 > 0$) with an input disturbance d_i and output y

$$\ddot{y} = K_s(u_r + d_i) - a_0(y) \; ; \;\; \ddot{y} = d^2y/dt^2 \tag{1}$$

are frequently considered e.g. in motion control. For example, such a constrained continuous-time pole assignment control considering a saturated input

$$U_{r1} \leq u_r \leq U_{r2} \tag{2}$$

has been applied in [4] to control a propeller pendulum that represents a core module of an autonomous paracopter. Attractiveness of this problem increased lately due to new results achieved in the controller tuning by the performance portrait method and in a modular design and tuning of filtered controllers [3,5–7]. Results of this paper will later allow to show several advantages of the

© Springer International Publishing Switzerland 2015
R. Moreno-Díaz et al. (Eds.): EUROCAST 2015, LNCS 9520, pp. 64–71, 2015.
DOI: 10.1007/978-3-319-27340-2_9

constrained continuous-time pole assignment control design. The key property is its modularity, i.e. the possibility of a simple extension by an integral action based on disturbance observers for input, or output disturbances, an easy filter design, an extension by a dynamical feedforward control considering the control constraints, an extension to systems with a long dead time, or a relatively simple consideration of an additional loop dynamics (as e.g. given by the motor-propeller inertia in the propeller pendulum control [4]). Analytical formulation of the controller equations gives also a possibility to be generalized by a gain scheduling to nonlinear control.

2   Problem Formulation

For a given setpoint reference signal $r(t)$ and $\mathbf{x} = (y, \dot{y})^t$ being the plant state, it is usual to describe the system in terms of deviations

$$\bar{y}(t) = y(t) - r(t) \; ; \; \dot{\bar{y}}(t) = \dot{y}(t) - \dot{r}(t) \tag{3}$$

These move a reference point to the phase plane origin $\bar{\mathbf{w}} = [\bar{r}, \dot{\bar{r}}]^t = [0, 0]^t$ of a new coordinates system $\bar{\mathbf{x}} = [\bar{y}, \dot{\bar{y}}]^t$. In the new state coordinates $\bar{\mathbf{x}} = [\bar{y}, \dot{\bar{y}}]^t$

$$\ddot{\bar{y}}(t) = \ddot{y}(t) - \ddot{w}(t) = K_s(u_r + d_i) - a_0(y - w + w) - \ddot{w}$$

A new control variable $\bar{u}$ covering all inputs

$$\bar{u} = K_s(u_r + d_i) - a_0 w - \ddot{w} \tag{4}$$

allows a new simplified system description

$$\ddot{\bar{y}}(t) = \bar{u} - a_0 \bar{y}; \quad F(s) = \left[\frac{\overline{Y}(s)}{\overline{U}(s)} \right]_{d_i=0} = \frac{K_s}{s^2 + a_0} \tag{5}$$

A control design starts firstly with determining $\bar{u}$. Real control is then based on calculating u_r by means of an inverse transformation and saturation

$$u_r = sat((\bar{u} + a_1 \dot{w} + a_0 w + \ddot{w})/K_s - d_i) \tag{6}$$

2.1   Stability and Controllability

Admissible control range for the new input $\bar{U}_1 \leq \bar{u} \leq \bar{U}_2$ is limited by

$$\bar{U}_j = K_s(U_{rj} + d_i) - a_1 \dot{w} - a_0 w - \ddot{w} \; ; \; j = 1, 2 \tag{7}$$

One possible requirement on controllability of the constrained system (5) is that during transients it must always be possible to change the sign of $\ddot{\bar{y}}(t)$ by the input (4) with constraints (7). From this requirement, admissible inputs may be defined as reference setpoints w and input disturbances d_i of (1) satisfying $\bar{U}_1 \bar{U}_2 < 0$. To get a simple denotation, next we are going to work with the shifted variables (3) without the bar in the denotation, i.e. with $\mathbf{x} = [y, \dot{y}]^t$ and u

$$\dot{\mathbf{x}} = \mathbf{A}_0 \mathbf{x} + \mathbf{b}_0 u \; ; \; y = \mathbf{c}_0^t \mathbf{x} \tag{8}$$

$$\mathbf{A}_0 = \begin{bmatrix} 0 & 1 \\ -a_0 & 0 \end{bmatrix} \; ; \; \mathbf{b}_0 = \begin{bmatrix} 0 \\ 1 \end{bmatrix} ; \; \mathbf{c}_0^t = [1 \; 0]$$

2.2   Linear Pole Assignment PD Control for Real Poles

Similarly as in [8], for a closed loop system

$$\frac{d}{dt}\mathbf{x}(t) = \mathbf{A}\mathbf{x}(t); \ \mathbf{A} = \mathbf{A}_0 - \mathbf{b}_0 \mathbf{r}^t \tag{9}$$

and for real closed loop poles $\alpha_1, \alpha_2 < 0$ one gets the eigenvectors

$$\mathbf{A}\mathbf{v}_i = \alpha_i \mathbf{v}_i; \ \mathbf{v}_i = (\alpha_i \mathbf{I} - \mathbf{A})^{-1}\mathbf{b}; \ i = 1, \text{or } 2 \tag{10}$$

These define two eigenlines $L_i, i = 1, 2$ written by means of vectors $\mathbf{a_i} \perp \mathbf{v}_i$ as

$$L_i : \ \mathbf{a}_i^t \mathbf{x} = 0 \tag{11}$$

L_i represent invariant sets for the final phase of control transients. During the initial phase the controller has to decrease (oriented) distance from L_i

$$\rho_l \{\mathbf{x}(t)\} = \mathbf{a}_i^t \mathbf{x} \tag{12}$$

with a speed proportional to the pole α_2

$$\frac{d\rho_l \{\mathbf{x}(t)\}}{dt} = \alpha_2 \rho_l \{\mathbf{x}(t)\}; \ \rho_l \{\mathbf{x}(t)\} \neq 0; \tag{13}$$

During the motion along L_i, the controller task is to decrease the (oriented) distance from the origin $\rho_0 \{\mathbf{x}(t)\} = sign(y)abs(\mathbf{x})$ according to

$$\frac{d\rho_0 \{\mathbf{x}(t)\}}{dt} = \alpha_1 \rho_0 \{\mathbf{x}(t)\}; \ \rho_l \{\mathbf{x}(t)\} = \mathbf{a}_i^t \mathbf{x}(t) = 0 \tag{14}$$

Both these properties may be guaranteed by linear PD controller

$$u = -\mathbf{r}^t \mathbf{x}; \ \mathbf{r}^t = \frac{\mathbf{a}_i^t [\mathbf{A}_0 - \alpha_2 \mathbf{I}]}{\mathbf{a}_i^t \mathbf{b}_0} = [a_0 - \alpha_1 \alpha_2, \ \alpha_1 + \alpha_2] \tag{15}$$

2.3   Invariant Sets of Linear Control G_L

For some chosen $\mathbf{v} = \mathbf{v}_i$ and $\mathbf{z} \perp \mathbf{v}$ satisfying $\mathbf{r}^t \mathbf{z} = 0$, the proportional band of control defined by $sat(u) = u$ may be expressed as

$$P_b = \{\mathbf{x} = x_v \mathbf{v} + x_z \mathbf{z} | x_v \in \langle U_1, U_2 \rangle\} \tag{16}$$

For an undamped oscillator with $a_0 > 0$

$$\mathbf{v} = \begin{bmatrix} \frac{1}{\alpha_1^2 + a_0} \\ \frac{\alpha_1}{\alpha_1^2 + a_0} \end{bmatrix}; \ \mathbf{z} = \begin{bmatrix} \frac{(\alpha_1 + \alpha_2)\alpha_1}{(\alpha_1^2 + a_0)(\alpha_2^2 + a_0)} \\ \frac{\alpha_1(\alpha_1\alpha_2 - a_0)}{(\alpha_1^2 + a_0)(\alpha_2^2 + a_0)} \end{bmatrix} \tag{17}$$

Obviously, choice of "faster" poles ($\alpha_i \to -\infty$) leads to a fast decrease of the length of $\mathbf{z}$ and $\mathbf{v}$. P_b will be limited by two lines B_1 and B_2 parallel to $\mathbf{v}$ and corresponding to the limit control values U_1 and U_2. Thus, since an invariant set of linear control G_L consisting of fully linear trajectories must lie in P_b, its size may rapidly decrease and it become negligibly small. The linear pole assignment control gives acceptable results just in vicinity of the required states.

B_j; $j = 1, 2$ cross the chosen eigenline $L = L_i$; $i = 1, 2$ in points

$$X_0^j = \begin{bmatrix} x_0^j \\ \dot{x}_0^j \end{bmatrix} = \mathbf{v}U_j = \begin{bmatrix} \frac{1}{\alpha_1^2 + a_0} \\ \frac{\alpha_1}{\alpha_1^2 + a_0} \end{bmatrix} U_j \tag{18}$$

In these points still holds the distance decrease from the origin (14)

$$[dx/dt]_{\mathbf{x}=X_0^j} = \mathbf{A}\mathbf{v}U_j + \mathbf{b}U_j = \alpha_1 \mathbf{v}U_j \tag{19}$$

2.4   Reference Braking Curves RBC^j

RBC^j [8]; $j = 1, 2$ represent curves consisting from the line segments $0X_0^j$ and curves corresponding to limit braking with $u = U_j; j = 1, 2$ and finishing in X_0^j

$$\mathbf{x}(\tau)^j = \mathbf{A}(-\tau)X_0^j + \mathbf{b}(-\tau)U_j; \ i, j = 1, 2 \ ; \ \tau > 0 \tag{20}$$

After eliminating the time τ from (20) one gets linear and nonlinear segments of RBC^j: linear segments $0X_0^j$ (or $X_0^1 X_0^2$) represent targets for low velocities, nonlinear for high. Linear reference lines follow from $\dot{x}_0^j = \alpha_1 U_j/(\alpha_1^2 + a_0)$ as

$$y_b = \frac{\dot{y}}{\alpha_1} \ ; \ y < 0 \cap \dot{y} < \dot{x}_0^1 \cup y > 0 \cap \dot{y} > \dot{x}_0^2 \tag{21}$$

Nonlinear segments of RBC^j may be described as

$$y_b^j = \frac{U_j}{a_0} - sign(y)p \ ; \ p = \sqrt{\frac{\alpha_1^2 U_j^2}{(\alpha_1^2 + a_0)a_0^2} - \frac{\dot{y}^2}{a_0}} \tag{22}$$

$$j = \frac{3 + sign(y)}{2} \ ; \ \dot{p}_{max}^j = \frac{\alpha_1 U_j}{\sqrt{(\alpha_1^2 + a_0)a_0}}$$

$$y > 0 \cap \dot{p}_{max}^2 \leq \dot{y} \leq \dot{x}_0^2 \cup y < 0 \cap \dot{p}_{max}^1 \geq \dot{y} \geq \dot{x}_0^1 \tag{23}$$

2.5   Controllers Decreasing the Distance from RBC

The linear pole assignment control (15) decreasing distance from the reference eigenline L_i according to (13) will now be generalized for a constrained control decreasing the distance from RBC^j. The first problem to solve is, how to define a distance $\rho_1 \{\mathbf{x}(t)\}$ from RBC^j? It offers infinitely many solutions [8]: in direction of a normal to the RBC (too complicated), parallel to the y-axis, parallel to the $\dot{y}$-axis, under a chosen angle to the axes, etc. Which solution is "the best"? The best answer to this question seems to be: *the simplest one giving good results*.

2.6   Constrained PD Controller for Distance $\rho_l(\mathbf{x}) = y - y_b$

For the distance definition

$$\rho_1(\mathbf{x}) = y - y_b^j \tag{24}$$

the basic controller equation becomes

$$\frac{d\rho_l(\mathbf{x})}{dt} = \dot{y} - sign(y)\frac{\dot{y}}{a_0 p}(u - a_0 y) = \alpha_2\,\rho(\mathbf{x}) \tag{25}$$

For the considered plant and $\rho_l(\mathbf{x})$ (24) one gets for decreasing the distance from RBC^j a nonlinear PD controller

$$u = a_0 y + \frac{\alpha_2 p^2 a_0}{\dot{y}} + sign(y)(a_0 p + \alpha_2 p\frac{(U_j - a_0 y)}{\dot{y}}) \tag{26}$$

It is applied for

$$y > 0 \cap \dot{p}_{max}^2 \le \dot{y} \le \dot{x}_0^2 \cup y < 0 \cap \dot{p}_{max}^1 \ge \dot{y} \ge \dot{x}_0^1 \tag{27}$$

Both the linear (L) and nonlinear controller (NL) are followed by a saturation (Fig. 1 left) limiting the output to the limits (7).

2.7   Constrained PD Controller for Distance Definition $\rho_1(\mathbf{x}) = \dot{y} - \dot{y}_b$

The "linear" and "nonlinear" segments of RBC^j will now be expressed as

$$\dot{y}_b = \alpha_1 y\ ;\quad x_0^1 \le y \le x_0^2 \tag{28}$$

$$\dot{y}_b = -sign(y)p\ ;\quad p = \sqrt{-\left[y^2 a_0 + (x_0^j - 2y)U_j\right]} \tag{29}$$

$$j = (3 + sign(y))/2$$

The distance decrease concept is applicable just for

$$\left[1 - \frac{\alpha_1}{\sqrt{\alpha_1^2 + a_0}}\right]\frac{U_1}{a_0} \le y \le \left[1 - \frac{\alpha_1}{\sqrt{\alpha_1^2 + a_0}}\right]\frac{U_2}{a_0} \tag{30}$$

P_b of the constrained pole assignment controller includes just a segment of G_L constrained by switching lines running parallel to $\dot{y}$-axis and crossing points X_0^j; $j = 1, 2$ (Fig. 1).

At the border of the linear and nonlinear segments of P_b it is possible to identify points Z_0^j and Y_0^j, in which $u = 0$, or $u = U_{3-j}$. Both these points have the first coordinate $z_0^j = y_0^j = x_0^j$, when:

$$Z_0^j = \begin{bmatrix} \frac{\alpha_1(\alpha_1+\alpha_2)}{(\alpha_1^2+a_0)(\alpha_1\alpha_2-a_0)} \\ \frac{\alpha_1}{\alpha_1^2+a_0} \end{bmatrix} U_j; \quad \mathbf{r}^t Z_0^j = 0; \quad j = 1, 2 \tag{31}$$

$$Y_0^j = \begin{bmatrix} \frac{\alpha_1(\alpha_1+\alpha_2)-(\alpha_1^2+a_0)U_{3-j}/U_j}{(\alpha_1^2+a_0)(\alpha_1\alpha_2-a_0)} \\ \frac{\alpha_1}{\alpha_1^2+a_0} \end{bmatrix} U_j; \quad -\mathbf{r}^t Y_0^j = U_{3-j} \tag{32}$$

The basic region nonlinear (NL) controller equation becomes

$$u = a_0 y + \alpha_2 \dot{y} - sign(y)\left[(U_j - a_0 y)/p\dot{y} - \alpha_2 p\right] \tag{33}$$

The border of a full acceleration defined by $u = U_{3-j}$ corresponds to

$$\dot{y}_3^j = \frac{(U_{3-j} - sign(y)\alpha_2 p - a_0 y)}{\alpha_2 p - sign(y)(U_j - a_0 y)} p \tag{34}$$

This curve is singular in points

$$y_s^j = \left[1 + \frac{\alpha_1\alpha_2}{\sqrt{(\alpha_1^2 + a_0)(\alpha_2^2 + a_0)}}\right]\frac{U_j}{a_0}; \ j = 1, 2$$

For the control (33) these points limit the maximal usable deviations y. Due to $|\alpha_i|/\sqrt{\alpha_i^2 + a_0} < 1$ these borders are narrower than (30).

In NL segment the control changes its sign in points of the critical curve

$$\dot{y}_{cr}^j = -\frac{\alpha_2 sign(y)p + a_0 y}{\alpha_2 p - sign(y)(U_j - a_0 y)} p; \quad j = 1, 2$$

This formula is singular for (35). This curve crosses the y-axis in points

$$Z_1^j = \begin{bmatrix} \frac{\alpha_2}{a_0(\alpha_2^2+a_0)}\left(\alpha_2 - \sqrt{\frac{\alpha_1^2\alpha_2^2-a_0^2}{\alpha_1^2+a_0}}\right) \\ 0 \end{bmatrix} U_j; \quad j = 1, 2 \tag{35}$$

lying between y_s^1 and y_s^2. For a line running parallel to the $\dot{y}$-axis, its crosssections with $\dot{y}_{cr}^j$, RBC^j and $\dot{y}_3^j$ yield points, in which $u = 0$, $u = U_j$ and $u = U_{3-j}$

$$Y_1^j = \begin{bmatrix} \frac{\alpha_2}{a_0(\alpha_2^2+a_0)}\left(\alpha_2 - \sqrt{\frac{\alpha_1^2\alpha_2^2-a_0^2}{\alpha_1^2+a_0}}\right) \\ \dot{y}_1 \end{bmatrix} U_j \tag{36}$$

$$\dot{y}_1 = \frac{c_2 p^2 + c_1 p}{1}; \ c_2 = \alpha_2(\alpha_1^2 + a_0)(\alpha_2^2 + a_0);$$

$$c_1 = (\alpha_1^2 + a_0)(U_2(\alpha_2^2 + a_0) - \alpha_2^2 U_1) + \alpha_2 U_1\sqrt{(\alpha_1^2 + a_0)(\alpha_1^2\alpha_2^2 - a_0^2)}$$

$$X_1^j = \begin{bmatrix} \frac{\alpha_2}{a_0(\alpha_2^2+a_0)}\left(\alpha_2 - \sqrt{\frac{\alpha_1^2\alpha_2^2-a_0^2}{\alpha_1^2+a_0}}\right) \\ -\sqrt{\frac{2\alpha_1^2\alpha_2^2+\alpha_2^2 a_0-a_0^2-2\alpha_2\sqrt{(\alpha_1^2+a_0)(\alpha_1^2\alpha_2^2-a_0^2)}}{(\alpha_1^2+a_0)(\alpha_2^2+a_0)}} \end{bmatrix} U_j \tag{37}$$

Control out of the basic region may follow from continuity at the border of the basic region and it corresponds to a derivative (D) control

$$u = K_D \dot{y}; \quad K_D^{-1} = -\sqrt{\frac{2\alpha_1^2 \alpha_2^2 + \alpha_2^2 a_0 - a_0^2 - 2\alpha_2 \sqrt{(\alpha_1^2 + a_0)(\alpha_1^2 \alpha_2^2 - a_0^2)}}{(\alpha_1^2 + a_0)(\alpha_2^2 + a_0)}} \quad (38)$$

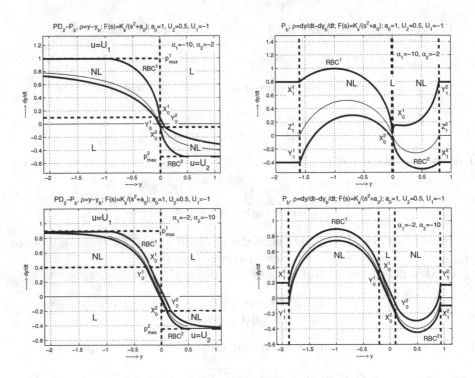

Fig. 1. Proportional band P_b and the switching lines (dashed) of the controller with the distance from RBC^j measured in direction of the y-axis (left) and of the $\dot{y}$-axis (right) for oriented closed loop pairs $-2, -10$ and $-10, -2$; $a_0 = 1$; $U_1 = -1$; $U_2 = 0.5$.

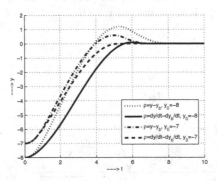

Fig. 2. Transients of a dead time system ($K_s = 1, T_d = 0.05, a_0 = 0.25, \alpha_{1,2} = -5.628$ with distance from RBC^j measured in direction of the y and $\dot{y}$-axis; $U_1 = -1, U_2 = 0.5$

3   Conclusions

New solution to the constrained pole assignment control problem for an undamped second order system has been presented. It has shown that the ambiguous character of a distance decrease concept may under constrained control be used for improving properties of the time delayed system control (Fig. 2). Here, the superior performance of the loops with controllers based on the distance measurement along the $\dot{y}$ axis follows from broader P_b (Fig. 1) enabling an adequate controller reaction. For larger initial conditions, transients cross P_b at higher velocities. For the controller based on the distance decrease measurement along the y axis, the P_b is too narrow at these velocities to give sufficient time to start the braking process.

Our future work will deal (similarly as in [5]) with deriving optimal tuning applicable to time delayed systems and with comparing transients achievable by the double integrator model with those corresponding to the oscillatory plant model (5) both by simulation and real time control.

Acknowledgment. Partially supported by the grants APVV-0343-12 Computer aided robust nonlinear control design and VEGA 1/0937/14 Advanced methods for nonlinear modeling and control of mechatronic systems.

References

1. Huba, M., Bisták, P.: Dynamic classes in the PID control. In: American Control Conference, San Diego (1999)
2. Huba, M., Sovisova, D., Oravec, I.: Invariant sets based concept of the pole assignment control. In: ECC 1999, Karlsruhe (1999)
3. Huba, M.: Performance measures, performance limits and optimal PI control for the IPDT plant. J. Process Control **23**, 500–515 (2013)
4. Huba, M., Malatinec, T., Huba, T.: Preparatory laboratory experiments for robust constrained UAVs control. In: 10th IFAC ACE, Sheffield, UK (2013)
5. Huba, M.: Tuning of a filtered pole assignment controller for an integral plant. In: 15th ICCC, Velke Karlovice, Czech Republic (2014)
6. Huba, M., Belai, I., Bistak, P.: Noise attenuation motivated controller design. part II: position control. In: Speedam Symposium, Ischia, Italy, pp. 1331–1336 (2014)
7. Huba, M., Belai, I.: Experimental evaluation of a DO-FPID controller with different filtering properties. In: IFAC World Congress, Cape Town, South Africa (2014)
8. Huba, M.: Constrained pole assignment control for a 2nd order integral system. In: 18th ICSTCC, Sinaia, Romania (2014)

Parallel and Distributed Metaheuristics

Czesław Smutnicki[✉] and Wojciech Bożejko

Wroclaw University of Technology, Wroclaw, Poland
czeslaw.smutnicki@pwr.edu.pl

Abstract. The paper deals with problems and ultramodern approaches recommended to solve various combinatorial optimization (CO) tasks, by using different types of computing environments, including various clouds (CC). A lot of new ideas have been proposed or at least outlined. Non-standard evaluation of the goal function value is also considered.

1 Introduction

CO problems derived from practice, by reasons of characteristic features of the domain, require relatively high calculation power in order to find a solution satisfactory for the user, [11]. This power is usually required in a relatively short slot of time, to hammer out the properly good solution, used next in practice in the long application period. The amount of calculations has tendency contrary to the quality of provided results.

Researchers' and practitioners' view on optimization tasks generated by CO problems to realize an on-line decision, resource usage balancing, production and/or transport planning, scheduling, timetabling, etc. significantly has changed in recent years. Huge effort has been done by scientist in order to reinforce power of solution methods and to fulfil expectations of practitioners. Metaheuristics, perceived as universal "medicine" for basic troubles of CO algorithms, have reached the limit in very recent years and are replaced by a new ultramodern approaches being as yet in the development phase. CO problems with unimodal, convex, differentiable scalar goal functions disappeared from research labs, because a lot of satisfactory efficient methods were already designed. There are still remained very hard cases: multimodal, multi-criteria, non-differentiable, NP-hard, discrete, with huge dimensionality, with exponential increase of the number of local extremes, without a priori information about data, etc. These practical tasks, generated by computer systems and networks, industry and market, evoke serious troubles in the process of seeking global optimum. Any success in algorithms development strike practitioners fancy, so permanent research in this area are still welcome.

2 Optimization Dilemmas

Practitioners usually want to evaluate solutions from various points of views, thus using a number of different criteria. Then, we refer hereinafter to the following

© Springer International Publishing Switzerland 2015
R. Moreno-Díaz et al. (Eds.): EUROCAST 2015, LNCS 9520, pp. 72–79, 2015.
DOI: 10.1007/978-3-319-27340-2_10

vector optimization task: find $x^* \in \mathcal{X}$, such that

$$K(x^*) = \min_{x \in \mathcal{X}} K(x), \tag{1}$$

where

$$K(x) = [K_1(x), \ldots, K_s(x)]^T \tag{2}$$

and x, x^*, $\mathcal{X}$ and $K(x)$ are solution, optimal solution, set of feasible solutions and vector of goal function, respectively. The forms of x, $\mathcal{X}$ and $K_i(x)$, $i = 1, \ldots, s$ depend on the type of optimization task. In practical CO conditions, we assume that $\mathcal{X}$ is discrete, $K_i(x)$ are nonlinear and non-differentiable, x is a combinatorial object or composition of objects, whereas the optimization problem is proved to be strongly NP-hard.

Problems (1)–(2) covers almost all discrete optimization cases. Assuming $s = 1$ one can obtain the classical well examined but still hard single criterion optimization. For $s > 1$, the 'min' operator in (1) does not specify any particular technology of minimization over the set of vectors, therefore we still need a method of vector comparison, which implies from user preferences expressed directly or indirectly. Up to now a lot of user expectations were proposed, examined and implemented, see surveys [6, 9, 10] or summary in [12]. The primary goal of multi-objective optimization is to model preferences of the decision maker, expresses as the importance of each particular criteria, see also [12].

As the result of long-time research, there have been recognized main disadvantages of the solution methods, namely features commonly observed in conventional sequencing computer environments and detected also in parallel and distributed calculation environments. Among mentioned disadvantages are: (a) inability of finding any feasible solution in a reasonable time, (b) NP-completeness of checking whether $\mathcal{X}$ is empty, (c) exponentially increasing calculation cost while searching optimum solution x^* in the set $\mathcal{X}$, (d) poor approximation and/or slow convergence to the Pareto frontiers, (e) high calculation cost for management of non-dominated solutions, (f) slow convergence to optimal or suboptimal solution not too worse from $K(x^*)$, (g) premature convergence to approximate solutions of poor quality, (h) search stagnation, (i) imprecise data of the instance. Up to now, there have been identified a few reasons, discussed below, considered as responsible for appearance of these faults, [11, 12]: (1) NP-hardness, (2) excessive (exponential) number of local extremes, (3) uneven distribution of local extremes, (4) deception points, (5) flat valley of extremes, (6) sequential character of calculations.

It becomes evident that the solution algorithm have to be adjusted or adapted to the type of landscape of the solution space in order to exploit fully acquired information about its structure, as well as uneven distribution of local extremes. Space landscape depends not only on the problem type, constraints on $\mathcal{X}$, form of $K(x)$, but also on the particular instance, i.e. data of the problem. Although the notion *landscape* is defined precisely, and can be perceived as "localization of solutions in the space depending on the distance among them", its refers indirectly to human's capability of interpreting 3D images in order to extract an information supporting the search. Unfortunately, solution spaces are usually multi-dimensional, which implies that landscape features are hardly transformed into search directions, trajectory, convexity, etc. in 3D. One expects, that the detection of several recognized up to now properties of the landscape allow us to design better solution algorithms. Although several parameters characterizing search space and landscape were detected, described, examined, there is still lack of general rules how to extract the knowledge, what kind of knowledge is important and how to utilize the knowledge in the solution method, see among others [12].

There are at least a few approaches of collecting and utilizing the knowledge about the features of the solution space: (1) static, (1.1) arbitrary defined in advance, (1.2) found through a trial space sampling, (2) dynamic, (2.1) passive adaptive, (2.2) active self-learned. In (1.1), while designing the solution algorithm we set by expert some parameters in advance on the base his knowledge. Regarding (1.2), we perform three steps in order: (A) automatic analysing (e.g. by random sampling) the structure of the space; (B) calculating parameters and tuning solution algorithm; (C) searching solution with already set configuration of the algorithm. In (2.1) we collect data about solution space during the search and then use this knowledge to control searching process. Approach (2.2) keeps long-term memory to collect and extract knowledge about all problems and instances solved in the history and continuously realizes process of self-learning in the spare time of IaaS. There exist a lot of *intermediate* constructions located between these approaches. Beside the pure search over the solution space along trajectories, one can find a need of some auxiliary, accompanying calculations, such as space sampling, collecting search history, tuning, etc., fully justified and recommended for realizing in enhanced parallel and distributed calculating environments.

3 Ultramodern Approaches

The evolution of solution methods for CO problems has long, rich and gripping history, see Fig. 1. Although directions in the figure refer essentially to single-criteria case, they have an application to solution methods used in multiple-criteria problems.

The philosophy of used approaches and appreciation of their significance have changing over the span of years. The common trend observed in long-time period of time switches from universal exact methods (like ILP) to universal meta-heuristics (like GA or SA), depending on the fashion. Between these extremely cases one can find numerous valuable particular solutions approaches with various solution technologies dedicated for a narrow classes of problems or even a narrow classes of instances of the same problem. The development of theory of NP-hardness allow us to set precisely the borderline between easy and hard problems. Algorithms for problems from the latter class usually employ special properties of the problem in order to improve algorithms' efficiency as much as possible. That's why a rich variety of the solution algorithms has been created

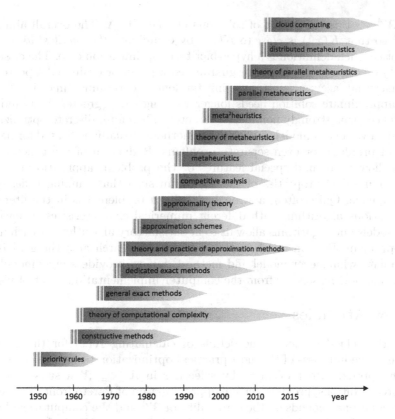

Fig. 1. Evolution of solving approaches in CO

and available now. "No free lunch" theorem clearly defines the possible areas of superiority of an algorithm over others.

Quite natural is to use model IaaS to reinforce virtual computational power by distributing calculations over virtual computing nodes distributed geographically widely. This approach requires possibility of making decomposition of CO into subproblems solved on independent nodes, however in cooperation. By using SaaS model, we have some choices: (1) homogenous engine with common interface (single method of solution) located in form of copies in calculation nodes, (2) various specialized algorithms located in different calculation nodes (own specialization) with common interface for various methods to solve the same problem.

Too high calculation cost observed for exact method forces us to use substitutes acceptable in practice. For a minimization problem *approximate algorithm* A provides solution x^A, so that

$$K(x^A) = \min_{x \in \mathcal{X}^A} K(x) \geq K(x^*) \tag{3}$$

where $\mathcal{X}^A \subset \mathcal{X}$ is the subset of solutions checked by A. The overall aim is to find x^A so that $K(x^A)$ is *close* to $K(x^*)$ by examining *the smallest as possible* $\mathcal{X}^A$. Notice, such definition is a hyper-bicriteria optimization case. The closeness to $K(x^*)$ (accuracy) can be either guaranteed a priori or evaluated a posteriori. It is clear that accuracy has opposing tendency to running time, i.e. finding better approximate solution needs longer running time (greater $\mathcal{X}^A$), and this dependence owns strongly nonlinear character. Therefore, discrete optimization manifests a variety of models and solution methods, usually dedicated for narrow classes of problems or even separate problems. Reduction of the generality of models allow us to find special features of the problem, application of which improve numerical properties of the algorithm such that running time, speed of convergence. Quite often, a strongly NP-hard problem has in the literature several various algorithms with different numerical characteristics. Knowledge about models and algorithms allow us to fit satisfactory algorithm for each newly stated problem. Bear in mind, in the considered research area the goal *is not* to formulate whatsoever model and method, but to provide *simply* model and solution method *reasonable* from the computer implementation point of view.

4 New Attitudes

Formulation (1) does not define details of calculating $K(x)$ for the given x. Because of the hardness of the most practical optimization tasks, one can expect that an approximate procedure, by selecting in $\mathcal{X}^A \subseteq \mathcal{X}$ a subset of non-dominated solutions, provides certain approximation of Pareto front. The cost of such calculations depends on the cardinality of $\mathcal{X}^A$ and the computational complexity of performing the basic step "for the given x find $K(x)$". In case of too high cost of calculations, one can either replace $K(x)$ by a cheapest its approximation $K'(x)$ or by limiting cardinality of $\mathcal{X}^A$. After an analysis we propose, by our previous paper [12], the following approaches: (1) x is deterministic, (1.2) $K(x)$ is given by an analytical formula, (1.2) $K(x)$ is given by a deterministic polynomial-time algorithm, (1.3) $K(x)$ is given by a deterministic exponential-time algorithm, (1.4) $K(x)$ is given by a deterministic algorithm provided in form of program code, (2) x is random variable, (2.1) $K(x)$ represents a statistical parameters of x or their estimators, (2.2) $K(x)$ is given by an algorithm, (2.3) $K(x)$ is a result of neural net activity, (3) x is fuzzy variable, (3.1) $K(x)$ represents certain defuzzified measure on x; (4) x is any variable, (4.1) $K(x)$ is given as the result of running simulation, (4.2) function $K(x)$ is given as the result of sensor measurement, (4.3) as previous one but in presence of noise. In any enumerated case $K(x)$ can be calculated precisely or approximately, depending on the computational complexity of required calculations, implying various requirements addressed for CC in aggregated or distributed environments.

5 Metaheuristics

New generation of metaheuristics, designed to work in parallel and distributed environments, offers powerful tool capable to overcome shortcomings observed in traditional approximate approaches, [4,5,7]. Dynamic development of the network as well as the development of Cloud Computing (CC) technology offer new advantageous properties to build in the newly designed efficient solution methods. CC can be perceived as an infrastructure accessible transparently, remotely and virtually through the network, which eliminates the need for maintaining single-handedly expensive computing resources, [13], kept by the user. By sharing the physical resources (hardware, software, broadband, communication links, etc.) of the strong power, provided by CC operator, among large number of users, CC offers not only a reduced cost of service but also allows on rational management of computing goods in case of solving very hard problems derived from science and practice. One can say that CC offers: for scientists - a cheaper alternative to clusters, grids, and supercomputers to solve hard problems computationally expensive; for users - the powerful tool to solve quickly applicative problems for the commercial and business usage.

6 Parallel Metaheuristics

In recent years the increase of computational power of computers evolves towards parallel architectures. Since the increase of the number of processors or cores in single computer or CUDA is still too slow comparing it with the increase of the number of solutions in the space, there is no hope to vanquish barrier of NP-hardness. Even cloud computing with the use of computer clusters does not offer good alternative, chiefly because of too high calculation cost. On the other hand, computer parallelism can improve significantly metaheuristics in terms of running time and quality, [2,3]. Thus parallel metaheuristics become the most desired class of algorithms, since they link excellent quality with a short running time. Sophisticated implementations of parallel algorithms require skilful application of a few fundamental elements linked with parallel programming theory, calculation models, and practical tools, see [12].

Sequential metaheuristics can be implemented in parallel calculation environments in different manner, providing variety of algorithms with different numerical properties. Let us consider, for example, SA approach, [1]. We can adopt this method as follows: (a) single thread, conventional SA, parallel calculation of the goal function value, fine grain, conventional theory of convergence, (b) single thread, pSA, parallel moves, subset of random trial solutions selected in the neighbourhood, parallel evaluation of trial solutions, parallel theory of convergence, (c) exploration of equilibrium state at fixed temperature in parallel, (d) multiple independent threads, coarse grain, (e) multiple cooperative threads, coarse grain. Similarly, for GS we have [2,8]: (a) single thread, conventional GA, parallel calculation of the goal function value, small grain, theory of convergence, (b) single thread, parallel evaluation of population, (c) multiple independent threads, coarse grain, (d) multiple cooperative threads, (e) distributed subpopulations, migration, diffusion, island models.

7   Distributed Metaheuristics

Rapid development of computer networks offers inhomogeneous computational resources distributed geographically widespread, offering IaaS, PaaS or SaaS in different business model. Long list of solution approaches dedicated for CO problems implies existence of many alternative solution algorithms with different numerical characteristics even for the same CO case. Collection of these algorithms provide certain knowledge being the best up to now research results. In this context, net nodes can offer "highly specialized" software developed in scientific laboratories accessible in the SaaS technology. Developing of such software need less cost (since no repetitions occur) and provided a variety of solution methods.

CO problems require for solving commitment of high computing resources in the relatively short time intervals. Assuming that a market firm would like to use CO to improve the competitiveness, it solves various CO instances periodically, depending on needs. In order to obtain sufficient efficiency, firm has to buy high capacity, high availability, expensive workstation, which will be utilize in the average rather weakly. On the contrary, dispersed CC is able to provide computing resources of required power in required time interval on demand. Moreover, due to possibility of net connections, CC may locate computing tasks with green energy and low expenditures, however unreliable because of the net features.

CC offers in natural way the infrastructure to realize parallel computing (especially, parallel metaheuristics) for application of CO solution methods in the form of independent or cooperative searching threads, running on various virtual machines (VM) somewhere in the cloud, depending on current workload of real and virtual machines inside the cloud, user preferences (quality of expected service), financial expenditure versus profits from implementation of the best solution found. Notice, cooperative threads require a technology of exchanging messages between virtual machines. From this point of view CC offers IaaS by providing pure calculation power, possibly homogenous and transparent, for the run of multiple copies of searching algorithm. One hope that quality of the best solution found increases with the increased number of checked solutions. For the user it is irrelevant where individual threads run, and whether all of them hopefully have finished. Thus one can imagine an unusual scenario, where some of initiated threads simply perished somewhere in the net (their results are provided with a probability) because of communication obstacles or because of limited access to VM. In terms of parallel CO methods, the proposed approach realizes coarse grain models, skipping consciously fine grain case leading to very precise programming on a low level. These threads can be performed in different technologies enumerated at the end of the previous sections.

8   Conclusions and Comments

The given survey of optimization methodologies does not provide all details necessary to make an universal algorithm or a repository of algorithms. It rather outlines crucial aspects important for the design and context of use of solution methods for the hard discrete optimization problems in the environment having rich variety of possible approaches. The present tendency prefer metaheuristics (sequencing as well as parallel) since they links high or good quality of generated solutions with relatively small or moderate calculation cost. Moreover they are resistant to local extremes. Real usefulness and applicability of each particular method depends on space landscape, roughness, big valley, distribution of solutions in the space and the problem balance between intensification and diversification of the search. Recent study suggests that efficient finding of Pareto from can be done by united force of a few different algorithms. If cost of calculations becomes high, for example for instances of greater size, there is recommended to consider parallel methods, possible to implement already on a PC with multicore processor or CUDA.

Acknowledgments. Paper is supported by funds of NCS, project DEC-2012/05/B/ST7/00102.

References

1. Aarts, E.H.L., van Laarhoven, P.J.M.: Simulated annealing: a pedestrian review of the theory and some applications. In: Deviijver, P.A., Kittler, J. (eds.) Pattern Recognition and Applications. Springer, Berlin (1987)
2. Alba, E.: Parallel Metaheuristics: A New Class of Algorithms. Wiley, Hoboken (2005)
3. Bozejko, W.: A New Class of Parallel Scheduling Algorithms. Oficyna Wydawnicza PWr, Wrocław, Poland (2010)
4. Corne, D., Dorigo, M., Glover, F. (eds.): New Ideas in Optimization. McGraw Hill, Cambridge (1999)
5. Dorigo, M., Stützle, T.: Ant Colony Optimization. Bradford Books, Bradford (2004)
6. Ghosh, A., Dehuri, S.: Evolutionary algorithms for multi-criterion optimization: a survey. Int. J. Comput. Inf. Sci. $2(1)$, 38–57 (2004)
7. Glover, F., Laguna, M.: Tabu Search. Kluwer Academic Publishers, Boston (1997)
8. Goldberg, D.E.: Genetic Algorithms in Search, Optimization and Machine Learning. Addison-Wesley, Boston (1989)
9. Marler, R.T., Arora, J.S.: Survey of multi-objective optimization methods for engineering. Struct. Multi. Optim. **26**, 369–395 (2004)
10. Nedjah, N., Coelho, L.S., de Mourelle, L.M. (eds.): Multi-objective Swarm Intelligent Systems. Studies in Computational Intelligence, vol. 261. Springer, Heidelberg (2009)
11. Smutnicki, C.: Optimization technologies for hard problems. In: Fodor, J., Klempous, R., Araujo, C.P.S. (eds.) Recent Advances in Intelligent Engineering Systems, pp. 79–104. Springer, Heidelberg (2011)
12. Smutnicki, C.: Optimization in CIS systems. In: Zamojski, W., Sugier, J. (eds.) Dependability Problems of Complex Information Systems. Advances in Intelligent Systems and Computing, vol. 307, pp. 111–128. Springer, Heidelberg (2015). doi:10.1007/978-3-319-08964-5_7
13. Vouk, M.A.: Cloud Computing - Issues, Research and Implementations. J. Comput. Inf. Technol. **16**, 235–246 (2008). doi:10.2498/cit.1001391

Dynamic Similarity and Distance Measures Based on Quantiles

Monica J. Ruiz-Miró and Margaret Miró-Julià[(✉)]

Departament de Ciències Matemàtiques i Informàtica,
Universitat de les Illes Balears, 07122 Palma de Mallorca, Spain
{monicaj.ruiz,margaret.miro}@uib.es

Abstract. Data Mining emerges in response to technological advances and considers the treatment of large amounts of data. The aim of Data Mining is the extraction of new, valid, comprehensible and useful knowledge by the construction of a simple model that describes the data and can also be used in prediction tasks. The challenge of extracting knowledge from data is an interdisciplinary discipline and draws upon research in statistics, pattern recognition and machine learning among others.

A common technique for identifying natural groups hidden in data is clustering. Clustering is a process that automatically discovers structure in data and does not require any supervision. The model's performance relies heavily on the choice of an appropriate measure. It is important to use the appropriate similarity metric to measure the proximity between two objects, but the separability of clusters must also be taken into account.

This paper addresses the problem of comparing two or more sets of overlapping data as a basis for comparing different partitions of quantitative data. An approach that uses statistical concepts to measure the distance between partitions is presented. The data's descriptive knowledge is expressed by means of a boxplot that allows for the construction of clusters taking into account conditional probabilities.

1 Introduction to Cluster Analysis

Cluster analysis divides data into meaningful or useful groups, called clusters, by identifying "natural" groups hidden in data. If meaningful clusters are the goal, then the resulting clusters should capture the "natural" structure of the data. A precise definition of what constitutes a cluster is not easy to formalize and, at times, clusters are not well separated from one another. Nonetheless, cluster analysis seeks as a result, a crisp partition of the data into non-overlapping groups. This partition depends strongly on the type of data and the desired results. Even though cluster analysis is a useful tool in many areas, it is only part of a solution to a larger problem which typically involves other steps and techniques. Clustering is a process that automatically discovers structure in data and does not require any supervision, it is an unsupervised learning method [1].

Objects are usually represented as points (vectors) in a multi-dimensional space, where each dimension represents a distinct attribute describing the object.

© Springer International Publishing Switzerland 2015
R. Moreno-Díaz et al. (Eds.): EUROCAST 2015, LNCS 9520, pp. 80–87, 2015.
DOI: 10.1007/978-3-319-27340-2_11

Data is the collection of attribute values describing the objects. A set of objects is represented as an $m \times n$ matrix, the data matrix, with m rows, one for each object, and n columns, one for each attribute. The attributes of the objects can be of different data types and can be measured on different data scales.

The different types of attributes are: binary (two values), discrete (a finite number of values) and continuous (an infinite number of values). The different data scales are: qualitative nominal (the values are just different names), qualitative ordinal (the values just reflect an ordering), quantitative by interval (the difference between values is meaningful), quantitative by ratio (the scale has an absolute zero so that ratios are meaningful). Data scales and types are important since the type of clustering used depends on the data scale and type.

Given a data set $\mathcal{D} = \{X_1, X_2, \ldots, X_N\}$, where each X_k is characterized by a set of attributes, clustering is the process of identifying and describing groups present within the data. The grouping is done in such a way that objects in the same group or cluster are more similar to each other than to those in other clusters. The determination of the clusters relies heavily on the concept of similarity or distance between the data. A good clustering method will produce high quality clusters in which the intra-cluster similarity is high and the inter-cluster similarity is low. The model's performance relies heavily on the choice of an appropriate measure; finding and implementing the correct measure is fundamental and results in more accurate data analysis.

Informally, the similarity within a cluster is a numerical measure of the degree to which the two objects are alike. It is important to use the appropriate similarity metric to measure the proximity between two objects, but the separability of clusters must also be taken into account. The goal is to find clusterings that satisfy homogeneity within each cluster as well as heterogeneity between clusters [2].

The similarity between two elements is a measure that quantifies the dependency between the data. A data point is represented by a vector $X_k = \{x_k^i, i = 1, 2, \ldots, n\}$, where n is the number of features. These features can be quantitative or qualitative descriptions of the object. Given two data points $X_k, X_j \in \mathcal{D}$, the similarity is measured by a function $s : \mathcal{D} \times \mathcal{D} \to [s_{min}, s_{max}] \subseteq \Re$ that satisfies:

1. $s(X_k, X_k) = s_{max}$ for all $X_k \in \mathcal{D}$.
2. Symmetry: $s(X_k, X_j) = s(X_j, X_k)$ for all $X_k, X_j \in \mathcal{D}$.

where s_{min} denotes minimal similarity and s_{max} the maximal similarity. A similarity measure with $s_{min} = 0$ and $s_{max} = 1$ is a dichotomous similarity function.

On occasions it is convenient to measure the dissimilarity of objects by their distance instead of defining a similarity measure. The distance is measured by a function $d : \mathcal{D} \times \mathcal{D} \to [d_{min}, d_{max}] \subseteq \Re$ that satisfies:

1. $d(X_k, X_k) = d_{min}$ for all $X_k \in \mathcal{D}$.
2. Symmetry: $d(X_k, X_j) = d(X_j, X_k)$ for all $X_k, X_j \in \mathcal{D}$.

where d_{min} denotes minimal distance and d_{max} the maximal distance. If in addition the distance fulfills $d_{min} = 0$ and $d_{max} = \infty$ and

1. Reflexivity: $d(X_k, X_j) = 0$ if and only if $X_k = X_j$ for all $X_k, X_j \in \mathcal{D}$.
2. Triangle Inequality: $d(X_k, X_j) + d(X_j, X_r) \geq d(X_k, X_r)$.

then the distance function is called a metric distance function.

Computing distances or measures of similarity can be problematic, since the different data scales and types of features are not comparable and one standard measure is not applicable. In practice, different distance measures are used for different features of heterogeneous data.

In descriptive statistics, when dealing with quantitative data sets, percentiles or quartiles provide information on how the data are spread [3]. A boxplot is a graph used to display patterns of quantitative data. A boxplot splits the data set into quartiles. The body of the boxplot consists of a "box" which goes from the first quartile (Q_1) to the third quartile (Q_3). Within the box, a line is drawn at the median of the data set (Q_2). Two vertical lines, called whiskers, extend from the bottom and top of the box. The bottom whisker goes from Q_1 to the lowest datum still within $1.5 \cdot IQR$ of the lower quartile (lower fence LF), and the top whisker goes from Q_3 to the highest datum still within $1.5 \cdot IQR$ of the upper quartile (upper fence UF). Data points falling beyond the whiskers are known as outliers. If the data set includes outliers, they are plotted on the graph separately as points. See Fig. 1.

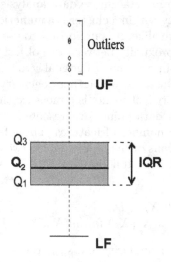

Fig. 1. Boxplot of a quantitative feature.

The clustering process depends on the specific similarity criterion used. When forming clusters it is not uncommon to find overlapping data. This paper addresses the problem of comparing two or more sets of overlapping data as a basis for comparing different partitions of quantitative data. An approach that uses statistical concepts to measure the distance between partitions is presented. The data's descriptive knowledge is expressed by means of a boxplot that allows for the construction of clusters taking into account conditional probabilities. In particular, quartiles and interquartile range are used in the calculation of a dissimilarity measure between clusters. The method presented is dynamical and allows for the adjustment of the measure's intensity, given by the percentiles, to improve the model's performance.

2 Dispersion and Multi-splits: Boxplot as a Similarity Measure

Boxplots display data variation without making any assumptions of the underlying statistical distribution. A boxplot is a convenient way to graphically display the data and identify outliers. Boxplots are useful when comparing data sets. Therefore, boxplots are a convenient tool to study overlapping data.

Given a data set $\mathcal{D} = \{X_1, X_2, \ldots, X_N\}$, we consider the dispersion of the data given by the boxplots as shown in Fig. 2.

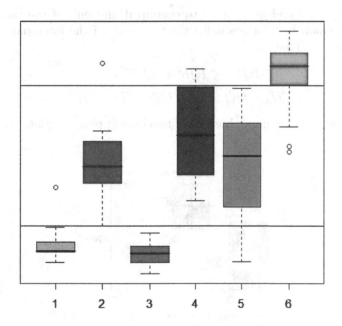

Fig. 2. Dispersion of the data given by the boxplots.

The box of a boxplot represents half of the data, the central 50 %. It's the most representative part of the attribute. The amplitude of the box is the interquartilic range $IQR = Q_3 - Q_1$, it represents the dispersion of the data. Observing the boxes in Fig. 2, it's clear that boxes 1 and 3 have similar dispersion. Same thing happens with boxes 2, 4 and 5. But the dispersion between boxes 1 and 3 is different from dispersion between boxes 2, 4 and 5. By definition, boxes 1 and 3 form a cluster whereas boxes 2, 4 and 5 form another one. Box 6 is a cluster on its own. The dispersion and Multi-split method studies possible clusters and calculates split values that separates the attribute into clusters in the most discriminatory manner.

2.1 Number of Clusters

Considering the data shown in Fig. 2, intuitively we appreciate that three clusters are formed. Two variables, more precisely, the dispersion of two variables are similar, when the boxes amplitudes are similar. Therefore, if the boxes overlap or intersect, the dispersion of the variable is similar and they belong to the same cluster. Given an attribute X_i with s overlapping boxplots, each limited by Q_1^i and Q_3^i, $i = 1, 2, \ldots, s$; the union boxplot consists of a "box" which goes from $Q_1^\cup$ the to $Q_3^\cup$ where:

$$Q_1^\cup = min(Q_1^1, Q_1^2, \ldots, Q_1^s)$$
$$Q_3^\cup = max(Q_3^1, Q_3^2, \ldots, Q_3^s)$$

Two boxplots l and m are said to overlap if and only if the interquartilic range of the union boxplot is smaller than the sum of the interquartilic ranges of boxes l and m. That is,

$$IQR^\cup \leq IQR^l + IQR^m$$
$$|Q_3^\cup - Q_1^\cup| \leq |Q_3^l - Q_1^l| + |Q_3^m - Q_1^m|$$

Figure 3 depicts the union boxplot of two overlapping boxplots l and m.

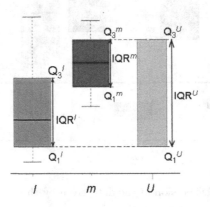

Fig. 3. Boxplot overlapping.

In the same way that an adjacent matrix of a graph can be constructed, an overlapping matrix $S = \{s_{lm}\}$ associated to attribute X_i can be constructed as follows:

$$s_{lm} = \begin{cases} 1 & \text{if boxes } l \text{ and } m \text{ overlap} \\ 0 & \text{otherwise} \end{cases}$$

The overlapping matrix S is binary and symmetric. It is also associated with a graph, where the nodes represent boxes and the edges represent overlapping boxplots. The number of connected subgraphs represents the number of clusters nc_i. See Fig. 4.

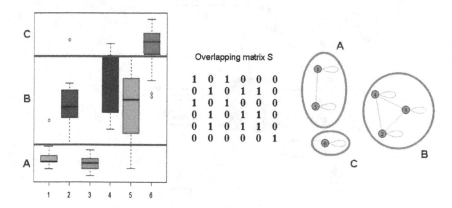

Fig. 4. Cluster analysis.

2.2   The Best Splits

When a variable appears in a split, it is hard to know if the variable is indeed the most important, or if the selection is due to bias. Unbiased multiway splits are studied in [4].

Given an attribute X_i, the interval o splitting points are those that better discriminate the clusters found though the overlapping matrix. Two cases are considered:

– Case 1: All g attributes have only one connected graph, $\sum_h nc_h = g$.

In this case, each of the attributes form one cluster, that is, every box overlaps with at least one other box. The elements of the splitting vector SP are the splitting points $SP = \{sp_k\}$, $k = 1, 2, \ldots, g - 1$. The middle point of the intersection of overlapping boxes form the splitting points. To simplify the notation, ordered boxes are considered $(Q_1^1 \leq Q_1^2 \leq \ldots)$, the splitting points are illustrated in Fig. 5 and calculated as follows:

$$sp_k = \frac{Q_3^k + Q_1^{k+1}}{2}$$

– Case 2: Some of the g attributes have more than one connected subgraph, $\sum_h nc_h > g$.

In this case, there is at least one attribute with more than one cluster. For each cluster, the union boxplot is considered. The elements of the splitting vector SP are the splitting points $SP = \{sp_k\}$, $k = 1, 2, \ldots, nc-1$. The middle point of the distance that separates each pair of union boxes form the splitting points. Once again, to simplify the notation, ordered boxes are considered, the splitting points are illustrated in Fig. 6 and calculated as follows:

$$sp_k = \frac{Q_3^k + Q_1^{k+1}}{2}$$

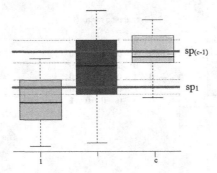

Fig. 5. Spitting vector for case 1.

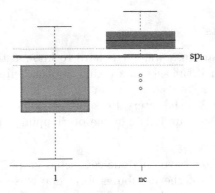

Fig. 6. Spitting vector for case 2.

3   Conclusion and Future Work

A method for cluster analysis and split construction has been presented. The clusters are formed using similarity measures based on boxplots. Boxplots are non-parametric, they display variation in the data of a statistical population without making any assumptions of the underlying statistical distribution. The spacings between the different parts of the box indicate the degree of dispersion and skewness in the data, and show outliers. A boxplot is a convenient way to graphically display the data and identify outliers. Boxplots are useful when comparing data sets. Therefore, boxplots are a convenient tool to study overlapping data. Once clusters are identified the multiway split selection is forthcoming. The number of splits depends on the number of clusters found.

This paper offers a limited vision of one of the many clustering methods available. The following aspects can be considered as future work: construction of splitting vectors that take into account datas skewness, study in depth case 1 $\sum_h nc_h = g$ and box l is completely contained in box m, extend the method to consider overlapping as a function of percentiles.

References

1. Cios, K.J., Pedrycz, W., Swiniarski, R.W., Kurgan, L.A.: Data Mining. A Knowledge Discovery Approach. Springer, New York (2007)
2. Grabmeier, J., Rudolph, A.: Techniques of cluster algorithms in data mining. Data Min. Knowl. Discov. **6**, 303–360 (2002)
3. Witte, R.S., Witte, J.S.: Statistics, 9th edn. Wiley, New Jersey (2010)
4. Kim, H., Loh, W.Y.: Classification trees with unbiased multiway splits. J. Am. Stat. Assoc. **96**, 589–604 (2001)

Eulerian Numbers Weigths in Distributed Computing Nets

Gabriel de Blasio[1]([⊠]), Arminda Moreno-Díaz[2], and Roberto Moreno-Díaz[1]

[1] Instituto Universitario de Ciencias Y Tecnologías Cibernéticas, ULPGC,
Las Palmas, Spain
gdeblasio@dis.ulpgc.es, rmoreno@ciber.ulpgc.es
[2] School of Computer Science, Madrid Technical University, Madrid, Spain
amoreno@fi.upm.es

Abstract. We explore the possibilities of Eulerian numbers to define weights in layered networks and model distributed computation at the level of neurons receptive fields. These networks are then compared to those defined by binomial coefficients (Newton filters). Their potential as structures for signals convergence, divergence and overlapping is also established.

1 Introduction

1.1 Convergent-Divergent Layered Nets

The existence of a convergent-divergent path in the structure of the neurons system of vertebrates is a fact that has been long demonstrated in both peripheral (sensory) and central parts [1,2].

Also, the retina as well as cortex, show a conspicuous layered anatomy, with interconnections among the units (neurons) of each layer and the following layers, always exist overlapping of input (or sensory) "fields" (zones), and thus, a double process of convergence and divergence of the input information and the outputs from the layers also exists.

In our representations, it is a type of distributed computation by a layered network of almost equally functional computing agents. This is illustrated in Fig. 1 for one dimensional ($x = x_1, x_2, \ldots, x_{20}$) input field. The value of the discrete inputs are x_i. Note that this representation is highly paradigmatic and that there is not a one-to-one correspondence between each of them and a real nervous structure.

The outputs of the nets are $\Omega_1, \ldots, \Omega_j$. Overlapping, convergence and divergence of signals are evident.

Assume we start with a net with m ($x_1, \ldots, x_m$) input signals. Then, in some cases (depending on the type of computation performed by the computing agents), there may exist an equivalent net of m layers, in which each computing

© Springer International Publishing Switzerland 2015
R. Moreno-Díaz et al. (Eds.): EUROCAST 2015, LNCS 9520, pp. 88–94, 2015.
DOI: 10.1007/978-3-319-27340-2_12

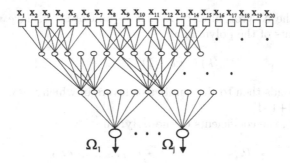

Fig. 1. A general three layers computing network.

agent have just two input lines. It is no difficult to show that the equivalent nets always exist for linear networks, that is for nets in which:

$$\Omega_j = \sum_k W_{jk} x_k$$

where W_{jk} is the weighting factor.

1.2 Newton-Hermite Filters

The name Newton filters was introduced in [3], and they were applied to linear filters in which the weights of the "zero order" and length m are given by the row of the m binomial (or Newton) coefficients, that is the coefficients of the polynomials:

$$P_m(0) = (x - 1)^m$$

As it has been shown ([3]) it corresponds to a layered structure of the type described in Fig. 2, in which all weights are +1.

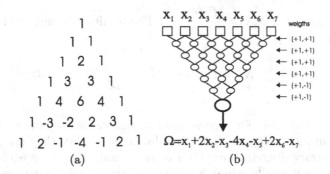

Fig. 2. (a) Triangular array for Newton filter $N_7(2)$. (b) Layered network performing the filter.

In general, the Newton filter of length m and order k, have weights which are the coefficients of the polynomial:

$$P_m(k) = (x-1)^{m-k}(x+1)^k$$

where k corresponds then to the number of layers in which the weights $(+1,+1)$ are changed to $(+1,-1)$.

In general [3], the coefficients of the polynomial:

$$P_m = (x - e_1)(x - e_2)\ldots(x - e_m)$$

correspond to a layered net in which the weights of the computing units of each layer are $(+1,e_1),(+1,e_2),\ldots(+1,e_m)$. And viceversa, any arbitrary row of weights , W_i, for a linear filter of m inputs, that is:

$$\Omega = \sum_{i=1}^m W_i X_i$$

corresponds to a layered net of m layers, each layer having the weights $(+1,e_i)$, where e_i are the roots of the polynomial:

$$P_m = \sum_{i=1}^m \frac{W_i}{W_1} x^i$$

The coefficients of the Newton Filters of a length m and order k can be arranged in a triangular array of numbers, starting $m = 1$ in the vertex. For $N_m(0)$ it corresponds to the Pascal Triangle. This is illustrated in Fig. 2(a) for $N_7(2)$, which is the so called "inverted Mexican hat" filter. Figure 2(b) shows the layered net for the filter having two "inhibitory layers". Notice that it is irrelevant where the "inhibitory layers" are, but their number.

Newton filters of order zero, $N_m(0)$, tend to a gaussian (after proper normalization) for $m \to \infty$. Also [4], Newton filters of order k, tend to Hermite functions of order k, $H(x,k) = \dfrac{d^k \left(e^{-x^2}\right)}{dx^k}$. The resulting kernels in the continuous formulation will be:

$$\underbrace{\Omega = \sum_{i=x}^m N_i(k)\, x_i}_{\text{Newton Filter}} \quad \to \quad \underbrace{\Omega = \int_{-\infty}^{+\infty} H(x,k)\, x\, dx}_{\text{Hermite Filter}}$$

Notice that the basis for representing a Newton array into an equivalent layered computing structure is its triangular nature, when they are generated. Also, any arbitrary discrete linear filter of real numbers have an equivalent layered network, so it finally admit a triangular array equivalent representation. Notice that also this applies to Eulerian Networks (next section).

2 Eulerian Numbers, Eulerian Networks and Eulerian Filters

Eulerian numbers appear normally in an apparent quite different context: the management of series [4,5]. A typical introduction [4] is through the successive derivatives of the identity:

$$\sum_{i=1}^{\infty} x^k = \frac{x}{1-x} \quad \text{for } |x| < 1$$

By repeatedly differentiating, multiplying by x, taking the coefficients of the polynomials of the resulting numerators and putting them into a triangular array, it results the Euler triangle.

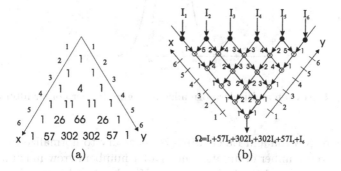

(a)   (b)

Fig. 3. (a) Triangular array for Eulerian numbers with superimposed coordinate system. Notices that x, y start at 1 (not 0). (b) Layered net representation of filter of length 6 and zero order, where the weights are the first 6 Eulerian numbers.

The array of the first 6 Eulerian numbers is shown in Fig. 3(a), with a convenient superimposed coordinate system. Notice that both x and y are integers starting in 1 (not in 0).

By this coordinate reference system, Eulerian numbers can be generated by the recurrence [5]:

$$E(x,y) = yE(x-1,y) + xE(x,y-1) \tag{1}$$

where $E(x, y)$ is the Eulerian number in position (x, y).

By inverting the triangle "upside down" the corresponding triangular layered network is obtained as illustrated in Fig. 3(b). As it can be seen, to obtain outputs in each layer which are a linear combination of the inputs, the local weights must be (from recurrence (1)):

$$W(\lambda, \rho) = (y, x)$$

that is, in position (x, y), the weight of the input coming from the left (λ) to each computing unit is the coordinate y, and that of the inputs coming from the right (ρ) is the coordinate x. This is illustrated in Fig. 3(b).

This is an important drawback when compared to Newton filters, since weights depend not only on the layer, but also on the rows of the computing unit. This will provoke a much stronger sensitivity the position of local scotomas, in relation to reliability. Also, for this, weights cannot be changed in position without more or less seriously changing the resulting computation.

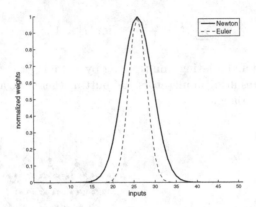

Fig. 4. Newton and Euler normalized weights for zero order filters.

To compare Newton and Euler filters is necessary to normalize to the center values for a given number of inputs, since Euler numbers grow much faster than Newton's. The output of the Eulerian filter of order 0 and length l is then:

$$\Omega_l(0) = e_1 I_1 + e_2 I_2 + \ldots + e_l I_l$$

where e_i are eulerian numbers normalized to the central value.

By appropriate re-scaling the (integer) indexes of the input lines [4], normalized Eulerian weights (numbers), approaches a gaussian (just as binomial coefficients). We shall consider re-scaling later, for the continuous filters. Figure 4 shows the plot of Newton and Euler weights for zero order filters of length 51, where the approaching to gaussian is already apparent.

As it is also apparent, Euler filters of order 0 have a narrower receptive field extension, which correspond to a higher spatial frequency averaging effect. Also, higher order filters will have a more sharp contrast detection effect and provide for narrower harmonic representation on input signals.

Higher order Euler filters $\Omega_l(k)$ should be obtained by analogy to the Newton filters, that is, changing the sign of the inputs left to right to each computing unit in k layers. However in this case, the change does not correspond to a kth discrete derivatives, because the weights are no longer all $+1$. What is more, the resulting filter weights depend on what layers we select to change signs, that is, in Newton Filter's terminology, what layers are inhibitory. This, obviously, means a much lower reliability to changes of the place of the inhibitions for Eulerian filters.

3   Higher Order Euler Filters and Hermitian Euler Formulation

To obtain higher order (higher derivatives) Eulerian filters, we may successively "move" the original filter of length l, one place to the right (or left), change the sign of the output and add a final new computing unit. This means that by every discrete derivative, we increase the supposed resolution by one, ending in effect in a filter of order k, but length $k + l$. Or viceversa, to obtain a filter of order k, and length l, we shall start with k Eulerian filters of order $l - k$ and add k inhibitory layers. For l large and k not very large (first derivatives), the effects are not different from the ones for Newton filters.

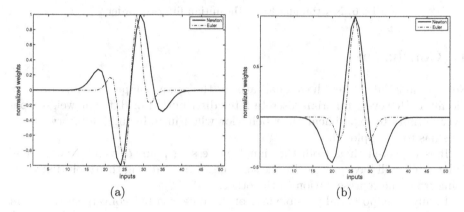

Fig. 5. (a) First derivatives Newton and Euler filter profiles. (b) The corresponding global weights profiles.

Figure 5(a) shows the filter profiles for $N_{51}(1)$ and $\Omega_{52}(1)$ (first derivatives) and Fig. 5(b) the corresponding Mexican hats. All weights have been normalized.

Again, the parallelism between Newton and Eulerian filters is very apparent. The receptive field for Eulerian filters is "narrower" than for Newton's filters, which again means more sensitivity to higher spatial frequencies.

As it has been already pointed out, normalized Eulerian filter of order 0 approaches a gaussian, but with a different σ (standard deviation) than the Newton's filter. This corresponds to:

$$W(0) = e^{-x^2} \quad \text{Newton}$$
$$\Omega(0) = e^{-kx^2} \quad \text{Euler}$$

where $\sqrt{k} \cdot x$ is the homothetic transformation of one set of kernels into the other. The value of k can be approximated by $k = 2\sqrt{2} = \sqrt{8}$. That is, an homothecy in the continuous input field of coordinate x that transforms Newton filters into Euler filters. The corresponding Hermitian filters (Newton's and Euler) of order 2 are shown in Fig. 6.

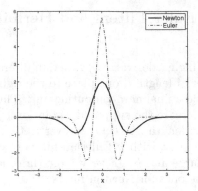

Fig. 6. Newton and Euler Hermitian filters of order 2.

4   Conclusion

Newton and Euler filters have qualitatively the same "shape", for any order of the filter. However, Eulerian discrete filter distribution of different weights per layer permits to experiment their behavior when introducing inhibitory layers. This has to be explored.

It is expected that, from the signal processing point of view, Newton and Euler filters will have practically the same effect as changing the resolution when going from one representation to the other.

In any case, potential possible uses of these neuron-like convergent-divergent networks is still under study by computer simulation of larger networks.

Acknowledgments. This work has been supported, in part, by Spanish Ministry of Science projects MTM2011-28983-CO3-03 and MTM2014-56949-C3-2-R.

References

1. Leibovic, K.N.: Principles of brain function: information processing in convergent and divergent pathways. In: Pichler, F., Trappl, R. (eds.) Progress in Cybernetics and Systems, vol. VI, pp. 91–99. Hemisphere, Washington, D.C. (1982)
2. Moreno-Díaz, A., de Blasio, G., Moreno-Díaz Jr. R.: Distributed, layered and reliable computing nets to represent neuronal receptive fields. Math. Biosci. Eng. **11**(2), 343–361 (2014)
3. Moreno-Díaz Jr., R.: Computación paralela y distribuida: relaciones estructura-función en retinas. Ph.D thesis, Universidad de Las Palmas de Gran Canaria (1993)
4. http://www.mathpages.com/home/kmath012/kmath012.htm
5. Carlitz, L., Kurtz, D.C., Scoville, R., Stakelber, O.P.: Asymptotic properties of Eulerian numbers. Zeitschrift für Wahrscheinlichkeitstheorie und Verwandte Gebiete **23**(1), 47–54 (1972)

Autonomous Paracopter Control Design

Tomáš Huba[(✉)] and Mikuláš Huba

Slovak University of Technology in Bratislava,
Ilkovičova 3, 812 19, Bratislava, Slovakia
{tomas.huba,mikulas.huba}@stuba.sk
http://uamt.fei.stuba.sk

Abstract. This paper deals with introduction to the design of a motorized paraglider control. This device known also as a paracopter, parafoil delivery system, or powered parachute aircraft may be considered as a special type of Unmanned Aerial Systems (UAVs). Due to several degrees of freedom, a highly nonlinear and unstable dynamics with internal couplings and strong external disturbances, its control represents a challenging problem. Thus, its education requires corresponding learning approaches. One possible controller tuning method based on relay identification is treated and applied to the propeller pendulum representing motion typical for one degree of freedom of the paracopter control.

Keywords: Paracopter · Propeller pendulum · Relay identification

1 Introduction

At the university level, UAVs are frequently used to demonstrate different aspects of automation and control design. Thereby, due to the complexity of their flight dynamics, the paracopter control is not as popular as other types of UAVs, for example the quadrocopters. In practice, it has been deeply studied in several military applications, or by NASA as a transport mean for evacuation of the International Space Station (ISS) [1–6].

On the other hand, the paracopter dynamics brings several advantages and it may also be useful in demonstrating several advanced control concept. Due to its unstable character, in its control design, one of the basic problems is given by a reliable and safe identification. The unstable system character, together with its strongly variable and nonlinear dynamics significantly constraint the spectrum of applicable identification methods. Experience shows that the considered controllers and identification methods have to be limited to the simplest ones offering the highest possible tracking performance and robustness together with excellent disturbance compensation. When wishing to approach this problem systematically, it is recommended to start with identification and control of a propeller pendulum that may represent a simplified version of the paracopter systems. This paper will extend information published in [9,10] and discuss experience gained in relay experiments based controller tuning (based on a phase plane limit cycle analysis [7,8]) verified by a subsequent controller design.

© Springer International Publishing Switzerland 2015
R. Moreno-Díaz et al. (Eds.): EUROCAST 2015, LNCS 9520, pp. 95–102, 2015.
DOI: 10.1007/978-3-319-27340-2_13

2   Propeller Pendulum

The propeller pendulum systems represents a simplified approximation of the paracopter systems allowing motion with one degree of freedom. This is used in initial design phases to profit from a safe environment for mastering several paracopter functionalities, its sensorics and control design aspects [10].

Since the system represents a weakly damped oscillator, it could be expected to be approximated as a second order oscillator. But, when wishing to simplify the still complex theoretical framework wrapped around the oscillatory system with a propeller subsystem, an ultralocal double integrator model extended by a dead time may be used instead. Thereby, the propeller subsystem inertia may be approximated by the first order linear model.

3   Relay System Identification

Similarly as an identification of unstable UAVs, also the pendulum identification around an unstable operating point requires a closed loop identification with a stabilizing controller. Thereby, a relay identification may be used, when a controller + filter subsystem necessary for the derivative action is considered as

$$R_f(s) = R(s)F(s) = K_P \frac{1 + T_D s}{(1 + T_n s)^n} = \frac{K_P + K_D s}{(1 + T_n s)^n}; \ n = 1, 2, 3, \ldots \quad (1)$$

The simplest system model (including possibly also the necessary filters) is

$$S(s) = \frac{K_s e^{-T_d s}}{s^2} \quad (2)$$

For the paracopeter or pendulum identification one has to use a relay with offset

$$u = M_{00} + M \, sign(u_{PD}) \quad (3)$$

Traditionally, the most frequently used method for a relay identification is the describing function method. However, when applied to the loop with a second order plant and a stabilizing PD controller, due to the relative degree one of the resulting transfer function it does not yield sufficiently precise results. Thus, we are going to use an identification method based on a phase plane analysis of the generated limit cycles [8]. Consideration of a relay controller output with an offset M_{00} that may be combined with an unknown input disturbance into the offset M_0 yields two limit control signal values

$$U_1 = M_0 - M; \ \ U_2 = M_0 + M \quad (4)$$

In general $M_0 \neq M_{00}$ is unknown.

Due to the output relay, the PD controller equation may be simplified to

$$R(s) = U(s)/Y(s) = -(s + a); \ \ u_{PD} = -\dot{y} - ay; \ \ y = y_f - w \quad (5)$$

$w=$ piecewise constant reference variable, $y_f=$ the filtered output and $\dot y = \dot y_f =$ its derivative. In a phase plane $(y, \dot y)$, such a controller followed by an output relay may be interpreted as a switching line

$$L : \; \dot y = -ay \tag{6}$$

This separates the areas with $u = U_1$ and $u = U_2$. Due to the dead time, after crossing L the trajectory changes appear with the delay T_d (Fig. 1).

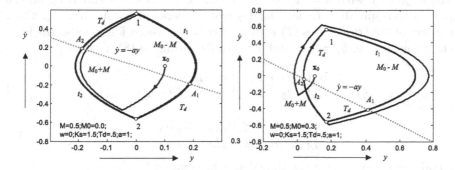

Fig. 1. Symmetrical and unsymmetrical oscillations of a delayed double integrator

For $u = U = const$ the phase plane trajectories are described as

$$\dot y(t) = \dot y_0 + K_s U t; \quad y(t) = y_0 + \dot y_0 t + K_s U t^2/2$$
$$\dot y^2 - \dot y_0^2 + 2K_s U (y - y_0) = 0 \tag{7}$$

They are symmetric with respect to y axis.

Let us consider a stable limit cycle, where the representing points returns after one period of oscillation back to the original position. The assumption of a steady-state cycle implies zero mean derivative value. For an initial point "1" taken as the trajectory vertex with a positive derivative value, it must hold

$$K_s U_1 (t_1 + T_d) + K_s U_2 (t_2 + T_d) = 0 \tag{8}$$

The time intervals corresponding to the positive U_2 and negative limit input values U_1 will be denoted as

$$t^+ = t_2 + T_d; \quad t^- = t_1 + T_d \tag{9}$$

Their sum gives the limit cycle duration

$$P_u = t^+ + t^- = 2T_d + t_1 + t_2 \tag{10}$$

Their ratio used later in the identification will be denoted as

$$\epsilon = t^+/t^- = -\frac{M_0 + M}{M_0 - M} \tag{11}$$

According to the above equation, for known limit cycle parameters P_u, M and ϵ it is firstly possible to calculate the offset

$$M_0 = -M\frac{1-\epsilon}{1+\epsilon} \tag{12}$$

By determining M_0 we get the limit values (4).

The vertex at the begin of the trajectory segment corresponding to $u = U_1$ (Fig. 1) let us denote with the index "1" and similarly the vertex at the begin of the trajectory with $u = U_2$ as "2". Points at the line (6) and lying on the segments corresponding to U_1 and U_2 will be denoted as A_1 and A_2. From symmetry of the trajectories (7) with respect to the y-axis follows also the limit cycle symmetry, i.e. $\dot{y}_1 = -\dot{y}_2$ and $y_1 = y_2$. According to (8) it holds

$$\begin{aligned} \dot{y}_1 &= -K_sU_1(t_1 + T_d)/2 = -K_sU_1t^-/2 \\ \dot{y}_2 &= -K_sU_2(t_2 + T_d)/2 = -K_sU_2t^+/2 = -\dot{y}_1 \end{aligned} \tag{13}$$

$$\begin{aligned} \dot{y}_{A1} &= \dot{y}_2 - K_sU_1T_d = -ay_{A1} \\ \dot{y}_{A2} &= \dot{y}_1 - K_sU_2T_d = -ay_{A2} \end{aligned} \tag{14}$$

Intervals swept out during the time delays are limited by the points

$$\begin{aligned} y_1 &= y_{A2} + \dot{y}_{A2}T_d + K_sU_2T_d^2/2 \\ y_2 &= y_{A1} + \dot{y}_{A1}T_d + K_sU_1T_d^2/2 \end{aligned} \tag{15}$$

which for $y_1 = y_2$ yields

$$y_{A1} - y_{A2} + \dot{y}_{A1}T_d - \dot{y}_{A2}T_d + K_sU_1T_d^2/2 - K_sU_2T_d^2/2 = 0 \tag{16}$$

From (14)

$$\dot{y}_{A1} - \dot{y}_{A2} = \dot{y}_2 - \dot{y}_1 - K_sU_1T_d + K_sU_2T_d = -a(y_{A1} - y_{A2}) \tag{17}$$

Then, from (16)

$$y_{A1} - y_{A2} = \frac{K_sT_d^2}{2}\frac{U_2 - U_1}{1 - aT_d}; \quad \dot{y}_{A1} - \dot{y}_{A2} = -a\frac{K_sT_d^2}{2}\frac{U_2 - U_1}{1 - aT_d} \tag{18}$$

and from (17) with $\dot{y}_2 = -\dot{y}_1$

$$\dot{y}_1 = \frac{1}{4}K_sT_d(U_2 - U_1)\frac{2 - aT_d}{1 - aT_d} \tag{19}$$

From (13) follows

$$t^- = -\frac{2\dot{y}_1}{K_sU_1}; \quad t_+ = \frac{2\dot{y}_1}{K_sU_2} \tag{20}$$

and

$$P_u = \frac{2\dot{y}_1}{K_s}\frac{U_1 - U_2}{U_1U_2} = -\frac{T_d}{2}\frac{aT_d - 2}{aT_d - 1}\frac{(U_2 - U_1)^2}{U_1U_2} \tag{21}$$

Solving this equation according to T_d yields the dead time estimate

$$T_d = -\frac{P_u a U_1 U_2 - (U_2 - U_1)^2 + \sqrt{(U_2 - U_1)^4 + (P_u U_1 U_2 a)^2}}{a(U_2 - U_1)^2} \tag{22}$$

that might yet be corrected by the contribution $\Delta T_d \approx n T_f$ of the filter used for the PD implementation.

Parameter K_s may be determined from (21) as

$$K_s = \frac{2\dot{y}_1}{P_u} \frac{U_1 - U_2}{U_1 U_2} \tag{23}$$

4 Application to the Propeller Pendulum Control

The experiments have been carried out under Linux with a pendulum system controlled by a BeagleBone processor by a cape including all required sensorics, communications and actuators. The pendulum angle measurement used signal from the complementary filter processed and additionally filtered by an independent program thread. Another program thread has been used for measurement of the propeller angular velocity.

Firstly, the time constant of the propeller subsystem T_p [10] has been determined by measuring speed step responses of a fixed pendulum generated by step changes of the propeller power supply. From noisy and quantized signals one gets $T_p \approx 0.3 - 0.4\,$s. In following calculations, $T_p = 0.4\,$s has been used.

When defining the pendulum angle y_p as the controlled output and the propeller power u as the input, the considered system dynamics has a relative degree equal to 3. Thus, in order to decrease the relative order and to get a nearly 2nd order oscillatory system, new state variables have to be used

$$y = y_f + T_p \dot{y}_f; \quad \dot{y} = \dot{y}_f + T_p \ddot{y}_f \tag{24}$$

The required signals $y_f, \dot{y}_f$ and $\ddot{y}_f$ are produced from the measured pendulum output y_p taken from the complementary filter by means of a 3rd order binomial filter $F(s)$ considered in (1). The new output and its derivative are fed to the PD controller (5) with $K_P = K_D = 1$ ($a = K_D/K_P = 1$) and a relay output levels $U_{min} = 5$ and $U_{max} = 20$ yielding $M = (U_{max} - U_{min})/2 = 7.5$.

Transients have been carried out with the sampling period $T_s \approx 8\,$ms. Since the applied solution without a real time kernel does not guarantee fixed sampling period values, in filter difference equations, actual sampling period has been used. The filter time constant has been set to $T_f = 32\,$ms. Results of a relay experiment in Fig. 2 show strong effect of the measurement and quantization noise. The phase plane trajectories corresponding to U_{max} and U_{min} (Fig. 2 right) are shown in red and blue.

By analyzing particular limit cycles one gets values P_u, t^+ and t^- shown in Fig. 3 left. Identified limit cycle periods range from $2T_s$ to $60T_s$. Their mean value is $P_{um} = 0.1302 \approx 16T_s$. From $\epsilon = 1.1760$ one gets $M_0 = 0.6067; U_1 = -6.8933; U_2 = 8.1067$.

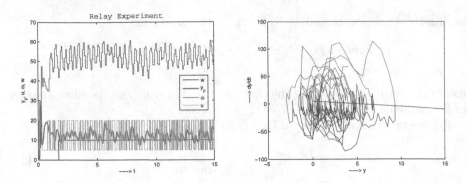

Fig. 2. Relay experiment: time responses (left) and phase plane trajectories (right); $T_p = 0.4$s, $U_{min} = 5$, $U_{max} = 20$, $K_P = K_D = 1$ (Color figure online)

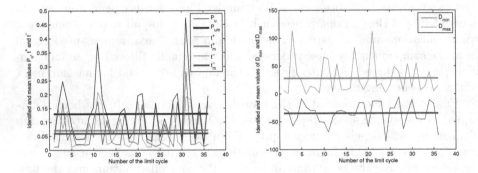

Fig. 3. Identified and mean values P_u, t^+ and t^- from the identification experiment (left); $D_{max} \equiv \dot{y}_1$, $D_{min} \equiv \dot{y}_2$ and their mean values (right)

An improved identification precision could be expected by excluding the extreme limit cycle values influenced evidently by the measurement noise, or by other Linux tasks. Due to the time quantization, the mean derivative values of particular limit cycles are not exactly zero, which causes their permanent drifting [7]. Neither their mean values (Fig. 3 right, bold) are symmetric. From $D_{max} \equiv \dot{y}_1 = 27.9188$ then follows $T_d = 0.0318$ and $K_s = 115$.

The identified model parameters have been verified by the linear pole assignment PD controller with a static feedforward u_0 (determined experimentally)

$$u = K_P(w - y) - K_D\dot{y} + u_0; \ K_P = \alpha_1\alpha_2/K_s; \ K_D = -(\alpha_1 + \alpha_2)/K_s \quad (25)$$

The identified dead time is respected by the closed loop poles [10]

$$\alpha_{1,2} = (-0.231 \pm j0.161)/T_d \quad (26)$$

which after substituting into (25) yield

$$K_P = 0.079/(K_sT_d) = 0.678 \ ; \ K_D = 0.461/(K_sT_d^2) = 0.126 \quad (27)$$

Achieved transient responses in Fig. 4 confirm fast dynamics and do not significantly depend on $T_p \in (0.3, 0.4)$ s. However, due to the control signal constraint $u \geq 0$ the linear controller is not fully able to carry out the intrinsically considered active damping. Thus, the output step response have relatively strong overshooting that may not be simply eliminated by a modified tuning. Its elimination could be achieved by using the constrained controller described in [10].

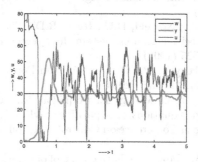

Fig. 4. Transients corresponding to the identified PD controller with static feedforward

5 Conclusions and Future Work

New simple and robust procedure for a reliable PD controller tuning has been shown. Based on a relay experiment with a stabilizing controller, it is appropriate also for unstable UAVs. In order to examine basic features of this new identification method based on the phase plane limit cycle analysis, it has been used in the simplest possible framework decreasing the achievable loop performance. In controller programming, use of a real time kernel could increase regularity in the sampling and together with a finer complementary filter tuning to decrease the measurement noise. In identification, a precision increase could be achieved by excluding parameters of the extreme limit cycles and by modifying the identification formulas to include both extreme limit cycle parameters $\dot{y}_1$ and $\dot{y}_2$, or to include also their amplitudes in the y axis. Higher attention could also be paid to the influence of the implementation filters (1) and their optimal tuning [11]. With respect to the results shown in [12] it could also be interesting to evaluate effect of higher order filter degrees.

Effect of the control signal constraint $u \geq 0$ given by the system construction could be eliminated by using the constrained controller [10].

The static feedforward used with the basic PD controller could be replaced by a disturbance observer based integral action [11]. Yet before application to the paracopter control it might yet be interesting to compare the presented design with other similar approaches as, for example, the exact linearization [14] method, the model-free control [15], or the back calculation method [13].

References

1. Puranik, A., Parker, G., Passerello, Ch., Bird, III, J.D., Yakimenko, O., Kaminer, I.: Modeling and simulation of a ship launched Glider cargo delivery system. In: AIAA Guidance, Navigation, and Control Conference and Exhibit. AIAA, Keystone, pp. 2006–6791 (2006)
2. Jann, T.: Development and flight testing of an autonomous parafoil-load system demonstrator. In: 25th international congress of the aeronautical sciences ICAS 2006, Hamburg (2006)
3. Sim, A.G., Murray, J.E., Neufeld, D.C., Reed, R.D.: The development and flight test of a deployable precision landing systems for spececraft recovery. NASA Technical Memorandum 4525 (1993)
4. Yamauchi, B., Rudakevych, P.: Griffon: A Man-Portable Hybrid UGV/UAV. Industrial Robot **31**(5), 443–450 (2004)
5. Cumer, C., Toussaint, C., Le Moing, T., Poquillon, E., Coquet, Y.: Simulation of generic dynamics flight equations of a parafoil/payload system. Preprints of the 2012 20th Mediterranean Conference on Control & Automation (MED), Barcelona, Spain, 3–6 July 2012
6. Slegers, N., Costello, M.: Model predictive control of a parafoil and payload system. J. Guidance Control Dyn. **28**(4), 816–821 (2005)
7. Huba, M.: Digital time optimal controller with a variable structure. PhD. thesis (in Slovak). EF SVŠT, Bratislava (1981)
8. Huba, M.: Theory of automatic control 3: constrained PID control (in Slovak). Vydavateľstvo STU v Bratislave (2006)
9. Huba, T., Pestun, I., Huba, M.: Learning by pleasure - powered paraglider and other UAVs control. In: 14th International Conference on Interactive Collaborative Learning (ICL), pp. 548–552, Piestany (2011)
10. Huba, M., Malatinec, T., Huba, T.: Laboratory Experiments for Robust Constrained UAVs Control. In: 10th IFAC Symposium on Advances in Control Education (ACE), Sheffield (2013)
11. Huba, M.: Modular PID-controller design with different filtering properties. In: 39th Annual Conference of the IEEE Industrial Electronics Society (IECON). IEEE, Vienna (2013)
12. Huba, M.: Filter choice for an effective measurement noise attenuation in PI and PID controllers. In: IEEE/IES International Conference on Mechatronics, ICM 2015, Nagoya (2015)
13. Adamy, J.: Nichtlineare Regelungen. Springer, New York (2009)
14. Isidori, A.: Nonlinear Control Systems, 3rd edn. Springer, New York (1995)
15. Fliess, M., Join, C.: Model-free control. Int. J. Control **86**(12), 2228–2252 (2013)

A Class of 3-D Distributed Modular Computing Nets

Arminda Moreno-Díaz[1]($\boxtimes$), Gabriel de Blasio[2], and Roberto Moreno-Díaz[2]

[1] School of Computer Science, Madrid Technical University, Madrid, Spain
amoreno@fi.upm.es
[2] Instituto Universitario de Ciencias Y Tecnologías Cibernéticas, ULPGC,
Las Palmas, Spain
gdeblasio@dis.ulpgc.es, rmoreno@ciber.ulpgc.es

Abstract. The class of flat triangular and layered nets of simple computing units, which gives rise to Newton and Hermite filters in two dimensions are extended to 3-D by means of two natural discrete ways. First, by means of the so called Pascal Pyramids; and second, by introducing a rectangular grilled "retina", which leads to a kind of Newton quadrangular pyramids and to 3-D Newton Filters and Nets. Both cases can be extended to the continuous in the form of 2-D Hermite functions and filters of different orders (degree of derivatives). Preliminary results and examples are presented.

1 Introduction and Objectives

Natural neural nets are frequently three dimensional structures, apparent in many parts of the central nervous system, though there are also many instances of strings and surfaces of neurons [1]. The 3-D structure is obvious in case of handling two-dimensional signals, such as in the visual system. However neuron-like networks of computing units are scarcely developed for 3-D, except perhaps for pseudo-3D visual processing applications.

The classical theory of McCulloch-Pitts formal neurons was never focused on a strict 3-D structural point of view; the main argument was that nets can formally always be "flattened" into a plane [2]. Only Pitts seems to have treated formal 3-D neural nets, according to a testimony by Lettvin. However, in committing his "social suicide", Pitts burned all his manuscripts [3,4].

Newton and Hermite formulation of receptive fields are very attractive and successful formal representations of linear receptive fields for higher vertebrate retinal quasi-linear ganglion cells [5,6]. However they are based in one dimensional receptive fields (two dimensional "flat" computing nets).

When extending the two dimensions (for more real receptive fields) it is required a kind of artificial "rotational symmetry" and operations afterwards on rectangular coordinates. This results in the lost of the advantages of the original Newton-Hermite, which relates micro-structures to global functions. That is, the possibilities to introduce local micro non-linearities and local changes in the

© Springer International Publishing Switzerland 2015
R. Moreno-Díaz et al. (Eds.): EUROCAST 2015, LNCS 9520, pp. 103–109, 2015.
DOI: 10.1007/978-3-319-27340-2_14

structure of the net to investigate their effect in the global functions and check for reliability under local scotomas, are lost.

To overcome this, we start here with a restricted class of neuron-like structures which, at least partially, can be approximated by a linear relation of the type (see introduction in [7]):

$$\Omega_j = \sum_{k=1}^{m} W_{jk} x_k$$

where W_{jk} is a weighting factor and x_i the m external input signals. As it is shown in [6] this class of nets can be represented by an m-layered network of $m(m-1)/2$ computing units having two inputs-one output each, the weights per layer being all equals to $1, e_i$, where e_i are the roots of the normalized polynomials having the W_{ij}'s as coefficients. We shall call this a "triangular flat net". The simplest case is when all two inputs weights are equal to $+1$. That corresponds to the so called "Newton filter" of order zero, which is generalized to the continuum to a gaussian (or Hermite function of order zero). Notice that the l layer's (counted from bottom up) weights on the output units for Newton filters of order zero and length m corresponds to the l layer's numbers (counted from up-down) in Pascal or Tartaglia triangle.

The extension of Newton filters of order zero and higher to "3-D Newton Filters" and Nets can be done more naturally preserving the connection rules and properties of the "flat 2-D filters", as it is shown in the sections that follow.

2   From Pascal Pyramids to Pascal Filters and Nets

A natural way to extend the Pascal or Tartaglia Triangle to a three dimensional array of numbers are the so called Pascal Pyramids [8]. For the Newton's binomial in terms of y_0, y_1, the expansion (z, non negative integer is):

$$(y_0 + y_1)^z = \sum_{m=0}^{z} \binom{z}{m} y_0^{z-m} y_1^m$$

By denoting the trinomial coefficients by $(z; x, y)$, where z, x and y are non-negative integers and setting:

$$P_z(x, y) = \frac{z!}{(z-x)!(x-y)!y!}$$

the expansion of the trinomial takes the form:

$$(y_0 + y_1 + y_2)^z = \sum_{x=0}^{z} \sum_{y=0}^{z} P_z(x, y) y_o^{z-x} y_1^{x-y} y_2^y$$

The trinomial coefficients $P_z(x, y)$ orders in the Pascal Pyramid and their cross sections are shown in Fig. 1a [8].

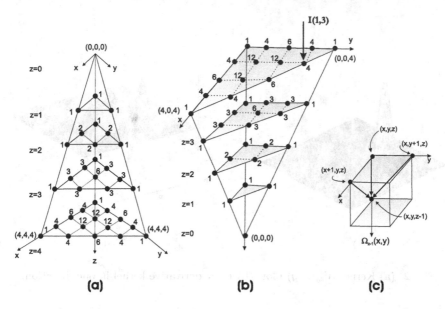

Fig. 1. (a) Pascal Pyramid for trinomial coefficients. (b) Illustration of a Pascal Net of order 0 (all weights are +1); $z_0 = 4$. (c) Illustration of the three inputs converging in one computing unit.

It is not difficult to show that the trinomial coefficients satisfy the recurrence relation:

$$P_{z+1}(x, y) = P_z(x, y) + P_z(x - 1, y) + P_z(x, y - 1)$$

Notice that in this recurrence, the "weight" of each element from layer z to layer $z + 1$ is just +1, as in the Pascal triangle.

The 3-D Pascal Net or filter is obtained by drawing the Pascal Pyramid "upside-down", the lower single unit being the output unit. The computing units, of three inputs each, are placed in the nodes of the pyramid, being connected to the three units immediately above in the prior layer, as shown in Fig. 1b.

By using cartesian coordinates as shown in said figure, recurrent relation between the outputs of each unit and its three inputs from above is (from the recurrent relations of trinomial coefficients):

$$\Omega_{z-1}(x, y) = \Omega_z(x, y) + \Omega_z(x + 1, y) + \Omega_z(x, y + 1)$$

Local weights are all +1 (excitatory) for the net of order zero. The rule is similar the one for Newton filters of order zero, just increased in one input. Figure 3b shows the outputs of the three units impinging in each unit of the next layer. Notice that x, y, z are positive integers starting at 0. In the coordinate system chosen, the origin is the point $(0,0,0)$ (where the output unit is). The inputs to computing units at layer $z - 1$ are as illustrated in Fig. 3b. Denoting by $I(x, y)$ the inputs, they run from $I(0, 0)$ to $I(0, z_0)$ and $I(z_0, 0)$; that is, there are $z_0(z_0 + 1)/2$ input lines, forming a kind of triangular retina. The sides of the

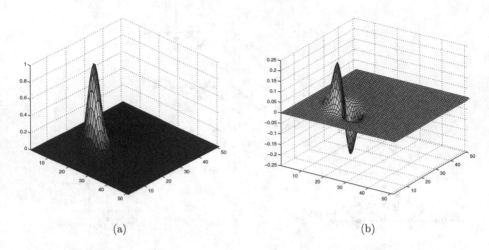

Fig. 2. (a) Kernel $W_{z_0}(x,y)$ plot. (b) First derivative kernel in one direction.

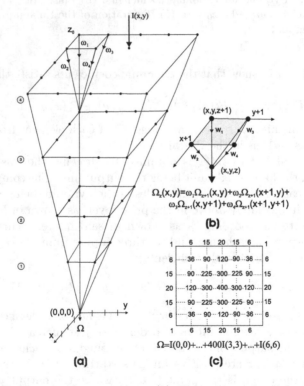

Fig. 3. (a) 3-D Newton Net structure. (b) Illustration of weights to each unit. (c) Overall weights (kernel) for $w_i = 1$ and $z_0 = 6$.

Net are Newton filters of order zero and length $z_0 + 1$. The output of the net is then

$$\Omega = \sum_{x=0}^{z_0} \sum_{y=0}^{z_0} W_{z_0}(x, y) I(x, y) \quad \text{for } x + y \leq z_0$$

where $W_{z_0}(x, y)$ (the weights) are the corresponding numbers of the z_0th Pascal pyramid layer.

The kernel $W_{z_0}(x, y)$ has a Gauss profile (Fig. 2(a)) more apparent in a coordinate system where x and y subtend an angle of $\pi/3$ instead of the cartesian $pi/2$ (triangular equilateral coordinates).

First discrete derivatives can be obtained by "moving" the net along one of the three sides of the output kernel triangle and subtracting. Since weights are all $+1$, a derivative effect is also to be expected by changing weights $(+1,+1,+1)$ or $(+1,+1,-1)$, in a way similar to 2-D Newton filters. The corresponding derivatives will correspond to higher order 3-D Pascal Nets. The kernel of an order one net for a first derivative in one direction is shown in Fig. 2(b).

In the extension to the continuum to obtain Hermite type Nets, results similar to the one presented in next section are to be obtained, because the "gaussian" profiles for nets of order zero, very clearly manifest in triangular equilateral coordinates.

3   Newton and Newton-Hermite 3-D Filters and Nets

A better and more manageable way to extend "triangular flat nets" of m layers to 3-D nets in cartesian coordinates is to start with two flat nets on (x, z) and (y, z) axis, and complete up to an square input grill, as illustrated in Fig. 3a (This generalization was introduced in [5] but was not developed). Figure 3b shows the convergence recurrent rules for the four inputs to each computing unit.

The simplest case is Newton 3-D Net of order zero, where all weights w_i are $+1$. In this case Newton (or Pascal) quadrangles are obtained as weights. The convergence recurrence rule for each weight is similar to Pascal Pyramid, but now the addition is for the four numbers up and behind. That is, counting weight layers from bottom $z = 0$, to top z_0:

$$W_z(x, y) = W_{z-1}(x, y) + W_{z-1}(x + 1, y) + W_{z-1}(x, y + 1) + W_{z-1}(x + 1, y + 1)$$

These weights can be arranged in square grills formed by the coefficients of the Newton's double binomial:

$$(1 + a)^2 (1 + b)^2 = \sum_{z=0}^{z} \sum_{z=0}^{z} \binom{z}{x} a^x \binom{z}{y} b^y$$

Some cases of the squares are sometimes called "squared Pascal triangles" [9]. Again, the sides of the 3-D Newton Net are four Newton filters of length $z_0 + 1$.

The weights associated to each point of the input retina at z are simply:

$$W_z(x,y) = \binom{z}{x}\binom{z}{y} = W_z(x,0)W_z(0,y) \quad \text{(factorization of kernel)}$$

The output of the 3-D Newton net of order zero is then:

$$\Omega = \sum_{x=0}^{z_0}\sum_{y=0}^{z_0} \binom{z_0}{x}\binom{z_0}{y} I(x,y)$$

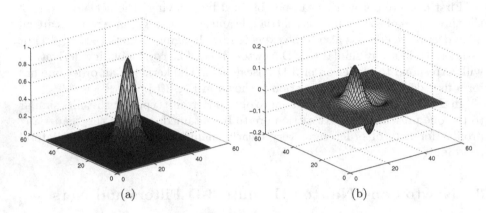

(a)   (b)

Fig. 4. (a) Output of the 3-D Newton Net of order zero. (b) First derivative kernel in x direction.

A variety of locations for "inhibitory weights" (-1) are now possible, giving some kind of different orders of "oriented" Nets. A net of order 1 is easily obtained from a discrete derivative in one direction x or y, as illustrated in Fig. 4(b).

The extension to the continuum is straightforward by the Central Limit Theorem. By proper normalization:

$$\Omega = \sum\sum \binom{z_0}{x}\binom{z_0}{y} I(x,y) \rightarrow \Omega = \int\int e^{-(x^2+y^2)} I(x,y)dx\,dy$$

By denoting $H_0(x,y) = e^{-(x^2+y^2)}$ (two-dimensional Hermite function of order zero), a variety of higher order Hermite kernels are obtained by derivatives in the directions x and y. For example:

$$H_{xx} + Hyy = \frac{\partial^2 H(x,y)}{\partial x^2} + \frac{\partial^2 H(x,y)}{\partial y^2} = -4(1-r^2)e^{-r^2} \quad ; \quad r^2 = x^2 + y^2$$

This is a second order Hermite in two dimensions corresponding to the known Marr's optimal filter [10]. Notice that the Second Radial Hermite is $\frac{d^2 H(r)}{dr^2} = -2(1-2r^2)e^{-r^2}$ [6], which can be shown to result in more intense and wider inhibitory ring.

4   Conclusion

3-D distributed Modular Nets of identical computing units are interesting structures that somehow mimic natural processing networks. Their properties and the effect of including local inhibitions and non-linearities are to be investigated, both for the discrete and their "quasi-Hermitian" continuous counterparts. Higher order 3-D Hermite filters also provide for new tools for visual signal analysis.

Acknowledgments. This work has been supported, in part, by Spanish Ministry of Science projects MTM2011-28983-CO3-03 and MTM2014-56949-C3-2-R.

References

1. Nolte, J.: The Human Brain: An Introduction to its Functional Anatomy. Elsevier Health Sciences Pub. (2008)
2. Moreno-Díaz, R., McCulloch, W.S.: Circularities in nets and the concept of functional matrices. In: Proctor, L. (ed.) Biocibernetics of the Central Nervous System, pp. 145–150. Little & Brown, MA (1969)
3. Lettvin, J.: Warren and Walter. In: McCulloch, R. (ed.) Collected Works of W.S. McCulloch, vol. II, chap. 56, pp. 514–530. Intersystems Pub. (1969)
4. Sánchez, C.: Un genio vagabundo amante de la lógica (2015). http://www.eldiario.es/hojaderouter/ciencia/Walter_Pitts-McCulloch-pioneros-cibernetica-inteligencia_artificial_0_367814000.html
5. Moreno-Díaz, Jr., R.: Computación Paralela y Distribuida: Relaciones Estructura-Función en Retinas. Ph.D thesis, Universidad de Las Palmas de Gran Canaria (1993)
6. Moreno-Díaz, A., de Blasio, G., Moreno-Díaz Jr., R.: Distributed, layered and reliable computing nets to represent neuronal receptive fields. Math. Biosci. Eng. **11**(2), 343–361 (2014)
7. de Blasio, G., Moreno-Díaz, A., Moreno-Díaz, R.: Eulerian numbers weigths in distributed computing nets. In: Moreno-Díaz, R., Pichler, F., Quesada-Arencibia, A. (eds.) Computer Aided Systems Theory. LNCS, pp. 88–94, Springer, Heidelberg (2015)
8. Bondarenko, B.A.: Generalized Pascal triangles and pyramids. The Fibonacci Association Pub. (Translated from Russian by R.C. Bollinger), chapter 1.5 (1993)
9. Brannen, C.: Pascal Triangle and Lisi's E8 Quantum Numbers (2008). https://carlbrannen.wordpress.com/2008/03/03/pascals-triangle-and-lisis-e8-quantum-numbers/
10. Marr, D.: Vision. Freeman and Company, San Francisco (1982)

Standardized Mapping Model for Heritage Preservation and Serendipity in Cloud

Lucia Carrion Gordon[✉], Zenon Chaczko, and Germano Resconi

FEIT Faculty of Engineering and IT, UTS University of Technology,
Sydney, NSW, Australia
{Lucia.CarrionGordon,Zenon.Chaczko}@uts.edu.au,
resconi@speedyposta.it

Abstract. In this research the proposal of a model covers and explanation of how to construct and decide an accurate framework for Data Preservation. The relation between Preservation and Digital patterns of Heritage is well related because of the two aspects to consider: Accessibility and Context.

They cover the conceptualization of real digital preservation. However availability, contextualization and value of the information are the principal matters to focus. First in the introduction we can find the context and the description of the initial scenario. Second the process of preservation with the modelling applications and implementation of patterns. Finally the conclusions and future projects based on the findings. The principal objective is the integration between models and standardization for sustainable solution.

1 Introduction

Digital Data and Heritage Preservation as concepts are related to data management, contextualization and storage. There are many issues and concerns around it. This research explores the precise definition, context and the need of patterns of heritage. The relations, interpretation and context give us the appropriate methods to keep information for a long term use. The management of massive amounts of critical data involves designing, modeling, processing and implementation of accurate systems. The methods to understand data have to consider two dimensions that this research has to focused on: access dimension and cognitive dimension. Both of these dimensions have relevance to get results because at the same time, ensure the correct data preservation.

Our cultural heritage, documents and artefacts increase regularly and place Data Management as a crucial issue. The first stage involves exploration and approaches based on review of recent advances. The second stage involves adaptation of architectural framework and development of software system architecture in order to build the system prototype. Increasing regulatory compliance mandates are forcing enterprises to seek new approaches to managing reference data. Sometimes the approach of tracking reference data in spreadsheets and doing manual reconciliation is both time consuming and prone to human error. As organizations merge and businesses evolve, reference data must be continually mapped and merged as applications are linked and integrated, accuracy and consistency, realize improved data quality, strategy lets organizations adapt reference data as the business evolves.

R. Moreno-Díaz et al. (Eds.): EUROCAST 2015, LNCS 9520, pp. 110–117, 2015.
DOI: 10.1007/978-3-319-27340-2_15

1.1 Context of Preservation and Serendipity Concepts

Serendipity is also a process which leads to a serendipitous finding, and here the insight is the key element. Serendipity as a process starts with something unexpected or odd happening an event, result, encounter or situation/context that triggers insight. And when this insight will eventually leads to value creation for the individual, community or company, then we are witnessing serendipity. In the global business world great insights are rare and therefore so valuable. The competitive edge can often be achieved by only one single insight well executed. Therefore understanding serendipity in all forms becomes a vital part of expertise in tomorrow's business climate [5] (Fig. 1).

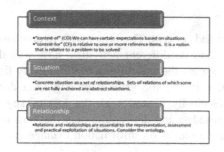

Context, Situation, Relationship

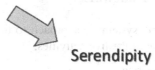

Serendipity

Fig. 1. Context [1]

1.2 Quality Attributes

The quality attributes and the approaches around Digital Data Preservation are:

1. Performance and Scalability
2. Dependability
3. Manageability
4. Data Access

For the formulation of the Hypothesis the relation between keywords and statements is important consideration for improvement of the proposal model (Table 1).

The relation between Software Architecture, and Serendipitous Heritage is going to improve Data Preservation Heritage oriented meta-data for improving the real usage of the information.

The inclusion of Serendipitous Heritage improves performance, scalability, dependability. manageability and data access for Digital Data Preservation Mechanisms in Big Data Architectural solutions. The important knowledge, exactly the

Table 1. Quality attributes: Lucia Carrion 2014

Performance and Scalability	Dependability	Manageability	Data Access
Data Ingest	High Availability	Management Tools	File System Access
Metadata Architecture	MapReduce HA	Volume Support	File I/O
Database Performance	Upgrading	Alerts	Security ACLs
Applications	Replication	Integration	Wire-Level Authentication
	Snapshots	Data and Job Placement Control	
	Disaster Recovery		

context situation relationship and concept. The best way is to demonstrate, validate and show the benefits. The mankind do different activities, how well the Serendipitious Heritage concept will help to grow the meaning of Data in every field.

The massive amount of data and the growth of Big Data drive the society to preserve the information principally related with the lost of key information. The protagonism in the role of metadata and the requirement that data has to be keep in a long term open the alternative to focus on information management (Fig. 2).

2 Architectural Framework

Introduce a consolidated, systematic approach to the redesign of a business enterprise. The methodology includes the five activities:

- Prepare for reengineering.
- Map and Analyse As-Is process.
- Design To-be process.
- Implement reengineered process
- Improve continuously

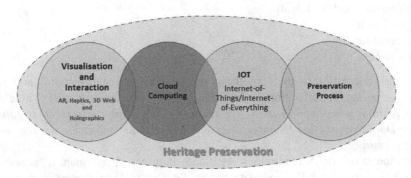

Fig. 2. Computer processing

3 Architecture Vision

The formatting of information provides the unique result as a digital age of the information. Other objective is the knowledge management and Ontology as techniques for analysing information. Also could develop a system could give a result and next steps with a specific process. One concern of digitalization would be the format, standards and migration of the data. It should be solved with the use of Architectural Methodology and with the development of a fast prototype. This requires the definition of the sequential process.

First, should be considering a Framework as a whole front end and for reception of the information in a basic way. Using the Open Group Architectural Framework (TOGAF) it is found to be more suitable as a result of dissemination of the data. Meanwhile, it is associated with an Ontology and Knowledge Management terms to be more specific and with a deep sense of definition. Second the Methodology with an architectural vision using concepts of Architectural Development Method (ADM). It has been identified in terms of enterprise description for validating information of several types of data. Third, the conceptualization of patterns for a centralization f the preservation knowledge providing a unique result: the digital age of the data. The connection is also with the artefacts and the correct use of them. The recovering of the information is another issue has to considering between the techniques used for this purpose like: migration and emulation. The challenges and constraints shown by the type of data classified as structured and unstructured information are rejected in the requirements of each field.

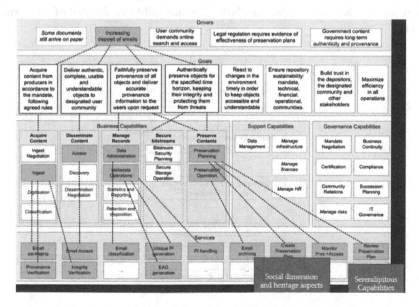

Fig. 3. Functional entities of the OAIS reference model [2]

The evaluation is based on PRIST model denying by Privacy, Rights, Integrity, Security and Trust across PC considerations related with Physical and Cognitive characteristic of data.

The authenticity of the information and the reliability of the same is the principal challenge of the study. The concepts of e-infrastructure are useful for the evaluation of requirements in specific cultural matters like Libraries. According to the author the correct use of the interface and the exact generation of metadata, are the key considerations to follow around the process of optimal data preservation TOGAF + ADM + PRIST (Fig. 3).

4   Evaluation Methods

Based on the exposed statements, the basic techniques are related with genetic and biological cases of study. The relationship between these terms is given for the behaviour and the treatment of data. There are examples referenced by known authors. The sustainability of the preservation of the information give us the discussion about the appropriate resources infrastructure.

5   Cost Model for Digital Preservation

We have applied the OAIS functional entities Ingest, Archival Storage, Data Management, Administration, Preservation Planning, Access, and Common Services. Furthermore we have included the OAIS roles of Producer, Consumer, and Management, as placeholders for external cost factors, which influence the cost of preservation (Fig. 4).

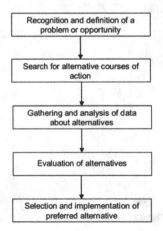

Fig. 4. Rational economic model of decision making [3]

- Producer who performs the dance La Bomba
- Entities cost-critical activities
- The basic formula for an activity is the effective time required to complete an activity (measured in pw) multiplied by the wage level, plus purchases (monetary value) [9].

Bottom Up. The bottom-up design methodology is known for producing autonomous, scalable and adaptable systems often requiring minimal (or no) communication. The design process consists of three steps: Synthesis, Modeling and Analysis, and Optimization.

Cost equations

$$Costperactivity = (Time \times Wage) + Purchase \tag{1}$$

$$c(a) = \sum_{i-0}^{N1} t_i * \sum_{i-0}^{N1} W_i + P \tag{2}$$

Costing Preservation Planning and Digital Migrations while the goal is to model the whole lifecycle of digital preservation. The first version of the model only deals with the cost of Preservation Planning and digital migrations.

- The amount of documentation (number of pages) is one of the principal factors
- The complexity of the documentation (low, medium, high)
- The quality of the documentation (low, medium, high),

FI means Formal Interpretation.

$$FI = \#pages \times timeperpage \times complexity \times quality. \tag{3}$$

6 Future Projects

Data preservation: Digitalization of the Heritage, the result of proposal is to have like a result of the experimental work, a reliable Framework for measure the digital age of the information and patterns that qualified usability and accessibility of the data. The best pathway for commercialization could be some of them.

- Commercial Business Structure like a Partnership assuming the cost of the investment and the taxes that generate the buying of the equipment for implementation of the scanning in the digitalization.
- Initial Public Offering IPO, because the application of the data preservation could be focus on Entities from Government and Historical materials and artifacts that sometimes have to be preserved with a public responsibility.

– This research could have through the market with POCs proof of concepts, showing the advantages and challenges of the new solution. In this case the relationship between the process and the final patterns there is a model.

7   Conclusion

– The context, relation and situation of the Serendipitous Heritage are impressive relevant in the research because it gives the sense of the future of the Knowledge in the World. Through the Socio - Technical, Cultural fields, the process of Preservation will do a contribution for the Memories of the World.
– The use of tools like Hadoop, Softwarch, Archimate and Bonitasoft, the concepts of Software Architecture will have a real approach and meaningful characteristics for the relevance of the investigation.
– The context, relation and situation of the Serendipitous Heritage are impressive relevant in the research because it gives the sense of the future of the Knowledge in the World. Through the Socio - Technical, Cultural fields, the process of Preservation will do a contribution for the Memories of the World.
– The Business Process Management give us a good approach to the development of Performance and Data Preservation. Through process the increase of data can be justified.
– According to this consideration it is important to mention the type and structure of data. Through the time preserving digital information has a process for designing a practical system for managing massive amounts of critical data. The way to improve the understanding of the methodology, the information has to consider two dimensions: access dimension and cognitive dimension. Both of them have the level of importance in terms of the results. As a methodology of treatment digital preservation, it could be risky even when the strategy could develop a clear idea of digital resources and digital artefacts. The approaches related with other authors have similarities and differences in opinion.
– The context, relation and situation of Heritage are impressive relevant in the research because it gives the sense of the future of the Knowledge in the World. Through medical process of Preservation will do a contribution for society advances.

References

1. Thalmann, S., Seeber, I., Maier, R., Ren, P., Pawlowski, J.M., Hetmank, L., Kruse, P., Bick, M.: Ontology-based standardization on knowledge exchange in social knowledge management environments. In: Proceedings of the 12th International Conference on Knowledge Management and Knowledge Technologies, pp. 1–8. ACM, Graz, Austria (2012)

2. Strodl, S., Becker, C., Neumayer, R., Rauber, A.: How to choose a digital preservation strategy: evaluating a preservation planning procedure. In: Proceedings of the 7th ACM/IEEE-CS Joint Conference on Digital Libraries, pp. 29–38. ACM, Vancouver, BC, Canada (2007)
3. Kaner, M., Karni, R.: A capability maturity model for knowledge-based decision-making. Inf. Knowl. Syst. Manag. **4**(4), 225–252 (2004)
4. Challa, S., Gulrez, T., Chaczko, Z., Paranesha, T.N.: Opportunistic information fusion: a new paradigm for next generation networked sensing systems. In: 2005 8th International Conference on Information Fusion, vol. 1, p. 8 (2005)
5. McCay-Peet, L.: Investigating work-related serendipity, what influences it, and how it may be facilitated in digital environments (2014)
6. Olson, J.M., Janes, L.M.: Asymmetrical impact: vigilance for differences and self-relevant stimuli. Eur. J. Soc. Psychol. **32**, 383–393 (2002)
7. Gulden, J.: Methodical support for model-driven software engineering with enterprise models, Universität Duisburg-Essen (2013)
8. Strodl, S., Becker, C., Neumayer, R., Rauber, A.: How to choose a digital preservation strategy: evaluating a preservation planning procedure. Paper Presented to the Proceedings of the 7th ACM/IEEE-CS Joint Conference on Digital Libraries, Vancouver, BC, Canada (2007)
9. Neumann, A., Miri, H., Thomson, J., Antunes, G., Mayer, R., Beigl, M.: Towards a decision support architecture for digital preservation of business processes. In: Proceedings of the 9th International Conference on Digital Preservation (iPres 2012) (2012). Cite-seer: Addison-Wesley, Harlow, England, 1999

Structuring the Model of Complex System Using Parallel Computing Techniques

Jan Nikodem[✉]

Department of Computer Engineering,
Wrocław University of Technology, Wrocław, Poland
jan.nikodem@pwr.edu.pl

Abstract. The contribution of this paper is to present a results of applications of set theory and relations in modeling a complex distributed systems, based on parallel computing platform. The advantages of using the set theory are: the possibility of a formal examination of the local problems, and the possibility to organize individuals as elements of the considered classes, defined globally. To govern the collective behavior we propose three key relations and mappings determined taxonomic order on them. That can insulate us from reductionism and single-cause thinking, as people deal with complexity before. On three examples, we show how take advantage of the new parallel programming tools to obtain more effective multiple inputs in parallel way, than assigning sequentially single causes for any outputs.

Keywords: Modeling of complex system · Parallel computing · Relations

1 Introduction

There are many systems in nature that we can undoubtedly name it as a complex system. Very often, however, calling something as complex, we generally think how complex is its model, not exactly the system itself. For creating a model we employ the conceptual frameworks from the fields of mathematics, physics, chemistry etc. It is obvious, that the selection of these concepts/abstractions significantly determines the nature and complexity of the resulting model.

Because of selectively revealing only some aspects of the complex system, the models are always a restriction of the observed reality. Agreeing with these selectivity of transition from system to its model, we should decide what properties of real system should characterize well-suited projection of mapping the reality. If the behavior of complex system is really *complex* to our mind, the models we develop are certainly complicated, but they will become simpler when we understand it better. It turns out that *complexity* reflects inability to develop *simple* models to describe the behavior of these systems.

Another issue is the choice of tools suitable to model and to analyze complex systems. Along with creating better models, we must also figure out how to

© Springer International Publishing Switzerland 2015
R. Moreno-Díaz et al. (Eds.): EUROCAST 2015, LNCS 9520, pp. 118–125, 2015.
DOI: 10.1007/978-3-319-27340-2_16

evaluate success when choosing tools for working on them. The proper selection of system modeling tools, results in transparent model and facilitates its further analysis. Ill-suited selection of methods and tools leads to increased complexity of the model and indirectly will be a reason of future problems that undoubtedly will appear during analysis of its behavior.

2   Complex Systems Properties

Modern development of computer technology allows for extensive use of parallel computing techniques for modeling a behavior of complex systems. New GPUs and streaming multiprocessor's card, assisted by the parallel programming technology opens a wide range for their use.

One of the areas, where these new technologies especially comes in handy, is the modeling of complex systems. However, the definition of a complex system is still the basic problem. We can find, in the literature, a lot of opinions what is a complex system. Some papers discuss the relativity of this idea, claiming that; the same system, that by one may be seen as complex and unpredictable, by another may be seen as simple and easily understood. Another researches state that, complexity is a measure of the observer misunderstanding what system is being examined. Before going any further, in this paper we follow Corning, Lloyd, Northrop [3,5,9] who argue that complexity generally possess three attributes:

(a) a complex system has many parts (items, units, parameters, variables),
(b) there are many relationships, interactions between the parts,
(c) the parts produce combined effects (synergies) that are not easily foreseen and may often be novel, surprising, unexpected, chaotic.

There are many examples of complex system characterized by having many parts, parameters or states that are functionally interconnected and generally leading to non-intuitive system behavior. For our purpose let us consider a few of them.

3   Computational Complexity

Mathematics occupies special place in the development of the complex systems models. For centuries, mathematicians has been attempting to develop tools to study these problems. So, at the beginning, we start with a pure mathematical example with intricacy measure classified as computational complexity. The problem is referred to as the *problem of n-queens* and may be formulated as follows: How can N queens be placed on an $N \times N$ chessboard, so that no two of them attack each other? For the sake of a full problem formulation, it must be recalled that a chessboard queens can attack horizontally, vertically, and diagonally.

The considered problem has no counterparts in nature or technology. Its peculiarity is that the relationships between elements are very clear and simple.

One simple sentence surely was enough to describe these relationships precisely. Moreover, it is difficult to find any complex and unpredictable behavior as a whole. Even if the we assume that someone has no computational background and very little mathematical background, essentially it is not difficult to explain him what the problem is. So, where lies the complexity of this issue? The answer is: the multitude of solutions necessary to be checked makes this issue computationally hard. Even if we skillfully perform this check (not brute force), the number of operations required, soared with increasing number of chessboard fields.

Today, $N = 26$ is the maximum value for which we know the number of N-queens problem solutions. It is an order of magnitude of $2 \cdot 10^{16}$.

The number of all squares in $N \times N$ chessboard (CB) is defined as $card(CB) = N^2 = 26^2 = 676$, while the number of all subsets of CB is $Pow(CB) = 2^{card(CB)} = 2^{(N \cdot N)} = 2^{676} \simeq 3 * 10^{203}$. This is an awfully big number. We reduce it, putting the requirement that every solution must consist of $N = 26$ elements, although we know that for $N = 8$ the *domination number* (minimum number) of queens that meet the required condition is 5. As a result we obtain the reduction of the search space to the value of $N! = 26! \simeq 4 \cdot 10^{26}$. It's still a very large number, so we are looking for an algorithms which exploit the idea of propagation and backtracking.

Implementing a backtracking algorithm, and using tree pruning techniques of the state space, the algorithm will examine only a fraction 1% of the entire state space. It sounds optimistic, but 1% means that obtained reduction of the entire problem is an order of magnitude 10^2, but this is meager compared with the enormous number 10^{26} of states.

So, we are still on the road! Neither the implementation of parallel computing, nor application of special hardware, can improve this situation. Let us remember about the rules governing the parallelization of algorithms (e.g. Amdahl's rule) and the fact, that even we had an infinite number of cores, we can reach all solutions in linear time. Alas, we do not have an infinite number of cores. Therefore, in this way we can only obtain an speed-up of computation, but not solution of the problem.

Mathematics, while attempting to develop tools to study these (NP-hard) problems, will be sought new conceptual frameworks. The first signal we have already. In complex systems relationships and topological properties play an important role. Considering propagation and backtracking algorithms; they work in state space tree locally (neighborhood is a topological abstraction) using such relations as: subordination (parent-child), tolerance (promising node) and collision (dead end node). To cope with complexity we tend to use both, a wide variety of mathematical techniques (e.g., combinatorial or arithmetic functions and differential equations) as well as topological, relational and set theory frameworks. The latter possess substantive advantages over their analytical counterparts, and are devoid of profound assumptions and some limitations.

4   Structuring a Complex Systems Models

Let us consider water distribution network as another example of a complex system possesses (a), (b) attributes from the Corning, Lloyd, Northrop [3,5,9] list presented above.

Water distribution network is a technical system with a large degree of complexity, both structural, technological and computational. It extends over large areas, so it is geographically distributed system. Moreover, it is distributed due to decision-making. The spatial distribution of water consumers demand varies in time. Decisions on this matter are taken by consumers individually. When pressure in network will increase, the consumer reduce tap water, what locally decrease the flow, and affects the activity of whole system. Also, decisions about supply parameters although coordinated, however, strongly depend on the local conditions that temporary prevail in neighborhood of reservoirs and pumping stations.

Multi-loop structure of the pipeline network, multitude and diversity of components (pipes, nodes, valves, tanks, pumps, fittings) entails the diversity of relationships between system elements. So, we have fulfill locally both, functions (especially for pipe sections) as well as relationships which can be calculated from the nomograph of a transit function (in case of fittings). Good knowledge of local physical rules provide us:

 (i) Darcy-Weisbach equation for a head loss due to the friction along a given length of pipe segment, to the average velocity of the water flow.
 (ii) Hazen-Williams equation which relates the flow of water in a pipeline with the physical properties of the pipeline and the pressure drop caused by friction.
(iii) Mannings equation estimating the average velocity of a water flowing in an open channel (i.e. driven by a gravity).
(iv) Hydraulic Grade Line, the sum of pressure head and elevation head
 (v) Velocity profile in a pipeline, which generally is greatest at the center of the pipe.

Topological properties of a pipeline network as a whole (so globally) are described by incidence matrix $A_{[m \times n]}$ (where m denotes the number of nodes, and n is number of pipe segments) and by loop matrix $B_{[n \times o]}$ (where o represents the number of loops). First and second Kirchhoff's laws forming two global relationships in whole water distribution network. The first law - material continuity at a node

$$A \cdot y = \sigma. \tag{1}$$

where $y \in R^n$ and $\sigma \in R^m$ is a vector of consumer demands.

The second law - loop equations

$$B \cdot x = 0; \quad 0 \in R^n \tag{2}$$

where x is a vector of head difference between two ends of a pipeline segment.

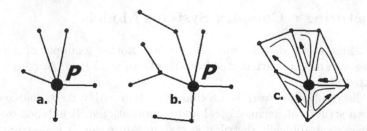

Fig. 1. Three examples of node P topological neighborhood (a.- nodes-edges, first order, b.- nodes-edges, second order, c.- loops-edges neighborhood.)

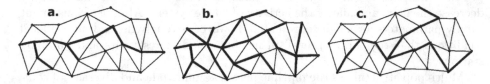

Fig. 2. Different type of tree structure according to global ordering relation (a.- for chosen pipe diameters, b.- minimum spanning tree, c.- trunk pipeline).

The model of water distribution network consists of set of Eqs. (1)–(2), determining the global relationships, extended with plenty of local dependencies (i)–(v). While modeling water distribution network [1,6,7,12] we could tackle it using sequential programing. In such a case, putting the expressions (i)–(v) into Eqs. (1)–(2) cause that these latter become nonlinear. Moreover, using sequential approach we have to treat network as a whole, although it is evident that water distribution network consists of many divers elements. Consequently, even when something changes locally, we should re-calculate the model of all network. So, in that case a global perspective overshadow local activity, evoking a number of undesirable computational consequences.

Local and global activities are not actually in competition, because the best approach is to combine them. That is what we would like to do using parallel programing techniques. Having at our disposal many (hundreds or thousands) cores (Fig. 3), we can harnessed many of them to calculate local dependencies within neighborhoods. Simultaneously, other cores can support the process of casting some global laws (Kirchhoff's) from the whole network area to the neighborhood.

The incidence (A) and loop (B) matrices reflect a topological properties of the whole pipeline network. Employing the theories of sets and relations, we can shape the neighborhood abstraction, according to individual requirements of modeling (Figs. 1 and 2). The number of possible neighborhoods is huge. More than enough to model (using this topological framework) a very diverse situations that can occur in the water supply network.

5 Modeling of Collective Animal Behavior

Presented in the previous section the water distribution system, despite the high degree of complexity is (as a technical layout) fully predictable. Its mathematical model consisting of set of nonlinear equations, can exhibit unstable, chaotic behavior. However, this chaotic behavior is, in fact, deterministic. Its occurrence, at first may appear random, but for example, the conditions of high frequency oscillation in pipeline are very well known. Not all complex systems possess such a property. In many of occurring in nature complex systems [14] we can observe such features as chaotic behavior and a tipping points. How to model the chaotic behavior?

Flocking starlings is a good example of a natural complex system with collective chaotic behavior, so it is worth to spend some time on it. The papers dealing with complexity of a natural complex systems appear regularly in journals. Plenty of them raises the issue of collective animal behavior.

At first glance it seems that flocking birds or shoaling fish, using the classification outlined in Chapter 2, should be characterized by all three attributes $(a), (b), (c)$. It means; has many parts; there are many relationships between the parts; and the parts produce combined effects that are not easily foreseen and may often be novel, surprising, unexpected, chaotic. However, the most authors emphasize that in these collectivizes there are no many relationships between the members.

One of the best known model of the birds collective behavior was proposed by Reynolds [11]. He claims that, in order to properly model the collective behavior

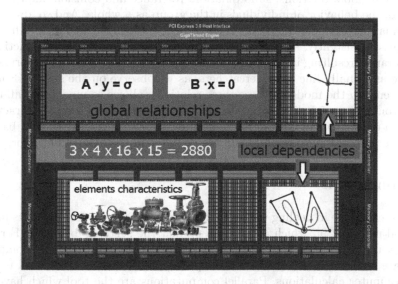

Fig. 3. Structuring the water supply network model using multicores structure (Kepler GK110, $3 \cdot 4 \cdot 16 \cdot 15 = 2880$ cores).

of birds, is sufficient to consider three types of local interactions between individuals forming the flock. Each bird should follow three rules:

- *Dispersion*, as a result of the collision avoidance. The bird maintains a minimum distance from other birds thereby avoid collisions with the neighbors.
- *Alignment*, as a result of the velocity matching, i.e. birds matches its own velocity (as a vector) with the neighbors.
- *Cohesion*, as attraction toward the birds within the neighborhood. The bird steer to move toward the average position of local flockmates.

Remarkably, these three very simple rules govern the local interactions between neighbors to each other, and produce a realistic-looking flocking behavior. The Craig model confirms that complex behavior, like flocking, need not have many and complex rules.

Craig's work has shown, how the control of local activity has an impact on the behavior of the whole, but only for one, selected (starlings) group of birds. Craig's model does not explain how a delta of ducks or V-shaped formation of geese [13] are formed. To do this, we use parallel programming, the set theory [4], and relations defined on them.

If we use the topological abstractions, we can structure the flock (using ordering relation), and to obtain the encountered in the nature, well shaped structures of birds flock. Usage of the relations; subordination (π), tolerance (ϑ) and collision ($\varkappa$) is indirect descendant of Craig's ideas. Indeed, subordination is global exemplification of *Alignment* while both global tolerance and collision are analogue to local *Cohesion*, and *Dispersion*.

A three global relations; subordination, tolerance and collision allow coordination of the behavior of individuals in the group as a whole. And so, dwindling subordination produces the effects of chaos noticeable in the behavior of flocking starlings. Consistently, strengthen coordination with simultaneous reduction in the tolerance, resulting in the formation as delta of ducks or V-shaped formation of geese and finally line of oystercatchers, as we observe on the sky [8]. Finally, the presence in the model of these three relations, allows to model the influence of environmental stimuli on whole group behavior. Predator - prey interactions like flash expansions of flocking birds forming eddies on the sky or bait balls of schooling fish cruising parabolas [10] are good examples of such behavior.

6   Conclusion

A major challenge in dealing with complex system is, how to formulate its mathematical model [2,9], which allow us to predict the system's behavior. For this purpose, unprecedented technological progress in the construction of computer hardware realizing highly paralleled computing, has given us a new tool to perform computer calculations. Parallel computations are the tool which have the biggest impact on complex system modeling.

Parallel computing tools accelerate calculation in case of problem that's hard because of computational complexity, but above all that, with its help we can more accurately model real complex systems. Having at our disposal a computer operating parallel, we are looking for solutions tailored just for such equipment.

As a result, now we can model distributed system, using neighborhood relation in natural way, as a set of distributed elements cooperating with each other. Moreover, we can use relations to insulate us from reductionism and single-cause thinking, as people deal with complexity before. Our experience has indicated that (for complex, distributed systems) it is generally more effective to try multiple inputs in parallel way, than assigning single causes for any outputs.

References

1. Arsene, C., Bargiela, A., Al-Dabass, D.: Simulation of network systems based on loop flows algorithms. Int. J. Simul. Syst. Sci. Technol. **5**(1–2), 61–72 (2004)
2. Box, G.E.P., Draper, N.R.: Empirical Model Building and Response Surfaces. Wiley, New York (1987)
3. Corning P.A.: Synergy and self-organization in the evolution of complex systems. Syst. Res. **12**(2), 89–121 (1995). doi:10.1002/sres.3850120204 (Wiley)
4. Kuratowski, K., Mostowski, M.: Set Theory, with introduction to descriptive set theory. In: Studies in Logic and the Foundations of Mathematics, vol. 86. PWN-Warsaw, North- Holland- Amsterdam, New York, Oxford (1976)
5. Lloyd, S.: Measures of complexity: a nonexhaustive list. IEEE Control Sys. Mag. **21**(4), 7–8 (2001). doi:10.1109/MCS.2001.939938
6. Marques, J., Cunha, M.C., Sousa, J., Savic, D.: Robust optimization methodologies for water supply systems design. Drinking Water Eng. Sci. **5**(1), 31–37 (2012). doi:10.5194/dwes-5-31-2012
7. Nikodem, J., Klempous, R.: Smart water distribution system, cloud computing. In: ICIT 2013, The 6th International Conference on Information Technology, Amman/Jordan, Al-Dahoud. Al-Zaytoonah University of Jordan, Amman (2013)
8. Nikodem, J.: Modelling of collective animal behavior using relations and set theory. In: Moreno-Díaz, R., Pichler, F., Quesada-Arencibia, A. (eds.) EUROCAST. LNCS, vol. 8111, pp. 110–117. Springer, Heidelberg (2013)
9. Seiffertt, J., Wunsch, D.C.: Introduction. In: Seiffertt, J., Wunsch, D.C. (eds.) Unified Computational Intell. for Complex Sys. ALO, vol. 6, pp. 1–17. Springer, Heidelberg (2010)
10. Parrish, J.K., Viscido, S.V., Grunbaum, D.: Selforganized fish schools: an examination of emergent properties. Biol. Bull. **202**, 296–305 (2002)
11. Reynolds, C.W.: Flocks, herds, and schools: a distributed behavioral model. In SIGGRAPH 1987 Conference Proceedings, Computer Graphics, vol. 21, no. 4, pp. 25–34 (1987)
12. Siew, C., Tanyimboh, T.: Augmented gradient method for head dependent modeling of water distribution networks. World Environmental and Water Resources Congress (2009). doi:10.1061/9780784410363
13. Speakman, J.R., Banks, D.: The function of flight formations in Greylag Geese Anser anser; energy saving or orientation? Department of Zoology, University of Aberdeen, Aberdeen AB24 2TZ. Scotland, UK, IBIS **140**(2), 280–287 (1998). doi:10.1111/j.1474-919X.1998.tb04390.x
14. Sumpter, D.J.T.: The principles of collective animal behaviour. Phil. Trans. R. Soc. B **361**, 5–22 (2006). doi:10.1098/rstb.2005.1733

The Evolution of Models: Uncovering the Path of Model Improvement

Markus Schwaninger[✉]

University of St. Gallen, Dufourstrasse 40a, 9000 St. Gallen, Switzerland
markus.schwaninger@unisg.ch

Abstract. The purpose of this contribution is to learn from the theory of evolution in order to improve the design of modeling processes. The aim of the chapter is to advance the understanding of the evolutionary structural characteristics of modeling processes which lead to better models, and to find design rules for systematically achieving higher model quality. We use a simulation approach, building a System Dynamics model. The simulation-based analysis uncovers several surprising, counterintuitive results and useful insights. These deliver lessons for advancing the design of model-building processes.

Keywords: Modeling and simulation · Model-building · Evolutionary process · Model quality

1 Purpose

The assumption underlying this paper is that the modeling process leading to model quality is driven by the evolutionary "mechanisms" of variation, selection and retention (Aldrich 1999). Assuming that the evolution of models can be influenced, the research questions, then, are how and to what extent this can be done. We intend to learn from the nature of general processes of evolution how we can better design modeling processes.

The principles of evolution have been studied extensively in the biological-ecological realm (Darwin 1859; Jablonka and Lamb 2005). In the technical domain, the principles of evolution have been used to amplify the improvement of technical objects (e.g., Rechenberg 1973; Price et al. 2005). Also, the evolution of social systems – societies, economies and organizations – in both structural and cultural terms, have been explained in terms of the theory of evolution (Campbell 1965; Mesoudi et al. 2006; Aldrich 2008; Dopfer and Potts 2008). Qualitative models of the substantive evolution of models have been published (e.g., Wartick and Cochran 1985), and quantitative model systems for experimental evolution have been built (e.g., Collins et al. 2014).

To the author's knowledge, however, until now modeling processes have not been studied quantitatively in a way that allows one to learn how to improve them by applying the general principles of evolution. We will refer to computer models as used for the purpose of simulation.

To answer the research questions, we are building a simulation model of an idealized modeling process. We are using the System Dynamics (SD) methodology

© Springer International Publishing Switzerland 2015
R. Moreno-Díaz et al. (Eds.): EUROCAST 2015, LNCS 9520, pp. 126–132, 2015.
DOI: 10.1007/978-3-319-27340-2_17

developed by Prof. Jay Forrester at the Massachusetts Institute of Technology (Forrester 1961; Sterman 2000). SD models represent complex systems with two kinds of variables, stocks and flows, and their interrelationships. These structures are simulated as continuous processes, with feedbacks and delays. The dynamic behavior of the system under study results from the interactions of the variables, and is nonlinear.

2 A Generic Model of the Modeling Process

The model built here reflects the structure of evolutionary processes. However, we refrain from using the commonly adopted sequential representation. The model consists of causal feedback loops for each one of the evolutionary "mechanisms". These mechanisms are interdependent, and they converge at the construct "Model Quality" (MQ). MQ is the variable in focus that expresses the degree to which the maturity of a model has evolved. Given its embeddedness in three causal circuits, it can grow, but it can also shrink.

The stock-and-flow diagram, which represents the modeling process, is shown in Fig. 1. The logic of the three causal loops in the diagram is as follows:

1. *Variation Loop:* The variety of available models is generated by the introduction of new models into the process. The quantity of new models inserted depends on the current level of model quality. These new models are subject to a first validation. The validated models can, but do not necessarily, increase model quality. They also have to stand up to the competition from current models-in-process, i.e., those models which are already in the improvement process ("models-in-process").

2. *Selection Loop:* A selection criterion determines the level of errors upon which the decision is made either to use a model-in-process or to adopt one of the new models (from loop 1). Model quality then is changed either by an improved, current model or by the use of a new model. This loop is closed by the connection of model quality, tests and errors.

3. *Retention Loop:* A comparison between the model quality standard and the actual quality of models-in-process results in a gap. The gap determines the frequency of tests: the greater the gap, the more tests there will be. Errors discovered in these tests and subsequent error corrections cause changes in model quality.

Stocks are represented by boxes and flows by valves. The orthogonal dashes on several arrows denote delays. The arrows marked with negative polarities ("−") represent a causality in which more of the cause leads to less of the effect, and vice versa. All other variables are assumed to have a positive polarity, with more (less) of the cause leading to more (less) of the effect. The overall polarity of a loop is the product of the signs on the arrows constituting that loop. For example, in the case of the Retention Loop: "−" * "+" * "+" * "+" * "+" * "+" = "−". The simulation model is made up of equations and constants. The accumulation of stocks is captured in differential equations.

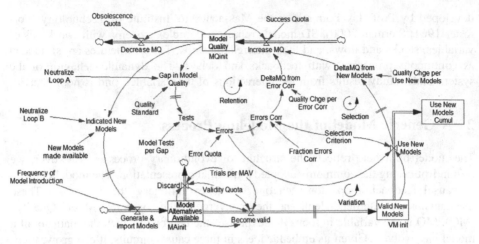

Fig. 1. Stock-and-flow diagram of the simulation model

A more parsimonious representation of this quantitative model, at a macro-level, is captured in formula (1):

$$OPT\{M : M \in gen(Processes)\} = \int_{t=0}^{tfinal} S[Coupling(Var, Sel, Ret)]dt, \qquad (1)$$

where M denotes model(s), and S an event-coupling system of cyclic processes. *Var*, *Sel*, *Ret* are dynamically coupled processes, with *Var* standing for Variation, *Sel* for Selection, and *Ret* for Retention.

Two crucial micro-level equations are in formulas (2) and (3). First, Model Quality is the accumulation of all net flows:

$$Model\ Quality = \int_{t=0}^{tfinal} (IncreaseMQ - DecreaseMQ)dt \qquad (2)$$

Second, a formula from the Selection Loop incorporates the focal decision between the options (A) to continue working on the same model, and (B) to use a new model. A Selection Criterion defines the determinant threshold: the minimal number of errors upward from which a new model must be used [Use New Model], instead of carrying on with the correction of errors on the current model. The formula is:

$$Use\ New\ Models = Min(Valid\ New\ Models/AT,$$
$$Min(IF\ THEN\ ELSE(Errors > Selection\ Criterion, 1, 0), \qquad (3)$$
$$INTEGER((valid\ New\ Models))/AT)),$$

where *AT* is an adaptation delay.

3 Simulation Results

The variable in focus here is [Model Quality]. Plotted over time, it shows the following pattern in the base run (Fig. 2).

The pattern is oscillatory. In the long term it varies: over 300 weeks the variable *MQ* [Model Quality] shows a period between 23 and 40 weeks, i.e., an average period of 30 weeks (~7 months) and an amplitude between 0.98 and 1.73 *Qual*. *Qual* is the unit of measurement for *MQ*. Average MQ, in the base run, converges to an equilibrium of 4.7 *Qual/week*.

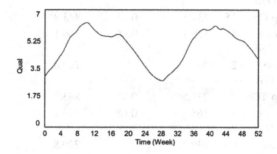

Fig. 2. Pattern of model quality (time horizon: one year, i.e., 52 weeks)

To ascertain the impact of changes in parameter values, elasticities e_i^j are calculated for cumulative MQ, i.e., Q_{cum}, and cumulative oscillations of MQ, i.e., O_{cum}, over 52 weeks. The formula for the elasticities eq and e_o is:

$$e_i^j = \frac{\frac{J_i^j - J_i^b}{J_i^b}}{\frac{P_i^j - P_i^b}{P_i^b}}, \tag{4}$$

where J_i are outcomes, either Q_{cum} or O_{cum}. Pi, $i = 1, ..., 6$ denotes the parameters. b stands for the base value of a parameter, and j stands for parameter changes, - u, up, and d, down. $j = 1, 2, 3$ indexes the three scenarios for parameter values at b, u, and d.

Oscillations of MQ, o and O_{cum} are calculated as follows:

$$Q_{cum} = \int_{t=0}^{t_{final}} q \cdot dt, \ \bar{q} = \frac{Q_{cum}}{t_{final}}, \ o = q - \bar{q}, \ O_{cum} = \int_{t=0}^{t_{final}} |o| \cdot dt, \tag{5}$$

where variable q stands for MQ, o for oscillations of MQ, and $\bar{q}$ for average MQ.

The parameters Pi, analyzed in Table 1, are:

- For the Retention Loop: Selection Criterion (SC), Quality Standard (QS), Tests of Model per Gap (TG), Obsolescence (OB).

Table 1. Scenario settings, outcomes and elasticities

Parameters	Parameter values		MQ cumulated at t = 52	Elasticity for MQ	Oscillations MQ cumulated at t = 52	Elasticity for oscillations MQ
Selection criterion	Base SCb	8	249.7		729.8	
	Up SCu	12	260.1	0.08	273.5	−1.25
	Down SCd	4	231.5	0.15	843.9	−0.31
Quality standard	Base QSb	10	249.7		729.8	
	Up QSu	15	231.5	−0.15	843.9	0.31
	Down QSd	5	129.4	0.96	106.1	1.71
Model tests per gap	Base TGb	2	249.7		729.8	
	Up TGu	3*	231.5	−0.15	843.9	0.31
	Down TGd	1	165	0.68	95.2	1.74
Obsolescence	Base OBb	0.1	249.7		729.8	
	Up OBu	0.15	223.3	−0.21	545.4	−0.51
	Down OBd	0.05	340.6	−0.73	471.4	0.71
New models made available	Base NMb	4	249.7		729.8	
	Up NMh1	6	259.8	0.08	556.2	−0.48
	Up NMh2	8	268.2	0.07	557.4	−0.24
	Up NMh3	10	276.6	0.07	432.6	−0.27
	Down NMl	2	97.35	1.22	1353	−1.71
Frequency of model introduction	Base FIb	1	249.7		729.8	
	Up FIh	1.5	259.8	0.08	556.2	−0.48
	Down FIl	0.5	97.35	1.22	1353	−1.71

*same results for TG = 4.00 (saturation)
Correlation MQ cum/Osc cum: −0.36

- For the Variation Loop: New Models Made Available (NM), and Frequency of Model Introduction (FI). The results for these two variables are equal, as changing them has the same effect in both cases. They are kept separate because they represent two distinct policies.

As far as the elasticities for MQ are concerned, if these move in the same direction as parameter changes, then a general assumption would be that most negative values represent unexpected results.

Summarizing the results:

1. It is generally difficult to improve MQ. The only improvements are visible in the small elasticities e_q with SC, NM and FI.
2. MQ and Oscillations are negatively correlated, i.e., there is a tradeoff between the two. Low levels of MQ are often associated with high oscillation levels.
   There are ways of reducing oscillations, but they are often associated with lower MQ, as in the case of parameters QS, TG, and OB.
3. Quality Standard (QS): Stretching parameter QS too high lowers MQ.[1]
4. Testing: Neither an increase nor a decrease in the number of model tests can raise MQ: both damage MQ. We have an inverted-U-relationship here.
5. Obsolescence: Increasing obsolescence should «refresh» MQ, but it does not. What it does is reduce both MQ and Oscillations substantially.

Conclusively, we derive the following insights and implications:

- The best way to reduce MQ is by enhance keeping the number of New Models introduced or the Frequency of Introduction high. With both procedures the necessary redundancy of options is created to enable better models. → Provide redundancy!
- High levels of obsolescence damage MQ. → Do not abandon models-in-process too early!
- Both too many and too few tests are detrimental. → Find a reasonable level of test intensity; avoid over- and under-testing!
- Quality is difficult to increase but easy to lose: Erosion of quality is very dangerous. → Keep Quality Standard high, but do not exaggerate!

4 Conclusion

At the outset, we posed two parallel research questions: if the evolution of models can be influenced, then how and to what extent can this be done? This study has demonstrated that such evolutionary modulation can be accomplished, and that a number of parameters are appropriate to influencing model evolution in both level and direction.

Given a number of unexpected results found via the simulations, certain clues for the improvement of modeling processes have been identified. These findings deliver both conceptual value, further instructing us about the "anatomy" of modeling processes, and also economic potential, in terms of quality and productivity improvements.

The model presented here is structurally validated, but has not been tested yet on the basis of empirical data. For the time being it is a generic model with didactic

---

[1] q_{QS}^b was already set at a demanding level, but q_{QS}^u was overstretched.

benefits, providing insights about generic patterns of system behavior. Adding more detail could lead to outcomes different in degree but not distinct in kind. Fitting the model to real life could be useful in making it a steering tool for model-builders.

Acknowledgement. The author wishes to thank Profs. Franz Pichler and Stefan Ott for their precious comments and encouragement.

References

Aldrich, H.: Organizations Evolving. Sage Publications, Thousand Oaks (1999)

Aldrich, H.E.: Organizations and Environments. Stanford University Press, Stanford (2008)

Campbell, D.T.: Variation and selective retention in socio-cultural evolution. In: Barringer, H.R., Blanksten, G.I., et al. (eds.) Social Change in Developing Areas: A Reinterpretation of Evolutionary Theory, pp. 19–49. Schenkman, Cambridge (1965)

Wartick, S.L., Cochran, P.L.: The evolution of the corporate social performance model. Acad. Manage. Rev. **10**, 758–769 (1985)

Collins, S., Rost, B., Rynearson, T.A.: Evolutionary potential of marine phytoplankton under ocean acidification. Evol. Appl. **7**, 140–155 (2014)

Dopfer, K., Potts, J.: The General Theory of Economic Evolution. Routledge, London (2008)

Darwin, C.: On the Origin of Species. Harvard University Press, Cambridge (1859). (Facsimile edition 1964)

Forrester, J.W.: Industrial Dynamics. MIT Press, Cambridge (1961)

Jablonka, E., Lamb, M.J.: Evolution in Four Dimensions. Genetic, Epigenetic, Behavioral, and Symbolic Variation in the History of Life. MIT Press, Cambridge (2005)

Mesoudi, A., Whiten, A., Laland, K.N.: Towards a unified science of cultural evolution. Behav. Brain Sci. **29**, 329–383 (2006)

Price, K.V., Storn, R.N., Lampinen, J.A.: Differential Evolution: A Practical Approach to Global Optimization. Springer, Berlin (2005)

Rechenberg, I.: Evolutionsstrategie. Frommann, Stuttgart (1973)

Sterman, J.D.: Business Dynamics. Systems Thinking and Modeling for a Complex World. Irwin/Mc Graw-Hill, Boston (2000)

Modelling Biological Systems

Some Remarks on First-Passage Times for Integrated Gauss-Markov Processes

Marco Abundo and Mario Abundo$^{(\boxtimes)}$

Tor Vergata University, Rome, Italy
marco.abundo@gmail.com, abundo@mat.uniroma2.it

Abstract. It is considered the integrated process $X(t) = x + \int_0^t Y(s)ds$, where $Y(t)$ is a Gauss-Markov process starting from y. The first-passage time (FPT) of X through a constant boundary and the first-exit time of X from an interval (a, b) are investigated, generalizing some results on FPT of integrated Brownian motion.

Keywords: Diffusion · Gauss-Markov process · First-passage-time

1 Introduction

First-passage time (FPT) problems for integrated Markov processes arise both in theoretical and applied Probability. For instance, in certain stochastic models for the movement of a particle, its velocity, $Y(t)$, is modeled as Ornstein-Uhlenbeck (OU) process, which is indeed suitable to describe the velocity of a particle immersed in a fluid; as the friction parameter approaches zero, $Y(t)$ becomes Brownian motion B_t (DM). More generally, the particle velocity $Y(t)$ can be modeled by a diffusion. Thus, particle position turns out to be the integral of $Y(t)$, and any question about the time at which the particle first reaches a given place leads to the FPT of integrated $Y(t)$. The study of $\int_0^t Y(s)ds$ has interesting applications in Biology, in Queueing Theory, in Economy and in Finance (see [1] and references therein).

FPT problems of integrated BM (namely, when $Y(t) = B_t$) through one or two boundaries, attracted the interest of a lot of authors (see e.g. [4,6,8,9,11] for single boundary, and [7,12,13] for double boundary).

Let $m(t)$, $h_1(t)$, $h_2(t)$ be C^1-functions of $t \geq 0$, such that $h_2(t) \neq 0$ and $\rho(t) = h_1(t)/h_2(t)$ is a non-negative and monotonically increasing function, with $\rho(0) = 0$. If $B(t) = B_t$ denotes standard Brownian motion (BM), then

$$Y(t) = m(t) + h_2(t)B(\rho(t)), \ t \geq 0, \tag{1}$$

is a continuous Gauss-Markov (GM) process with mean $m(t)$ and covariance $c(s,t) = h_1(s)h_2(t)$, for $0 \leq s \leq t$.
Throughout the paper, Y will denote a GM process of the form (1), starting from $y = m(0)$.

© Springer International Publishing Switzerland 2015
R. Moreno-Díaz et al. (Eds.): EUROCAST 2015, LNCS 9520, pp. 135–142, 2015.
DOI: 10.1007/978-3-319-27340-2_18

Besides BM, a noteworthy case of GM process is the OU process, and in fact any continuous GM process can be represented in terms of a OU process (see e.g. [14]); for examples of integrated GM processes, see [1].

Given a continuous GM process Y, we consider its integrated process, starting from $X(0)$, i.e. $X(t) = X(0) + \int_0^t Y(s)ds$. For a given boundary a, we study the FPT of X through a, with the conditions that $X(0) = x < a$ and $Y(0) = y$, that is, $\tau_a(x,y) = \inf\{t > 0 : X(t) = a|X(0) = x, Y(0) = y\}$; moreover, for $b > a$ and $x \in (a,b)$, we also study the first-exit time of X from the interval (a,b), with the conditions that $X(0) = x$ and $Y(0) = y$, that is, $\tau_{a,b}(x,y) = \inf\{t > 0 : X(t) \notin (a,b)|X(0) = x, Y(0) = y\}$.

In our investigation, an essential role is played by the representation of X in terms of BM, which was previously obtained by us in [2]. This allows to avoid the use of Kolmogorov's equations; our approach is based on the properties of BM and continuous martingales and it has the advantage to be quite simple, since the problem is reduced to the FPT of a time-changed BM. Actually, for $Y(0) = y = 0$ we present explicit formulae for the density and the moments of the FPT of the integrated GM process X, both in the one-boundary and two-boundary case; in particular, in the two-boundary case, we are able to express the nth order moment of the first-exit time as a series involving only elementary functions.

2   Main Results

We recall from [2] the following:

Theorem 1. *Let Y be a GM process of the form (1); then $X(t) = x + \int_0^t Y(s)ds$ is normally distributed with mean $x + M(t)$ and variance $\gamma(\rho(t))$, where $M(t) = \int_0^t m(s)ds$, $\gamma(t) = \int_0^t (R(t) - R(s))^2 ds$ and $R(t) = \int_0^t h_2(\rho^{-1}(s))/\rho'(\rho^{-1}(s))ds$. Moreover, if $\gamma(+\infty) = +\infty$, then there exists a BM $\widehat{B}$ such that $X(t) = x + M(t) + \widehat{B}(\widehat{\rho}(t))$, where $\widehat{\rho}(t) = \gamma(\rho(t))$. Thus, the integrated process X can be represented as a GM process with respect to a different BM.* □

Example 1. (integrated Brownian motion)
Let be $Y(t) = y + B_t$, then $m(t) = y$, $h_1(t) = t$, $h_2(t) = 1$ and $\rho(t) = t$. Moreover, $R(t) = \int_0^t ds = 1$ and $\gamma(t) = \int_0^t (t - s)^2 ds = t^3/3$. Thus, $\widehat{\rho}(t) = t^3/3$, $\gamma(+\infty) = +\infty$, and so there exists a BM $\widehat{B}$ such that $X(t) = x + yt + \widehat{B}(t^3/3)$.

Example 2. (integrated OU process)
Let $Y(t) = \beta + e^{-\mu t}[y - \beta + \widetilde{B}(\rho(t))]$, where $\widetilde{B}$ is BM and $\rho(t) = \frac{\sigma^2}{2\mu}\left(e^{2\mu t} - 1\right)$. Y is a GM process with $m(t) = \beta + e^{-\mu t}(y - \beta)$, $h_1(t) = \frac{\sigma^2}{2\mu}\left(e^{\mu t} - e^{-\mu t}\right)$, $h_2(t) = e^{-\mu t}$ and $c(s,t) = h_1(s)h_2(t)$. After calculating the functions M, R and γ of Theorem 1, we conclude that $X(t) = x + \int_0^t Y(s)ds$ is normally distributed with mean $x + M(t)$ and variance $\widehat{\rho}(t) = \gamma(\rho(t))$. Moreover, as easily seen, $\lim_{t \to +\infty} \gamma(t) = +\infty$, so there exists a BM $\widehat{B}$ such that $X(t) = x + M(t) + \widehat{B}(\widehat{\rho}(t))$.

In the following, we suppose that $Y(t) = y + h_2(t)B(\rho(t))$, namely, $m(t) = y$ is constant, and $\gamma(+\infty) = +\infty$, so the integrated process is of the form $X(t) = x + yt + \widehat{B}(\widehat{\rho}(t))$, where $\widehat{\rho}(t) = \gamma(\rho(t))$ and $\widehat{B}$ is a suitable BM. Notice however, that the integrated OU process belongs to this class only if $y = \beta$.

2.1 FPT Through One Boundary

Under the previous assumptions, let a be a fixed constant boundary; for $x < a$ and $y \in \mathbb{R}$, the FPT of X through a can be written as $\tau_a(x, y) = \inf\{t > 0 : x + yt + \widehat{B}(\widehat{\rho}(t)) = a\}$. Thus, if we set $\widehat{\tau}_a(x, y) = \widehat{\rho}(\tau_a(x, y))$, we get $\widehat{\tau}_a(x, y) = \inf\{t > 0 : \widehat{B}_t = h(t)\}$, where $h(t) = a - x - y\widehat{\rho}^{-1}(t)$, and so we reduce to consider the FPT of BM through a curved boundary. For $x < a$ and $y \geq 0$, since the function $h(t)$ is not increasing, we can conclude that $\tau_a(x, y)$ is finite with probability one. More difficult is to find the distribution of $\widehat{\tau}_a(x, y)$, and then that of $\tau_a(x, y)$. However, if $h(t)$ is either convex or concave, then lower and upper bounds to the distribution of $\widehat{\tau}_a(x, y)$ can be obtained by considering a "polygonal approximation" of $h(t)$ by means of a piecewise-linear function (see e.g. [3]), but in general, it is not possible to find the distribution of $\widehat{\tau}_a(x, y)$ exactly.

For $y = 0$ we can find the density of $\tau_a(x, 0)$ in closed form; in fact, $\widehat{\tau}_a(x, 0)$ is the FPT of BM $\widehat{B}$ through the level $a - x > 0$, and so its density is

$$\widehat{f}_a(t|x) := \frac{d}{dt}P(\widehat{\tau}_a(x, 0) \leq t) = \frac{a - x}{\sqrt{2\pi} \, t^{3/2}}e^{-(a-x)^2/2t}, \tag{2}$$

from which the density of $\tau_a(x, 0) = \widehat{\rho}^{-1}(\widehat{\tau}_a(x, 0))$ follows:

$$f_a(t|x) := \frac{d}{dt}P(\tau_a(x, 0) \leq t) = \widehat{f}_a(\widehat{\rho}(t)|x)\widehat{\rho}'(t) = \frac{(a - x)\, \widehat{\rho}'(t)}{\sqrt{2\pi}\, \widehat{\rho}(t)^{3/2}}e^{-(a-x)^2/2\widehat{\rho}(t)}. \tag{3}$$

If X is integrated BM, we have $X(t) = x + \widehat{B}(\widehat{\rho}(t))$, with $\widehat{\rho}(t) = t^3/3$, so we get (cf. [6]):

$$f_a(t|x) = \frac{3^{3/2}(a - x)}{\sqrt{2\pi}\, t^{5/2}}e^{-3(a-x)^2/2t^3}. \tag{4}$$

If X is integrated OU process, the density of $\tau_a(x, 0)$ can be obtained by inserting in (3) the function $\widehat{\rho}(t)$ deducible from Example 2, but it takes a more complex form.

Remark. Formula (3) implies that the nth order moment of the FPT is finite if and only if the function $t^n\widehat{\rho}'(t)/\widehat{\rho}(t)^{3/2}$ is integrable in $(0, +\infty)$.

Now, let us suppose that there exists $\alpha > 0$ such that $\widehat{\rho}(t) \sim const \cdot t^\alpha$, as $t \to +\infty$; then, in order that $E(\tau_a^n(x, 0)) < \infty$, it must be $\alpha = 2(n + \delta)$, for some $\delta > 0$. For integrated BM, we have $\alpha = 3$, then for $n = 1$ the last condition holds with $\delta = 1/2$, so we obtain the finiteness of $E(\tau_a(x, 0))$. If X is integrated OU process, we have $\rho(t) \sim const \cdot e^{2\mu t}$, $\gamma(t) \sim const \cdot \ln(2\mu t/\sigma^2)$, as $t \to +\infty$, and so $\widehat{\rho}(t) = \gamma(\rho(t)) \sim const \cdot t$, as $t \to +\infty$, namely $\alpha = 1$ and the condition above is not satisfied with $n = 1$; therefore $E(\tau_a(x, 0)) = +\infty$.

As for the second order moment of the FPT of integrated BM, instead, we obtain $E\left[(\tau_a(x, 0))^2\right] = +\infty$, since the equality $\alpha = 2(n + \delta)$ with $\alpha = 3$ and $n = 2$ is not satisfied, for any $\delta > 0$.

From (2) we get that the nth order moment of $\tau_a(x, 0)$, if it exists finite, is explicitly given by:

$$E\left[(\tau_a(x, 0))^n\right] = E\left[(\widehat{\rho}^{\,-1}(\widehat{\tau}_a(x, 0)))^n\right] = \int_0^{+\infty} (\widehat{\rho}^{\,-1}(t))^n \frac{a - x}{\sqrt{2\pi t^{3/2}}} e^{-(a-x)^2/2t} dt.$$
(5)

For instance, if X is integrated BM, one has:

$$E(\tau_a(x, 0)) = E((3\,\widehat{\tau}_a(x, 0))^{1/3}) = \int_0^{+\infty} (3t)^{1/3} \frac{a - x}{\sqrt{2\pi t^{3/2}}} e^{-(a-x)^2/2t} dt$$

$$= \left(\frac{3}{2}\right)^{1/3} \Gamma\left(\frac{1}{6}\right) \frac{(a - x)^{2/3}}{\sqrt{\pi}}.$$
(6)

We introduce now a randomness in the starting point, replacing $X(0) = x$ with a random variable η, having density $g(x)$ whose support is the interval $(-\infty, a)$; the corresponding FPT problem is particularly relevant in contexts such as neuronal modeling, where the reset value of the membrane potential is usually unknown (see e.g. [10]). If X is integrated BM and $y = 0$, one gets from (6) that the average FPT through the boundary a, over all initial positions $\eta < a$, is $\overline{T}_a = \int_{-\infty}^a E(\tau_a(x, 0))g(x)dx = \left(\frac{3}{2}\right)^{1/3} \frac{\Gamma(\frac{1}{6})}{\sqrt{\pi}} \int_{-\infty}^a (a - x)^{2/3} g(x)dx$. For instance, if $a - \eta$ has Gamma distribution with parameters $\alpha, \lambda > 0$, by calculations we get $\overline{T}_a = \frac{(\frac{3}{2\lambda^2})^{1/3}}{\sqrt{\pi}} \cdot \frac{\Gamma(\frac{1}{6})\Gamma(\alpha+\frac{2}{3})}{\Gamma(\alpha)}$.

2.2 FPT in the Two-Boundary Case: First Exit Time from an Interval

Assume, as always, that $\gamma(+\infty) = +\infty$; for $x \in (a, b)$ and $y \in \mathbb{R}$, the first-exit time of X from the interval (a, b) is $\tau_{a,b}(x, y) = \inf\{t > 0 : x + yt + \widehat{B}(\widehat{\rho}(t)) \notin (a, b)\}$. Set $\widehat{\tau}_{a,b}(x, y) = \widehat{\rho}(\tau_{a,b}(x, y))$, then $\widehat{\tau}_{a,b}(x, y) = \inf\{t > 0 : x + \widehat{B}_t \leq a - y\widehat{\rho}^{-1}(t)$ or $x + \widehat{B}_t \geq b - y\widehat{\rho}^{-1}(t)\}$. If $\widehat{\tau}_{a,b}(x, y)$ is finite with probability one, also $\tau_{a,b}(x, y)$ is so. In the sequel, we will focus on the case when $y = 0$, namely we will consider $\tau_{a,b}(x, 0) = \widehat{\rho}^{-1}(\widehat{\tau}_{a,b}(x, 0))$, where $\widehat{\tau}_{a,b}(x, 0) = \inf\{t > 0 : x + \widehat{B}_t \notin (a, b)\}$; as it is well-known, $\widehat{\tau}_{a,b}(x, 0)$ is finite with probability one and its moments are solutions of Darling and Siegert's equations (see [5]). The following result holds (for the proof, see [1]).

Proposition 1. *If $\widehat{\rho}$ is convex, then $E\left(\tau_{a,b}(x, 0)\right) < \infty$; moreover, if there exist constants c, $\delta > 0$, such that $0 \leq \widehat{\rho}^{-1}(t) \leq c \cdot t^\delta$, then $E\left(\tau_{a,b}(x, 0)\right)^n < \infty$, for* any integer n. In particular, if $a = -\alpha$, $b = \alpha$, $\alpha > 0$, then, for $x \in (-\alpha, \alpha)$ we have:

$$E\left[(\tau_{a,b}(x,0))^n\right] = E\left[(\tau_{-\alpha,\alpha}(x,0))^n\right] = E\left[\left(\widehat{\rho}^{-1}(\widehat{\tau}_{-\alpha,\alpha}(x,0))^n\right)\right] = \sum_{k=0}^{\infty} A_{n,k}(x),$$

(7)

where

$$A_{n,k}(x) = \frac{\pi}{\alpha^2}(-1)^k \left(k + \frac{1}{2}\right) \cos\left(\left(k + \frac{1}{2}\right)\frac{\pi x}{\alpha}\right) \times$$

$$\int_0^{+\infty} e^{-(k+1/2)^2\pi^2 t/2\alpha^2} \left(\widehat{\rho}^{-1}(t)\right)^n dt.$$

(8)

$\square$

Remark. The condition $0 \le \widehat{\rho}^{-1}(t) \le c \cdot t^\delta$ is satisfied e.g. for integrated BM, since $\widehat{\rho}^{-1}(t) = 3^{1/3}t^{1/3}$, and for integrated OU process, because $c_1 t \le \widehat{\rho}^{-1}(t) \le c_2 t$, for suitable $c_1, c_2 > 0$ which depend on μ and σ (see [1]).

Now, we carry on explicit computations of $E\left[\tau_{a,b}(x,0)\right]$ and $E\left[(\tau_{a,b}(x,0))^2\right]$, in the case of integrated BM. Inserting $\widehat{\rho}(t) = t^3/3$, $(\widehat{\rho}^{-1}(y) = (3y)^{1/3})$, and $n = 1,2$ in (7), (8), after some calculations we obtain:

$$E\left[\tau_{a,b}(x,0)\right] = \frac{3^{1/3}2^{7/3}\Gamma(\frac{4}{3})(b-a)^{2/3}}{\pi^{5/3}} \times$$

$$\sum_{k=0}^{\infty} \frac{(-1)^k}{(2k+1)^{5/3}} \cos\left[\frac{\pi(2k+1)}{b-a}\left(x - \frac{a+b}{2}\right)\right].$$

(9)

$$E\left[(\tau_{a,b}(x,0))^2\right] = \frac{12(b-a)^4}{\pi^4} \sum_{k=0}^{\infty} \frac{(-1)^k}{(2k+1)^4} \cos\left[\frac{\pi(2k+1)}{b-a}\left(x - \frac{a+b}{2}\right)\right].$$

(10)

Notice that, in [12,13], it was obtained a formula for $E(\tau_{a,b}(x,0))$ in terms of hypergeometric functions. The two series in (9), (10) converge fast enough, so to obtain "good" estimates of the moments, it suffices to consider a few terms of them. As for $E\left[\tau_{a,b}(x,0)\right]$, it appears to be fitted very well by the square root of a quadratic function (see Fig. 1).

In the Fig. 2, we plot the second order moment of $\tau_{a,b}(x,0)$ and its variance.

As in the one boundary case, we introduce a randomness in the starting point, replacing $X(0) = x \in (a,b)$ with a random variable η, having density $g(x)$ whose support is the interval (a,b); for $y = 0$ the average exit time over all initial positions $\eta \in (a,b)$ is $\overline{T}_{a,b} = \int_a^b E(\tau_{a,b}(x,0))g(x)dx$. In the case of integrated BM, $\overline{T}_{a,b}$ can be calculated by using the expression of $E(\tau_{a,b}(x,0))$ given by (9). In the special case when g is the uniform density in the interval (a,b), we get $\overline{T}_{a,b} = \frac{3^{1/3}2^{10/3}\Gamma(\frac{4}{3})(b-a)^{2/3}}{\pi^{8/3}} \sum_{k=0}^{\infty} \frac{1}{(2k+1)^{8/3}}$. Thus, $\overline{T}_{a,b} = const \cdot (b-a)^{2/3}$ which confirms the result by Masoliver and Porrà (see [12]).

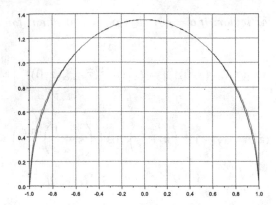

Fig. 1. Plots of the mean exit time, $E(\tau_{-1,1}(x,0))$, of integrated BM from the interval $(-1,1)$ (lower curve), and of the function $z(x) = 1.35 \cdot (1 - x^2)^{1/2}$ (upper curve), as functions of $x \in (-1,1)$; the two curves appear to be almost undistinguishable.

As for integrated OU process, the moments of $\tau_{a,b}(x,0)$ can be found again by formula (7), whit the corresponding $\widehat{\rho}(t)$; however, it is not possible to calculate explicitly the integral which appears in the expression of $A_{n.k}(x)$, so it has to be numerically computed. In the Fig. 3 we have plotted, for comparison, the numerical evaluation of the mean exit time of integrated OU process with $y = \beta = 0$, from the interval $(-1,1)$, as a function of $x \in (-1,1)$, for $\sigma = 1$ and several values of μ; in the Fig. 4 we we have plotted the numerical evaluation of second order moment.

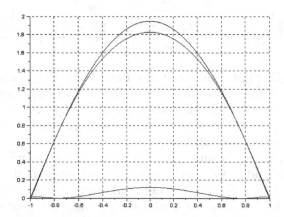

Fig. 2. From top to bottom: plot of the second moment (first curve), the square of the first moment (second curve), and the variance of the first-exit time $\tau_{-1,1}(x,0)$ (third curve) of integrated BM from the interval $(-1,1)$, as functions of $x \in (-1.1)$.

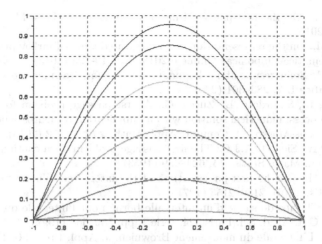

Fig. 3. Plot of numerical evaluation of the mean exit time, $E\left(\tau_{-1,1}(x,0)\right)$, of integrated OU with $\beta = y = 0$, from the interval $(-1,1)$, as a function of $x \in (-1,1)$, for $\sigma = 1$ and several values of μ. From top to bottom, with respect to the peak of the curve: $\mu = 2; 1.8; 1.6; 1.4; 1.2; 1$.

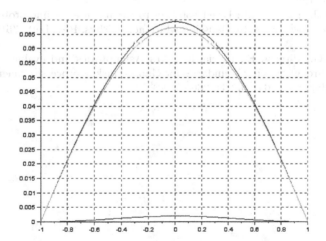

Fig. 4. From top to bottom: plot of the second moment (first curve), the square of the first moment (second curve), and the variance of the first-exit time $\tau_{-1,1}(x,0)$ (third curve) of integrated OU with $y = \beta = 0$, from the interval $(-1,1)$, as a function of $x \in (-1,1)$, for $\sigma = 1, \mu = 1$.

References

1. Abundo, M.: On the first-passage time of an integrated Gauss-Markov process. Preprint (2015)
2. Abundo, M.: On the representation of an integrated Gauss-Markov process. Scientiae Mathematicae Japonicae Online e-2013, pp. 719-723 (2013)
3. Abundo, M.: Some results about boundary crossing for Brownian motion. Ricerche di Matematica L 2, 283–301 (2001)
4. Benedetto, E., Sacerdote, L., Zucca, C.: A first passage problem for a bivariate diffusion process: numerical solution with an application to neuroscience when the process is GaussMarkov. J. Comput. Appl. Math. 242, 41–52 (2013)
5. Darling, D.A., Siegert, A.J.F.: The first passage problem for a continuous Markov process. Ann. Math. Statis. 24, 624–639 (1953)
6. Goldman, M.: On the first-passage time of the integrated Wiener process. Ann. Math. Statis. 42(6), 2150–2155 (1971)
7. Lachal, A.: Temps de sortie d'un intervalle borné pour l'intégrale du mouvement Brownien. C.R. Acad. Sci. Paris 324, serie I, pp. 559–564 (1997)
8. Lachal, A.: L'integrale du mouvement Brownien. J. Appl. Prob. 30, 17–27 (1993)
9. Lachal, A.: Sur le premier instant de passage de l'integrale du mouvement Brownien. Annales de l' I.H.P. B, 27(3), pp. 385–405 (1991)
10. Lansky, P.: The effect of a random initial value in neural first- passage-time models. Math. Biosci. 93(2), 191–215 (1989)
11. Lefebvre, M.: Moment generating function of a first hitting place for the integrated Ornstein-Uhlenbeck process. Stoch. Proc. Appl. 32, 281–287 (1989)
12. Masoliver, J., Porrà, J.M.: Exact solution to the exit-time problem for an undamped free particle driven by Gaussian white noise. Phys. Rev. E 53(3), 2243–2256 (1996)
13. Masoliver, J., Porrà, J.M.: Exact solution to the mean exit-time problem for free inertial processes driven by Gaussian white noise. Phys. Rev. Lett. 75(2), 189–192 (1995)
14. Nobile, A.G., Pirozzi, E., Ricciardi, L.M.: Asymptotics and evaluations of FPT densities through varying boundaries for Gauss-Markov processes. Scientiae Mathematicae Japonicae 67(2), 241–266 (2008)

A Sequential Test for Evaluating Air Quality

Giuseppina Albano[✉] and Cira Perna

Department of Economics and Statistics, University of Salerno,
Via Giovanni Paolo II, 84084 Fisciano, SA, Italy
{pialbano,perna}@unisa.it

Abstract. The present paper provides a simple sequential test for evaluating air quality, to verify a relative higher health risk of some area. The proposed procedure is based on the identification of a Poisson process representing the number of a particular pollutant at day t in a given year. A maximized sequential probability ratio test based on a composite alternative hypothesis has been implemented. The test is performed on emissions of air pollutants in the area of Salerno in which only partial data are available.

Keywords: Sequential analysis · Poisson process · Air pollutants

1 Introduction

The incidence of diseases caused by some pollutants as well as death rates from cancer have significantly increased in some areas over the last few years. For example, in the town of Taranto in Italy, an increment of some illnesses has been observed and many studies report association between this increase and air pollution due to the presence of steelworks. Moreover, in some areas of Campania region (the so called Triangle of Death or Land of Fire) (see, for example, [1,2,6]), some municipalities have recently experienced higher mortality rates for cancer and other diseases relative to the Italian average rates. Again, this increase is thought to be mainly caused by pollution from illegal waste disposal. Since variations in cancer mortality rate among different zones exist anyway (due, for example, to different lifestyles), to properly assess the significance on a difference in average, accurate statistical evaluations are required. However, data on air quality are not always accurate and updated, especially when small area are considered.

The present paper provides a simple test for evaluating air quality in the presence of partial data, to verify an increase risk for health in some area with respect other areas. In particular, focusing on a particulate matter, the proposed procedure is essentially based on the preliminary identification and estimation of a Poisson process representing the number of exceedances (with respect to a fixed limit L generally established by European Union) of an air pollutant at day t in a given year. The test verifies the null hypothesis that in a fixed area the number of exceedances of the limit L for the considered pollutant is equal to that in other neighboring areas.

© Springer International Publishing Switzerland 2015
R. Moreno-Díaz et al. (Eds.): EUROCAST 2015, LNCS 9520, pp. 143–149, 2015.
DOI: 10.1007/978-3-319-27340-2_19

In order to detect as early as possible an abnormal number of exceedances of the considered pollutant, a near-continuous monitoring is obtained by using a sequential test. The alternative hypothesis H_A is chosen to be composite in order to have a rejection region that does not depend on a particular value specified under H_A. Finally, since the distribution of the test statistic does not have a closed form, the critical values can be obtained by Monte Carlo simulations.

The paper is organized as follows. In Sect. 2 the test procedure is proposed and discussed. In order to validate the approach, an application to real data has been considered. The analysis focuses on a particular matter, PM_{10} observed in a small area of Salerno. In particular, in Sect. 3 the data are described while in Sect. 4 the results of the analysis are shown and discussed. Some remarks close the paper.

2   The Proposed Methodology

Let C_t be the number of exceedances of a given indicator y at day t in a given year and let c_t the corresponding observed value.

Under the null hypothesis (H_0) C_t follows a Poisson distribution with mean λ_t, where λ_t is a known function reflecting the mean number of exceedances of the indicator y at the day t. Under (H_A) the mean number of exceedances for y is instead $RR\lambda_t$, where RR is the increased relative risk in the area object of our study. In order to detect a health risk increase as early as possible, the test is performed continuously at every time point $t > 0$ as additional data are collected. For such continuous sequential analysis, the traditional approach generally used in the statistical literature is the Wald sequential probability ratio test (SORT). A signal is generated if the likelihood ratio exceeds a set value, and the observation ends if the likelihood falls below another predetermined lower bound. The key aspect of this method is that the p-values change when more data are added.

One problem with Wald's classical sequential probability ratio test is that the result is highly dependent on the relative risk used to specify the alternative hypothesis (see, for example, [5]). We propose instead the use of a maximized sequential probability ratio test (MaxSPRT), where the alternative hypothesis is composite rather than simple, with the relative risk defined as being greater than one rather than a specific value. Therefore, the hypotheses to test are:

$$H_0 : RR = 1$$
$$H_A : RR > 1$$

The MaxSPRT likelihood ratio based test statistic is

$$LR_t = \max_{H_A} \frac{P[C_t = c_t \mid H_A]}{P[C_t = c_t \mid H_0]} = \max_{RR>1} e^{(1-RR)\lambda_t}(RR)^{c_t}.$$

The maximum likelihood estimate of RR is c_t/λ_t when $c_t \geq \lambda_t$, so the test statistic becomes

$$LR_t = \begin{cases} e^{\lambda_t - c_t}(c_t/\lambda_t)^{c_t} & \text{if } c_t \geq \lambda_t \\ 1 & \text{otherwise.} \end{cases}$$

Equivalently, when defined using the log-likelihood ratio

$$LLR_t = \ln(LR_t) = \begin{cases} (\lambda_t - c_t) + c_t \ln(c_t/\lambda_t) & \text{when } c_t \geq \lambda_t \\ 0 & \text{otherwise.} \end{cases}$$

Note that the maximum likelihood estimate is unique and that it is also the minimum variance unbiased estimator.

Unfortunately, the distribution of the test statistic LLR_t does not have a closed form, so the critical values are obtained by Monte Carlo simulations. In particular the following procedure is implemented:

- For all t simulate N samples from a Poisson distribution with parameter λ_t, obtaining c_t;
- Plug in c_t in the log-likelihood LLR_t;
- Fix α and obtain the critical value $z_{\alpha t}$ as the $(1 - \alpha)$ percentile of the sample distribution of LLR_t.

Finally, we reject H_0 if it exists a value t for which LLR_t is greater than the corresponding critical value $z_{\alpha t}$.

3   The Data

The aim of the present section is to test if in the area near Salerno, that is Fratte, the rate of exceedances of air pollutants are higher than those in other areas of the city.

The first step of the analysis is to choose an indicator to measure air quality. The indicators commonly used are nitrogen dioxide NO_2, carbon monoxide CO, ozone O_3 and particle pollution (also known as "particulate matter") $PM_{2.5}$ and PM_{10}. These latter indexes are particle pollution less than 2.5 micrometers in diameter ($PM_{2.5}$) and between 2.5 and 10 micrometers in diameter (PM_{10}).

In this analysis, we focus on the concentration of PM_{10} since numerous studies have demonstrated its negative effect on human health (see, for example, [3] and [4]). Current European Union legislation regulating the PM_{10} concentration in ambient air is given in the EU directive 1999/30/EC. It states that for PM_{10} two binding limit values are to be respected as from 1 January 2005:

- a daily limit of $50\,\mu g/m^3$ not to be exceeded on more than 35 days within a calendar year
- an annual mean value of $40\,\mu g/m^3$.

While new policies in Europe have contributed to significant decreases in air pollution over the past several decades, an estimated 80 % of Europe's urban population is still exposed to PM levels above World Health Organization air quality guidelines, and several areas in the Campania region still experience PM levels exceeding the air quality limit values set by European Union laws, according to the European Environment Agency.

The data have been collected from the website of Agenzia Regionale per la protezione Ambientale in Campania (ARPAC), a regional agency which develops monitoring, prevention and control activities aimed at protecting Campania area.

The control of the parameters of air quality is one of the main institutional activities of the Agency. It manages the monitoring network which consists of twenty monitoring stations located in the five provincial capitals of Campania. As part of the monitoring activities related to the areas near industrial centers, ARPAC manages three stations named $SA21$, $SA22 - ASL2$ and $SA23 - Fratte$ in Salerno which monitor the air parameters. In particular, from the ARPAC website (see [7]) we can find data series from SA21 and SA22, but only partial data from SA23. In Fig. 1 we have some partial hourly data from the station of Fratte, in which the limit $50\,\mu g/m^3$ for PM_{10} is almost always overcrossed. Our results are based on daily values of PM_{10} in the stations SA21 and SA22 in the years 2011, 2012, 2013 and 2014 and on daily values of PM_{10} in Fratte from 29 October 2014- 8 December 2014.

Report libero dal: 26/nov/2014 al: 27/nov/2014Aggregazione dati: Nessuna [Vista: MMB]

GIORNO	ORA	SO2 (MED) ug/m3	H2S (MED) ug/m3	NO (MED) ug/m3	NO2 (MED) ug/m3	NOx (MED) ppb	CO (MED) mg/m3	O3 (MED) ug/m3	Benzene (MED) ug/m3	Toluene (MED) ug/m3	M-Xylene (MED) ug/m3	CH4 (MED) ug/m3	NMHC (MED) ug/m3	PM2_5 (MED) ug/m3	PM10 (MED) ug/m3
01/12/2014	1.00	0,5	0,4	7,1	23,5	18,2	0,3	18,2	0,1	0,2	0	277,2	918,5	45,2	89,5
01/12/2014	2.00	0,8	0,7	20,8	34,8	35,5	0,5	5,5	0,1	0,2	0	277	887,6	45,2	86,7
01/12/2014	3.00			8,7	20,5	18	0,6		0,2	0,2	0	281,6	903,6	45,2	79,3
01/12/2014	4.00		0	7,7	18	15,9	0,6	14,3	0,1	0,1	0	282,8	947,2	41,8	79,3
01/12/2014	5.00		0	9,8	19,2	18,1	0,3	15,7	0	0,2	0	276,5	897,1	41,5	79,3
01/12/2014	6.00			3,8	17,7	12,5	0,3	19,2	0	0,1	0	258,2	863,8	41,5	79,3
01/12/2014	7.00		0,1	10	25	21,5	0,2	15,5	0	0	0	243,6	810,5	41,5	79,3
01/12/2014	8.00	0	0,3	22,4	34,4	36,6	0,5	13,5	0	0,1	0	238	765	41,5	79,3
01/12/2014	9.00	0,3	0,4	18,1	35,3	33,5	0,3	19,6	0,1	0,2	0	242,8	763,4	41,5	79,3
01/12/2014	10.00	1,6	0,7	29,9	46,6	49	0,5	12,9	0,1	0,2	0	236,3	771,9	41,5	79,3
01/12/2014	11.00	2,1	1,3	48,2	51,1	66,3	0,7	6,5	0,1	0,3	0	241,1	819,5	41,5	79,3
01/12/2014	12.00	1,8	0,8	24,5	36,5	39,2	0,6	22,3	0,1	0,4	0	253,6	847,3	41,5	79,3
01/12/2014	13.00	4,2	1	36,8	50,8	56,9	0,6	16,5	0,1	0,3	0,1	263,7	897,1	41,5	79,3
01/12/2014															
01/12/2014	15.00	4,5	1,3	53,5	53	71,7	0,7	11,2	0,2	0,3	0,1			41,5	79,3
01/12/2014	16.00	5,5	1,8	77,6	67,3	98,9	0,9	3,5	0,2	0,4	0,2			41,5	79,3
01/12/2014	17.00	5,2	1,7	70	76,9	97,7	0,8	2,4	0,2	0,4	0,2			41,5	79,3
01/12/2014	18.00	5,2	1,8	83,4	76,3	108,5	0,9	3,5	0,2	0,5	0,3			41,5	79,3
01/12/2014	19.00	5	1,5	79,6	75,4	104,8	0,9	4,5	0,5	1,2	0,2			41,5	79,3
01/12/2014	20.00	5,2	1,7	88,3	74,8	111,6	1,1	2,5	0,3	0,7	0,1			41,5	79,3
01/12/2014	21.00	4,2	1,5	80,3	68,1	101,4	1	1	0,4	1,5	0			41,5	79,3
01/12/2014	22.00	4,2	1,4	74,2	53	88,4	0,9	0,4	0,5	1,5	0			41,5	79,3
01/12/2014	23.00	0,5	0,6	25,1	43,6	43,5	0,6	3,3	0,3	1	0			41,5	79,3
01/12/2014	24.00.00		0,6	6,9	30,5	21,8	0,3	23,1	0,2	0	0			41,5	79,3
02/12/2014	1.00		0,3	3,4	19,7	13,3	0,3	37,2						41,5	79,3
02/12/2014	2.00		0	3,7	19,2	13,2	0,2	31,6						41,5	106,9
02/12/2014	3.00			2,5	15,4	10,2	0,2							41,5	180,5
02/12/2014	4.00		0,4	15,9	25,8	26,6	0,3	5,9						52	180,5
02/12/2014	5.00		0,6	13	25,4	24,1	0,2	4,3						53,1	180,5
02/12/2014	6.00		0,3	6,9	24,4	18,6	0,2	24,7						53,1	180,5
02/12/2014															

Fig. 1. Hourly data from the station of Fratte from 1 to 2 December 2014. In the last column PM_{10} emissions are shown.

4   Results

To test if in some areas there is a health risk increase due to higher concentrations of a particulate matter in the air, we focus on the number of exceedances of PM_{10}

per year. Clearly, the procedure we suggest can be applied for $PM_{2.5}$ as well, or also in other contexts, such as an increased death rate. Our procedure is essentially based on

- the identification and the estimate of a Poisson process representing the number of exceedances of PM_{10} at day t in a given year;
- a test evaluating an increased risk for health.

Let C_t be the number of exceedances of PM_{10} at day t in a given year and let c_t the corresponding observed value. In order to apply the methodology illustrated in Sect. 2, it is necessary to verify if the assumption $C_t \sim Pois(\lambda_t)$ can be supported from data. To this aim, a Chi-Square test is performed; the results, which are not reported for the sake of brevity, show the plausibility of the assumption.

For our procedure, we assume that λ_t generally changes day by day. We estimate λ_t from the daily values of PM_{10} in the stations SA21 and SA22 in the years 2011, 2012, 2013 and 2014. In particular, by using the probability of increments for the Poisson process C_t

$$P[C_{t+h} - C_t = 1] = \lambda_t h + o(h),$$

where h is the minimum number of days to observe at least an increment in C_t, we obtain the estimated λ_t, $\hat{\lambda}_t$. The time-plot is reported in Fig. 2.

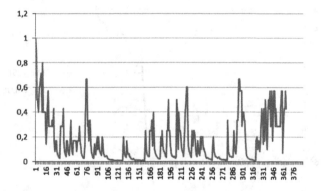

Fig. 2. Estimated λ_t by daily values of PM_{10} in the stations SA21 and SA22 in the years 2011, 2012, 2013 and 2014.

Finally, the test for evaluating an increase in the number of measured exceedances of PM_{10} in the area of Fratte, can be formulated as:

H_0 : the number of exceedances of limit $50\,\mu g/m^3$ for PM_{10} in Fratte is equal to the number of exceedances in the areas near the other two stations in Salerno,

H_A : the number of exceedances of limit $50\,\mu g/m^3$ for PM_{10} in Fratte is greater than the number of exceedances in the areas near the other two stations in Salerno.

Daily values of PM_{10} in Fratte from 29 October 2014- 8 December 2014 are used to perform the previous test. In particular, the test statistic is obtained as:

$$TS := \begin{cases} (\hat{\lambda}_t - c_t) + c_t \ln(c_t/\hat{\lambda}_t) & \text{when } c_t \geq \hat{\lambda}_t \\ 0 & \text{otherwise.} \end{cases}$$

The critical values are obtained by Monte Carlo simulations implementing the procedure suggested in Sect. 2. More specifically,

- For all t simulate 1000 samples from a Poisson distribution with parameter $\hat{\lambda}_t$, obtaining c_t;
- Plug in c_t in TS;
- Fix $\alpha = 0.05$ and obtain the critical value $z_{\alpha t}$ as the $95th-$percentile of the sample distribution of TS.

In Fig. 3 the test statistic and its critical value are reported for all values of t. From 29 October to 28 November 2014 the test statistic is zero since the observed exceedances are always less than the estimated values of λ_t. Starting from 29 November 2014 the test rejects the null hypothesis that the number of exceedances of limit $50\,\mu g/m^3$ for PM_{10} in Fratte is equal to the number of exceedances in the areas near the other two stations in Salerno.

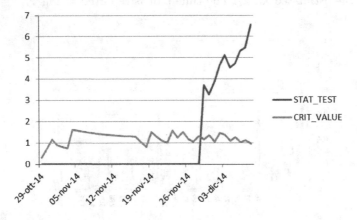

Fig. 3. Time-plot of the test statistic and the corresponding critical value for the number of exceedances of limit $50\,\mu g/m^3$ for PM_{10} in the area of Salerno.

5   Some Concluding Remarks

In the paper a simple test for evaluating air quality is provided and discussed. The test is based on the identification and estimate of a Poisson process and uses a maximized sequential probability ratio test, so the test statistic is monitored over the time. An application to emissions of PM_{10} in the area of Salerno shows the ability of the proposed procedure to correctly identify a significant difference in mean PM values among the monitoring stations.

However, some issues still remain open. For example, environmental data are not always accurate and updated, so criteria for evaluating their accuracy are needed. Moreover a peculiarity of datasets concerning air quality is the presence of missing data due to many factors such as machine failure, routine maintenance and human errors, so methods to "recostruct" such time series are needed.

Acknowledgements. This work was supported in part by University of Salerno grant program "Sistema di calcolo ad alte prestazioni per l'analisi economica, finanziaria e statistica (High Performance Computing - HPC)- prot. ASSA098434, 2009.

References

1. Senior, K., Mazza, A.: Italian "Triangle of death" linked to waste crisis. Lancet. Oncol. **5**(9), 525–527 (2004)
2. Rendina, D., Gennari, L., De Filippo, G., Merlotti, D., de Campora, E., Fazioli, F., Scarano, G., Nuti, R., Strazzullo, P., Mossetti, G.: Evidence for increased clinical severity of familial and sporadic paget's disease of bone in Campania, Southern Italy. J. Bone Miner. Res. **21**(12), 1828–1835 (2006)
3. Samoli, E., Peng, R., Ramsay, T., Pipikou, M., Touloumi, G., Dominici, F., Burnett, R., Cohen, A., Kreswski, D., Samet, J.: Acute effects of ambient particulate matter on mortality in Europe and North America: results from the APHENA study. Environ. Health Perspect. **116**, 1480–1486 (2008)
4. Zanobetti, A., Schwartz, J.: The effect of fine and coarse particulate air pollution on mortality: a national analysis. Environ. Health Perspect. **117**, 1–40 (2009)
5. Kuldorff, M., Davis, R.L., Kolczak, M., Lewis, E., Lieu, T., Platt, R.: A maximazed sequential probability ratio test for drug and vaccine safety surveillance. Sequent. Anal. Desgn Meth. Appl. **30**(1), 58–78 (2011)
6. Raaschou-Nielsen, O., et al.: Air pollution and lung cancer incidence in 17 European cohorts: prospective analyses from the European study of cohorts for air pollution effects (ESCAPE). Lancet Oncol. **14**(9), 813–822 (2013)
7. Website of ARPAC (Agenzia Regionale per la Protezione Ambientale in Campania). www.arpac.it

Population Models and Enveloping

Paul Cull[✉]

Computer Science, Kelley Engineering Center, Oregon State University,
Corvallis, OR 97331, USA
pc@cs.orst.edu

Abstract. One dimensional nonlinear difference equations are commonly
used to model population growth. Although such models can display wild
behavior including chaos, the common models have the interesting property that they are globally stable if they are locally stable. We show that a
model with a single positive equilibrium is globally stable if it is *enveloped*
by a self-inverse function. In particular, we show that the standard population models are enveloped by linear fractional functions which are self-
inverse. Although enveloping by a linear fractional is sufficient for global
stability, we show by example that such enveloping is not necessary. We
extend our results by showing that *enveloping implies global stabilty* even
when $f(x)$ is a discontinuous multifunction, which may be a more reasonable description of real biological data. We also show that our techniques
can be applied to situations which are not population models. Finally, we
mention some extensions and open questions.

1 Introduction

Many years ago, population biologists fit nonlinear models to various real or
hypothetical data and after demonstrating that a model was locally stable, they
then used the model as if it were globally stable. Pleasantly, they never ran into
any difficulty. The problem for mathematicians was to explain why the biologists
were "lucky". In a series of papers from 1981 [6] through 2007 [7], we investigated
this question and concluded that biologists used models that looked "smooth"
in a free-hand drawing, and further that this intuition could be mathematically
caputured by the idea of *enveloping* by a *linear fractional*.

In Fig. 1, we give examples of population models. The usual assumptions are
that the model has the form $x_t = f(x_{t-1})$ with f being a function which starts
at $f(0) = 0$ proceeds to a maximum, and then decreases. We assume that f has
a single positive fixed point which we normalize to 1. The model on the Left is
enveloped by the linear fractional $2 - x$ which represented by the dotted line.

We define a Population Model as a first order difference equation

$$x_{t+1} = f(x_t)$$

with the conditions:

- $f(x)$ maps **positives** to **positives**, or to **nonnegatives**

© Springer International Publishing Switzerland 2015
R. Moreno-Díaz et al. (Eds.): EUROCAST 2015, LNCS 9520, pp. 150–157, 2015.
DOI: 10.1007/978-3-319-27340-2_20

- $f(x)$ has a single Hump
- single positive equilibrium {normalized at $x = 1$, $f(1) = 1$ }
- { If needed: 3 times continuously differentiable}
- { May be 0 for all $x \geq x_{max}$ }

We define two types of *stability* for such models:

Global Stability: $\forall x \in (0, x_{max})$ $\lim_{t \to \infty} f^{(t)}(x) = 1$

Local Stability: for all x near 1, $f(x)$ is nearer 1, (which implies $|f'(1)| \leq 1$.)

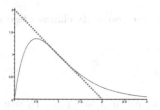 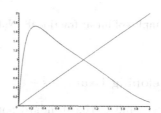

Fig. 1. Left: a population model which is both *locally* and *globally* stable. Right: a population model which is *locally* but not *globally* stable.

2   Enveloping

If one plots the functions $2 - x$ and x between 0 and 2, the resulting picture looks like the back of an envelope and this suggests the name *enveloping* for the following definition.

$\phi(x)$ **ENVELOPS** $f(x)$ iff

$$\phi(x) > f(x) \quad \text{for} \quad x \in (0, 1)$$
$$\phi(x) < f(x) \quad \text{for} \quad x > 1 \quad \text{and} \quad f(x) > 0$$
$$f(x) > x \quad \text{for} \quad x \in (0, 1)$$
$$f(x) < x \quad \text{for} \quad x \in (1, \infty)$$

Theorem 1 (Enveloping Theorem). *If a population model $f(x)$ is enveloped by a monotone decreasing, self-inverse $\phi(x)$ then the model is globally stable.*

$$\lim_{t \to \infty} f^{(t)}(x) = 1 \quad for\ all \quad x \quad with \quad f(x) > 0.$$

Theorem 2 (Stability by Enveloping). *If $f_1(x)$ is enveloped by $f_2(x)$ and $f_2(x)$ is globally stable, then $f_1(x)$ is globally stable.*

2.1   Linear Fractionals

$$\phi(x) = \frac{1 - \alpha x}{\alpha + (1 - 2\alpha) x} \qquad \begin{array}{c} \alpha \in [0, 1) \\ \text{Monotone Decreasing} \\ \text{Self-Inverse} \end{array}$$

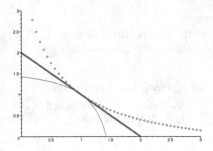

Fig. 2. Examples of linear fractionals. Notice how the concavity changes as α goes from 1 to 0.

2.2 Enveloping Examples

To envelope some of the standard population models, we have to use different linear fractionals because the "shape" of the models will depend on on the parameters. For example, as the following figure shows $f(x) = \frac{r\,x}{1+(r-1)\,x^c}$ can be enveloped by $1/x$ when $c \leq 2$, but for larger c the enveloping function is $\frac{(c-1)-(c-2)x}{(c-2)-(c-3)x}$ and specifically $(3-x)/(1+x)$ when $c = 2.5$, $r = 5$.

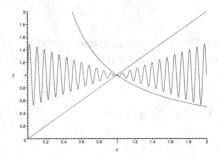

By assumption all of our population models have the One-Hump form, but enveloping and particularly enveloping by linear fractionals can show global stability for highly oscillatory functions, e.g.

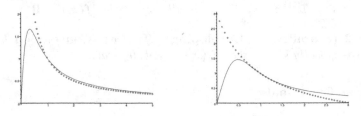

2.3 Enveloping by a Linear Fractional is only Sufficient

Here we want to give a simple model which has global stability, but cannot be enveloped by any linear fractional. Define $f(x)$ by

$$f(x) = \begin{cases} 6x & 0 \leq x < 1/2 \\ 7 - 8x & 1/2 \leq x < 3/4 \\ 1 & 3/4 \leq x. \end{cases}$$

then $x_{t+1} = f(x_t)$ has $x = 1$ as its globally stable equilibrium point because if $x_t \geq 1$ then $x_{t+1} = 1$, for $x_t \in [1/2, 1)$, $x_{t+1} > 1$ and $x_{t+2} = 1$, and for $x_t \in (0, 1/2)$, the subsequent iterates grow by multiples of 6 and eventually surpass $1/2$. This $f(x)$ cannot be enveloped by a linear fractional because $f(1/2) = 3$ which implies that the linear fractional would have $\alpha \leq -1$ and hence have a pole in $(0, 1)$ and thus it could not envelop a positive function. On the other hand, the self-inverse function

$$\phi(x) = \begin{cases} 5 - 4x & x \leq 1 \\ (5 - x)/4 & x > 1 \end{cases}$$

does envelop $f(x)$ and so demonstrates global stability.

2.4 Other Enveloping Functions

Although we will use linear fractionals as the enveloping functions for our example population models, other function can also serve as enveloping functions.

For our set-up, we can take any function $g(x)$ so that $g(1) = 1$ and $g(x)$ is monotone decreasing on $(0, 1)$, and then construct an enveloping function $e(x)$ given by:

$$e(x) = \begin{cases} g(x) & 0 < x \leq 1 \\ g^{-1}(x) & 1 \leq x < g(0) \end{cases}$$

As a very specific example, let $g(x) = (3 - x^2)/2$ then

$$e(x) = \begin{cases} (3 - x^2)/2 & 0 < x \leq 1 \\ \sqrt{3 - 2x} & 1 \leq x < 3/2 \end{cases}$$

Clearly $e(x)$ is continuous and monotone decreasing. It is also twice continuously differentiable, but the third derivative is not continuous.

Let us concoct a population model that can be enveloped by this $e(x)$.

$$f(x) = \begin{cases} x(3 - 2x) & 0 < x \leq 1 \\ \sqrt{2 - x} & 1 \leq x < 2 \end{cases}$$

is a population model since it is unimodal with a maximum at $x = 3/4$. While $f(x)$ and its first derivative are continuous, the 2nd derivative has a discontinuity at $x = 1$. It is easy to see that this $f(x)$ is enveloped by this $e(x)$. We conclude that $x = 1$ is the globally stable fixed point for $f(x)$, i.e. for all $x \in (0, 2)$, $\lim_{n \to \infty} f^{(n)}(x) = 1$.

3   Techniques $\mathcal{A}$ and $\mathcal{B}$

The following two techniques can be used to show that the common population models are enveloped by linear fractionals. (see Summary Table.)

Technique $\mathcal{A}$: If $f(x) = xh(1 - x)$ and

$$h(1 - z) = \sum_{i=0}^{\infty} h_i z^i$$

$$h_0 = 1, \quad h_1 = 2$$

$$\forall n \geq 1 \quad h_n \geq h_{n+1}$$

$$\forall n \geq 2 \quad h_n - 2h_{n+1} + h_{n+2}$$

THEN $f(x)$ is enveloped by the linear fractional with

$$\alpha = \frac{3 - h_2}{4 - h_2} \geq \frac{1}{2}$$

and $f(x)$ is globally stable.

Technique $\mathcal{B}$: $\phi(x) = A(x)/B(x)$ **envelopes** $f(x) = C(x)/D(x)$
if $G(x) = A(x)D(x) - B(x)C(x)$ and

$$G(1) = 0 \text{ and } G'(1) = 0$$

$$G''(x) > 0 \text{ on } (0, 1)$$

$$G''(x) < 0 \text{ for } x > 1.$$

4   General Theorem

Although our enveloping method was devised for the population models discussed above, the method can also be applied to other iterations. Not all iterations are normalized so that the fixed point is at $x = 1$. In many cases, the iteration is designed to compute the fixed point.

Theorem 3. *If the iteration $x_{t+1} = f(x_t)$ obeys*

$$f(x) > x \qquad\qquad on \qquad (a, p)$$

$$f(x) < x \qquad\qquad on \qquad (p, b)$$

where $f(x)$ may be a discontinuous multifunction but has p as its only limit point on the straight line $y = x$ and if there is a self-inverse function $\phi(x)$ so that

$$\phi(x) > f(x) \qquad\qquad on \qquad (a, p)$$

$$f(x) > \phi(x) \qquad\qquad on \qquad (p, b)$$

and p is the only limit point of $f(x)$ which is on $\phi(x)$ then $\lim_{k \to \infty} f^{(k)}(x_0) = p$ for every $x_0 \in (a, b)$.

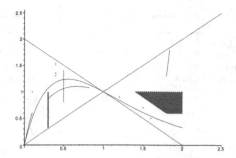

Fig. 3. A multifunction enveloped by the linear fractional $2 - x$.

4.1   Multifunctions

A multifunction is a function which maps each element of its domain to a non-empty set of values in its range. In this picture, the curve, the block, the points, and the "vertical" lines indicate values (Fig. 3).

4.2   Multidimensional

One of the major reasons to consider multifunctions is that they allow us to use 1-dimensional methods on multi-dimensional models.

A multi-dimensional model can have the form

$$x_t = f(x_{t-1}, \ldots, x_{t-k})$$

with the population size depending on the last k population sizes, or even on the whole history of sizes. We can consider such a model to be a 1-dimensional multifunction by using $x_t = g(x_{t-1})$ where the set of values for g will depend on the values of $x_{t-1}, \ldots, x_{t-k}$ which are considered to be unknown or perhaps known to be within a certain range.

For example,

$$x_t = 1 + .9(1 - x_{t-1})\cos(y),$$

can be considered to be a 1-dimensional multifunction when y is allowed to be any function of $x_{t-1}, \ldots, x_{t-k}$. Since $\cos(y)$ will be bounded between $+1$ and -1, it is easy to show that this model is enveloped by $2 - x$, and will display global stability.

5   Summary Table

The following Table shows a number of commonly used population models and their regions of global stability together with the techniques used to show stability. (See Sect. 3 for $\mathcal{A}$ and $\mathcal{B}$ and see [4] for negative Schwarzian $\mathcal{S}$.)

Model number	Function	Parameters	Techniques	Bounding linear fractionals
I	$f_1(x) = xe^{r(1-x)})$	$0 < r \le 2$	A, B, S	$2 - x$
II	$f_2(x) = x(1 + r(1 - x))$	$0 < r \le 2$	A, B, S	$(4 - 3x)/(3 - 2x)$
III	$f_3(x) = x(1 - r\ln x)$	$0 < r \le 2$	A	$(3 - 2x)/(2 - x)$
IV	$f_4(x) = x(\frac{1}{b+cx} - d)$	$\frac{d-1}{(d+1)^2} \le b < \frac{1}{d+1}$	A, S	$(11 - 8x)/(8 - 5x)$
V	$f_5(x) = \frac{(1+ae^b)x}{1+ae^{bx}}$	$0 < a, 0 < b,$ $a(b - 2)e^b \le 2$	B, S	$2 - x$ for $b \le 2$ $\frac{b-(b-1)x}{(b-1)-(b-2)x}$ for $b \ge 2$
VI	$f_6(x) = \frac{(1+a)^b x}{(1+ax)^b}$	$0 < a, 0 < b,$ $a(b - 2) \le 2$	B, Modified S	$1/x$ for $b \le 2$ $\frac{2(b-1)-(b-2)x}{(b-2)+2x}$ for $b \ge 2$
VII	$f_7(x) = \frac{rx}{1+(r-1)x^c}$	$r(c - 2) \le c$	B	$1/x$ for $c \le 2$ $\frac{c-1-(c-2)x}{c-2-(c-3)x}$ for $c \ge 2$

6 Conclusion

This paper has demonstrated that local stability implies global stability when the function is enveloped by a linear fractional function. In particular, this result covers a number of commonly used population models. Detailed discussion of these population models appears in [7]. That discussion is aimed at biologists, a discussion aimed at mathematicians appears in Hirsch [10].

Even though enveloping is based on 1-dimensional models, we pointed out that it can also be used to show stability for multi-dimensional models with suitable form. Enveloping can also deal with more complicated cases as shown in Wright's recent thesis [9].

Other techniques like Lyapunov functions [5] and Schwarzian Derivative [4] can be used to show global stability, but the Lyapunov calculation is rather complicated and the Schwarzian technique cannot be applied to all the models in the above Table.

This paper shows that under reasonable hypotheses, population models display global stability, but with other hypotheses (see [1–3]) much more complicated behavior (including chaos) is possible for even seemingly simple population models.

Finally, there are still some unanswerd questions suggested in [8]. Can there still be stability in the face of chaos? Would stability from a open interval be more meaningful than stability for all positives? We hope that others might find answers to these questions.

References

1. Cull, P., Flahive, M., Robson, R.: Difference Equations: From Rabbits to Chaos. Springer, New York (2005)
2. Li, T.-Y., Yorke, J.: Period three implies chaos. Am. Math. Mon. **82**, 985–992 (1975)
3. Sarkovskii, A.: Coexistence of cycles of a continuous map of a line to itself. Ukr. Mat. Z. **16**, 61–71 (1964)

4. Singer, D.: Stable orbits and bifurcation of maps of the interval. SIAM J. Appl. Math. **35**, 260–267 (1978)
5. Fisher, M.E., Goh, B.S., Vincent, T.L.: Some stability conditions for discrete-time single species models. Bull. Math. Biol. **41**, 861–875 (1979)
6. Cull, P.: Global stability of population models. Bull. Math. Biol. **43**, 47–58 (1981)
7. Cull, P.: Population models: stability in one dimension. Bull. Math. Biol. **69**, 989–1017 (2007)
8. Cull, P., Walsh, K., Wherry, J.: Stability and of instability in one dimension population models. Scientiae Mathematicae Japonicae Online **e–2008**, 29–48 (2008)
9. Wright, J.P.: Periodic Dynamical Systems of Population Models, Ph.D. thesis, North Carolina State University (2013)
10. Hirsch, M.: Dynamics of acyclic interval maps (preprint. mhirsch@chorus.net)

Fractional Growth Process with Two Kinds of Jumps

Antonio Di Crescenzo[✉], Barbara Martinucci, and Alessandra Meoli

Dipartimento di Matematica, Università di Salerno, Via Giovanni Paolo II, n. 132,
84084 Fisciano, SA, Italy
{adicrescenzo,bmartinucci,ameoli}@unisa.it

Abstract. We consider a suitable fractional jump process describing growth phenomena, that may be viewed as a counting process characterized by 2 kinds of jumps with size 1 and 2. We obtain the probability generating function and the probability law of the process, expressed in terms of the generalized Mittag-Leffler function. The mean, variance, and squared coefficient of variation are also provided.

Keywords: Fractional poisson process · Mittag-Leffler functions · Fractional equations

1 Introduction

Fractional calculus has gained considerable popularity and importance during the last decade, mainly due to its applications in several fields of science and engineering (see, for instance, Tenreiro Machado [16]). One of the main features of fractional-order differential equations is their nonlocal property. Indeed, the definition of fractional derivative involves an integration which is a non-local operator. Hence, fractional order differential equations play a relevant role in the modeling of memory-dependent phenomena which emerge in biological systems.

Specifically, we recall that the fractional calculus has been employed to describe complex dynamics in biological tissues. For instance, Magin [10] illustrates various areas of bioengineering research where fractional calculus is applied to build new mathematical models. Moreover, a generalization of the classical logistic equation based on fractional calculus has been used in Varalta *et al.* [17] for the description of cancer tumor growth. Fractional derivatives are also considered in El-Sayed [5] to embody essential features of the behavior of the pattern formation in bacterial colonies.

In some biological contexts the existence of power-law behavior is observed also in spatial structures rather than in temporal patterns. For instance, Muiño *et al.* [11] found that specific cancer types show a power-law in interoccurrence distances, instead of the expected exponential distribution as for Poisson process.

In some recent papers (Garra *et al.* [6], Orsingher and Polito [12,13] and Orsingher *et al.* [14]) some fractional birth-death processes were introduced and studied. These processes generalize the classical birth-death processes, with the

© Springer International Publishing Switzerland 2015
R. Moreno-Díaz et al. (Eds.): EUROCAST 2015, LNCS 9520, pp. 158–165, 2015.
DOI: 10.1007/978-3-319-27340-2_21

Caputo fractional derivative replacing the integer-order derivative in the difference-differential equations governing the state probabilities. Also, Garra and Polito [7] devote attention to the role of fractional birth-death processes with linear rates in epidemic models with empirical power law distribution of the events. A multiple birth-death process with fractional birth probabilities in the form $\lambda_i(\Delta t)^\alpha + o((\Delta t)^\alpha), 0 < \alpha < 1$, has been studied in Jumarie [9]. The usefulness of such process in biology is found in the description of cell replicas.

The need of dealing with processes exhibiting power-law behavior and multiple occurrences of events in biology applications stimulates us to investigate fractional Poisson-type processes subject to multiple kinds of jumps. Specifically, in Sect. 2 we recall some preliminary results both on the fractional Poisson process and on a basic continuous-time growth process which performs two kinds of jumps. In Sect. 3, on the ground of the given preliminaries, we introduce the fractional growth process of interest, characterized by jumps with size 1 and 2. We obtain the probability distribution and the relevant moments of such process. The extension to more than 2 jumps is presented in Di Crescenzo et al. [4].

2   Background and Preliminary Results

This section is devoted to useful notions. We first recall the (two-parameter) Mittag-Leffler function and the generalized Mittag-Leffler function, defined as

$$E_{\alpha,\beta}(x) = \sum_{r=0}^{\infty} \frac{x^r}{\Gamma(\alpha r + \beta)}, \qquad E_{\alpha,\beta}^{\gamma}(x) = \sum_{r=0}^{\infty} \frac{(\gamma)_r}{r!} \frac{x^r}{\Gamma(\alpha r + \beta)}, \qquad x \in \mathbb{R}, \quad (1)$$

respectively, for $\alpha, \beta, \gamma \in \mathbb{C}, Re(\alpha), Re(\beta), Re(\gamma) > 0$, with $(\gamma)_0 = 1$ and $(\gamma)_r := \gamma(\gamma+1)\ldots(\gamma+r-1)$ for $r = 1, 2, \ldots$.

2.1   Fractional Poisson Process

Consider the fractional Poisson process (see Beghin and Orsingher [3]).

$$\{N_\lambda^\nu(t); t \geq 0\}, \qquad \nu \in (0, 1], \lambda \in (0, \infty). \tag{2}$$

This is a renewal process with i.i.d. interarrival times $\mathcal{U}_j$ distributed according to the following density, for $j = 1, 2, \ldots$

$$f_1^\nu(t) = \mathbb{P}\{\mathcal{U}_j \in dt\}/dt = \lambda t^{\nu-1} E_{\nu,\nu}(-\lambda t^\nu), \qquad t \in (0, \infty). \tag{3}$$

Let $T_k = \sum_{j=1}^{k} \mathcal{U}_j$ be the waiting time of the k-th event; the density function and the corresponding distribution function are given respectively by (see [3])

$$f_k^\nu(t) = \mathbb{P}\{T_k \in dt\}/dt = \lambda^k t^{k\nu-1} E_{\nu,k\nu}^k(-\lambda t^\nu), \qquad t \in (0, \infty), \tag{4}$$

and

$$F_k^\nu(t) = \mathbb{P}\{T_k < t\} = \lambda^k t^{k\nu} E_{\nu,k\nu+1}^k(-\lambda t^\nu), \qquad t \in (0, \infty). \tag{5}$$

We point out that the density (3) of the interarrival times $\mathcal{U}_j$ is completely monotone, and therefore log-convex. Indeed, for $\lambda > 0$, the function $t^{\beta-1} E_{\alpha,\beta}^{\gamma}(-\lambda t^{\nu})$ is completely monotone if and only if $0 < \alpha, \beta \leq 1$ and $0 < \gamma \leq \beta/\alpha$ (cf. Chap. 5 of Gorenflo et al. [8]). We recall that random variables with log-convex densities are also said to have the decreasing likelihood ratio (DLR) property.

Taking into account (5), the probability mass function of the process $N_\lambda^{\nu}(t)$ can be easily computed as follows (see, also, Eq. (2.21) of [3]):

$$\mathbb{P}\{N_\lambda^{\nu}(t) = n\} = \mathbb{P}(T_n \leq t < T_{n+1}) = (\lambda t^{\nu})^n E_{\nu,n\nu+1}^{n+1}(-\lambda t^{\nu}), \qquad t \in (0, \infty).$$

Moreover, the probability generating function of the process $N_\lambda^{\nu}(t)$ can be expressed as (see Eq. (2.29) of [3]) $G_\nu(u, t) = E_{\nu,1}(\lambda(u-1)t^{\nu})$, $|u| \leq 1$, $t > 0$. Consequently, its moment generating function is given by

$$M_\nu(s, t) = G_\nu(e^s, t) = E_{\nu,1}(\lambda(e^s - 1)t^{\nu}), \quad |s| \leq s_0, \ s_0 > 0.$$

Finally, the mean and the variance of $N_\lambda^{\nu}(t)$ read (see Eqs. (2.7) and (2.8) of [2])

$$\mathbb{E}[N_\lambda^{\nu}(t)] = \frac{\lambda t^{\nu}}{\Gamma(\nu+1)}, \quad \text{Var}[N_\lambda^{\nu}(t)] = \frac{2(\lambda t^{\nu})^2}{\Gamma(2\nu+1)} - \frac{(\lambda t^{\nu})^2}{(\Gamma(\nu+1))^2} + \frac{\lambda t^{\nu}}{\Gamma(\nu+1)}.$$

2.2 Jump Process with 2 Kinds of Jumps

We consider a jump process $\{\mathcal{N}(t); t \geq 0\}$ with rates λ_1 and λ_2, $(\lambda_1, \lambda_2 > 0)$, defined by means of the following rules:

1. $\mathcal{N}(0) = 0$ a.s.;
2. $\mathcal{N}(t)$ has stationary and independent increments;
3. $\mathbb{P}\{\mathcal{N}(t) = k\} = \lambda_k t + o(t)$, $k = 1, 2$;
4. $\mathbb{P}\{\mathcal{N}(t) \geq 3\} = o(t)$.

Clearly, this is a suitable extension of the Poisson process. The probabilities $p_j(t) = \mathbb{P}\{\mathcal{N}(t) = j\}$ satisfy the difference-differential equations

$$\begin{cases} \dfrac{dp_0(t)}{dt} = -(\lambda_1 + \lambda_2)p_0(t) \\ \dfrac{dp_1(t)}{dt} = \lambda_1 p_0(t) - (\lambda_1 + \lambda_2)p_1(t) \\ \dfrac{dp_k(t)}{dt} = \lambda_2 p_{k-2}(t) + \lambda_1 p_{k-1}(t) - (\lambda_1 + \lambda_2)p_k(t), \qquad k = 2, 3 \ldots, \end{cases} \tag{6}$$

with Kronecker-delta initial condition

$$p_k(0) = \delta_{k,0} = \begin{cases} 1, & k = 0, \\ 0, & k \geq 1. \end{cases} \tag{7}$$

The probability generating function $G(z, t)$ of $\mathcal{N}(t)$ can be derived from (6) and (7) using a rather standard technique. Indeed, it is immediate to check that it coincides with the solution of the differential equation

$$\frac{\partial}{\partial t} G(z, t) = [-\lambda_1(1 - z) - \lambda_2(1 - z^2)]G(z, t),$$

subject to the initial condition $G(z,0) = 1$. In light of this, the probability generating function can be expressed as

$$G(z,t) = e^{-\left[\lambda_1(1-z)+\lambda_2(1-z^2)\right]t}, \qquad z \in [0,1], \ t \geq 0. \tag{8}$$

We now use this result to derive the probability mass function of $\mathcal{N}(t)$.

Proposition 1. *The solution $p_j(t)$, for $j = 0, 1, \ldots$ and $t \geq 0$, of the Cauchy problem (6)-(7) is given by*

$$p_j(t) = e^{-(\lambda_1+\lambda_2)t} \sum_{k=\lceil \frac{j}{2} \rceil}^{j} \binom{k}{j-k} \frac{t^k}{k!} \lambda_1^k \left(\frac{\lambda_2}{\lambda_1}\right)^{j-k}. \tag{9}$$

Proof. By expanding $e^{(\lambda_1 z+\lambda_2 z^2)t}$ in (8) into its MacLaurin series, and performing some algebraic manipulations, we get the result. □

From (8) and (9) it is easy to infer that $p_j(t)$ represents a proper probability distribution. Thanks to the probability generating function (8) we can obtain the mean and the variance of process $\mathcal{N}(t)$:

$$\mathbb{E}\left[\mathcal{N}(t)\right] = t\left(\lambda_1 + 2\lambda_2\right), \qquad \text{Var}\left[\mathcal{N}(t)\right] = t\left(\lambda_1 + 4\lambda_2\right).$$

Remark 1. Process $\mathcal{N}(t)$ can be seen as a proper compound Poisson process, i.e.

$$\mathcal{N}(t) \stackrel{d}{=} \sum_{i=1}^{N_{\lambda_1+\lambda_2}(t)} X_i,$$

where $N_{\lambda_1+\lambda_2}(t)$ is a homogeneous Poisson process with rate $\lambda_1 + \lambda_2$. Moreover, $\{X_n : n \geq 1\}$ is a sequence of i.i.d. random variables, independent of $N_{\lambda_1+\lambda_2}(t)$, such that for any positive integer n

$$X_n \stackrel{d}{=} X = \begin{cases} 1, & \text{w.p. } \frac{\lambda_1}{\lambda_1+\lambda_2}, \\ 2, & \text{w.p. } \frac{\lambda_2}{\lambda_1+\lambda_2}. \end{cases} \tag{10}$$

Note that $N_{\lambda_1+\lambda_2}(t)$ and X_n depend on the same parameters λ_1 and λ_2.

3   Fractional Growth Process

In this section we examine a fractional extension of the recursive differential equations (6) and explore the main properties of the resulting stochastic process. We consider the following system of fractional difference-differential equations

$$\begin{cases} \dfrac{d^\nu p_0^\nu(t)}{dt^\nu} = -(\lambda_1 + \lambda_2)p_0^\nu(t) \\[2mm] \dfrac{d^\nu p_1^\nu(t)}{dt^\nu} = \lambda_1 p_0^\nu(t) - (\lambda_1 + \lambda_2)p_1^\nu(t) \\[2mm] \dfrac{d^\nu p_k^\nu(t)}{dt^\nu} = \lambda_2 p_{k-2}^\nu(t) + \lambda_1 p_{k-1}^\nu(t) - (\lambda_1 + \lambda_2)p_k^\nu(t), \quad k = 2, 3 \ldots \end{cases} \tag{11}$$

together with the Kronecker-delta initial condition

$$p_k(0) = \delta_{k,0}, \tag{12}$$

obtained by replacing in (6) the standard derivatives by the fractional derivatives, i.e.

$$\frac{d^\nu f(t)}{dt^\nu} = \begin{cases} \frac{1}{\Gamma(1-\nu)} \int_0^t \frac{(d/ds)f(s)}{(t-s)^\nu} \, ds, & 0 < \nu < 1, \\ f'(t) & \nu = 1. \end{cases}$$

Hereafter we obtain the solution to (11) in terms of the generalized Mittag-Leffler function (1) and show that it represents a true probability distribution of a certain jump process, which we will denote by $M^\nu(t)$. Hence, we write

$$p_k^\nu(t) = \mathbb{P}\left\{M^\nu(t) = k\right\}.$$

Proposition 2. *The solution $p_k^\nu(t)$, for $k = 0, 1, \ldots$ and $t \geq 0$ of the Cauchy problem (11)-(12) is given by*

$$p_k^\nu(t) = \sum_{j=\lceil \frac{k}{2} \rceil}^{k} \binom{j}{k-j} \lambda_1^j \left(\frac{\lambda_2}{\lambda_1}\right)^{k-j} t^{j\nu} E_{\nu,j\nu+1}^{j+1}(-(\lambda_1 + \lambda_2)t^\nu). \tag{13}$$

Proof. By taking the Laplace transform of Eq. (11), together with the condition (12), we have

$$\mathcal{L}\left\{p_k^\nu(t); s\right\} = \sum_{j=\lceil \frac{k}{2} \rceil}^{k} \binom{j}{k-j} \lambda_1^j \left(\frac{\lambda_2}{\lambda_1}\right)^{k-j} \frac{s^{\nu-1}}{(s^\nu + \lambda_1 + \lambda_2)^{j+1}}.$$

Hence, Eq. (13) can be obtained by using formula (2.5) of [15], i.e.

$$\mathcal{L}\left\{t^{\gamma-1}E_{\beta,\gamma}^\delta\left(\omega t^\beta\right); s\right\} = \frac{s^{\beta\delta-\gamma}}{(s^\beta - \omega)^\delta} \tag{14}$$

(where $Re(\beta) > 0$, $Re(\gamma) > 0$, $Re(\delta) > 0$ and $s > |\omega|^{\frac{1}{Re(\beta)}}$) for $\beta = \nu$, $\delta = k+1$ and $\gamma = k\nu + 1$. □

Some plots of probabilities (13) are shown in Figs. 1 and 2. We remark that the use of the Caputo fractional derivative permits us to avoid fractional initial conditions since, in general, $\mathcal{L}\left\{f^\nu; s\right\} = s^\nu \mathcal{L}\left\{f; s\right\} - s^{\nu-1}f\big|_{x=0}$, $\nu \in (0,1]$. From (11), we can easily infer that the probability generating function of $M^\nu(t)$,

$$\widehat{G}(u,t) = \mathbb{E}[u^{M^\nu(t)}] = \sum_{i=0}^{\infty} u^i p_i^\nu(t), \qquad |u| \leq 1, \, 0 < \nu \leq 1, \, t > 0,$$

satisfies the Cauchy problem

$$\begin{cases} \dfrac{\partial^\nu \widehat{G}(u,t)}{\partial t^\nu} = [-\lambda_1(1-u) - \lambda_2(1-u^2)]\widehat{G}(u,t), & |u| \leq 1, \, 0 < \nu \leq 1, \\ \widehat{G}(u,0) = 1. \end{cases} \tag{15}$$

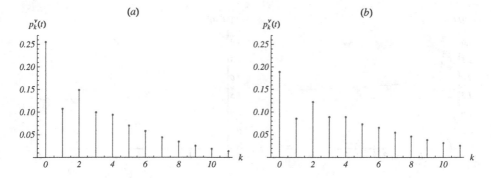

Fig. 1. Probability distribution of $M^{\nu}(t)$, given in (13), for $k = 0, 1, \ldots, 11$, with $\nu = 0.5$, $\lambda_1 = \lambda_2 = 1$, (a) $t = 1$ and (b) $t = 2$. The displayed probability mass is (a) 0.967153 and (b) 0.908498.

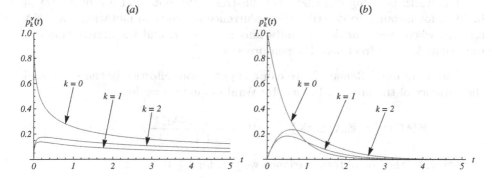

Fig. 2. Probability distribution of $M^{\nu}(t)$, given in (13), for $0 \leq t \leq 5$, $\lambda_1 = \lambda_2 = 1$, (a) $\nu = 0.5$ and (b) $\nu = 1$.

By taking the Laplace transform of (15) and making use of (14), we obtain

$$\widehat{G}(u,t) = E_{\nu,1}\left(\left(-\lambda_1\left(1-u\right) - \lambda_2\left(1-u^2\right)\right)t^{\nu}\right). \tag{16}$$

Since $E_{\nu,1}(0) = 1$, formula (16) is useful in checking that $p_j^{\nu}(t)$ represents a true probability distribution.

Remark 2. The process $M^{\nu}(t)$ can be seen as a special case of the process defined by Beghin and Macci in Eq. (7) of [1]. Specifically, one can check that

$$M^{\nu}(t) \stackrel{d}{=} \sum_{i=1}^{N_{\lambda_1+\lambda_2}^{\nu}(t)} X_i, \qquad t \geq 0, \tag{17}$$

where $N_{\lambda_1+\lambda_2}^{\nu}(t)$ is a fractional Poisson process, defined as in (2), with intensity $\lambda = \lambda_1 + \lambda_2$ ($\lambda_1, \lambda_2 > 0$). Moreover, $\{X_n : n \geq 1\}$ is a sequence of independent random variables, independent of $N_{\lambda_1+\lambda_2}^{\nu}(t)$, distributed as in (10).

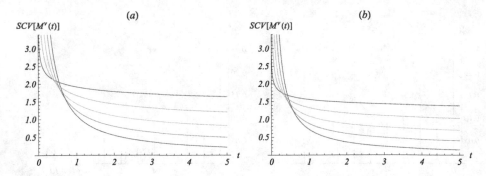

Fig. 3. Squared coefficient of variation of $M^\nu(t)$, given in (20), for $\nu = 0.2, 0.4, 0.6,$ 0.8 and 1 (from top to bottom for large t), $\lambda_1 = 0.5$, (a) $\lambda_2 = 0.5$ and (b) $\lambda_2 = 1$.

It is worth pointing out that (17) illustrates the potential use of $M^\nu(t)$ in biology, for instance to describe the occurrence of multiple mutations in DNA regions, where single or double mutations may occur, and the arrival times of mutations follow a fractional Poisson process.

Bearing in mind Remark 2, we can compute more effortlessly the mean and the variance of the process. In fact, by Wald's equation we have

$$\mathbb{E}\left[M^\nu(t)\right] = \mathbb{E}[X]\,\mathbb{E}\left[N^\nu_{\lambda_1+\lambda_2}(t)\right] = \frac{(\lambda_1 + 2\lambda_2)\,t^\nu}{\Gamma(\nu+1)}, \qquad t \geq 0. \qquad (18)$$

Moreover, by the law of total variance we get, for $t \geq 0$,

$$\begin{aligned}
\text{Var}\left[M^\nu(t)\right] &= \text{Var}\left[X\right]\,\mathbb{E}\left[N^\nu_{\lambda_1+\lambda_2}(t)\right] + (\mathbb{E}\left[X\right])^2\,\text{Var}\left[N^\nu_{\lambda_1+\lambda_2}(t)\right] \\
&= \frac{(\lambda_1 + 4\lambda_2)\,t^\nu}{\Gamma(\nu+1)} + (\lambda_1 + 2\lambda_2)^2\,t^{2\nu}\,Z(\nu),
\end{aligned} \qquad (19)$$

where

$$Z(\nu) := \frac{1}{\nu}\left(\frac{1}{\Gamma(2\nu)} - \frac{1}{\nu\Gamma^2(\nu)}\right).$$

It follows that the process $M^\nu(t)$ is overdispersed, i.e. $\text{Var}\left[M^\nu(t)\right] > \mathbb{E}\left[M^\nu(t)\right]$, since $Z(\nu) > 0$ for all $\nu \in (0,1)$ and $Z(1) = 0$. Furthermore, from (18) and (19) we have that the squared coefficient of variation of $M^\nu(t)$, $t > 0$, is given by

$$\text{SCV}\left[M^\nu(t)\right] = \frac{\text{Var}\left[M^\nu(t)\right]}{(\mathbb{E}\left[M^\nu(t)\right])^2} = \frac{(\lambda_1 + 4\lambda_2)}{(\lambda_1 + 2\lambda_2)^2}\,\Gamma(\nu+1)\,t^{-\nu} + (\Gamma(\nu+1))^2\,Z(\nu).$$

$$(20)$$

Finally, some plots of $\text{SCV}\left[M^\nu(t)\right]$ are provided in Fig. 3.

Acknowledgements. This research is partially supported by GNCS-Indam and Regione Campania (Legge 5).

References

1. Beghin, L., Macci, C.: Fractional discrete processes: compound and mixed Poisson representations. J. Appl. Prob. **51**, 19–36 (2014)
2. Beghin, L., Orsingher, E.: Fractional Poisson processes and related planar random motion. Electron. J. Prob. **14**, 1790–1826 (2009)
3. Beghin, L., Orsingher, E.: Poisson-type processes governed by fractional and higher-order recursive differential equations. Electron. J. Prob. **15**, 684–709 (2010)
4. Di Crescenzo A., Martinucci B. and Meoli A., A fractional counting process and its connection with Poisson process. submitted
5. El-Sayed, A.M.A., Rida, S.Z., Arafa, A.A.M.: On the solutions of time-fractional bacterial chemotaxis in a diffusion gradient chamber. Intern. J. Nonlin. Sci. **7**, 485–492 (2009)
6. Garra, R., Orsingher, E., Polito, F.: State-dependent fractional point processes. J. Appl. Prob. **52**, 18–36 (2015)
7. Garra, R., Polito, F.: A note on fractional linear pure birth and pure death processes in epidemic models. Physica A **390**, 3704–3709 (2011)
8. Gorenflo, R., Kilbas, A.A., Mainardi, F., Rogosin, S.V.: Mittag-Leffler Functions, Related Topics and Applications. Springer Monographs in Mathematics. Springer, Heidelberg (2014)
9. Jumarie, G.: Fractional multiple birth-death processes with birth probabilities $\lambda_i(\Delta t)^\alpha + o((\Delta t)^\alpha)$. J. Franklin Inst. **347**, 1797–1813 (2010)
10. Magin, R.L.: Fractional calculus models of complex dynamics in biological tissues. Comput. Math. Appl. **59**, 1586–1593 (2010)
11. Muiño, J.M., Kuruoğlu, E.E., Arndt, P.F.: Evidence of a cancer type-specific distribution for consecutive somatic mutation distances. Comput. Biol. Chem. **53**, 79–83 (2014)
12. Orsingher, E., Polito, F.: On a fractional linear birth-death process. Bernoulli **17**, 114–137 (2011)
13. Orsingher, E., Polito, F.: Fractional pure birth processes. Bernoulli **16**, 858–881 (2010)
14. Orsingher, E., Polito, F., Sakhno, L.: Fractional non-linear, linear and sublinear death processes. J. Stat. Phys. **141**, 68–93 (2010)
15. Prabhakar, T.R.: A singular integral equation with a generalized Mittag Leffler function in the kernel. Yokohama Math. J. **19**, 7–15 (1971)
16. Tenreiro Machado, J.A.: And I say to myself: "What a fractional world!". Fract. Calc. Appl. Anal. **14**, 635–654 (2011)
17. Varalta, N., Gomes, A.V., Camargo, R.F.: A prelude to the fractional calculus applied to tumor dynamic. TEMA Tend. Mat. Apl. Comput. **15**, 211–221 (2014)

Towards Stochastic Modeling of Neuronal Interspike Intervals Including a Time-Varying Input Signal

Giuseppe D'Onofrio[1]([✉]), Enrica Pirozzi[1], and Marcelo O. Magnasco[2]

[1] Dipartimento di Matematica e Applicazioni, Università di Napoli Federico II,
Monte S. Angelo, 80126 Napoli, Italy
{giuseppe.donofrio,enrica.pirozzi}@unina.it
[2] Laboratory of Mathematical Physics, The Rockefeller University,
New York, NY 10021, USA
magnasco@rockefeller.edu

Abstract. We construct a LIF-type stochastic model for interspike times of the firing activity of a single neuron subject to a time-varying input signal. By using first passage time densities some numerical evaluations of ISI densities and comparisons with simulation results are given.

1 Introduction

Motivated by the investigations carried out in some recent papers ([1–13] and references therein) in the context of the stochastic modeling, we consider the problem of the description of successive spike times and interspike intervals (ISIs) of the membrane potential of a single neuron. In particular, we refer to the non homogeneous Leaky Integrate-and-Fire (LIF) neuronal model

$$dV(t) = \{-\alpha(V(t) - V_{rest}) + I(t)\}\, dt + \sigma dW(t), \quad t \geq 0, \quad V(0) = v_0, \quad (1)$$

where $I(t)$ describes the time-varying input signal (current), with $\alpha > 0$, $\sigma > 0$, $v_0 \in \mathbb{R}$. The parameter $1/\alpha$ is the characteristic (decay) time of the membrane potential, V_{rest} is the resting potential, v_0 is the initial (reset) value, σ represents a constant intensity of the noise and $W(t)$ the standard Brownian motion.

The dynamics of the neuronal membrane potential is described by the stochastic process $V(t)$ and evolves in the presence of a constant boundary S (the firing threshold). The first passage time (FPT) of $V(t)$ through S, i.e.

$$T_1 = \inf_{t \geq 0}\{t : V(t) \geq S\} \quad \text{with} \quad V(0) = v_0 < S,$$

is used to model the first spike time. After the first spike, the process $V(t)$ is instantaneously reset to the initial value, i.e. $V(T_1) = v_0$ that means for $T_1 = t_1$

This paper is partially supported by G.N.C.S.- INdAM, Programme STAR of Compagnia di San Paolo and Project "Metodi, Modelli, Algoritmi e Software per le Scienze di Base ed Applicate", and Campania Region.

© Springer International Publishing Switzerland 2015
R. Moreno-Díaz et al. (Eds.): EUROCAST 2015, LNCS 9520, pp. 166–173, 2015.
DOI: 10.1007/978-3-319-27340-2_22

then $V(t_1) = v_0$, and its evolution restarts again obeying to the SDE (1) but without any reset of the input signal $I(t)$.

The successive spike times T_k for $k = 2, 3 \ldots, n$ are described by the successive passage times of the process $V(t)$ through S, i.e. by the following ordered random variables:

$$T_k = \inf_{t \geq 0} \{t \geq T_{k-1} : V(t) \geq S\} \quad \text{with} \quad V(T_{k-1}) = v_0 < S. \tag{2}$$

The randomness of the reset times in (2), considered as initial conditions for the SDE (1) after each firing time, and the time-dependence of the current $I(t)$ make extremely difficult the determination of the solution of the SDE (1). Nevertheless, it is possible to provide simulations of random paths of the process $V(t)$. In [12, 13] extensive simulations of an analogous model, suitable converted in an Ornstein-Uhlenbeck process in the presence of a time-varying threshold, were performed. Here, in a preliminary investigation, we apply the Euler discretization method to the SDE (1) and obtain estimations of the probability density function (pdf) of the successive firing times $T_1, T_2 \ldots, T_n$, by histograms of samples of simulated successive passage times of $V(t)$ through S. This enables us to build also histograms of successive ISIs $T_k - T_{k-1}$, for $k = 1, 2, \ldots, n$ with $T_0 = 0$.

In this paper our aim is to provide an alternative stochastic model for successive spike times and ISIs based on tractable SDEs by which we are able to carry out some numerical approximations for pdfs of firing densities. In particular, in the next Section we explain our model and in Sect. 3 we give our numerical evaluations specifically for the first, the second firing times and the corresponding ISI with a specified time-varying current. We finally compare these evaluations with the simulation results of the original model (1).

2   The Model

Our model to describe the occurrence of the successive firing times $T_0, T_1, \ldots, T_n$ (with $T_0 = 0$) is based on the idea of representing the firing times by means of FPTs $\mathcal{T}_1, \mathcal{T}_2, \ldots, \mathcal{T}_n$ of stochastic processes $\{V_1(t), V_2(t), \ldots, V_n(t)\}$ through the constant threshold S. Moreover, for modeling the successive ISIs $T_k - T_{k-1}$ for $k = 1, 2, \ldots, n$, we consider the FPTs $\Theta_1, \Theta_2, \ldots, \Theta_n$ of stochastic processes $\{Y_1(t), Y_2(t), \ldots, Y_n(t)\}$ through S. The processes $\{V_1(t), V_2(t), \ldots, V_n(t)\}$ are linked to each other, while each process $Y_k(t)$ is linked to the process $V_k(t)$ for $k = 1, 2, \ldots, n$.

Successive Firing Times. Specifically, we model the behavior of the neuronal membrane potential by using the diffusion processes $\{V_1(t), V_2(t), \ldots, V_n(t)\}$ solutions of the system of SDEs (LIF-type), for $k = 1, 2, \ldots, n$,

$$dV_k(t) = \left\{ -\alpha V_k(t) + \alpha \left[V_{rest} + \frac{I(t)}{\alpha} \right] \mathbb{P}(\mathcal{T}_{k-1} \leq t) \right\} dt + \sigma dW(t), t > 0, V_k(0) = v_0 \tag{3}$$

with $\mathbb{P}(\mathcal{T}_0 = 0) = 1$ and $\mathbb{P}(\mathcal{T}_{k-1} \leq t)$ is the probability that the FPT $\mathcal{T}_{k-1}$ of the process V_{k-1} has already occurred. The other involved parameters in (3) have the same meaning of those in (1).

The successive firing times are described by using the corresponding FPTs

$$\mathcal{T}_k := \inf_{t \geq 0}\{t : V_k(t) \geq S\}, \quad V_k(0) = v_0 < S \quad (k = 1, 2, \dots, n)$$

characterized by pdf

$$g_{V_k}(S, t | v_0, 0) := \frac{d\mathbb{P}(\mathcal{T}_k \leq t)}{dt}.$$

Note that each process $V_k(t)$ is linked to the previous one $V_{k-1}(t)$ because of the presence in (3) of the term $\mathbb{P}(\mathcal{T}_{k-1} \leq t)$. From this kind of dependency between the processes $V_k(t)$ it is possible to derive the stochastic ordering between the corresponding FPTs $\mathcal{T}_k$ (see [7]).

InterSpike Intervals (ISI). For modeling the ISIs $T_k - T_{k-1}$, for $k = 1, 2, \dots, n$, we now consider the following SDEs

$$dY_k(t) = \left\{ -\alpha Y_k(t) + \alpha \left[V_{rest} + \frac{I(t)}{\alpha} \right] \mathbb{P}(\mathcal{T}_k > t) \right\} dt + \sigma dW(t), t > 0, Y_k(0) = v_0,$$
(4)

where the process $Y_k(t)$ obeys to a similar dynamics of the process $V_k(t)$ except for the probability term $\mathbb{P}(\cdot)$ in (4). In particular, $Y_k(t)$ is linked to the process $V_k(t)$, because the dynamics (4) of $Y_k(t)$ depends on the probability distribution function of the FPT $\mathcal{T}_k$ of $V_k(t)$. We use the process $Y_k(t)$ to mimic the behavior of the membrane potential *before* the occurrence of $\mathcal{T}_k$, taking into account that $\mathcal{T}_{k-1}$ is already occurred. Then, we model the ISIs by using the FPTs of $Y_k(t)$, i.e.

$$\Theta_k := \inf_{t \geq 0}\{t : Y_k(t) \geq S\}, \quad Y_k(0) = v_0 < S,$$

with the pdf

$$g_{Y_k}(S, t | v_0, 0) := \frac{d\mathbb{P}(\Theta_k \leq t)}{dt}.$$

We refer to the paper [7] for the explanation of the origin and the motivation of this kind of model. Here, we can say that the proposed LIF-type SDEs (3) and (4) are mathematically tractable and some our results about the evaluations of the corresponding FPTs can be exploited as shown in the following.

In particular, here, we consider the input current $I(t)$ with the following form:

$$I(t) = \mu + \lambda e^{-\beta t} \quad \text{with } \beta > 0, \mu, \lambda \in \mathbb{R}, \quad t \geq 0. \tag{5}$$

According to [1], and for the specified current (5), we set for $k = 1, 2, \dots, n$ and for $0 \leq \tau \leq t$

$$\mathcal{M}_{V_k}(t | \tau) = [\alpha V_{rest} + \mu] e^{-\alpha t} \int_\tau^t \mathbb{P}(\mathcal{T}_{k-1} \leq \xi) e^{\alpha \xi} d\xi + \lambda e^{-\alpha t} \int_\tau^t \mathbb{P}(\mathcal{T}_{k-1} \leq \xi) e^{(\alpha - \beta)\xi} d\xi,$$
(6)

and

$$\mathcal{M}_{Y_k}(t|\tau) = [\alpha V_{rest} + \mu] e^{-\alpha t} \int_\tau^t \mathbb{P}(\mathcal{T}_k > \xi) e^{\alpha \xi} d\xi + \lambda e^{-\alpha t} \int_\tau^t \mathbb{P}(\mathcal{T}_k > \xi) e^{(\alpha - \beta)\xi} d\xi.$$
(7)

Therefore, the Gauss-Markov (GM) processes $V_k(t)$ and $Y_k(t)$, for $k = 1, 2, \ldots, n$, have the following mean functions, for $t \geq 0$,

$$m_{V_k}(t|v_0, 0) = v_0 e^{-\alpha t} + \mathcal{M}_{V_k}(t|0), \quad m_{Y_k}(t|v_0, 0) = v_0 e^{-\alpha t} + \mathcal{M}_{Y_k}(t|0), \quad (8)$$

and they have the same covariance function for $k = 1, 2, \ldots, n$

$$c_k(s, t) = \frac{\sigma^2}{2\alpha} e^{-\alpha t} \left[e^{\alpha s} - e^{-\alpha s} \right] \qquad (0 \leq s \leq t).$$
(9)

Furthermore, the normal transition pdf $f_k(x, t|y, \tau)$, for $k = 1, 2, \ldots, n$, of $V_k(t)$ and $Y_k(t)$ is

$$f_k[x, t|y, \tau] = \frac{\sqrt{\alpha}}{\sqrt{\pi \sigma^2 (1 - e^{-2\alpha(t-\tau)})}} \exp \left\{ -\alpha \frac{\left[x - y e^{-\alpha(t-\tau)} - \mathcal{M}_k(t|\tau) \right]^2}{\sigma^2 \left(1 - e^{-2\alpha(t-\tau)} \right)} \right\}$$
(10)

for $\mathcal{M}_k(t|\tau) = \mathcal{M}_{V_k}(t|\tau)$ and for $\mathcal{M}_k(t|\tau) = \mathcal{M}_{Y_k}(t|\tau)$, respectively.

About the FPT problem of the GM processes through a constant threshold S, we are able to provide a numerical approximation of the FPT pdf $g_k(S, t|v_0, 0)$ solving, by a numerical procedure [1], the following non singular second kind Volterra integral equation:

$$g_k(S, t|v_0, 0) = -\Psi_k[S, t|v_0, 0] + \int_0^t \Psi_k[S, t|S, \tau] g_k(S, \tau|v_0, 0) d\tau$$
(11)

for $k = 1, 2, \ldots, n$, with

$$\Psi_k[S, t|y, \tau] = f_k[S, t|y, \tau] \left\{ -S\alpha \frac{1 + e^{-2\alpha(t-\tau)}}{1 - e^{-2\alpha(t-\tau)}} + \frac{2\alpha y e^{-\alpha(t-\tau)}}{1 - e^{-2\alpha(t-\tau)}} \right.$$
$$\left. -\alpha \left[V_{rest} + \frac{\mu + \lambda e^{-\beta t}}{\alpha} \right] \mathbb{P}_k(t) + \frac{2\alpha \mathcal{M}_k(t|\tau)}{1 - e^{-2\alpha(t-\tau)}} \right\}.$$
(12)

The procedure is here applied to the integral equation (11) for $g_k(S, t|v_0, 0) = g_{V_k}(S, t|v_0, 0)$, setting $\mathbb{P}_k(t) = \mathbb{P}(T_{k-1} \leq t)$, $\mathcal{M}_k(t|\tau) = \mathcal{M}_{V_k}(t|\tau)$ and $f_k[S, t|y, \tau] = f_{V_k}[S, t|y, \tau]$ in the function $\Psi_k[S, t|y, \tau]$ of (12), in such a way to provide numerical estimations of the FPT pdf of $\mathcal{T}_k$. (In this case, we write $\Psi_{V_k}[S, t|y, \tau]$ for $\Psi_k[S, t|y, \tau]$). We point out that for solving the integral equation (11) for $g_{V_k}(S, t|v_0, 0)$ it is required to solve firstly the equations (11) for $g_{V_{k-1}}(S, t|v_0, 0)$, because the function $\Psi_{V_k}[S, t|y, \tau]$ is defined by means of

$$\mathbb{P}_k(t) = \mathbb{P}(T_{k-1} \leq t) = \int_0^t g_{V_{k-1}}(S, \xi|v_0, 0) d\xi.$$
(13)

Hence, the numerical procedure for solving the Eq. (11) has to be applied orderly respect to k for $k = 1, 2, \ldots, n$, giving also a numerical evaluation of the (13), for $t \geq 0$, useful for the successive FPT (successive value of k).

Then, the procedure is applied to the integral equation (11) for $g_k(S, t|v_0, 0) = g_{Y_k}(S, t|v_0, 0)$ setting $\mathbb{P}_k(t) = \mathbb{P}(T_k > t)$, $\mathcal{M}_k(t|\tau) = \mathcal{M}_{Y_k}(t|\tau)$ and $f_k[S, t|y, \tau] = f_{Y_k}[S, t|y, \tau]$ in the function $\Psi_k[S, t|y, \tau]$ of (12), in such a way to provide numerical estimations of the FPT pdf of Θ_k. (We write $\Psi_{Y_k}[S, t|y, \tau]$ for $\Psi_k[S, t|y, \tau]$). In this case, for solving the integral equation (11) for $g_{Y_k}(S, t|v_0, 0)$ it is required to solve at first the Eq. (11) for $g_{V_k}(S, t|v_0, 0)$, because the function $\Psi_{Y_k}[S, t|y, \tau]$ is defined by means of $\mathbb{P}_k(t) = \mathbb{P}(T_k > t) = 1 - \mathbb{P}(T_k \leq t)$.

Taking into account that $T_0 = 0$ and $\Theta_1 \equiv T_1$, in the next Section we provide some results for the first passage times T_1, T_2 and for Θ_2 in order to compare our numerical approximations with the simulation results of (1) for the first and second spike times T_1, T_2 and the second interspike interval $T_2 - T_1$, respectively.

3   Some Numerical and Simulation Results

In order to make easier to handle the numerical iterative procedure for solving the integral Eq. (11) for $k = 1$ and then for $k = 2$, we now give a closed form expression for $\mathcal{M}_{V_2}(t|\tau)$ to use in place of (6) with $k = 2$. In such a way, no preliminary numerical evaluations of $g_{V_1}(S, t|v_0, 0)$ and of $\mathbb{P}(T_1 \leq t)$ are required to obtain $\mathcal{M}_{V_2}(t|\tau)$.

3.1   An Asymptotic Approximation for $g_{V_1}(S, t|v_0, 0)$

Along the lines of [1], for $t > 1/\alpha$, if $S - \sup\limits_{t \geq 0} m_{V_1}(t|v_0, 0) > \sqrt{\sigma^2/\alpha}$ and having, from (5), that $\lim_{t \to +\infty} I(t) = \mu$ then the following exponential approximation for $g_{V_1}(S, t|v_0, 0)$ holds:

$$g_{V_1}(S, t|v_0, 0) \approx \widetilde{g}_{V_1}(t) = h_{V_1} e^{-h_{V_1} t} \tag{14}$$

with

$$h_{V_1} = - \lim_{t \to +\infty} \Psi_{V_1}(S, t|y, \tau) =$$
$$= \alpha \sqrt{\frac{\alpha}{\pi \sigma^2}} \left[S - \left(V_{rest} + \frac{\mu}{\alpha} \right) \right] \exp \left\{ -\frac{\alpha}{\sigma^2} \left[S - \left(V_{rest} + \frac{\mu}{\alpha} \right) \right]^2 \right\}. \tag{15}$$

Therefore, we can use the following expression for

$$\mathbb{P}(T_1 \leq t) \approx \widetilde{\mathbb{P}}(T_1 \leq t) = 1 - e^{-h_{V_1} t}. \tag{16}$$

Then, using (16) in (6) for $k = 2$, we have for the process $V_2(t)$ the following mean

$$\widetilde{m}_{V_2}(t|v_0, 0) = v_0 e^{-\alpha t} + \widetilde{\mathcal{M}}_{V_2}(t|0) \tag{17}$$

with

$$\widetilde{\mathcal{M}}_{V_2}(t|0) = \left[V_{rest} + \frac{\mu}{\alpha}\right]\left(1 - e^{-\alpha t}\right) + \frac{(\alpha V_{rest} + \mu)}{h_{V_1} - \alpha}\left[e^{-h_{V_1}t} - e^{-\alpha t}\right]$$

$$+ \frac{\lambda}{\alpha - \beta}\left[e^{-\beta t} - e^{-\alpha t}\right] - \frac{\lambda}{\alpha - \beta - h_{V_1}}\left[e^{-h_{V_1}t - \beta t} - e^{-\alpha t}\right]. \quad (18)$$

Hence, the numerical procedure can be applied to solve the integral equation (11) for $k = 2$ and specifically for $V_2(t)$, providing numerical evaluations of $g_{V_2}(S, t|v_0, 0)$ and of $\mathbb{P}(\mathcal{T}_2 \leq t)$. These evaluations are then used for solving again the integral equation (11) with $k = 2$ now for the process $Y_2(t)$. Indeed, the required $\mathbb{P}(\mathcal{T}_2 > t) = 1 - \mathbb{P}(\mathcal{T}_2 \leq t)$ has been numerically obtained for $V_2(t)$ and now it is possible to construct the function $\mathcal{M}_{Y_2}(t|0)$, as in (7) for $k = 2$, and also the function $\Psi_{Y_2}[S, t|y, \tau]$ as in (12). Finally, a numerical evaluation of the pdf of ISI Θ_2 is provided.

3.2 Some Comparisons

First of all, we note that the SDEs (1) and (3) are the same for $k = 1$, being $\mathbb{P}(\mathcal{T}_0 \leq t) = 1 \ \forall t \geq 0$ in (3). Here we do not compare our numerical FPT pdf $g_{V_1}(S, t|v_0, 0)$ with histograms of the first firing time T_1 obtained from simulations of SDE (1), but we refer to [2,5] for the excellent agreement between those kinds of approximations. Furthermore, for suitable choices of the involved parameters, we can exploit the asymptotic approximation (14) for $g_{V_1}(S, t|v_0, 0)$ and also in this case the agreement between the numerical and simulation results is quite satisfactory [2,5].

Now, we focus our attention on the second spike time T_2 and the ISI $T_2 - T_1$. Following our strategy we are able to give numerical approximations for pdfs of T_2 and Θ_2, plotted as blue curves in Figs. 1, 2, 3 and 4, respectively. The histograms of second spike times T_2 for $V(t)$ of the simulated SDE (1) are shown in Figs. 1 and 2, while those of $T_2 - T_1$ in Figs. 3 and 4. We point out that, for

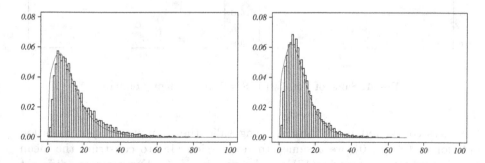

Fig. 1. Approximations for the pdf of T_2. Numerical evaluations of $g_{V_2}(S, t|v_0, 0)$ (blue) and histograms of 10^4 second passage times T_2 of simulated paths of $V(t)$ by (1), with time discretization step 10^{-4}, $\lambda = 0.25$, $\mu = 0.25$, $\alpha = 1$, $V_{rest} = 0.2$, $v_0 = 0$, $\sigma = 1$, $S = 1.8$, $\beta = 0.1$ (on the left) and $\beta = 0.01$ (on the right) (Color figure online).

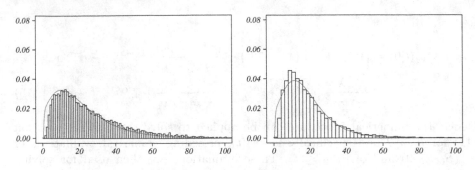

Fig. 2. Same of Fig. 1 with $S = 2$ (Color figure online)

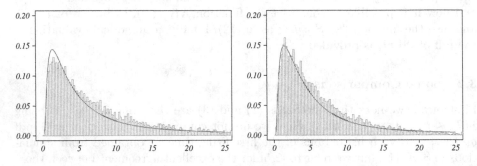

Fig. 3. Approximations for the ISI pdf of $T_2 - T_1$. Numerical evaluations of $g_{Y_2}(S, t|v_0, 0)$ (blue) and histograms of 10^4 ISI times $T_2 - T_1$ of $V(t)$ by simulations of (1), with time discretization step 10^{-4}. $S = 1.8$ and $\beta = 0.1$ (on the left) and $\beta = 0.01$ (on the right), other parameters as in Fig. 1 (Color figure online).

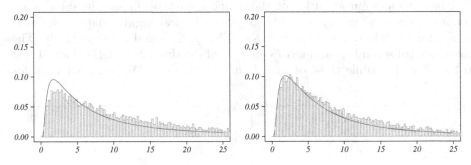

Fig. 4. Same of Fig. 3 with $S = 2$. (Color figure online)

the cases considered in all figures, being valid the asymptotic approximation (14) for $g_{V_1}(S, t|v_0, 0)$, we assumed the expression (18) to construct the mean function $m_{V_2}(t|v_0, 0)$ as in (17) for the process $V_2(t)$. Furthermore, different values are assigned to parameter β for considering characteristic times of the current greater than those of the neuronal membrane; but also different values are assigned to the firing threshold to validate the asymptotic regime for the first passage time T_1.

Finally, referring to a future paper for more extensive validations of our model and for more detailed comparisons, here we point out the agreement between our numerical results and the simulations of (1), although our approximations derive from averaged manipulations.

References

1. Buonocore, A., Caputo, L., Pirozzi, E., Ricciardi, L.M.: The first passage time problem for gauss-diffusion processes: algorithmic approaches and applications to lif neuronal model. Methodol. Comput. Appl. Prob. **13**, 29–57 (2011)
2. Buonocore, A., Caputo, L., Pirozzi, E., Ricciardi, L.M.: On a stochastic leaky integrate-and-fire neuronal model. Neural Comput. **22**, 2558–2585 (2010)
3. Buonocore, A., Caputo, L., Pirozzi, E., Carfora, M.F.: Gauss-diffusion processes for modeling the dynamics of a couple of interacting neurons. Math. Biosci. Eng. **11**, 189–201 (2014)
4. Buonocore, A., Caputo, L., Nobile, A.G., Pirozzi, E.: Gauss-Markov processes in the presence of a reflecting boundary and applications in neuronal models. Appl. Math. Comput. **232**, 799–809 (2014)
5. Buonocore, A., Caputo, L., Nobile, A.G., Pirozzi, E.: Restricted Ornstein-Uhlenbeck process and applications in neuronal models with periodic input signals. J. Comput. Appl. Math. **285**, 59–71 (2015)
6. Buonocore, A., Caputo, L., Nobile, A.G., Pirozzi, E.: Gauss-Markov processes for neuronal models including reversal potentials. Adv. Cognitive Neurodynamics (IV) **11**, 299–305 (2015)
7. D'Onofrio, G., Pirozzi, E.: Successive spike times predicted by a stochastic neuronal model with a variable input signal, Math. Biosci. Eng. (2015)
8. Giorno, V., Spina, S.: On the return process with refractoriness for a non-homogeneous Ornstein-Uhlenbeck neuronal model. Math. Biosci. Eng. **11**(2), 285–302 (2014)
9. Lánský, P., Ditlevsen, S.: A review of the methods for signal estimation in stochastic diffusion leaky integrate-and-fire neuronal models. Biol. Cybern. **99**, 253–262 (2008)
10. Kim, H., Shinomoto, S.: Estimating nonstationary inputs from a single spike train based on a neuron model with adaptation. Math. Bios. Eng. **11**, 49–62 (2014)
11. Taillefumier, T., Magnasco, M.O.: A fast algorithm for the first-passage times of Gauss-Markov processes with Holder continuous boundaries. J. Stat. Phys. **140**(6), 1130–1156 (2010)
12. Taillefumier, T., Magnasco, M.O.: A phase transition in the first passage of a Brownian process through a fluctuating boundary: implications for neural coding. PNAS **110**, E1438–E1443 (2013). doi:10.1073/pnas.1212479110
13. Taillefumier, T., Magnasco, M.O.: A transition to sharp timing in stochastic leaky integrate-and-fire neurons driven by frozen noisy input. Neural Comput. **26**(5), 819–859 (2014)

A Cancer Dynamics Model for an Intermittent Treatment Involving Reduction of Tumor Size and Rise of Growth Rate

Virginia Giorno[1] and Serena Spina[2]([✉])

[1] Dipartimento di Studi e Ricerche Aziendali (Management and Information Technology), Università di Salerno, Via Giovanni Paolo II, 132, Fisciano, SA, Italy
giorno@unisa.it
[2] Dipartimento di Matematica, Università di Salerno, Via Giovanni Paolo II, 132, Fisciano, SA, Italy
sspina@unisa.it

Abstract. We propose a model of tumor dynamics based on the Gompertz deterministic law influenced by jumps that occur at equidistant time instants. This model consents to study the effect of a therapeutic program that provides intermittent suppression of cancer cells. In this context a jump represents an application of the therapy that shifts the cancer mass to a fixed level and it produces a deleterious effect on the organism by increasing the growth rate of the cancer cells. The objective of the present study is to provide an efficient criterion to choose the instants in which to apply the therapy by maximizing the time in which the cancer mass is under a fixed control threshold.

1 Introduction

In the last decades great attention has been payed to the formulation and analysis of models describing the cancer dynamics. Among various models the Gompertz process plays an important role because it seems to fit experimental data in a reasonable precise way in several contexts (see, for instance, [3,7]). Recently, some models have been proposed to describe the tumor dynamic under the effect of therapies that instantly reduce an intrinsic factor of the tumor at predefined levels. In particular, in [2,6], models describing the growth of prostate tumor under intermittent hormone therapy have been studied. In this direction, assuming the tumor size as the intrinsic factor to control, in [1,5], stochastic models with jumps have been considered. Each jump represents the effect of a therapeutic application that shifts the process to a certain return value. Specifically, in [1] we analyzed a Gompertz diffusion process with jumps occurring at random time instants. Whereas in [5] we assumed that each therapeutic application involves a reduction of the tumor mass, but it also implies an increase of the growth speed and we proposed a strategy, based on the first passage time of the process through a control boundary, to select the inter-jump intervals.

This paper is partially supported by G.N.C.S. - INdAM and Campania Region.

R. Moreno-Díaz et al. (Eds.): EUROCAST 2015, LNCS 9520, pp. 174–182, 2015.
DOI: 10.1007/978-3-319-27340-2_23

In the present work we consider a deterministic Gompertz process with jumps to analyze the effect of a therapeutic program that provides intermittent reduction of the tumor size and a rise of the growth rate. A therapy is applied at equidistant time instants, it resets the process at a fixed state from which the cancer mass re-starts with a gradually increased growth rate, depending on the number of applications and on a constant representing aggressiveness of the therapy. We assume the growth rate increases after each application to take into account that when a therapy is applied there is a selection event in which only the most aggressive clones survive; for example, this perspective could be applied to targeted drugs that have a much lower toxicity for the patient. The combined effects, reduction of tumor size and rise of growth rate, put the problem of finding a compromise between these two aspects. We focus on the time in which the cancer mass reaches a control threshold and we provide an efficient criterion to maximize this instant. The paper is organized as it follows. In Sect. 2 we construct the model. In Sect. 3 we study some analytical properties of the model to choose the appropriate instants of therapeutic applications. Finally in Sect. 4 an extensive numerical analysis is performed to support the proposed criterion and to examine the role of the involved parameters.

2 The Model

We propose a mathematical model to analyze the effect of a therapeutic program that provides intermittent suppression of cancer cells. Each therapeutic application shifts the cancer mass to a return state $\rho > 0$ and it produces a deleterious effect on the organism by increasing the growth rate of the cancer cells. We suppose that the return state ρ is equal to the initial tumor mass. We denote by $\zeta > 0$ the width of inter-jump intervals.

Let $x(t)$ be the process describing the dynamic of tumor cells under the effect of the intermittent therapy. It consists of cycles described by deterministic Gompertz processes with different growth rates. In particular, starting from $\rho > 0$ at time $t = 0$, the process evolves in according to the Gompertz law with parameters $\alpha_0 = \alpha$ and β, where $\alpha > 0$ and $\beta > 0$ are the natural regulator parameters of the cancer growth. After the time ζ a therapy is applied, its effect is, on the one hand to reduce the tumor size to ρ, and the other one to increase the growth rate of a term γ. So, the evolution restarts with a new birth parameter $\alpha_1 = \alpha + \gamma$. Thus proceeding, after the k-th application, occurring at time $t_k = k\zeta$, the process will evolve from the state ρ with the growth parameter $\alpha_k = \alpha + k\gamma$. The constant $\gamma > 0$ describes the harmful effect of the therapy, that is it is greater in correspondence of more aggressive therapies.

Since $x(t)$ consists of cycles $x_k(t)$ described by Gompertz processes with different growth rate, the cancer size at time t can be described by using the indicator function

$$1_A(t) = \begin{cases} 1, & t \in A \\ 0, & t \notin A. \end{cases}$$

Indeed, if N denotes the number of therapeutic applications, one has:

$$x(t) = \sum_{k=0}^{N} x_k(t) 1_{[t_k, t_{k+1})}(t),$$ (2.1)

with $x(t_k^-) = x_{k-1}(t_k)$, $x(t_k) = \rho$, $t_0 = 0$, $t_k = k\zeta$, $t_{N+1} = +\infty$ and where

$$x_k(t) = \exp\left\{\frac{\alpha_k}{\beta} + \left(\log\rho - \frac{\alpha_k}{\beta}\right) e^{-\beta(t-t_k)}\right\}, \quad x_k(t_k) = \rho,$$ (2.2)

with $\alpha_k = \alpha + k\gamma$.

Denoting by S a control threshold, we require that $x(t) < S$ as long as possible during the treatment. Since the effectiveness of an intermittent treatment depends on the amplitude of the inter-jump intervals, in the following we propose a criterion to choose ζ in order to increase the crossing threshold time.

Specifically, we consider the couples $(t_k, x_{k-1}(t_k))$, for $k = 1, 2, \ldots$, where $t_k = \zeta k$ represents the time of the k-th therapeutical application and $x_{k-1}(\zeta k)$ is the corresponding cancer mass at this time. We note that $(\zeta k, x_{k-1}(\zeta k))$, the red points in Fig. 1, are the maximum of $x_{k-1}(t)$.

Let $y(t)$ be the curve interpolating the points $(\zeta k, x_{k-1}(\zeta k))$ for $k = 1, 2, \ldots$. One has:

$$y(t)\big|_{t=k\zeta} = x_{k-1}(t)\big|_{t=k\zeta} = x_{t/\zeta-1}(k\zeta),$$

from which it follows:

$$y(t) = \exp\left\{\frac{\alpha + \gamma\left(\frac{t}{\zeta}-1\right)}{\beta}\left(1 - e^{-\beta\zeta}\right)\right\} \rho^{e^{-\beta\zeta}}, \quad t \geq \zeta.$$ (2.3)

The curve $y(t)$ is useful in order to understand where the tumor mass is in a certain instant or when it reaches the control threshold $S > \rho$. Indeed, an alarm time for the patient, whose illness is described by $x(t)$, is given by the intersection point t^* between S and the curve $y(t)$. For example, in Fig. 1 the process $x(t)$ (black line), the curve $y(t)$ (red curve) and the threshold S (blue line) are plotted for $\alpha = 6.46$, $\beta = 0.314$, $\gamma = 0.5$, $\zeta = 1/4$, $\rho = 10^8$, $S = 8 \cdot \times 10^8$ and t^* is represented by the magenta circle. To determine the time t^* we solve the equation $y(t) = S$; in particular, from (2.3), one has:

$$t^* = \zeta\left[1 - \frac{\alpha}{\gamma} + \frac{\beta}{\gamma(1 - e^{-\beta\zeta})}\left(\log S - e^{-\beta\zeta}\log\rho\right)\right].$$ (2.4)

Note that t^* is not the time in which the cancer mass reaches the threshold, but it gives an alarm, indeed before the successive application of the therapy the cancer mass crosses S; in other words, if $t^* \in [(k-1)\zeta, k\zeta]$, then $x_k(t)$ crosses S. To know the time $\bar{t}$ of such crossing, represented by the green circle in Fig. 1, we will consider the intersection of the involved curve $x_k(t)$ with S. In the following Section we analyze some properties of t^* in order to provide the criterion to locate the application times and then we determine $\bar{t}$.

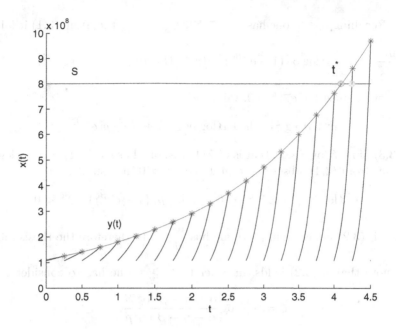

Fig. 1. The process $x(t)$ (black lines), the curve $y(t)$ (red curve) and the threshold S (blue line) with $\alpha = 6.46, \beta = 0.314, \gamma = 0.5, \zeta = 1/4, \rho = 1.074 \times 10^8, S = 8 \cdot 10^8$. The magenta circle is $y(t^*)$ and the green circle is $y(\bar{t})$, with t^* and $\bar{t}$ given in (2.4) and (3.9), respectively (Color figure online).

3 Some Remarks

First of all, we focus on maximizing t^*. Note that parameters α, β, S and ρ are fixed because they are specific of cancer or of patient's organism, hence we can analyze and, eventually, modify only the kind of therapy and the frequency of applications. In other words, we want to determine a strategy, i.e. a couple (γ, ζ), in order to delay the threshold's crossing.

We consider t^* as a function of γ and ρ. For each fixed ζ, t^* is decreasing with respect to γ, that is, if the toxicity of the drug increases, the alarm time t^* decreases. Hence, if we are forced to use a fixed ζ, it is better to apply the most delicate possible therapies.

Instead, for each fixed γ it is not evident the monotony of t^* with respect to ζ, thus we need to pay more attention on the analytic form of t^* by using its derivative with respect to ζ. From (2.4), setting $r = \gamma - \alpha$, one has:

$$\frac{dt^*}{d\zeta} = (r + \beta \log S) \left(1 - e^{-\beta\zeta}\right) - (r + \beta \log \rho) \left(1 - e^{-\beta\zeta}\right) e^{-\beta\zeta} + \zeta\beta^2 e^{-\beta\zeta} \log \frac{\rho}{S}.$$
(3.1)

Proposition 1. *If*

$$\gamma < \alpha - \beta \log S,$$
(3.2)

then the alarm time t^* is a decreasing function of ζ.

Proof. Recalling $\rho < S$, one has $\zeta \beta^2 e^{-\beta \zeta} \log \frac{\rho}{S} < 0$, hence, from (3.1) it follows:

$$\frac{dt^*}{d\zeta} < (r + \beta \log S) \left(1 - e^{-\beta \zeta}\right) - (r + \beta \log \rho) \left(1 - e^{-\beta \zeta}\right) e^{-\beta \zeta}. \qquad (3.3)$$

Moreover, since $1 - e^{-\beta \zeta} > 0$, we have

$$|r + \beta \log S| > |r + \beta \log \rho| > |r + \beta \log \rho| e^{-\beta \zeta}. \qquad (3.4)$$

From (3.3), if $r + \beta \log S < 0$, that is (3.2) holds, one has $r + \beta \log \rho < r + \beta \log S < 0$. So that, from (3.4), observing that $1 - e^{-\beta \zeta} > 0$, it results

$$(r + \beta \log S) \left(1 - e^{-\beta \zeta}\right) < (r + \beta \log \rho) \left(1 - e^{-\beta \zeta}\right) e^{-\beta \zeta} < 0.$$

Thus, if (3.2) holds, from (3.3) one has $\dfrac{dt^*}{d\zeta} < 0$, therefore the thesis follows.

We note that if (3.2) holds, in order to $t^* \geq 0$ one has to consider $\zeta < \bar{\zeta}$, where

$$\bar{\zeta} = -\frac{1}{\beta} \log \frac{\alpha - \gamma - \beta \log S}{\alpha - \gamma - \beta \log \rho}. \qquad (3.5)$$

From Proposition 1, if $\gamma < \alpha - \beta \log S$, we can conclude that t^* decreases with ζ; hence to have a longer crossing time it is better using the smallest plausible $\zeta < \bar{\zeta}$, that is, one should apply the therapies as frequently as possible.

However, (3.2) is only a sufficient condition and it would be interesting to analyze what happens in other cases. In particular, in the following, we determine conditions on γ such that t^* is an increasing function of ζ. To this purpose we consider the following lemma.

Lemma 1. *For all $x > 0$ the function*

$$G(x) = \frac{\beta \log \rho \left(1 - e^{-\beta x}\right) e^{-\beta x} - \beta \log S \left(1 - e^{-\beta x}\right) - \beta^2 x e^{-\beta x} \log \frac{\rho}{S}}{\left(1 - e^{-\beta x}\right)^2} \qquad (3.6)$$

is decreasing.

Proof. The derivative of $G(x)$ with respect to x is:

$$\frac{dG(x)}{dx} = \frac{e^{-\beta x} \log \frac{S}{\rho}}{\left(1 - e^{-\beta x}\right)^2} \left(2 - \beta x \frac{1 + e^{-\beta x}}{1 - e^{-\beta x}}\right).$$

To study the sign of $\dfrac{dG(x)}{dx}$, we note that $\dfrac{e^{-\beta x} \log \frac{S}{\rho}}{\left(1 - e^{-\beta x}\right)^2} > 0$, so we need to pay more attention on the sign of the function $2 - \beta x \dfrac{1 + e^{-\beta x}}{1 - e^{-\beta x}}$ depending only on sign of the function

$$f(y) = 2 \left(1 - e^{-y}\right) - y \left(1 + e^{-y}\right)$$

that is smaller than zero for $y > 0$. Indeed, $f(y)$ is null for $y \to 0$ and it is a decreasing function because, making use of from Bernoulli's inequality $e^y > 1+y$, one has:

$$\frac{df(y)}{dy} = (1+y)e^{-y} - 1 < 0 \qquad y > 0.$$

Hence, the thesis follows.

Proposition 2. *Let ζ_0 be the smallest plausible ζ. If*

$$\gamma > \alpha + G(\zeta_0), \tag{3.7}$$

with $G(\cdot)$ given in (3.6), then the alarm time t^* is a increasing function of ζ.

Proof. From (3.1), we have that $\dfrac{dt^*}{d\zeta} > 0$ if

$$\gamma > \alpha + G(\zeta).$$

Therefore, recalling that $G(\zeta)$ is decreasing respect to ζ, we obtain the thesis.

When condition (3.7) is satisfied, t^* is an increasing function of ζ, so that it is better applying the treatment infrequently.

Once chosen ζ and γ in order to maximize the time t^*, we calculate the crossing time $\bar{t}$ of $x(t)$ with S to understand how long the cancer mass is below the threshold.

To obtain the crossing time $\bar{t}$ we have to calculate k such that $t^* \leq \zeta k$ and then we have to solve the equation $x_k(t) = S$ in the variable t. In particular, taking into consideration the expression of t^* given in (2.4), one has $(k-1)\zeta < t^* \leq \zeta k$ for $k = \bar{k}$ with

$$\bar{k} = \left\lfloor 1 - \frac{\alpha}{\gamma} + \frac{\beta}{\gamma(1 - e^{-\beta\zeta})} \left(\log S - e^{-\beta\zeta} \log \rho \right) \right\rfloor, \tag{3.8}$$

where $\lfloor x \rfloor$ is the largest integer not greater than x. Then, considering this particular $\bar{k}$, that represents the maximum number N of applications, we obtain $\bar{t}$ by solving $x_{\bar{k}}(t) = S$. Hence, the crossing time $\bar{t}$ is:

$$\bar{t} = -\frac{1}{\beta} \log \left[\frac{\log S - \frac{\alpha + \bar{k}\gamma}{\beta}}{\log \rho - \frac{\alpha + \bar{k}\gamma}{\beta}} \right] + \zeta \bar{k}. \tag{3.9}$$

Moreover, we require that at least one application is made, that is $N \geq 1$. To compute the value $\hat{\zeta}$ such that $N \geq 1$, we solve the inequality $\bar{k} \geq 1$ respect to ζ, so from (3.8) we obtain:

$$\zeta \leq -\frac{1}{\beta} \ln \left(\frac{\alpha - \beta \ln S}{\alpha - \beta \ln \rho} \right) = \hat{\zeta}. \tag{3.10}$$

In conclusion, fixed γ, we have the following criterion to decide what is better to do:

- one should apply the therapy as frequently as possible if (3.2) is verified, by choosing $\zeta < \min\{\bar{\zeta}, \hat{\zeta}\}$, with $\hat{\zeta}$ and $\bar{\zeta}$ given in (3.5) and (3.10), respectively;
- one should apply the therapy as infrequently as possible if (3.7) holds, by choosing $\zeta < \hat{\zeta}$, with $\hat{\zeta}$ given in (3.10).

4   Numerical Analysis

To support the provided criterion and to analyze the role of the involved parameters we refer to the parathyroid tumor. Following [4], we consider $\alpha = 6.46 \ year^{-1}$, $\beta = 0.314 \ year^{-1}$ and $\rho = 10^8$. In particular, $\rho = 10^8$ is representative of a 0.1 g tumor mass and corresponds to the clinical threshold namely the smallest diagnosable mass. Since for this kind of tumor the mortality threshold is $9.3438 \cdot 10^8$, we choose $S = 6 \cdot 10^8$.

In Table 1 we show the alarm time t^* obtained from (2.4), the number of application $N = \bar{k}$ determined in (3.8) and the crossing time $\bar{t}$ given in (3.9) for various values of ζ by choosing two therapies with different toxicities; specifically, $\gamma = 0.1$ in the table on the left and $\gamma = 0.6$ on the right table. For $\gamma = 0.1$, one has $\gamma < \alpha - \beta \log S = 0.113294$, so our study suggests to apply the therapy as frequently as possible, with $\zeta < \bar{\zeta} = 12.0021$. The results on the left of Table 1 support this, since longer times are obtained in correspondence of more frequent applications ($\zeta = 1/12$). For $\gamma = 0.6$, one has $\gamma > \alpha + G(\zeta) = 0.404641$, so our study suggests to apply the therapy as infrequently as possible. The results on the right of Table 1 confirm this, since the longest time is obtained for the most infrequent application, that corresponds to $\zeta = 5.6$. We do not consider larger value of ζ because for $\zeta = 5.7$ one has $N = 0$.

Table 1. The alarm times t^* and $\bar{t}$ and the number of applications N are computed for $\alpha_k = 6.46 + \gamma k$, $\beta = 0.314$, $S = 6 \cdot 10^8$, $\rho = 10^8$, $\gamma = 0.1$ on the left, $\gamma = 0.6$ on the right and various choices of ζ.

$\gamma = 0.1$	$\zeta = \frac{1}{12}$	$\zeta = \frac{1}{4}$	$\zeta = \frac{1}{2}$	$\zeta = 1$
t^*	17.67	17.19	16.48	15.11
N	212	68	32	15
$\bar{t}$	17.74	17.24	16.49	15.95

$\gamma = 0.6$	$\zeta = 3$	$\zeta = 4$	$\zeta = 5$	$\zeta = 5.6$
t^*	4.23	4.78	5.28	5.63
N	1	1	1	1
$\bar{t}$	4.85	5.85	6.85	7.45

Now we analyze what happens for values of γ such that $\alpha - \beta \log S < \gamma < \alpha + G(\zeta)$. Note that in these cases we do not have analytical results, so only a numerical analysis can provide an efficient criterion to choose the application times. To this reason, in Table 2 we consider the same parameters of Table 1 with $\gamma = 0.3$ (on the left) and $\gamma = 0.4$ (on the right). For the chosen parameters, from Table 2 one has that if $\gamma = 0.3$ it is better to apply the therapy as frequently as possible, whereas if $\gamma = 0.4$ it is better to apply the therapy infrequently.

Finally, we analyze what happens for different values of the threshold. In Table 3 we consider $\gamma = 0.1$, $\zeta = 1/12$ and we compute N and $\bar{t}$. Obviously, for decreasing values of S the values of N and $\bar{t}$ decrease.

Table 2. The times t^*, $\bar{t}$ and the number of applications N are computed for the same value of Table 1 with $\gamma = 0.3$ on the left, $\gamma = 0.4$ on the right and for various choices of ζ.

$\gamma = 0.3$	$\zeta = \frac{1}{4}$	$\zeta = \frac{1}{2}$	$\zeta = 1$	$\zeta = 2$
t^*	5.89	5.82	5.70	5.53
N	23	11	5	2
$\bar{t}$	5.99	5.98	5.95	5.85

$\gamma = 0.4$	$\zeta = \frac{1}{4}$	$\zeta = \frac{1}{2}$	$\zeta = 1$	$\zeta = 2$
t^*	4.48	4.49	4.52	4.65
N	17	8	4	2
$\bar{t}$	4.49	4.49	4.90	5.52

Table 3. The times $\bar{t}$ and the number of applications N are listed for $\gamma = 0.1$, $\zeta = 1/12$ and various values of S.

S	$6 \cdot 10^8$	$3 \cdot 10^8$	$1.5 \cdot 10^8$
$\bar{t}$	17.74	10.66	3.66
N	212	127	43

Conclusion and Future Developments

We have proposed a deterministic model based on the Gompertz growth to describe the cancer dynamics subject to an intermittent treatment. The therapy is applied at constant intervals and each application shifts the cancer size to a specified value. After the therapeutic application, the process re-starts with an increased parameter of growth. The aim of our study has been to provide an efficient scheduling to maintain the cancer size under a control threshold as long as possible. For some values of the toxicity of the therapy analytical results have been provided, in the other cases we have used a numerical analysis to choice the therapeutic application times in the most appropriate way.

Some developments are possible. Specifically, since there is often a discrepancy between the clinical data and the theoretical predictions, the notion of growth in random environment would be considered. So, starting from the study of the deterministic process, we would analyze the correspondent stochastic model. Moreover, we would infer on the parameters because the choice of times in which to apply the therapy depends on the parameters involved in the model that can be known via statistical procedures. Future study would consist the inclusion of delay times after each therapeutic application. Indeed, it is reasonable to think that the effect of an application is not instantaneous, but it needs a time interval to observe the effect of the treatment. Such interval can have random duration imagining that the reaction times are different for different individuals. Finally, different scheduling would be compared in order to evaluate what is the best strategy in a specified context.

References

1. Giorno, V., Spina, S.: A stochastic gompertz model with jumps for an intermittent treatment in cancer growth. In: Moreno-Díaz, R., Pichler, F., Quesada-Arencibia, A. (eds.) EUROCAST. LNCS, vol. 8111, pp. 61–68. Springer, Heidelberg (2013)

2. Hirata, Y., Bruchovsky, N., Aihara, K.: Development of a mathematical model that predicts the outcome of hormone therapy for prostate cancer. J. Theor. Biol. **264**, 517–527 (2010)
3. Migita, T., Narita, T., Nomura, K.: Activation and therapeutic implications in non-small cell lung cancer. Cancer Res. **268**, 8547–8554 (2008)
4. Parfitt, A.M., Fyhrie, D.P.: Gompertzian growth curves in parathyroid tumors: further evidence for the set-point hypothesis. Cell Prolif. **30**, 341–349 (1997)
5. Spina, S., Giorno, V., Román-Román, P., Torres-Ruiz, F.: A stochastic model of cancer growth subject to an intermittent treatment with combined effects: reduction of tumor size and rise of growth rate. Bull. Math. Biol. **76**, 2711–2736 (2014). doi:10.1007/s11538-014-0026-8
6. Tanaka, G., Hirata, Y., Goldenberg, S.L., Bruchovsky, N., Aihara, K.: Mathematical modelling of prostate cancer growth and its application to hormone therapy. Phil. Trans. R. Soc. A **368**, 5029–5044 (2010)
7. Wang, J., Tucker, L.A., Stavropoulos, J.: Correlation of tumor growth suppression and methionine aminopetidase-2 activity blockade using an orally active inhibitor, Global pharmaceutical Research and Development, Abbott Laboratories. Edit by Brian W. Matthews, University of Oregon; Eugene, OR (2007)

On Time Non-homogeneous Feller-Type Diffusion Process in Neuronal Modeling

Amelia G. Nobile[1]($\boxtimes$) and Enrica Pirozzi[2]

[1] Dipartimento di Studi e Ricerche Aziendali
(Management and Information Technology), Università di Salerno,
84084 Fisciano, SA, Italy
nobile@unisa.it
[2] Dipartimento di Matematica e Applicazioni, Università di Napoli Federico II,
Monte S. Angelo, 80126 Napoli, Italy
epirozzi@unina.it

Abstract. Time non-homogeneous Feller-type and Ornstein-Uhlenbeck diffusion processes are considered for modeling the neuronal activity in the presence of time-varying input signals. In particular, the first passage time (FPT) problem is analyzed for both processes and the averages of FPT through a constant boundary are compared for a constant input signal and for different choices of involved parameters.

1 Diffusion Neuronal Models

Diffusion processes play an important role in the description of input-output behavior of single neurons (see, for instance, [1–11]). In particular, great attention has been dedicated to investigate the Leaky Integrate-and-Fire (LIF) neuronal models when an additional input in the drift is included (cf., for instance, [3,6,7,9]). Several alternative models have been proposed in the literature that take into account the existence of the reversal potential, which restricts the state space of the diffusion process from below (see, [2,4,8,10]).

In Sect. 1.1 we consider a time non-homogeneous Feller-type neuronal model $X(t)$ with the state space $[\nu, +\infty)$, where the lower boundary ν can be viewed as the neuronal reversal hyperpolarization potential. Instead, in Sect. 1.2 we consider an inhomogeneous LIF diffusion model $Y(t)$, described by a suitable Ornstein-Uhlenbeck process. For both models, firing densities are determined as solutions of specified Volterra integral equations and some asymptotic approximations are provided. For constant input signals and constant firing threshold, in Sect. 2 some theoretical and computational comparisons between the FPT averages of Feller and Ornstein-Uhlenbeck processes are carried out.

1.1 Feller-Type Process

A time non-homogeneous Feller-type neuronal model is defined as the diffusion process $\{X(t), t \geq 0\}$, characterized by the following drift and infinitesimal variance:

This paper is partially supported by G.N.C.S.- INdAM and Campania Region.

R. Moreno-Díaz et al. (Eds.): EUROCAST 2015, LNCS 9520, pp. 183–191, 2015.
DOI: 10.1007/978-3-319-27340-2_24

$$A_1(x,t) = -\frac{x-\varrho}{\vartheta} + \mu(t) \qquad A_2(x,t) = 2\xi\left[\frac{\varrho-\nu}{\vartheta} + \mu(t)\right](x-\nu), \qquad (1)$$

defined in the state space $[\nu, +\infty)$, with $\mu(t) \in C^1(0, +\infty)$, $\vartheta > 0$, $\xi > 0$, $\nu \in \mathbb{R}$, $\varrho > \nu$ and $(\varrho - \nu)/\vartheta + \mu(t) > 0$. The time constant ϑ governs the spontaneous decay of the membrane potential to the resting level ϱ, the function $\mu(t)$ represents the time-varying input signal to the neuron and the parameter ξ is an adimensional constant useful for tuning the noise. In the context of neuronal modeling, the lower boundary ν can be viewed as the neuronal reversal hyperpolarization potential.

The transition probability density function (pdf) $f(x,t|y,\tau)$ of $X(t)$ is solution of the following Fokker–Planck equation

$$\frac{\partial f}{\partial t} = -\frac{\partial}{\partial x}\left\{\left[-\frac{x-\varrho}{\vartheta} + \mu(t)\right]f\right\} + \xi\left[\frac{\varrho-\nu}{\vartheta} + \mu(t)\right]\frac{\partial^2}{\partial x^2}\{(x-\nu)f\},$$

with the zero–flux boundary condition at $x = \nu$ and the initial delta condition

$$\lim_{x\downarrow\nu}\left\{\left[-\frac{x-\varrho}{\vartheta} + \mu(t)\right]f\right\} - \xi\left[\frac{\varrho-\nu}{\vartheta} + \mu(t)\right]\frac{\partial}{\partial x}\{(x-\nu)f\} = 0,$$

$$\lim_{t\downarrow\tau} f(x,t|y,\tau) = \delta(x-y),$$

respectively. For $t \geq \tau$, one has:

$$f(x,t|y,\tau) = \frac{1}{\xi\,\Phi(t|\tau)}\exp\left\{-\frac{x-\nu+(y-\nu)e^{-(t-\tau)/\vartheta}}{\xi\,\Phi(t|\tau)}\right\}\left[\frac{x-\nu}{y-\nu}e^{(t-\tau)/\vartheta}\right]^{\frac{1-\xi}{2\xi}}$$

$$\times I_{\frac{1-\xi}{\xi}}\left(\frac{2\sqrt{(y-\nu)(x-\nu)e^{-(t-\tau)/\vartheta}}}{\xi\,\Phi(t|\tau)}\right) \qquad (x>\nu,\ y>\nu), \qquad (2)$$

with

$$\Phi(t|\tau) = (\varrho-\nu)\left(1 - e^{-(t-\tau)/\vartheta}\right) + e^{-t/\vartheta}\int_\tau^t \mu(z)\,e^{z/\vartheta}\,dz$$

and

$$I_\alpha(z) = \sum_{k=0}^{+\infty}\frac{1}{k!\,\Gamma(\alpha+k+1)}\left(\frac{z}{2}\right)^{2k+\alpha} \qquad (\alpha \in \mathbb{R})$$

denoting the modified Bessel function of the first kind. For the process $X(t)$ the boundary $x = \nu$ is a reflecting state if $\xi > 1$, whereas is an entrance boundary if $0 < \xi \leq 1$. The conditional mean and variance of $X(t)$ are:

$$E[X(t)|X(\tau) = y] = y\,e^{-(t-\tau)/\vartheta} + \varrho\left(1 - e^{-(t-\tau)/\vartheta}\right) + e^{-t/\vartheta}\int_\tau^t \mu(z)\,e^{z/\vartheta}\,dz$$

$$(y \geq \nu,\ 0 \leq \tau \leq t) \quad (3)$$

$$\mathrm{Var}[X(t)|X(\tau) = y] = \xi\left[(\varrho-\nu)\left(1 - e^{-(t-\tau)/\vartheta}\right) + e^{-t/\vartheta}\int_\tau^t \mu(z)\,e^{z/\vartheta}\,dz\right]$$

$$\times\left[(\varrho-\nu)\left(1 - e^{-(t-\tau)/\vartheta}\right) + e^{-t/\vartheta}\int_\tau^t \mu(z)\,e^{z/\vartheta}\,dz + 2(y-\nu)e^{-(t-\tau)/\vartheta}\right].$$

For the process $X(t)$ we assume that the neural firing takes place, and consequently an action potential (spike) is observed whenever the neuron's membrane potential $X(t)$ reaches the firing threshold $S(t)$. To this purpose, let $S(t)$ be a $C^1(0, +\infty)$-class function and denote by $g_X[S(t), t|y, \tau]$ the FPT pdf of $X(t)$ from $X(\tau) = y$ to the firing threshold $S(t)$. For $\nu \le y < S(\tau)$, the pdf $g_X[S(t), t|y, \tau]$ satisfies a non-singular second-kind Volterra integral equation (cf. [5]):

$$g_X[S(t), t|y, \tau] = -2\Psi_X[S(t), t|y, \tau] + 2\int_\tau^t g_X[S(u), u|y, \tau]\Psi_X[S(t), t|S(u), u]\,du,$$

where

$$\Psi_X[S(t), t|y, \tau] = \exp\left\{-\frac{S(t) - \nu + (y - \nu)e^{-(t-\tau)/\vartheta}}{\xi\,\Phi(t|\tau)}\right\}\left[\frac{S(t) - \nu}{y - \nu}e^{(t-\tau)/\vartheta}\right]^{\frac{1-\xi}{2\xi}}$$

$$\times \frac{1}{\xi\,\Phi(t|\tau)}\left\{\left[\frac{S'(t)}{2} + \frac{S(t) - \nu}{2\vartheta} + \left(\frac{\varrho - \nu}{\vartheta} + \mu(t)\right)\left(\frac{1}{2} - \frac{\xi}{4} - \frac{S(t) - \nu}{\Phi(t|\tau)}\right)\right]\right.$$

$$\times I_{\frac{1-\xi}{\xi}}\left(\frac{2\sqrt{[S(t) - \nu](y - \nu)}\,e^{-(t-\tau)/\vartheta}}{\xi\,\Phi(t|\tau)}\right) + \frac{\sqrt{[S(t) - \nu](y - \nu)}e^{-(t-\tau)/\vartheta}}{\Phi(t|\tau)}$$

$$\times\left.\left(\frac{\varrho - \nu}{\vartheta} + \mu(t)\right)I_{\frac{1}{\xi}}\left(\frac{2\sqrt{[S(t) - \nu](y - \nu)}\,e^{-(t-\tau)/\vartheta}}{\xi\,\Phi(t|\tau)}\right)\right\}. \qquad (4)$$

Feller-Type Process with Constant Input Signal. If we set $\mu(t) = \mu$ in (1), the process $X(t)$ admits the steady-state density:

$$W_X(x) = \lim_{t\to+\infty} f_X(x, t|y, \tau) = \frac{1}{\Gamma\left(\frac{1}{\xi}\right)}\frac{(x - \nu)^{(1-\xi)/\xi}}{[\xi(\varrho - \nu + \mu\vartheta)]^{1/\xi}}\exp\left\{-\frac{x - \nu}{\xi(\varrho - \nu + \mu\vartheta)}\right\}$$

$$(x > \nu), \qquad (5)$$

from which the asymptotic mean is $m_X = \varrho + \mu\vartheta$ and the asymptotic variance is $v_X = \xi(\varrho - \nu + \mu\vartheta)^2$. When $\xi \ge 1$ (ν is a regular boundary) $W_X(x)$ is a decreasing function of $x > \nu$; instead, for $0 < \xi < 1$ (ν is an entrance boundary) $W_X(x)$ presents a maximum in $\varrho + \mu\vartheta - \xi(\varrho - \nu + \mu\vartheta)$, that is equal to the asymptotic mode. Hence, if $0 < \xi < 1$ the asymptotic mode is always lower than the asymptotic mean m_X.

If $\mu(t) = \mu$ and $S(t) \equiv S > y \ge \nu$, the FPT probability $P(S|y) = \int_0^{+\infty} g_X(S, t|y)\,dt$ is unity and the mean FPT of the Feller process is (cf. [11]):

$$t_1(S|y) = \vartheta\left\{\frac{S - y}{\varrho - \nu + \mu\vartheta} + \sum_{k=1}^{+\infty}\frac{(S - \nu)^{k+1} - (y - \nu)^{k+1}}{(k + 1)(\varrho - \nu + \mu\vartheta)^{k+1}\prod_{i=1}^{k}(1 + i\xi)}\right\}. \qquad (6)$$

Furthermore, if $S > y \ge \nu$ for large threshold S the firing density $g_X(S, t|y)$ of the Feller process admits an exponential behavior:

$$g_X(S, t|y) \simeq R_X(S)\,e^{-R_X(S)t} \qquad (S > \varrho + \mu\vartheta > \nu, \varrho - \nu + \mu\vartheta > 0), \qquad (7)$$

where, by virtue of (4) and (5), one has:

$$R_X(S) = -2 \lim_{t \to +\infty} \Psi_X(S, t|y) = \left[\frac{S - (\varrho + \mu\vartheta)}{\vartheta} + \frac{\xi(\varrho - \nu + \mu\vartheta)}{2\vartheta} \right] W_X(S).$$

1.2   Ornstein-Uhlenbeck Process

A time non-homogeneous Ornstein-Uhlenbeck (OU) neuronal model is defined as the diffusion process $\{Y(t), t \geq 0\}$, characterized by the following drift and infinitesimal variance:

$$B_1(x, t) = -\frac{x - \varrho}{\vartheta} + \mu(t) \qquad B_2(t) = \sigma^2(t) \qquad (\vartheta > 0, \varrho \in \mathbb{R}), \qquad (8)$$

defined in the state space $(-\infty, +\infty)$, where $\mu(t)$, $\sigma(t) \in C^1(0, +\infty)$, with $\sigma(t) > 0$. Differently from the Feller-type process, in the OU process the infinitesimal variance is not state-dependent, while the drift preserves its linearity.

In the context of neuronal models, (8) characterize an inhomogeneous LIF diffusion process $Y(t)$, describing the evolution of the membrane potential, where $\sigma^2(t)$ gives the intensity of the noise.

The transition pdf $f_Y(x, t|y, \tau)$ of $Y(t)$ is normal with the following mean and variance:

$$E[Y(t)|Y(\tau) = y] = y e^{-(t-\tau)/\vartheta} + \varrho \left(1 - e^{-(t-\tau)/\vartheta}\right) + e^{-t/\vartheta} \int_\tau^t \mu(z) e^{z/\vartheta} \, dz$$

$$(y \in \mathbb{R}, \ 0 \leq \tau \leq t) \quad (9)$$

$$\mathrm{Var}[Y(t)|Y(\tau) = y] = e^{-2t/\vartheta} \int_\tau^t \sigma^2(z) e^{2z/\vartheta} \, dz.$$

When $y \geq \nu$, from (3) and (9) we note that the conditional mean of the Feller process (1) is identical to the conditional mean of the OU process (8), whereas the conditional variances are different.

For the process $Y(t)$ let $g_Y[S(t), t|y, \tau]$ be the FPT pdf of $Y(t)$ to the firing threshold $S(t) \in C^1(0, +\infty)$ starting from $Y(\tau) = y$. As shown [5], $g_Y[S(t), t|y, \tau]$ satisfies a non-singular second-kind Volterra integral equation

$$g_Y[S(t), t|y, \tau] = -2\Psi_Y[S(t), t|y, \tau] + 2 \int_\tau^t g_Y[S(u), u|y, \tau] \Psi_Y[S(t), t|S(u), u] \, du,$$

with $y < S(\tau)$, where

$$\Psi_Y[S(t), t|y, \tau] = \left\{ \frac{S'(t) - m'(t)}{2} + \frac{S(t) - m(t)}{2} \left[\frac{1}{\vartheta} - \frac{\sigma^2(t) e^{2t/\vartheta}}{\int_\tau^t \sigma^2(\xi) e^{2\xi/\vartheta} \, d\xi} \right] \right.$$

$$\left. + \frac{y - m(\tau)}{2} \frac{\sigma^2(t) e^{(t+\tau)/\vartheta}}{\int_\tau^t \sigma^2(\xi) e^{2\xi/\vartheta} \, d\xi} \right\} f_Y[S(t), t|y, \tau]. \qquad (10)$$

OU Process with Constant Input Signal. We assume that the input signal, the intensity of the noise and the threshold are constant, i.e.

$$\mu(t) = \mu, \quad \sigma^2(t) = \sigma^2, \quad S(t) = S. \tag{11}$$

If we set $\mu(t) = \mu$ and $\sigma^2(t) = \sigma^2$ in (8), the process $Y(t)$ admits a normal steady-state density with mean $m_Y = \varrho + \mu\vartheta$ and variance $v_Y = \sigma^2\vartheta/2$:

$$W_Y(x) = \lim_{t\to+\infty} f_Y(x,t|y,\tau) = \frac{1}{\sigma\sqrt{\pi\vartheta}} \exp\left\{-\frac{(x - \varrho - \mu\vartheta)^2}{\sigma^2\vartheta}\right\} \quad (x \in \mathbb{R}). \tag{12}$$

Under the assumptions (11), for $S > y$ the first passage time probability $P(S|y) = \int_0^{+\infty} g_Y(S,t|y,0)\, dt$ is unity and the mean FPT of the OU process is (cf. [11]):

$$t_1(S|y) = \vartheta\left\{\sqrt{\pi}\sum_{k=0}^{\infty} \frac{(S - \varrho - \mu\vartheta)^{2k+1} - (y - \varrho - \mu\vartheta)^{2k+1}}{(2k+1)\,k!\,(\sigma\sqrt{\vartheta})^{2k+1}}\right.$$
$$\left. + \sum_{k=0}^{\infty} \frac{2^k\,[(S - \varrho - \mu\vartheta)^{2k+2} - (y - \varrho - \mu\vartheta)^{2k+2}]}{(k+1)\,(2k+1)!!\,(\sigma\sqrt{\vartheta})^{2k+2}}\right\} \quad (y < S). \tag{13}$$

Moreover, if $S > y$ for large threshold S the firing density $g_Y(S,t|y)$ of the OU process admits an exponential behavior:

$$g_Y(S,t|y) \simeq R_Y(S)\, e^{-R_Y(S)\,t} \quad (S > \varrho + \mu\vartheta), \tag{14}$$

obtained from (10) and (12), with

$$R_Y(S) = -2 \lim_{t\to+\infty} \Psi_Y(S,t|y) = \frac{S - \varrho - \mu\vartheta}{\vartheta}\, W_Y(S).$$

Under the assumptions (11), the models (1) and (8) have identical drifts involving parameters ϑ, ϱ and μ. Infinitesimal variances are instead different from one another, both functionally and in terms of the involved parameters. In order to compare the two models, we consider the parameters in the Feller model $(\xi, \nu, \vartheta, \varrho, \mu)$ as fixed and determine σ^2, appearing in OU model, by imposing the equality of the asymptotic variances, i.e. $v_Y = v_X$, so that

$$\sigma^2 = \frac{2\xi}{\vartheta}(\varrho - \nu + \mu\vartheta)^2 \quad (\varrho - \nu + \mu\vartheta > 0). \tag{15}$$

Under the assumption (15), in Fig. 1 the steady-state densities (5) and (12) are compared for $\vartheta = 5$, $\mu = 0.5$, $\varrho = -2.5$, $\nu = -5.5$, with $\xi = 0.2$ on the left and $\xi = 1.2$ on the right. By virtue of (15), for $\xi = 0.2$ one has $\sigma^2 = 2.42$, whereas for $\xi = 1.2$ results $\sigma^2 = 14.52$. Moreover, under the assumption (15), in Fig. 2 the asymptotic firing densities (7) and (14) for the Feller and OU processes are plotted for $\xi = 0.2$ on the left and $\xi = 1.2$ on the right.

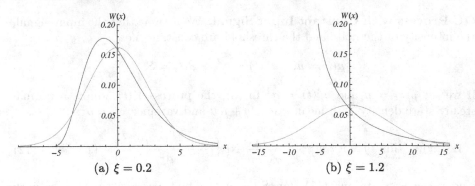

Fig. 1. Steady-state densities for the OU process (red curves) and for the Feller process (blue curves) are plotted for $\vartheta = 5$, $\mu = 0.5$, $\varrho = -2.5$ and $\nu = -5.5$ (Color figure online).

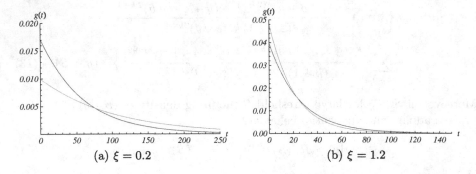

Fig. 2. For OU (red curves) and for Feller (blue curves) processes, (7) and (14) are plotted as function of t for $\vartheta = 5$, $\nu = -5.5$, $\varrho = -2.5$, $\mu = 0.5$, $y = -0.4$ and $S = 6$ (Color figure online).

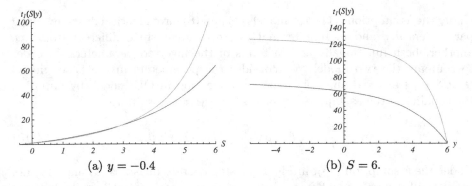

Fig. 3. $t_1(S|y)$ for the OU process (red curves) and for the Feller process (blue curves) is plotted as functions of the threshold S in (a) and as function of the initial value y in (b) for $\vartheta = 5$, $\xi = 0.2$, $\mu = 0.5$, $\varrho = -2.5$ and $\nu = -5.5$ (Color figure online).

2   Some Comparisons

In this section, assuming that (11) and (15) hold, some theoretical and computational results on $t_1(S|y)$ are indicated. First of all, for both the models $t_1(S|y)$ increases as S increases and it decreases as y increases (see Fig. 3). For OU and Feller models, $t_1(S|y)$ decreases as ξ increases. Indeed, since ξ appears as a multiplicative parameter only in the infinitesimal variance of the two models, on the average reaching the firing threshold S becomes most likely when ξ increases. Furthermore, for the Feller model one has

$$\xi_\infty = \lim_{\xi \to +\infty} t_1(S|y) = \frac{\vartheta(S - y)}{\varrho - \nu + \mu\vartheta},$$

whereas for the OU model $t_1(S|y)$ approaches 0 as ξ diverges (cf. Fig. 4(a)). Moreover, for OU and Feller models, $t_1(S|y)$ decreases as μ increases (cf. Fig. 4(b)).

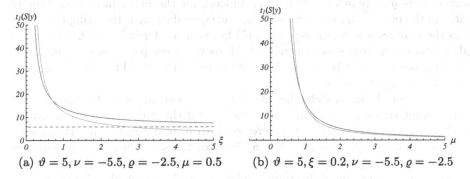

(a) $\vartheta = 5, \nu = -5.5, \varrho = -2.5, \mu = 0.5$ (b) $\vartheta = 5, \xi = 0.2, \nu = -5.5, \varrho = -2.5$

Fig. 4. For the OU process (red curves) and for the Feller process (blue curves) $t_1(S|y)$ is plotted as function of ξ on the left and as function of μ on the right for $y = -0.4$ and $S = 6$. The dashed line in Fig. 4(a) indicates the asymptotic value $\xi_\infty = 5.5$ (Color figure online).

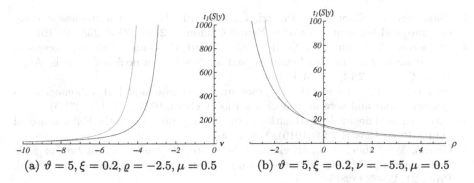

(a) $\vartheta = 5, \xi = 0.2, \varrho = -2.5, \mu = 0.5$ (b) $\vartheta = 5, \xi = 0.2, \nu = -5.5, \mu = 0.5$

Fig. 5. For the OU process (red curves) and for the Feller process (blue curves) $t_1(S|y)$ is plotted as function of ν on the left and as function of ρ on the right for $y = -0.4$ and $S = 6$.

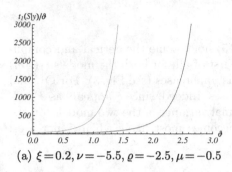 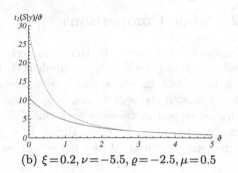

(a) $\xi = 0.2, \nu = -5.5, \varrho = -2.5, \mu = -0.5$ (b) $\xi = 0.2, \nu = -5.5, \varrho = -2.5, \mu = 0.5$

Fig. 6. For the OU process (red curves) and for the Feller process (blue curves), $t_1(S|y)/\vartheta$ is plotted as function of ϑ for $y = -0.4$ and $S = 1$.

Furthermore, for both models, $t_1(S|y)$ increases with ν (cf. Fig. 5(a)) and it decreases as ϱ increases (cf. Fig. 5(b)). Indeed, for the Feller model the sample paths of the process are progressively more attracted towards the firing threshold S as the boundary ν decreases; since (15) holds, a similar behavior holds for the OU model (σ^2 increases as ν decreases). Moreover, since $\varrho + \mu\vartheta$ is an equilibrium point for the two models, the reaching of the firing threshold becomes more and more likely as ϱ increases.

For OU and Feller models, the ratio $t_1(S|y)/\vartheta$ is constant in ϑ in the absence of the input signal ($\mu = 0$); instead, when $\mu > 0$ the ratio $t_1(S|y)/\vartheta$ decreases as ϑ increases, whereas this ratio increases with ϑ for a negative input signal μ. This behavior of $t_1(S|y)/\vartheta$ is shown in Fig. 6 for the same choices of parameters ξ, ν, ϱ, y, S and for $\mu = -0.5$ on the left and for $\mu = 0.5$ on the right.

The analysis of the Feller-type model when the input signal $\mu(t)$ decays exponentially or is a periodic function of time will be the object to future works.

References

1. Buonocore, A., Caputo, L., Pirozzi, E., Ricciardi, L.M.: On a stochastic leaky integrate-and-fire neuronal model. Neural Comput. **22**(10), 2558–2585 (2010)
2. Buonocore, A., Caputo, L., Nobile, A.G., Pirozzi, E.: Gauss-Markov processes in the presence of a reflecting boundary and applications in neuronal models. Appl. Math. Comput. **232**, 799–809 (2014)
3. Burkitt, A.N.: A review of the integrate-and-fire neuron model. II. Inhomogeneous synaptic input and network properties. Biol. Cybern. **95**(2), 97–112 (2006)
4. Ditlevsen, S., Lánský, P.: Estimation of the input parameters in the Feller neuronal model. Phys. Rev. E **73**(061910), 1–9 (2006)
5. Giorno, V., Nobile, A.G., Ricciardi, L.M., Sato, S.: On the evaluation of first-passage-time probability densities via non-singular integral equation. Adv. Appl. Prob. **21**, 20–36 (1989)
6. Giorno, V., Spina, S.: On the return process with refractoriness for a non-homogeneous Ornstein-Uhlenbeck neuronal model. Math. Biosci. Eng. **11**(2), 285–302 (2014)

7. Giraudo, M.T., Sacerdote, L.: Effect of periodic stimulus on a neuronal diffusion model with signal-dependent noise. BioSystems **79**, 73–81 (2005)
8. Inoue, J., Doi, S.: Sensitive dependence of the coefficient of variation of interspike intervals on the lower boundary of membrane potential for leaky integrate-and.fire neuron model. BioSystems **87**, 49–57 (2007)
9. Kobayashi, R., Shinomoto, S., Lánský, P.: Estimation of time-dependent input from neuronal membrane potential. Neural Comput. **23**, 3070–3093 (2011)
10. Lánský, P., Ditlevsen, S.: A review of the methods for signal estimation in stochastic diffusion leaky integrate-and-fire neuronal models. Biol. Cybern. **99**, 253–262 (2008)
11. Ricciardi, L.M., Di Crescenzo, A., Giorno, V., Nobile, A.G.: An outline of theoretical and algorithmic approaches to first passage time problems with applications to biological modeling. Math. Japonica **50**(2), 247–322 (1999)

Intelligent Information Processing

A Practical Experience on Reusing Problem-Solving Methods for Assessment Tasks

Abraham Rodríguez-Rodríguez[1]([⊠]), Gilberto Martel-Rodríguez[2],
Miguel Márquez-Marfil[2], and Francisca Quintana-Domínguez[1]

[1] Instituto Universitario de Ciencias y Tecnologías Cibernéticas,
Universidad de Las Palmas de Gran Canaria, Campus de Tafira,
35017 Las Palmas, Spain
{abraham.rodriguez,francisca.quintana}@ulpgc.es
[2] Departamento de Agua, Instituto Tecnológico de Canarias, Playa de Pozo
Izquierdo, s/n, 35119 Saint Lucia, Gran Canaria, Spain
{gmartel,mmarquez}@itccanarias.org

Abstract. Problem-solving methods (PSMs) facilitate the development of knowledge-based systems (KBSs), which provide an initial scheme to model both the domain knowledge and the inference process. However, the actual benefits of reusing PSMs are still unclear because most of the specifications omit how the structure must be adapted to fit into the current problem. This article describes our experience in the development of a KBS for the selection of wastewater treatment technologies by reusing a well-known PSM from the CommonKADS library. We describe how the adaptation process was performed, which involved both the simplification of the original inference template and the inclusion of new basic inferences.

Keywords: Problem-solving method · Knowledge-based system · Wastewater treatment technology

1 Introduction

The CARMAC Project consists of several initiatives with the common objective of improving the quality of the coastal environment in the European Macaronesian (which consists of the Canary, Azores and Madeira archipelagos) and particularly highlights the protection of hydrological resources in the coastal areas. One of the main objectives has been to provide support and advice on wastewater technologies, products, systems and companies to anyone interested in this topic. A knowledge-based system (KBS) has been developed as a part of this goal, which proposes a combination of technologies for wastewater treatment in an environment with up to 2000 population equivalent spill flow.

Wastewater treatment (WWT) involves physical, biological, and chemical processes, which ensure that the resultant pollution levels of treated effluent are within the applicable legal limits, and assumed in a sustainable manner by the operator and the environment. In general, small settlements and installations present the greatest

© Springer International Publishing Switzerland 2015
R. Moreno-Díaz et al. (Eds.): EUROCAST 2015, LNCS 9520, pp. 195–202, 2015.
DOI: 10.1007/978-3-319-27340-2_25

deficiencies in WWTs. Sewage treatment often cannot be solved using the same technologies as in medium and large-scale cases [1, 2]. However, decentralized wastewater solutions open a range of alternative technologies and combinations to achieve the desired level of performance. One of the main problems is the lack of knowledge of these possibilities by the stakeholders who make the final decision regarding the solutions. Within this context, accessible and comprehensive decision-making supporting tools used in the selection between different techniques and combinations according to the local conditions would be useful in resolving this constraint. Our tool will try to present the knowledge and alternatives to non-expert decision makers and to place them into contact with experts.

1.1 Problem-Solving Methods

The field of KBS is a long-established research area with several success cases. However, it is also known that the development of these types of systems must overcome multiple difficulties, making it a high-cost technology with a large number of failed developments. Some model-based methodologies, such as VITAL [3], MIKE [4] or CommonKADS [5], stress the use of generic components to facilitate the reuse of knowledge, Problem-Solving Methods (PSM) and code.

PSM are high-level structures that demonstrate how to reason using knowledge to achieve a goal [6]. PSM usually implements some type of generic task, such as diagnosis, assessment, or planning, and it provides a set of inferences and knowledge descriptions that enable the generation of a solution without any reference to specific domain elements. Thus, PSMs function at the knowledge-level as defined by Newell [7] in 1982. Clancey [8] validated some of Newell's ideas with his work on Heuristic Classification, which were later evolved by Chandrasekaran's works on Generic Tasks [9]. Model-based methodologies consider PSMs to be essential structures that are useful for controlling the methodological activities that must be performed to build an expertise model. PSMs claim to be valuable pieces to build KBS because they enforce the reutilisation of proven problem-solving strategies, and also facilitate organising and structuring a knowledge base via the use of knowledge structures (sometimes referred to as knowledge-roles).

Despite the optimism that can be deduced from some conclusions appearing in [10], PSM-based techniques have not achieved the expected success Some reasons that may have prevented the widespread adoptions of PSMs are discussed in (some reasons were discussed in [11–14]). However, as indicated by Brown [6], "*it was as if the people in the knowledge systems and engineering community totally lost their memory when they turned to the Web.*" In this sense, we are convinced that there are many interesting research issues that have been yet to be explored. We concur with those who view the use of PSMs as an approach to manage complexity, not only in the design and implementation of software systems, as argued in [15], but also in the analysis stage, where PSMs play an essential role to facilitate the integration of heterogeneous knowledge sources and domain perceptions. This article will describe our experience reusing a PSM and how the initial approach had to be modified to accommodate the specific characteristics of the actual task.

2   An Assessment Task for the Selection of Wastewater Treatment Technologies

The primary goal of this project was to *design* a combination of treatment technologies that complies with the requirements supplied by the user. However, we have reformulated the problem in the following manner: *to assess to what extent a particular combination of treatment technologies fits into the characteristics of the spill described by the user*, and how it iterates over a pre-defined set of plausible combinations of treatment systems. By doing so, we have transformed the type of generic task from synthesis to analysis, thus avoiding the inherent complexity of np-complex problems in favour of a simpler type. Among the types of analytical systems, as defined in the CommonKADS methodology [5], the assessment tasks fitted well with our project objectives and, as a consequence, we thought that the assessment model could give us a head start in domain modelling (Fig. 1).

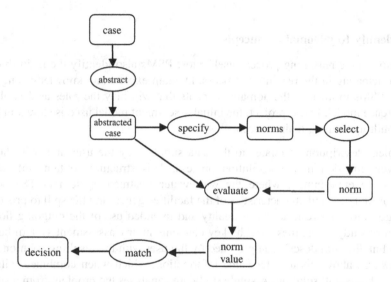

Fig. 1. Inference structure of the CommonKADS assessment method.

According to the generic task definition, the goal consisted of finding a decision category for a case, based on a set of domain specific norms. The default method usually starts by abstracting some of the case data. Next, depending on the case data, all of the relevant norms/criteria are selected for evaluation. The actual evaluation of every norm is made in the evaluate inference using the case data, and produces a qualitative value for each norm. In simple systems, this process produces a true/false value for the norm. The match inference will then confirm whether the results from the evaluation process lead to a decision.

Although the solving method described by any PSM tries to mimic human reasoning, that process is not always so simple. In our experience, the gap between these two resolution methods may cause difficulties during the entire development process, particularly when modelling expert knowledge. To overcome this risk, a balance must be found between both models of inference. The generated PSM method should maintain the main elements of the original assessment, while integrating new inferences to reflect the processes identified by human experts. In our case, the PSM was used to set a common sandbox that enables us to work with several human experts, while facilitating the integration of heterogeneous knowledge that is derived from multiple sources and written in different languages.

Once the type of task has been identified, the developing process was structured into two stages:

1. Describe the domain key elements and map them over the inference scheme, as defined in the PSM.
2. Adapt the PSM and operationalise the inferences, which involved making major changes to the PSM and detailing how all of the inference processes were to be implemented.

2.1   Identify Key Domain Concepts

In addition to the reasoning process itself, most PSMs also identify the main dynamic roles participating in the resolution process. Domain experts and knowledge engineers will use PSMs to identify the domain elements that will play the roles as described in the inference model. In our project, the initial assessment model used is shown in Fig. 1 and is built upon three main concepts:

- Problem description: it relates to the data supplied by the user and will play any relevant function in the resolution process. This structure contains information about the environment where the wastewater treatment system (WTS) will be deployed; types and characteristics of the facilities generating the spill to process; or the goals to achieve in terms of quality and intended use of the outgoing flow.
- A set of study areas: these are the key elements in any assessment system because they link the spill description provided by the user with the resulting solution. Each study area allows us to infer some information, which when combined will constitute the overall solution. A single study area analyses the problem from a specific dimension, such as odour generation, noise production, unusual overload, etc. The user input data are used to deduce the relevance of each study area or criteria. A WTS will be assessed only considering the relevance of the study areas and how the evaluated technologies fit (i.e., how well does a technology perform from the perspective of each study area).
- The solution structure: any solution represents a wastewater treatment system consisting of a set of linked technologies. In most cases, the resulting solution consists of a sequential combination of one technology from each category: preliminary, primary, secondary and tertiary. Each component is further parameterised by attributes and relationships, such as the required area (m^2) or performance (in terms of BOD^5 in the outgoing flow).

2.2   Adapt the PSM and Operationalise the Inferences

In this phase, the original PSM was modified to fit the actual inference process. It also included the description of the methods that will implement each stage of the PSM. The starting diagramme, shown in Fig. 1, was the original PSM, although the reasoning process of the human experts made necessary to delete, modify and include some reasoning steps. The resulting diagramme and its associated methods were used as a 'proof of concept,' which had to be assumed by all the human experts participating in the project. This new model also reflects how the key elements identified in the previous identifying step map into their inferences and roles.

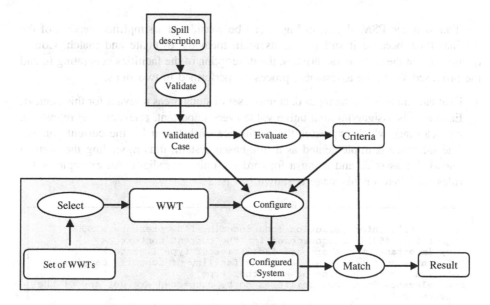

Fig. 2. Derived PSM.

The graded areas in Fig. 2 correspond to the added inferences and roles. The *validate* inference is used to confirm the coherence of the information provided by the user. Depending on the types of facilities (and their characteristics) that will be connected to the plant, the System is able to estimate the population equivalent, the incoming flow and the expected BOD^5.

The assessment process iterates over a set of WTS candidates. Each candidate is defined by the primary and/or secondary stages (i.e., septic tank + facultative lagoon). The list was elaborated by the expert and limits the combination to those that are feasible. The current version considers 28 combinations with the technologies considered. The Select inference selects the next combination in the list and passes it forward.

The Configure inference will try to complete the WTS with preliminary stages and configure each technology according to the user's requirements (mainly required area and performance). The preliminary stage is selected considering the technologies that have already been set for the other stages and the contextual information of the user's input. List 1 shows one of the rules used to set the preliminary stage.

```
Set the preliminary stage to Overflow cannel + screening + degritter
+ degreasing
When
The population equivalent is between 1000 and 2000 And
The secondary treatment is in (Bacteria Bed, Rotating biological con-
tactor)
```

List 1

The modified PSM shown in Fig. 2 can be considered a simplified version of the original PSM because it still retains its main methods: evaluate and match. Consequently, given the spill characteristics, the description of the facilities generating it, and the proposed WTS, the assessment process is performed in two steps:

1. Evaluate: transforms the input data into a set of study areas relevant for this context. Each area is assigned a qualitative value (very important, relevant, low relevance, not relevant), which expresses the pertinence of that area for the current context. The inference is implemented as a rule-based system, thus modelling the domain knowledge as rules and using a forward reasoning paradigm. An example of the rules modelled for this stage is shown in List 2.

```
The criteria "high pollution (the incoming flow presents a BOD5
higher than 450)" is considered for the current context as
Very important when there are facilities of type livestock.
Relevant when there is at least one facility of schools, camping or
hotels and more than one of any other type.
Low relevance when the facilities to be connected are not any of the
previous criteria.
Not relevant when the deduced BOD5 is lower than 450.
```

List 2

2. Match: This inference receives two inputs. The first input is a set of study areas and their relevance to the current problem. The second input is a complex structure that describes the wastewater treatment system in all of its stages (further details will be provided below). The relevance of each technology to the current problem is calculated considering the relevance of the study areas and their relationship with the technologies included in the WTS. This is implemented using an associative table, which uses the criteria and the technologies referenced in the WTS as the keys to the table. These values are later combined into a global result value using a nearest-neighbour formula.

The qualitative values of both the criteria relevance (as deduced in step 1) and how a technology complies with a single criterion (as defined in the associative table) are translated into numerical values using a predefined scale. The actual values of these parameters were empirically adjusted using a set of test scenarios.

The formula is evaluated for every combination of the predefined systems skeletons, as previously stated. The best solution, which is defined as the one with the higher rank, is presented to the user together with a shortened version of some alternatives. The KBS is embedded into an Information System (IS), which was also implemented as part of the CARMAC project. The IS was conceived to provide access to technical information, expert advice and to encourage the collaboration between experts and services industries.

3 Conclusions

We have developed an assessment KBS which smoothly integrates into the main information portal, in such a way that no distinction is made between the solutions generated by the human experts or by the KBS. They will use the same input forms with similar information and appearance.

Although the PSM can be considered to be a developing guide for KBS, the balance between re-usability and usability can be difficult to achieve depending on the characteristics of the target domain. In this specific case, the original CommonKADS inference scheme was gradually simplified until only the most relevant inferences were retained, and at the same time, new specific components were integrated into the PSM to match specific domain tasks and knowledge types. Overall, the perceived benefits of re-using a PSM as a whole could be synthesized as follows:

- They provide guidelines for representing and structuring the domain knowledge.
- They make possible the scheduling of knowledge acquisition sessions, which could be focused on specific goals, such as obtaining validation rules for the problem description (tied in with the 'validate' inference) or determining the relevance of the criterion (linked with the 'evaluate' inference).
- They facilitate the initial understanding of the assessment task, for both domain experts and computer scientists, thus smoothing the communication process and the transition to the final versions of the PSM.

The experience gained during the development of this project and the derived PSM scheme is currently being applied to develop a practical standard classification targeted at the categorisation of the touristic facilities considering the technological services that they provide. Although this initiative is still in progress, some preliminary results confirming the applicability of the derived PSM has been previously published [16].

Acknowledgements. This work has been partially supported by the European Community's Transnational Cooperation Programme Madeira-Açores-Canarias (MAC) 2007–2013 through the project "*Mejora de la calidad de las aguas recreativas y costeras de la Macaronesia (CARMAC)*", ref. MAC/2/2011, and by the Instituto Universitario de Ciencias y Tecnologías Cibernéticas at the University of Las Palmas de Gran Canaria.

References

1. Salas, J., Martel, G., Vera, L., Sardón, N.: Fundamentos de los sistemas de depuración natural (SDN). Tecnologías disponibles. In: Gestiónn sostenible del agua residual en entornos rurales: Proyecto Depuranat, pp. 3–33. Netbiblo, Oleiros (2008)
2. Aragón, C., Salas, J., Ortega, E., Ferrer, Y.: Lacks and needs of R&D on wastewater treatment in small populations. Water Pract. Technol. **6**(2) (2011). doi:10.2166/wpt.2011.030
3. Domingue, J., Motta, E., Watt, S.: The emerging VITAL workbench. In: Aussenac, N., Boy, G., Gaines, B., Linster, M., Ganasica, J.-G., Kodratoff, Y. (eds.) EKAW 1993. LNAI, vol. 723, pp. 320–339. Springer, Heidelberg (1993)
4. Angele, J., Fensel, D., Studer, R.: Domain and task modeling in MIKE. In: Proceedings of the IFIP WG8.1/13.2 Joint Working Conference on Domain Knowledge for Interactive System Design, pp. 8–10, Hall (1996)
5. Schreiber, G.T., Akkermans, H.: Knowledge Engineering and Management: The CommonKADS Methodology. MIT Press, Cambridge (2000)
6. Brown, D.C.: Problem solving methods: past, present, and future. Artif. Intell. Eng. Des. Anal. Manuf. **23**(Special Issue 04), 327–329 (2009)
7. Newell, A.: The knowledge level. Artif. Intell. **18**, 87–127 (1982)
8. Clancey, W.J.: Heuristic classification. Artif. Intell. **27**, 289–350 (1985)
9. Chandrasekaran, B.: Generic tasks in knowledge-based reasoning: a level of abstraction that supports knowledge acquisition, system design and explanation. In: Proceedings of the ACM SIGART International Symposium on Methodologies for Intelligent Systems (1986)
10. Benjamins, V.R., Fensel, D., Chandrasekaran, B.: PSMs do IT! - summary of track on sharable and reusable problem-solving methods of the 10th KAW96, Banff, Canada. http://citeseer.ist.psu.edu/viewdoc/download;jsessionid=92FE14AF41B38DC2CB90A0078B0742B6?doi=10.1.1.42.6181&rep=rep1&type=pdf
11. Breuker, J., Van de Velde, W.: CommonKADS Library for Expertise Modelling: Reusable Problem Solving Components. IOS Press, Amsterdam (1994)
12. Motta, E., Rajpathak, D., Zdrahal, Z., Roy, R.: The epistemology of scheduling problems. In: Proceedings of the 15th European Conference on Artificial Intelligence (2002)
13. Rodríguez, A., Palma, J., Quintana, F.: Experiences in reusing problem solving methods – an application in constraint programming. In: Palade, V., Howlett, R.J., Jain, L. (eds.) KES 2003. LNCS, vol. 2774, pp. 1299–1306. Springer, Heidelberg (2003)
14. Chandrasekaran, B.: Problem solving methods and knowledge systems: a personal journey to perceptual images as knowledge. Artif. Intell. Eng. Des. Anal. Manuf. **23**(Special Issue 04), 331–338 (2009)
15. O'Connor, M.J., Nyulas, C., Tu, S., Buckeridge, D.L., Okhmatovskaia, A., Musen, M.A.: Software-engineering challenges of building and deploying reusable problem solvers. Artif. Intell. Eng. Des. Anal. Manuf. **23**(Special Issue 04), 339–356 (2009)
16. Rodriguez-Rodriguez, A., Tejera-Correa, S., Moreno-Díaz, R.J.: 5@: a standard specification for the technological services provided at touristic facilities. In: 14th International Conference on Computer Aided Systems Theory (EUROCAST 2013), Las Palmas de Gran Canaria (2013)

Requirements for Long-Term Preservation of Digital Videos and First Experiments with an XMT-Based Approach

Alexander Uherek$^{(\boxtimes)}$, Sonja Maier, and Uwe M. Borghoff

Computer Science Department, Universität der Bundeswehr München,
85577 Neubiberg, Germany
`{alexander.uherek,sonja.maier,uwe.borghoff}@unibw.de`

Abstract. In this paper, we deal with the emerging challenge of long-term preservation of digital videos. We focus on aspects that have to be considered for long-term preservation in general and identify requirements for long-term preservation of digital videos. We refine an XMT-based approach, which was introduced in [1], document the experiences we gained during the design and implementation of a first prototype and give details about some major advantages and challenges that result from the separation of different artifacts and the use of an XML wrapper.

Keywords: Long-term preservation · Digital video · Requirements · XMT

1 Introduction

Video is one of the most important types of media we use today. Not all, but surely a lot of video material should be preserved for future generations. Nevertheless, a standard format for long-term preservation of digital videos has not been found, yet. In many cases, RAW formats or video tapes are used for archiving, in order to keep as much information as possible for later use. Today, the growing masses of data and the ongoing evolution of system environments and formats make it necessary to establish standards, soon. Lots of videos or at least parts of it might get lost, when storage mediums get damaged, the video material cannot be processed by contemporary systems or simply the migration of the growing masses of videos gets too costly.

In the following, we will give an overview on the topic of long-term preservation. Afterwards, we give details about special requirements for long-term preservation of digital videos and have a look at infrastructures for preservation. In Sect. 2, we will sketch our envisioned approach for the long-term preservation of digital videos. We further describe a first prototype that we have designed for poof of concept and summarize the experiences that we gained. At the end, we will give an outlook of our future work.

© Springer International Publishing Switzerland 2015
R. Moreno-Díaz et al. (Eds.): EUROCAST 2015, LNCS 9520, pp. 203–210, 2015.
DOI: 10.1007/978-3-319-27340-2_26

1.1 Long-Term Preservation

First of all, we have to make clear that when we talk about long-term preservation of videos, we do not only talk about playing a video taken in the last few years or about processing movies taken at the beginning of this technology (about 100 years ago). We talk about the preservation that aims to keep videos processable even in the very far future. For long-term preservation in general, some approaches have been identified to tackle this problem. In [2], technical approaches for long-term preservation are categorized as follows:

Hardware museums try to preserve the original system environments with hard- and software for future use. This approach provides the highest degree of authenticity.

Emulation means that contemporary systems get specified and in the future machines their behavior is implemented on the new systems (i.e., as virtual machines). So, software and data can almost be processed like it is today. If we can access a machine that acts like the original one, it might even be possible that we can run a high number of the different original programs on it.

Migration has the aim to keep data processable by adapting or transcoding it whenever data formats get obsolete and are no longer supported. This procrastinates a lot of work to the future, because all the archived items that have the affected format need to be transcoded.

The main challenges we face in the context of long-term preservation are:

– the limited life-time and availability of hardware
– the high diversity and the rapidly changing system environments, data formats and applications (an overview of the evolution of video technology is given in [3])
– a lack of exact specifications to emulate the behavior of contemporary or legacy systems
– the effort for implementation of emulators or migration algorithms when system evolution steps forward
– the change or loss of information caused by every transformation or migration step
– and as the (maybe) most important aspect - **the massively growing amount of video data**

As a result of these challenges, all approaches have in common that they require a certain (very high) degree of standardization. Standardization is not an independent strategy. But, obviously, it leads to a reduction of the effort related to preservation because we need to handle a lower variety of formats and systems. A smaller number of formats and a lower diversity of systems decrease the effort and the costs for all these approaches. It should also be obvious that hardware cannot be preserved for productive use for decades or centuries. This is why we have to focus on emulation or migration and the approach of hardware museums cannot be followed in this context.

1.2   Requirements for the Preservation of Digital Videos

The goal of long-term preservation of videos is to provide a processable file or record that is as similar to the original video as possible. In addition, it should be based on formats and algorithms, which are independent of special hardware [4]. This is because of the limited life time of hardware that we have mentioned before. Requirements for digital preservation systems have also been defined in [5]. Interestingly, here, system diversity is named as a requirement for successful preservation, because extreme mono-cultures are more vulnerable to catastrophic failure. As a consequence of this argumentation, it might be sensible to archive videos not only in specific preservation formats, but also their original format.

In addition to general requirements for the preservation, the following criteria specifically apply for videos:

Quality - Videos must be preserved in with the highest possible quality level. To prevent loss of information, at least the relevant parts of the video must be stored in a high quality and should not be compressed with lossy algorithms.

Authenticity - Basic characteristics like color information or sound have to be preserved as well as additional features like subtitles, 3D or semantic elements (e.g., control of nonlinear videos). Future consumers should be able to experience videos like they were produced.

Robustness - When parts of a video are corrupted or get damaged, the rest of the video should still be processable. For example, the formats should carefully use mechanisms like inter-frame coding. The loss of a keyframe must not lead to the damage of bigger parts of the video.

Flexibility - A standard format for preservation of videos must be able to integrate new technologies. Innovations like 3D with related information have to be preserved, too. Maybe even exotic features like moving seats or sprinkling water, which we know from adventure parks, become usual elements of video.

Retrievability - We must not only preserve the video physically, but also engage consumers to find relevant videos in the future. Meta data like places, persons, events or key words related to the video or parts of it must be identified and preserved together with the video itself.

Comfort - Videos and contained information must be easily processable. E.g., the preservation formats should provide random access, because relevant parts could be accessed rapidly without processing the whole video.

Legal Aspects - Protection of intellectual property and copyrights play an important role, too. Copy protection mechanisms like watermarks have to be handled in the process of archiving. Transformations can destroy contained information that is used for this purpose.

Other requirements that do not focus on the videos themselves, but on financial, technical and organizational factors, have to be considered, too. The budgets for infrastructure and handling of data are limited. This is why data should be stored economically and in a way that avoids effort for migration, etc. Some

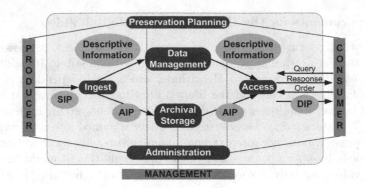

Fig. 1. The OAIS functional model

requirements (e.g., financial and quality issues) are conflicting. In most cases, we will have to make a trade-off to meet all of them in an acceptable degree. But, we have to keep in mind that due to the increasing amount of video material, there is a need for processes that procrastinate as little work as possible.

1.3   Archiving Infrastructure and Processes

For the design of our approach, we intend to rely on standards and best practices in preservation and archiving. Processes, roles and artifacts targeting the archiving of information are formalized by the Open Archive Information System (OAIS) [6]. The defined functional model helps us to illustrate the archiving infrastructure and procedures (Fig. 1).

Videos are delivered by the producers for archiving in submission information packages (SIP), get stored in archival information packages (AIP) and finally are sent to future consumers in dissemination information packages (DIP). The information packages contain the preserved video and additional information needed to process them. Descriptive information is used to manage archived videos and to find the videos matching consumers queries. Besides the video itself, all information packages contain additional pieces of information that is needed in their phase of the archiving process.

2   XMT-Based Approach for Archiving Digital Videos

With our envisioned approach that we sketched in [1] we try to make a step towards standardized long-term preservation of digital videos that meets the requirements named before. The approach is based on the Extensible MPEG-4 Textual Format (XMT) [7] and relies on the assumption that an abstract description of a video, which can be compiled to a playable video today is likely to be useable to be transformed into other future formats, if the content is still processable.

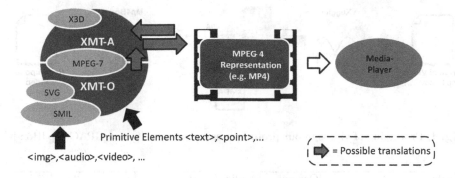

Fig. 2. Structure of XMT and handling of XMT data

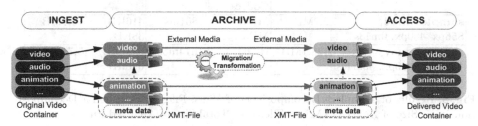

Fig. 3. Processing of archived videos

XMT is part of the MPEG4 standard and an XML format that is defined with
2 levels of abstraction (XMT-O and XMT-A). It integrates external standards
like SVG, SMIL and X3D and also allows to embed external media objects
(e.g., audio, images) into videos and compile playable video containers (MP4).
The structure of XMT and the handling of XMT data are illustrated in Fig. 2.

The overall idea (Fig. 3) of our approach is that the different elements of the
archived video get decomposed and are stored in individual standard preservation formats. In addition, an XMT file contains timing, meta information and
other artifacts that can be described in textual format. It also references the
extracted external content. For the dissemination of archived videos, a compiler
composes the relevant parts and generates videos in a contemporary format. The
processes and information structure are orientated on the OAIS reference model
that we introduced before.

2.1 Design and Implementation of a First Prototype

For proof of concept, we designed and implemented a first prototype (Fig. 4)
and experimented with it. Our experience shows that some existing tools can be
used for extraction and recompilation of different media types.

The tool, we implemented, whose purpose is to decompose the videos, uses
the *Xuggler*-Framework [8], which is Java-based, and which uses the *FFMpeg*[1]

---

[1] http://www.ffmpeg.org/.

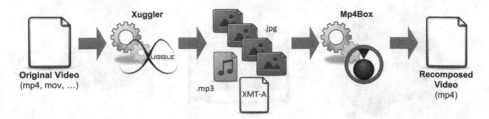

Fig. 4. Processing of videos in our prototype using Xuggler [8] and GPAC Mp4Box [9]

File	Orginal File Size	Audio-/ Video Codec	t_a	s_x	s_t
sample1.mp4, 856px*480px, 0m13s	2,7MB	MP4/ MP3	7861ms	416KB/ 38KB	15,7MB
sample2.mov, 1920px*1020px, 33m40s	128,1MB	H.264/ AAC	1h14m59s	69,5MB/ 6,4MB	5,74GB

Fig. 5. Results of exemplary Decomposition of Video Files. t_a = Time for Decomposition, s_x = Size of XMT-A/XMT-O File, s_t = Total Size of Archived Files

codec for decompression. At the moment, we only process video and audio data. For "archiving", the videos are stored in a set of image files (jpg), one audio file (mp3) and one XMT-A file, which was mentioned before. The named formats were chosen to ensure an easy recompilation. For productive use, the formats should be replaced by standards that fit best the purposes of preservation.

GPAC Mp4Box [9] is used to compile videos from the created XMT-A file and media resources. Because Mp4Box only supports XMT-A at the moment, we chose this kind of textual representation for archiving. The target format of the recompiled videos is mp4.

For our experiments, we chose two different sample video files. The first file (sample1.mp4) was a short video clip with lower resolution captured by a mobile device. The second file (sample2.mov) was a part of a Full-HD movie.

Besides some small technical problems, like flickering images or problems with bigger video files, we reached our goal to decompose exemplary videos successfully and compile processable videos from the generated artifacts. We believe that the approach is generally feasible and that problems can be solved by adaption or exchange of the frameworks. The results of our experiments are displayed in Fig. 5.

We can see that the space required by the video increased noticeably. This is caused by the loss of compression, when frames are stored separately. The size of the XMT files themselves can be reduced by compression and/or use of the corresponding XMT-O files, where possible. We experimentally generated XMT-O files, which were considerably smaller (about 10 times), due to their higher degree of abstraction. For instance, in XMT-O, the definition and disappearance of images is controlled by a single tag with a few attributes ("img"), while in XMT-A, this has to be handled much more complex.

2.2 Advantages of the Approach

The XMT-based approach provides some major advantages in the context of long-term preservation:

1. The approach eases the linking of meta data and keeps videos authorable for individual requests. XMT contains scene description formats that allow to condense and adapt the delivered content to the consumers' interests, depending on the query and the descriptive information linked to archived videos or parts of them.
2. The use of XMT makes it easy to integrate new technologies like interaction or new media formats. This is because we work on a very high level of abstraction. Only the individual extraction process and the compilers need to be adapted in order to integrate new content.
3. The high granularity leads to a radical reduction of effort related to migration. When standard preservation formats change (e.g., for audio), the relevant files can be migrated without the need to decode and process the whole video. The concentration on few specific formats will also reduce the effort for development, testing and maybe also preservation of migration algorithms and tools.

2.3 Challenges Related to the Approach

One challenge we face with our approach might be a conflict with one of the requirements listed in the introduction (Authenticity). Archived videos should be as similar as possible to the original video. Obviously, the decomposition and transformation of videos leads to severe changes in the format and surely slight changes in the contained information. This is because transformation always leads to a slight loss of parts of the information. But, from a pragmatic point of view, the reduction of necessary migration (transformation) steps caused by the standardization and the granularity will probably reduce the amount of unintended changes in the long term. For documentation of formats and contemporary technology, the additional preservation of videos in their original format may be sensible. They can be added to the archiving information packet to be available for future research and use.

Another aspect is the space required for the archived videos. An important factor for the comfortable, effective handling and exchange of video data in daily use are compression algorithms. Inter- and intra-frame coding are used for the compression of the frames of digital videos [10]. Depending on the quality requirements, intra-frame compression can still be used for separate frames. But, the decomposition of videos and the archiving with separate frames leads to the loss of the benefits that result from inter-frame compression. This is why the memory consumed by archived videos rises. If space is an issue, an unacceptable increase of memory usage can be tackled by choosing a format that uses inter-frame compression and does not store frames independently. Another solution could be the splitting of the visual parts of the video into sequences/chapters, which can also use inter-frame compression. At last, detailed predictions on the memory needed for preservation can not be made before the archiving formats and the required quality are defined.

3   Outlook and Conclusions

The described prototype has proven that the envisioned approach is generally feasible. In the future, the following is planned:

- Integration of all commonly used video formats
- Identification of formats that are suitable for long-term preservation
- Elicitation of performance and space requirements
- Improvement/ adaption of tools for decomposition/ recompiling
- Test of the approach with broadcasting stations and libraries that keep large amounts of videos
- Handling and linking of meta data
- Integration of additional media types and features to test extensibility

Last but not least, we'd like to benefit from the modularity and explore new application domains, such as extracting images from a collection of videos at a certain point of time.

References

1. Uherek, A., Maier, S., Borghoff, U.: An Approach for Long-Term Preservation of Digital Videos based on the Extensible MPEG-4 Textual Format. In: CTS 2014 Minneapolis (2014)
2. Borghoff, U., Rödig, P., Schmitz, L., Scheffczyk, J.: Long-Term Preservation of Digital Documents, pp. 12–19. Springer, Heidelberg (2003)
3. Schmidt, U.: Professionelle Videotechnik, pp. 1–15. Springer, Heidelberg (2009)
4. Neuroth, H., Oßwald, A., Scheffel, R., Strathmann, S., Jehn, M.: nestor Handbuch - eine kleine Enzyklopädie der digitalen Langzeitarchivierung - Kapitel 17.5 Video, Göttingen, Germany (2009)
5. Rosenthal, D., Robertson, T., Lipkis, T., Reich, V., Morabito, S.: Requirements for Digital Preservation Systems: A Bottom-Up Approach (2005). arXiv:cs/0509018v2
6. The Consultative Committee for Space Data Systems, Reference Model For an Open Archival Information System (OAIS) - Magenta Book, Washington DC, USA (2012)
7. Information technology - Coding of audio-visual objects - Part 11: Scene description and application engine (2013). ISO/IEC 14496–11:2005(E)
8. http://xuggle.com/xuggler
9. http://gpac.wp.mines-telecom.fr/mp4box/
10. Richardson, I.: The H.264 Advanced Video Compression Standard. Wiley, Chichester (2010)

Adaptive Flood Forecasting
for Small Catchment Areas

Bernhard Freudenthaler[✉] and Reinhard Stumptner

Data Analysis Systems, Software Competence Center Hagenberg,
Softwarepark 21, 4232 Hagenberg, Austria
{bernhard.freudenthaler,reinhard.stumptner}@scch.at

Abstract. In this paper a prototypical flood forecasting system for small catchment areas is presented. Due to the fact that flood forecasting models for small rivers normally not exist we developed an approach by combining a Continuous Situation Awareness (CSA) component with a workflow component. The CSA component permanently monitors sensor data and detects warnings which are presented to a decision maker. If the decision maker approves a warning, it is reported to the workflow component. The workflow component can dynamically react to changing situations and suggests preventive actions to a further user. That user can build a workflow and send tasks via a mobile client to emergency team leaders.

Keywords: Flood forecasting · Situation awareness · Dynamic workflow management · Decision tree · Disaster management

1 Introduction and Motivation

There are several sophisticated flood forecasting systems for large rivers like the Danube, the Rhine, the Main, and so on. Thereby, hydrological models are built by experts defined for a particular catchment area. But, large rivers generally have a larger warning time than small ones [4], which has to be considered when designing a flood forecasting system. The water gauge of small rivers can rise rapidly and dams as well as retention basins are sparsely available. Flood forecasting models for such small rivers are normally not available because the development of a flood forecasting system for each small river is too expensive. Therefore, within the project INDYCO[1] a prototypical flood forecasting system has been developed for small catchment areas. The INDYCO project provides an innovative approach based on dynamic workflows and integration as well as interpretation of sensor data in the frame of disaster management. The main goal was to develop a Decision Support System which can react rapidly and dynamically to changing situations during a disaster (for more information on dynamic workflows, see [11]).

The rest of this paper is organized as follows. In Sect. 2, we describe some related research. In Sect. 3, we present the flood forecasting system for small catchment areas

---

[1] "Integrated Dynamic Decision Support System Component for Disaster Management Systems", ERA-NET EraSME program under the Austrian grant agreement No. 836684 (FFG).

© Springer International Publishing Switzerland 2015
R. Moreno-Díaz et al. (Eds.): EUROCAST 2015, LNCS 9520, pp. 211–218, 2015.
DOI: 10.1007/978-3-319-27340-2_27

in detail. In Sect. 4, the prototype and results are shown. Finally, in Sect. 5 we conclude and show future work.

2 Related Research

In the domain of environmental research the forecasting problem is one which needs efficient computer support. Building predictive systems on environmental sensor networks mostly is challenging due to several reasons. Even when no events occur, the systems must stay online, must be able to handle different kinds of sensors and so on. Huang et al. [3] discuss a GIS-based approach for flood control which combines real-time precipitation and flow inspection, flood control administration, flood forecast and simulation, flood information dissemination, related damage evaluation and design a flood prevention decision support system in Quanzhou (China) for example.

In contrast to this contribution many environmental forecasting systems are based on neural models (e.g. Oprea and Matei [5]). The disadvantage of such approaches is that these models are not understandable for humans and thus often have problems with their acceptance in practice. Borrell et al. [2] describe a flash flood forecasting system by means of a flash flood evolution model. The model is designed to cope with a minimum amount of data (lacking data is a frequent problem), which is rainfall data from meteorological radar or soil properties viewed from space for that system. That particularly introduces interesting ideas concerning environmental observation. Basha et al. [1] describe an approach on river flood prediction allowing model-driven control to optimize the prediction capabilities of the system. Also, social media data can be a helpful data source in a disaster situation, as shown in [7]. However, trust plays a major role in this connection, but research shows that emergency responders by now already work with less than reliable information in offline practice and that they do use social media, but only within their known.

The approach presented in this work bases on a combined machine learned and expert defined model for flood forecasting. A continuous situation awareness component interprets sensor data and a learning component performs long-term analysis on sensor and operational data and tries to improve the models of the monitoring component, as shown in the following sections.

3 Flood Forecasting System for Small Catchment Areas

The main objective was to develop a model which can be adapted to small river environments as easily and fast as possible and thus be used like a template just being adjusted to new locations.

An overview of the system is illustrated in Fig. 2. First of all, different sensor data has to be rapidly integratable. Therefore, a generic data warehousing structure was developed, into which any available sensor data can be integrated in a short period of time (for more details see [6]). Such environmental sensor data could be actual and predicted rainfall, water gauge or soil humidity for instance (see Fig. 1).

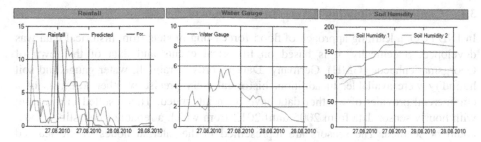

Fig. 1. Environmental sensors

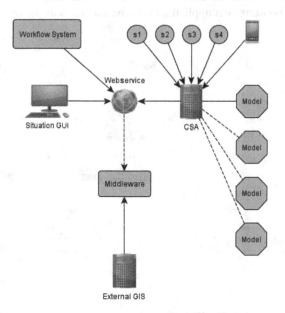

Fig. 2. System overview

Furthermore, multimedia sensor data (photos, videos ...) can be sent by mobile clients from the local emergency teams. These multimedia data are not interpreted automatically but support the decision maker in finding the right decisions.

In operation, a Continuous Situation Awareness (CSA) component permanently analyses these sensor data and provides warnings to decision makers. A warning could be for instance "A possible 30-year flood threats". A decision maker can take such warning including background information like weather forecast and geographical overview (GIS) into account and can then make a decision – the warning is valid or not. If a warning is approved by the decision maker, a dynamic workflow system, which provides possible measures, is triggered [8, 10]. The model for analyzing the sensor data is flexibly replaceable, e.g. decision trees, neural networks or Bayesian networks can be used. If historical data is not available expert knowledge has to be entered into a Bayesian network which then will be integrated in the CSA component.

3.1   Continuous Situation Awareness Component

In INDYCO, a learning approach of flood forecasting models from historical data was developed. Specifically, it is based on historical events and data of the town of Georgsmarienhuette (GMH), Germany. Data records of rainfall, water gauge and soil humidity were available. In addition, historical, very precise weather forecasts of a commercial provider of weather data have been integrated. This resulted in a dataset with hourly sensor data from 2005 until 2012 from which a reliable forecasting model could be learned. The sensors are represented in the internal nodes of the learned decision tree and the flood situations (from which should be warned) in the leaves. Figure 3 illustrates a decision tree for the flood forecasting of GMH[2]. As a Meta-Learner adaptive boosting was applied and the below tree was the one with the biggest weight.

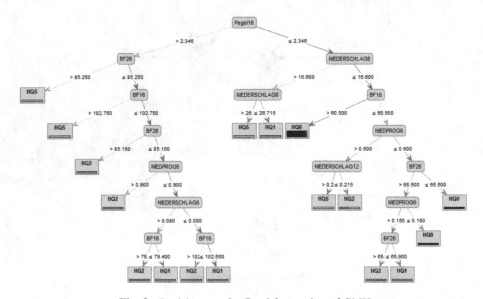

Fig. 3. Decision tree for flood forecasting of GMH

By using the learned model it can be warned of approximately six hours before flood situations appear. For each input vector consisting of the sensor data as described above, a forecast for the expected water gauge in six hours is calculated. The model has an overall accuracy of 95.21 % and is thereby able to predict the most correct water gauges. As already mentioned, adaptive boosting was used as meta-learning algorithm with decision trees as weak learner. Decision trees were chosen because they are intuitively understandable for domain experts and the generated warnings can be retraced. This is very important for a system in such a sensitive area as disaster

---

[2] Please note that Fig. 3 is in German because of usability for the domain experts.

management. The architecture of the CSA component is selected in a way that the models can be easily replaced depending on which disaster events should be monitored (floods, mudflows …). Such an approach is useful if no hydrological model (because development is too expensive) is available for a specific area. This applies to a lot of small rivers.

3.2 Dynamic Workflow Component

Immediately after a warning was detected by the CSA component and approved by the decision maker it is reported to a workflow system. The dynamic workflow component can dynamically adapt workflows (contingency plans) when situation changes changing situations occur and gives the possibility to build up new workflows.

Disaster situations are often characterized by a wide variety of variations, a multitude of previously unknown specifics and by a multitude of important data. There are many heterogeneous data sources for obtaining information such as diverse sensors, forecasting services, hydrographic and geological services, emergency control centers, control centers of neighboring cities, etc. Such a wide range of parameters and situations cannot be handled with traditional systems.

To efficiently support these complex situations, a so-called "mini story" concept was developed and prototypically implemented. A mini story is a semantically logical unit for the construction of complex workflows. The contingency plans were modeled as executable BPMN models (Business Process Model and Notation). The generated tasks are sent to the leaders of the emergency teams who execute them. Finished tasks and multimedia data are reported back to the INDYCO system. Detailed information about the workflow component can be found e.g. in [8–10].

4 Results

In the following, the prototype of the CSA component is described in more detail. The prototype consists of two modules: one that provides an overview of a specific large area (for the control center; see Fig. 4) and a second one that provides details of a clearly confined area (detailed view for the emergency team leaders; see Fig. 5). This clear split of the CSA component reflects the real distinction of responsibilities and decision-making competencies as it is usual under authorities and emergency services in real disaster events.

Based on incoming sensor data, the overview module provides detected "situations" respectively "warnings" and locates them on a geographical map. The detected warnings have to be approved by a decision maker before they are visible to the next level (leaders of the local emergency teams). If new situations occur existing information (photos, videos, reports …) are provided of the affected area (if exist in the database). Furthermore, also manually added warnings can be included (e.g. long-term warnings which would not be detected immediately from sensor data). Figure 4 exemplarily shows the overview module with detected warnings on the left side (with severity, name, date, approved or discarded) and a graphical overview on the right side

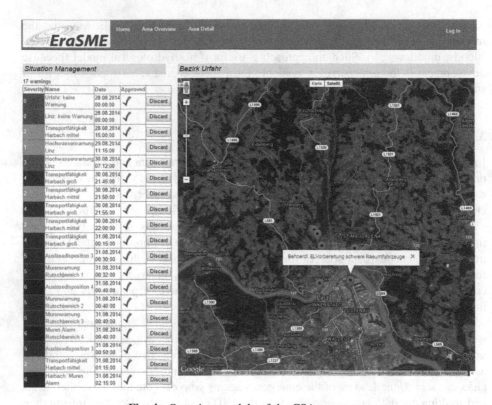

Fig. 4. Overview module of the CSA component

(with a graphical polygon of the affected areas and assigned tasks from the workflow component)[3].

If a warning is approved, further details can be provided (see Fig. 5). This includes local weather forecasts and severe weather warnings, environmental sensor data (rainfall, water gauge, etc.), approved warnings incl. assigned tasks and multimedia information from the mobile clients (local emergency team). This detailed view is intended for the use of emergency team leaders, whereby the control center can also consider this view. The detailed module shall give the best possible insight into the latest developments of a disaster event.

The developed models were trained and verified based on the real data set provided by the German town Georgsmarienhuette, which contained sensor data (rainfall, water gauge, soil humidity and weather prediction in five minutes intervals) starting from 1970 (see Fig. 1). After splitting these data into training and test set and adding weather predictions from 2005, the final performance of the learned model has an overall accuracy of 95.21 % (best class: 96.71 %, worst class: 58.82 %).

---

[3] Please note that some content in Figs. 4 and 5 is in German because of usability for the domain experts.

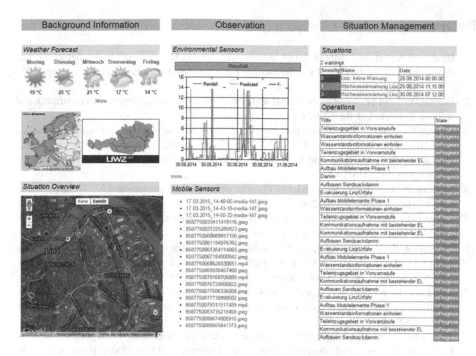

Fig. 5. Detailed module of the CSA component

5 Conclusion and Future Work

In this paper we have presented a prototypical flood forecasting system for small catchment areas to react dynamically and rapidly to changing situations. The prototype has been evaluated within a demonstration at the Upper Austrian firefighters association and has received positive feedback.

The results have shown that software systems can support the sensitive area of disaster management. The permanent monitoring of the sensor data with an overall accuracy of 95.21 % of the learned model underlines the potential of the CSA component. Furthermore, after detecting and approving warnings the workflow component suggests tasks, the user can build a workflow and send the tasks to the leaders of the emergency teams who give feedback to the control centers.

Additionally, the graphical overview of the current situation supports the control center when making decisions and give very important information to the leaders of the emergency teams.

As the model performs quite well in that environment, the next step will be to apply it to further environments to receive a more reliable evaluation of the adaptive flood forecasting system.

Acknowledgments. The research leading to these results has received funding from the ERA-NET EraSME program under the Austrian grant agreement No. 836684, project "INDYCO - Integrated Dynamic Decision Support System Component for Disaster Management Systems" and has been supported by the COMET program of the Austrian Research Promotion Agency (FFG).

References

1. Basha, E.A., et al.: Model-based monitoring for early warning flood detection. In: Proceedings of the 6th ACM Conference on Embedded Network Sensor Systems, pp. 295–308 ACM, Raleigh, NC, USA (2008)
2. Borrell, V.E., et al.: Development and application of computer techniques to environmental studies. Presented at the (2002)
3. Huang, Y., et al.: A decision support system based on GIS for flood prevention of Quanzhou city. In: Proceedings of the 2013 5th International Conference on Intelligent Human-Machine Systems and Cybernetics, vol. 01, pp. 50–53. IEEE Computer Society, Washington, DC, USA (2013)
4. Mahmoodi, O.: Hochwasser: Kleine Fluesse gefaehrlicher als grosse (2012). http://www.pressetext.com/news/20120123011
5. Oprea, M., Matei, A.: The neural network-based forecasting in environmental systems. WSEAS Trans. Syst. Control 5(12), 893–901 (2010)
6. Stumptner, R., Freudenthaler, B., Krenn, M.: BIAccelerator – a template-based approach for rapid ETL development. In: Chen, L., Felfernig, A., Liu, J., Raś, Z.W. (eds.) ISMIS 2012. LNCS, vol. 7661, pp. 435–444. Springer, Heidelberg (2012)
7. Tapia, A.H., Moore, K.: Good enough is good enough: overcoming disaster response organizations' slow social media data adoption. Comput. Supported Coop. Work 23(4–6), 483–512 (2014)
8. Thalheim, B., et al.: Application of generic workflows for disaster management. In: 23rd European-Japanese Conference on Information Modelling and Knowledge Bases XXV (EJC 2013), Nara, Japan, pp. 64–81, 3–7 June 2013
9. Tropmann-Frick, M., et al.: Generic workflows - a utility to govern disastrous situations. In: 24th International Conference on Information Modelling and Knowledge Bases XXVI (EJC 2014), Kiel, Germany, pp. 417–428, 3–6 June 2014
10. Tropmann-Frick, M., Ziebermayr, T.: Generic approach for dynamic disaster management system component. In: 25th International Workshop on Database and Expert Systems Applications, DEXA 2014, Munich, Germany, pp. 160–164, 1–5 September 2014
11. Ziebermayr, T., et al.: A proposal for the application of dynamic workflows in disaster management: a process model language customized for disaster management. In: Morvan, F., et al. (eds.) DEXA Workshops, pp. 284–288. IEEE Computer Society (2011)

A Scalable Monitoring Solution for Large-Scale Distributed Systems

Andreea Buga(✉)

Christian-Doppler Laboratory for Client-Centric Cloud Computing (CDCC),
Softwarepark 21, 4232 Hagenberg im Mühlkreis, Austria
andreea.buga@cdcc.faw.jku.at
http://www.cdcc.faw.jku.at/

Abstract. Applications running in large-scale distributed systems face
many challenges and difficulties. Constraints imposed to such systems
need to be thoroughly checked in order to ensure a proper service delivery to the client. The current paper proposes a monitoring solution for
large-scale distributed systems relying on abstract state machines. Data
gathered from the monitoring components are used in calculating metrics and establishing a diagnosis for the system. Emphasis is put on
failure detection and on ensuring non-functional requirements of the system such as fault-tolerance and resilience. The model introduced in this
paper will be integrated in a cloud-enabled large-scale distributed system. The novelty of the solution consists of finding the best integration
architecture for state-of-the-art algorithms and tools and refining them
to an efficient version for large-scale distributed systems.

Keywords: Large scale distributed systems · Monitoring · Decentralization · Formal modelling

1 Introduction

Cloud computing has its roots in the notion of utility computing [1] that was presented decades ago. The evolution of service-oriented applications and internet-
based solutions has favoured its expansion. Single clouds do not keep pace with
the requests of the clients, thus research is headed in the direction of designing and implementing interconnection of clouds. Like any other large-scale distributed systems, interconnected clouds face numerous challenges and real-time
constraints.

The aim of the monitoring framework is to provide meaningful information
about the whole system in order to efficiently adjust it towards optimal deployment and running. The monitoring components/monitors will be part of a larger
architecture and will work in close collaboration with the
adaptation component [2]. A special attention will be given to the context-
specific problems of CELDS such as failure detection, broken links, unavailability
and unresponsiveness.

© Springer International Publishing Switzerland 2015
R. Moreno-Díaz et al. (Eds.): EUROCAST 2015, LNCS 9520, pp. 219–227, 2015.
DOI: 10.1007/978-3-319-27340-2_28

The current paper introduces a formal model for the monitoring component of a cloud-enabled large scale distributed system (CELDS). The model is accompanied by a set of metrics built from collected data that will be used for establishing the state of the system. As the project is in its incipient stage, the current model focuses mostly on correctness and failure detection. The project will evolve in time with future refinements, optimization, and the integration in a bigger architecture. This paper presents only a proposal for the ground model which will be enhanced in several steps.

The rest of the paper is structured as follows. Section 2 introduces related work in the area of distributed systems and abstract state machines(ASMs). In Sect. 3, the current context and the problem definition of the project are offered. This section will help the reader in understanding the possible deployments of the model. Section 4 introduces the ground model of the monitoring component in terms of ASMs. The focus in Sect. 5 is twofold. On one hand, the data to be collected by the monitors is defined. On the other side, an example of an aggregated metric is presented. Section 6 discusses the state of the model and its future refinements. Conclusions are drawn in Sect. 7.

2   Related Work

The topic of monitoring distributed systems has already been introduced in the literature. Different approaches are tailored for either cloud or grid systems. In cloud systems, a special attention is given to the availability of the services [3–5], while in grids performance and reliability are carefully monitored [6]. Albeit these solutions are suitable for their proprietary services, they face the problem of vendor lock-in or they do not support reconfiguration.

Although there is a plethora of monitoring techniques, from the author's knowledge, there is none which attempts to solve the problems caused by the distributed nature of services. We aim to model a solution to handle the heterogeneity of the components and the distributed nature of processes through ASMs [7].

In building the model, we expect to minimize the gap between the real system and its formalization. Our aim is to extend existent distributed algorithms [8] that treat system failures (crash [9] and Byzantine failures [10]), for a correct and efficient run inside the CELDS. Due to the fact that such systems are exposed to many types of failures and constraints, it is important to thoroughly verify and validate their specification. Through the use of ASMs, properties of systems can be checked regardless of their intricate complexity [7,11–13].

3   System Description

Our work proposes the formalization of a novel decentralized monitoring architecture. Generally, monitoring solutions guarantee that the system behaves correspondingly to its specifications [14]. They are responsible for detecting abnormalities and disseminate the information throughout the system.

The ground model of the monitoring component is specified in terms of ASMs that can capture the intended requirements of the system. The model serves as a starting point for building executable code for various systems [7]. The first stage of the project includes an initial proposal of the ground model that will be further on refined in several steps. Verification of system properties is also planned as a future step.

The monitoring component is part of an architecture that envisions CELDS structured in a three-layered abstract machine model middleware in charge with normal service work flow, monitoring and adaptation. The proposed middleware aims to offer a unified interface for software services accessible via internet. System execution, monitoring and adaptation processes are distributed throughout the system. The monitors run in background with the normal execution of processes and collect data about the runtime. If data gathered by the probes indicate a critical situation (service unavailability, failures), the adaptation component is notified. A system recovery plan is proposed and executed so that the service execution is restored to normal mode. A special attention is oriented towards ensuring redundancy of components so that service availability is guaranteed. All work has been built up on previous research carried out in the area of cloud computing and ASM [7,15].

Before presenting the ground model, it is important to properly understand some properties of the monitoring components. In the context of CELDS, the monitors will run as normal processes, with an intended minimal intrusion. As the probes are exposed to the same problems as any other component, redundancy should be considered. Through redundancy, availability of data needed for establishing the state of the system is ensured. Collection of data should be done concurrently with the normal execution of the services.

Careful attention is given to consolidate our approach with state-of-the-art algorithms and tools [8]. Communication and interoperability remain open questions in CELDS. In addition, policy heterogeneity of different cloud providers overburdens their interconnection [6]. Detecting such problems and tackling them with proper techniques requires a robust monitoring solution.

The main focus of the monitoring components is directed towards failure detection and guaranteeing an efficient system deployment. Monitors gather information from assigned components and exchange it in order to offer an overview of the system. As collected data offers only low-level information, a set of aggregated metrics have been defined. Their purpose is to better evaluate system execution and to point towards the source of the problem, in case it exists.

4   Ground Model of the Monitoring Framework

As the project is still in its incipient phase, the first formalization of the model consists of the monitoring framework ground model. Definition of transition rules and constraints will be stated in the next development step. The current phase emphasizes the structure and work-flow inside the monitor framework and

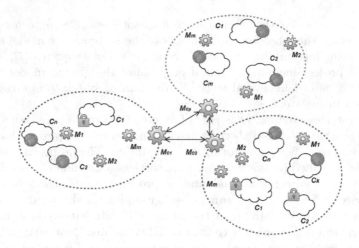

Fig. 1. Monitoring framework topology inside a CELDS

its collaboration with the middleware and the adaptation component [2]. The description of the framework starts from an ensemble view of the system, its integration and continues with a glimpse of the internal functioning.

Generally, in a distributed system, the topology and the interaction between components is very important. At the monitoring framework level, it is necessary to define the properties of its constituents. For each monitor we define its internal attributes, its topology in the framework and the information it gathers from the CELDS. The problem statement of our research can be defined in a more mathematical oriented way as follows:

Given a set of interconnected clouds

$$C = \{C_1, C_2, ..., C_n \mid \forall i, j \in \{1, 2, ..., n\}, i \neq j, C_i \neq C_j\}$$

and a set of monitoring components

$$M = \{M_1, M_2, ..., M_m\}$$

find the best topology and metrics for the monitoring components

$$config = \{(M_1, T_1, I_1), (M_2, T_2, I_2), ..., (M_m, T_m, I_m)\}^1$$

to obtain optimal runtime performance and thus, increased Quality of Service (QoS).

Above configuration favors the process of discovering the closest neighboring monitors according to the information they can provide to the system.

We decided to cluster clouds together with the probes responsible for their monitoring in order to reduce the communication overhead. Based on the topology, every cluster of clouds is assigned a group of monitors $\{M_1, M_2, ..., M_m\}$. Monitors will gather the data from their corresponding clouds, aggregate it into

---

[1] A tuple (M_k, T_k, I_k) refers to $(MonitoringComponent_k, Topology_k, MetricsSet_k)$.

more meaningful information and communicate with other monitors in case of abnormal situations.

The diagnosis of service execution is done hierarchically so that data transfer is diminished. Firstly, monitors detect anomalous runs of services in their designated cluster. In the next step they communicate with their pair monitors to check if the gathered data reflects the same interpretation. If the metrics locally collected correspond, the diagnosis is sent to the adaption component [2]. Otherwise, conflicts need to be solved by the elected leader monitor of the cluster, M_c. For the leader election processes, already existing algorithms [8] can be integrated. There are situations in which leader monitors of clusters can also fail. In this case, agreement through communication at leaders' level is needed. A possible topology of the system and collaboration between monitors can be depicted in Fig. 1.

For the beginning of the project, the focus was set on establishing the work flow of the monitoring framework. The associated ground model diagram is illustrated in Fig. 2. In the first state of the model, the configuration of the CELDS must be loaded. In case the information about the system is not complete, an additional request is sent. When this step is successfully completed, the monitoring probes are deployed. This part highly depends on distributed systems algorithms [8] and the initial configuration of the system. At the end of the probe deployment, leader election algorithms are run inside clusters. This step is followed by the monitoring processes in which data are collected by probes. Communication with the adaptation component [2] is also established.

Periodically, the framework checks the information gathered from the probes. If information are available and complete, they are further processed, analysed and logged. Based on the results a runtime usage model is defined. It notifies the presence of flaws and failures and/or establishes if the execution of services is correct and responsive. In case the monitoring framework detects abnormalities, a notification is sent to the adaptation component [2] which will be responsible for system reconfiguration.

If a probe cannot provide the monitoring information, there is a failure of either the monitored components, of the probe or of the two. Both probe and service provider components are checked and then the problem is sent to the adaptation component [2] which readjusts the system to a functioning state.

The first insight of the monitoring framework reveals mainly the work flow and ways in which data gathered by the probes can be used. Based on it relies the understanding of the role of the monitors and their interaction with other parts of the CELDS. The components should be completed with a formal description that should enforce real constraints imposed by either the environment or by the CELDS itself. In the next step of development, all the components will be formalized in terms of ASM rules and properties. Being described in specifications of formal models, the system properties can be easier checked. Flaws in logic can be detected in phases prior to actual code development.

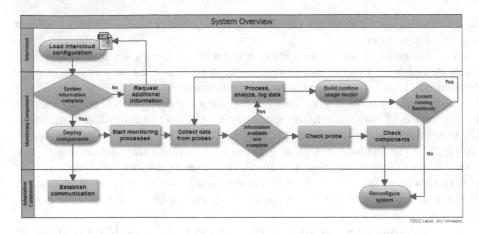

Fig. 2. Ground model of the monitoring framework

5 Monitoring Metrics

Monitoring framework is responsible for a proper deployment of the probes in the system, gathering and aggregation of data and communication with the adaptation component. In CELDS, it is assumed that services run in heterogeneous clouds which may or may not provide information about the system. In case the clouds provide monitoring information, the probes should be able to extract it and transform it to meaningful data. When there are no data from the environment, probes become responsible of data collection. In the first phase, emphasizing fault detection, the main base metrics to be analysed refer to system latency and responsiveness. Very important for our scope are also availability, network bandwidth and usage of resources. Nonetheless, there are other important metrics that need to be considered especially in the case of system reconfiguration or service migration.

High level metrics are built from base metrics for providing a deeper insight on the system. For instance, we consider the *process transfer effort*(PTE) as an aggregated metric who comprises several base metrics which helps in the case of service transfer. PTE encompasses process specific metrics (availability, performance and reliability), legislation issues, network bandwidth, costs and security concerns. If the migration of the process refers to an unavailable system or if it is not permitted by legislation issues then the value of the PTE is set to ∞. Otherwise, the metric is calculated with the aid of the following formula:

$$pte(i) = \frac{costs(i)}{max(costs(k))} \cdot \frac{1}{bdwidth(i)} \cdot \frac{max(perf(k))}{perf(i)} \cdot \frac{reliab(i)}{100} \cdot \frac{secure(i)}{100}. \quad (1)$$

Relevant metrics defined as description logic concepts or individuals [16] allow the representation of the system in terms of a knowledge base on top of which reasoning methods can be applied. Monitored data metrics are packaged in usage profiles further involved in the decision-making process. Based on them, the system applies reasoning methods so that an evaluation of the running-state is set. Usage profiles from individual components are consulted among each other to check for the best reconfiguration strategy. In this manner, the system is aware of the unavailability of monitoring components and of data and aims to find the best solution. Using real-time measurements and description language, rules and corresponding triggered actions are defined.

6 Future Refinements of the Model

The model presented in the current paper will be completed with rules and transitions expressed in terms of ASM modules. ASM formalization targets also the algorithms used for ensuring a correct runtime of the system, its robustness and reliability. Adapted versions of the leader election algorithm and of building a decentralized topology of the distributed system are expected for the next phase. Each step in the refinement process will be completed with a verification of system properties (correctness, safety, liveliness). In this way, errors can be discovered in an early phase.

Awareness of the global state of the components cannot be ensured in a decentralized system. Decisions have to be carried out only relying on partial information. Trust and dependency have to be carefully handled in order to reduce the possibility of an incorrect decision. A future refinement consists in modelling the Byzantine fault-tolerant behaviour of monitoring components. In such a system, agreement is reached when a sufficient number of participants establish and communicate the same result.

In future steps, additional components as loggers and metric processors need to be also formally defined. By ensuring their correctness the number of problems that can occur in the system is reduced.

7 Conclusions

The paper addresses a robust monitoring solution for CELDS. Importance of such a solution is even bigger for such systems because besides clients, cloud participants should be allowed to gather information about the whole system. Based on the collected information, the system should be able to decide feasible substitutes in case of a down-fall or detect untrustworthy parties. Our proposal enriches the existing monitoring techniques with its decentralized architecture formally defined and with the distributed usage profiles built upon basic and aggregated metrics.

Modelling the solution in terms of ASMs permits verification and validation of the models before starting the development of the code. Detected inconsistencies or incorrect specifications of the model can be tracked down, isolated and corrected correspondingly. Through incremental refinement, verification and validation, it is ensured that the solution meets the requirements while being correct.

The monitoring framework is part of a larger architecture that aims to ensure a decentralized CELDS. Distributing the control instead of keeping it centralized can improve the responsiveness, but in turn it brings many challenges that have to be overcome. Our approach handles in the current state of development failure detection and availability aspects.

References

1. Parkhill, D.F.: The Challenge of the Computer Utility. Addison-Wesley Publishing Company, Reading (1966)
2. Nemes, S. T.: Adaptation Engine for Large-Scale Distributed Systems. In: Computer Aided Systems Theory - EUROCAST 2015, To appear. Springer, Las Palmas (2015)
3. Kutare, M., Eisenhauer, G., Wang, C., Schwan, K., Talwar, V., Wolf, M.: Monalytics: online monitoring and analytics for managing large scale data centers. In: Proceedings of the 7th International Conference on Autonomic Computing, pp. 141–150. ACM (2010)
4. Rak, M., Venticinque, S., Mahr, T., Echevarria, G., Esnal, G.: Cloud application monitoring: the mOSAIC approach. In: 2011 IEEE Third International Conference on Cloud Computing Technology and Science (CloudCom), pp. 758–763. IEEE (2011)
5. Palmieri, R., di Sanzo, P., Quaglia, F., Romano, P., Peluso, S., Didona, D.: Integrated monitoring of infrastructures and applications in cloud environments. In: Alexander, M., D'Ambra, P., Belloum, A., Bosilca, G., Cannataro, M., Danelutto, M., Di Martino, B., Gerndt, M., et al. (eds.) Euro-Par 2011, Part I. LNCS, vol. 7155, pp. 45–53. Springer, Heidelberg (2012)
6. Massie, M.L., Chun, B.N., Culler, D.E: The ganglia distributed monitoring system: design, parallel computing, implementation and experience (2003)
7. Börger, E., Stärk, R.F.: Abstract State Machines: A Method for High-Level System Design and Analysis. Springer, Heidelberg (2003)
8. Lynch, N.: Distributed Algorithms. Morgan Kaufmann Publishers Inc., San Francisco (1996)
9. Hamid, B., Mosbah, M.: A formal model for fault-tolerance in distributed systems. In: Winther, R., Gran, B.A., Dahll, G. (eds.) SAFECOMP 2005. LNCS, vol. 3688, pp. 108–121. Springer, Heidelberg (2005)
10. Driscoll, K., Hall, B., Sivencrona, H., Zumsteg, P.: Byzantine fault tolerance, from theory to reality. In: Anderson, S., Felici, M., Littlewood, B. (eds.) SAFECOMP 2003. LNCS, vol. 2788, pp. 235–248. Springer, Heidelberg (2003)
11. Stärk, R.F., Schmid, J., Börger, E.: Java and the Java Virtual Machine: Definition, Verification, Validation. Springer, Heidelberg (2001)
12. Blass, A., Gurevich, Y.: Abstract state machines capture parallel algorithms: correction and extension. ACM Trans. Comput. Logic **9**(3), 19:1–19:32 (2008)
13. Glässer, U., Gu, Q.-P.: Formal description and analysis of a distributed location service for mobile ad hoc networks. In: Theoretical Computer Science (2005)
14. Rady, M., Lampesberger, H.: Monitoring of client-cloud interaction. In: Buchberger, B., Prinz, A., Schewe, K.D., Thalheim, B. (eds.) Correct Software in Web Applications and Web Services. Texts & Monographs in Symbolic Computation, pp. 177–228. Springer, Heidelberg (2014)

15. Bósa, K.: A formal model of a cloud service architecture in terms of ambient ASM. Technical report, Christian Doppler Laboratory for Client-Centric Cloud Computing (CDCC), Johannes Kepler University Linz, Hagenberg, Austria (2012)
16. Baader, F., Calvanese, D., McGuinness, D.L., Nardi, D., Patel-Schneider, P.F.: The Description Logic Handbook: Theory, Implementation, and Applications. Cambridge University Press, New York (2003)

Using Smart Grid Data to Predict Next-Day Energy Consumption and Photovoltaic Production

Stephan Dreiseitl[1](✉), Andreas Vieider[2], and Christoph Larch[2]

[1] Department of Software Engineering,
University of Applied Sciences Upper Austria, 4232 Hagenberg, Austria
stephan.dreiseitl@fh-hagenberg.at
[2] SYNECO Srl, 39100 Bolzano, Italy

Abstract. The rise of sustainable energy production is a challenge for grid operators, who need to balance consumer demand with an increasingly volatile supply that is heavily dependent on weather conditions and environmental factors.

Smart gird data provides fine-grained insight into consumer behavior as well as local renewable energy producers. We use data from an electric company in a region of South Tyrol to model both energy consumption as well as energy production. With a simple nearest-neighbor approach, we predict next-day load profiles for local power stations with relative error rates as low as 3 %. The energy production at these local power stations (in the form of photovoltaic power plants) can be predicted by adapting an ideal irradiation model to actual production data, stratified by varying weather conditions. Using this approach, we achieve relative errors in predicting next-day power production of 3–9 % for favorable weather conditions.

Keywords: Smart grid · Energy prediction · Photovoltaic power production

1 Introduction

In the last decade, energy production by renewable (sustainable) resources has been increasing by about 6 % annually in the European Union, and now accounts for 22.3 % of total energy production [1]. Of these 22.3 %, the majority (66 %) is contributed by biomass plants, with hydropower (16 %), wind power (10 %), and solar power plants (5 %) making up the rest. Although the latter two thus contribute only about 3 % of the total energy production in the EU, they are the fastest-growing form of renewable energy resource.

While wind and solar power plants thus help reduce the carbon footprint of energy consumption, their increased role as energy providers is not without drawbacks: Their energy production, and thus their contribution to the power grid, depends on local weather conditions. Their contribution is thus highly

© Springer International Publishing Switzerland 2015
R. Moreno-Díaz et al. (Eds.): EUROCAST 2015, LNCS 9520, pp. 228–235, 2015.
DOI: 10.1007/978-3-319-27340-2_29

volatile, making grid management (which seeks to balance consumption with production) much more complicated.

Recently, there have been several investigations into the use of predictive modeling algorithms for analyzing the supply and demand curves that arise in energy production and consumption. While some of these took advantage of the increasingly wide-spread use of smart meters to model the demand side, others have investigated how best to predict the supply side of sustainable energy power plants.

On the demand side, Gajowniczek and Zabkowski [2] used artificial neural networks (ANNs) and support vector machines to predict an individual household's next-day energy consumption based on smart meter data. A much more comprehensive investigation can be found in the work of Mirowski [3] et al., who used a variety of time-series modeling tools to predicted consumption levels at three time horizons (next hour, next day, next week) and four levels of data aggregation (from single customers up to system-wide).

On the production side, and in particular as regards photovoltaic (PV) power plants with their dependence on weather conditions, more research effort has been exerted: Voyant et al. [4] used ANNs to predict hourly global solar irradiation values for the next 24 h based on air pressure, nebulosity, and precipitation. They observed that the ANN approach outperformed a standard auto-regressive moving average time series modeling approach. Cococcini et al. [5] performed a similar analysis, also using ANNs to predict the next day's energy production based on irradiation data as input, and obtained error rates of less than 5 %. Mandal et al. [6] developed a system to predict the next hour's power output of a PV system using a wavelet transformation for data pre-processing, and an ANN system for modeling the dependence of the output on the independent variables irradiation and temperature. With this system, the authors also obtained errors in the range of 5 %. Using a variety of time-series modeling approaches, Pedro and Coimbra [7] studied how well a baseline model using no external inputs could predict next-hour output of a PV power plant. The errors they obtained ranged between 6 % and 27 %. Local similarity search in historical records is the basis of a prediction algorithm by Monteiro et al. [8]. Finally, reviews of current methods for forecasting solar irradiation as well as PV power plant output are given by Diagne et al. [9] and Inman et al. [10].

In this paper, we use data on energy consumption and photovoltaic energy (PV) production in a part of South Tyrol (northern Italy) to predict the next day's energy consumption and PV production. The data was collected in the region serviced by AEW, a small regional power company with about 175 000 customers.

2   Materials and Methods

The data available for modeling power consumption and production was as follows:

- Load profiles for all large consumers combined ($> 55\,\mathrm{kW}$ connection lines) at hourly resolution;
- Combined PV production for all units connected to a local power station at 15 min. resolution;
- weather forecast and actual weather conditions.

This data was available for each of 14 local power stations operated by AEW, and every day of the year 2013.

2.1 Predicting Load Profiles

As evidenced by the literature cited in Sect. 1, there are a number of algorithmic approaches to model the power consumption of customers, either individually or on an aggregate level. In this work, we decided to apply a simple method to contrast the more elaborate approaches found in the literature, and thus to investigate whether the additional modeling effort translates into tangible gains (i.e., increased modeling accuracy). The simple method we used was a nearest neighbor search on the time axis, with the reasoning being that load profiles change over time to reflect changes in the season (slowly) and the weather (more rapidly). We used $k = 3$ nearest neighbors—i.e., past days' load profiles—to predict the next day's load profile. At each hour, the predicted load profile consisted of the arithmetic mean of the corresponding hours' load in the profile of the nearest neighbors.

   To take discontinuities in the day-to-day changes in load profiles into account, we stratified them into workdays (regular Mondays through Fridays), pre-holidays (regular Saturdays and days before holidays), and holidays (Sundays and holidays). The predicted profile of a Sunday could thus be influenced by Sundays as far as three weeks prior. In South Tyrol in 2013, there were 243 workdays, 61 pre-holidays, and 61 holidays.

2.2 Predicting PV Power Production

PV power production is mainly influenced by two factors: weather conditions (cloud layer, sunshine) and sun elevation, which in turn depends on the day of the year. Although production data was available at 15 min. resolution, for our purposes it was sufficient to model the total daily PV electricity production at each of the 14 local power stations.

   Weather data was available as local next-day forecasts; each of the 14 power stations was mapped to the nearest local forecast. Forecasts were used to group days with similar weather conditions; for each of the power stations, we built a predictive models for each weather condition.

   Originally, the weather forecasts consisted of 26 different conditions ranging from "clear skies" to "overcast with thunderstorms and heavy snowfall". This proved to be too fine-grained to be useful in our prediction models, as there were too few cases in most categories to fit a model. We thus combined the 26 forecast categories, depending on the amount of cloud cover, into the 4 classes "clear skies", "sunny", "cloudy", and "overcast".

We then built predictive models for each combination of the 4 weather forecast classes and 14 power stations by referring to an ideal solar irradiation model for the latitude of South Tyrol. From this model, we obtained the maximum possible solar irradiation for each day of the year. This model was then transformed in a affine manner to best fit the observed PV production data in each combination of forecast classes and power station. Thus, for each power station, we obtained four prediction models that exhibit the same dependency on the sun elevation as the idealized situation, but are dampened to account for weather conditions.

3   Results

Since each of the 14 local power stations had slightly different load profiles, we only used each station's own data to predict the next day's load profiles. A typical example of an actual and a predicted load profile for one of the larger local stations is shown in Fig. 1.

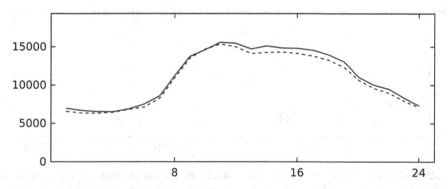

Fig. 1. 24-hour predicted load profile (dashed) vs. actual load profile (solid) for Thursday, April 11th, 2013. The predicted load profile is the arithmetic mean of profiles from April 8th through April 10th. Load units are in kWh; the prediction has absolute sum of errors of 9900 kWh, which corresponds to a relative error of 3.7 %.

For a total of 14 local power stations, and 3 categories of days (regular/pre-holiday/holiday), there are thus 42 combinations for which we can assess the quality of the predictions. A summary of this assessment is given in Table 1. One can observe that the errors are smallest for the weekdays, larger for the pre-holidays, and largest for the holidays. This is likely due to the nearest-neighbor nature of the load predictions, where the closest weekday is most often yesterday, whereas the closest pre-holidays and holidays may be some days prior. Furthermore, the relative prediction errors given in Table 1 are larger for the smaller power stations, as can be seen in Fig. 2. The power station with relative error of 21.6 % is one of the smallest stations, whereas the larger stations exhibit much smaller errors—down to 4 % and less for the two largest stations.

Table 1. The average relative errors of predicting next-day load profiles for stations # 1–14, stratified by day category. Errors were calculated as absolute differences between actual and predicted loads at 24 h in a day; averages were taken over all days in a day category.

#	Workdays	Pre-holidays	Holidays	#	Workdays	Pre-holidays	Holidays
1	3.1 %	5.9 %	7.9 %	8	7.3 %	13.2 %	12.3 %
2	4.3 %	5.5 %	7.8 %	9	10.2 %	10.5 %	16.0 %
3	3.7 %	6.8 %	8.0 %	10	5.5 %	7.8 %	10.3 %
4	8.2 %	13.5 %	17.5 %	11	4.0 %	5.7 %	9.0 %
5	7.3 %	10.7 %	12.0 %	12	21.6 %	38.5 %	42.3 %
6	6.4 %	8.7 %	12.7 %	13	8.0 %	9.7 %	11.8 %
7	7.0 %	8.5 %	12.0 %	14	7.0 %	13.4 %	14.4 %

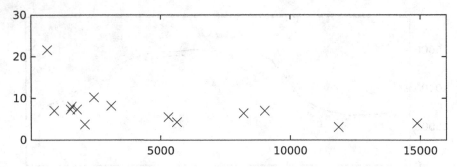

Fig. 2. Relative error in the prediction of load profiles (as percentage, on y-axis) vs. average load during workdays (as kWh, on x-axis) for each of the 14 local power stations.

The task of predicting PV power production was based on a combination of weather forecast data and an ideal irradiation model. The weather forecasts were grouped into four categories, with "clear skies" forecast for 38 to 52 days (depending on the location of the power station), "sunny" for 80 to 95 days, "cloudy" for 121 to 156 days, and "overcast" for 91 to 97 days of the year 2013. The forecast data was made available by *Südtiroler Informatik AG*[1].

We obtained the ideal irradiation data for South Tyrol from the Photovoltaic Geographic Information System [11], a service of the European Commission's Institute for Energy and Transport. Over the course of a calendar year, the ideal irradiation curve exhibits a pronounced inverted U-shape, with the maximal

---

[1] http://www.siag.it.

irradiation occurring during the summer months, and a drop-off to around 50 % of the maximum during the winter months. This curve, which was only available as 12 data points (one for every month), was linearly interpolated to have irradiation data for every day of the year. These daily values were then fit via an affine transformation $f(x) = ax + b$ so that the sum of squared errors between ideal irradiation and actual PV production was minimized. An example of such a curve fit is shown in Fig. 3.

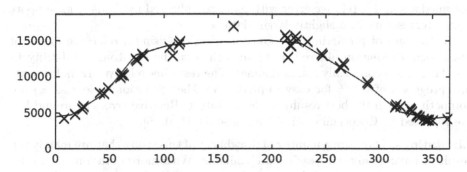

Fig. 3. Actual (crosses) and predicted (solid line) PV power production (in kWh, on x axis) for all 365 days in the year 2013 (on y axis). Data is for one of the larger stations and the weather forecast category "clear skies". The average relative error of predictions is 6 %.

Table 2. The average relative errors for predicting next-day PV power production for stations # 1–14, stratified by weather forecast conditions. Errors were calculated as absolute differences between actual and predicted PV power production for all days in a given forecast category.

#	Clear	Sunny	Cloudy	Overcast	#	Clear	Sunny	Cloudy	Overcast
1	6.0 %	9.4 %	18.7 %	39.9 %	8	4.5 %	6.6 %	23.8 %	47.8 %
2	5.4 %	8.5 %	18.0 %	33.8 %	9	4.6 %	8.7 %	21.5 %	38.6 %
3	5.0 %	8.0 %	19.3 %	40.4 %	10	6.8 %	7.1 %	21.3 %	30.0 %
4	7.2 %	7.2 %	20.7 %	36.6 %	11	8.7 %	8.9 %	18.0 %	34.5 %
5	4.6 %	6.9 %	18.1 %	32.9 %	12	9.4 %	12.1 %	25.5 %	47.6 %
6	4.0 %	5.8 %	21.0 %	38.7 %	13	4.7 %	8.7 %	19.7 %	37.4 %
7	2.9 %	6.2 %	19.9 %	39.1 %	14	3.4 %	6.5 %	22.3 %	46.9 %

A summary of the relative errors in predicting PV production across all 14 stations and 4 forecast categories is given in Table 2. One can observe that, as expected, more stable and favorable weather conditions lead to better predictions. The more volatile the weather condition, the worse the predictions become, with an increase of an order of magnitude between the "clear skies" and the "overcast" forecast categories.

4   Discussion

The results presented in the previous section show that the use of simple methods and algorithms can lead to results that are competitive with the best reported in the literature.

In the case of predicting next-day load profiles, a nearest-neighbor approach resulted in relative errors as low as 4 % for large power stations and workday load profiles. This is on par with results obtained by Mirowski et al. [3], who also obtained about 4 % relative error with more complicated methods (e.g., support vector regression) for a slightly larger data set.

In the case of predicting PV power production, using a reference model of ideal solar irradiation allowed us to smooth over the day-to-day volatility in the data in a theoretically sound manner. The resulting relative errors for next-day prognosis of 2–9 % for easy-to-predict weather situations (clear skies) are competitive with the best results in the literature: Relative errors of around 5 % are reported by Cococcini et al. [5] and Mandal et al. [6].

Limitations: There are a number of drawbacks of this study that are mainly the result of having only one year's data available. With more data, one could use the nearest-neighbor approach not just on the time axis, but also in profile space, in effect looking for similar profiles in several year's data. This may improve the predictive accuracy, in particular for the pre-holiday and holiday categories.

More data across several years would also benefit the PV power prediction task, because it would make more fine-grained weather conditions possible. Currently, we are using only four categories; more data would allow us to increase this number, and more finely adapt the ideal irradiation model to actual power production values in different weather conditions.

References

1. European Commission (Eurostat): EU Renewable Energy Statistics (2014). http://ec.europa.eu/eurostat/statistics-explained/index.php/Renewable_energy_statistics. Accessed 4 May 2015
2. Gajowniczek, K., Zabkowski, T.: Short term electricity forecasting using individual smart meter data. Procedia Comput. Sci. **35**, 535–576 (2014)
3. Mirowski, P., Chen, S., Ho, T., Yu, C.N.: Demand forecasting in smart grids. Bell Labs Technical J. **18**(4), 135–158 (2014)
4. Voyant, C., Randimbivololona, P., Nivet, M., Paoli, C., Muselli, M.: Twenty four hours ahead global irradiation forecasting using multi-layer perceptron. Meteorol. Appl. **21**(3), 644–655 (2013)
5. Cococcioni, M., D'Andrea, E., Lazzerini, B.: 24-hour-ahead forecasting of energy production in solar PV systems. In: Proceedings of the 11th International Conference on Intelligent Systems Design and Applications (ISDA), pp. 1276–1281 (2011)
6. Mandal, P., Madhira, S., Ul Haque, A., Meng, J., Pineda, R.: Forecasting power output of solar photovoltaic system using wavelet transform and artificial intelligence techniques. Procedia Comput. Sci. **12**, 332–337 (2012)
7. Pedro, H., Coimbra, C.: Assessment of forecasting techniques for solar power production with no exogenous inputs. Sol. Energy **86**, 2017–2028 (2012)

8. Monteiro, C., Fernandez-Jimenez, L.A., Santos, T., Ramirez-Rosado, I., Terreros-Olarte, M.: Short-term power forecasting model for photovoltaic plants based on historical similarity. Energies **6**, 2624–2643 (2013)
9. Diagne, M., David, M., Lauret, P., Boland, J., Schmutz, N.: Review of solar irradiance forecasting methods and a proposition for small-scale insular grids. Renew. Sustain. Energy Rev. **27**, 65–76 (2013)
10. Inman, R., Pedro, H., Coimbra, C.: Solar forecasting methods for renewable energy integration. Prog. Energy Combust. Sci. **39**, 535–576 (2013)
11. European Commission (Joint Research Centre, Institute for Energy and Transport): Photovoltaic Geographical Information System (PVGIS) (2015). http://re.jrc.ec.europa.eu/pvgis/. Accessed 4 May 2015

Sitting Property-Based Testing at the Desktop

Laura M. Castro [✉]

MADS Group – Department of Computer Science,
Universidade da Coruña, A Coruña, Spain
lcastro@udc.es

Abstract. The desktop ecosystem is full of software applications of all sizes that share a common space. From alarm clocks to agendas, chat programs, or volume widgets, these software applications are usually not regarded as highly critical software, but they are the kind of software used by millions of people every second. Their computer user experience depends heavily on how well these applications behave.

At the same time, these software applications are built using many different development frameworks, each of which has its own development and testing tools. This implies that novel verification approaches, such as property-based testing (PBT) will have a long way until they reach all of them, since technology-specific tools implementing PBT will need to be developed and adopted by their respective developers.

In this paper, we propose an alternative approach that will allow us to test desktop applications in a technology-agnostic manner. Taking advantage of the free and open-source project FreeDesktop, which enables interoperability at the desktop level, and specifically of its D-Bus interprocess communication system, we demonstrate the feasibility of performing automated property-based testing using a tool like QuickCheck, in a powerful, reusable, effort-effective way.

Keywords: FreeDesktop · D-Bus · Property-based testing · QuickCheck

1 Introduction

Research in software development is usually concerned about making big impact by addressing big problems, which are frequently identified with big applications, great amounts of data, or massive systems. However, end-user software is big in itself, in the sense that it is what defines, for millions of people, the user experience of using a computer on a daily basis.

For many people living in developed countries, an increasing amount of time each day is spent in front of a desktop computer, not only at work (cf. Fig. 1) but at home, performing simple leisure tasks, using software applications to write or talk to their friends or relatives, listen to music or watch videos, edit documents, or plan events (cf. Figs. 2 and 3). Even when a portion of these activities is migrating to the cloud, it is still the case that each of our desktops is full with small, often single-purpose applications.

© Springer International Publishing Switzerland 2015
R. Moreno-Díaz et al. (Eds.): EUROCAST 2015, LNCS 9520, pp. 236–243, 2015.
DOI: 10.1007/978-3-319-27340-2_30

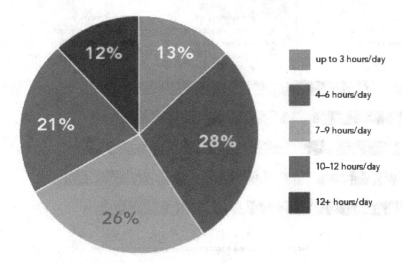

Fig. 1. Average use of computers at work (hours per day). (Source: http://www. theatlantic.com/health/archive/2012/09/how-to-keep-computer-screens-from-destroyi ng-your-eyes/263005/, Source: http://wearesocial.net/blog/2010/08/uks-media-consu mption-habits/)

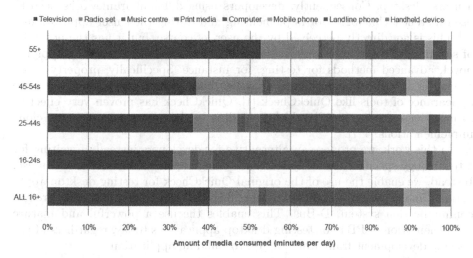

Fig. 2. Average use of computers for leisure (percentage of leisure time, per age group). (Source: http://wearesocial.net/blog/2010/08/uks-media-consumption-habits/)

At the same time, these software applications are built using many different development frameworks. For instance, the most famous desktops for Linux environments are GNOME and KDE, but there are many other Linux/UNIX GUI technologies, and this is unlikely to change. On the contrary, applications developed in different technologies and languages may very well live together in

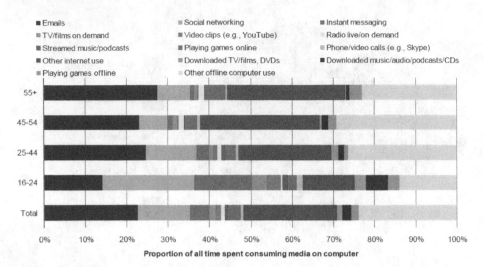

Fig. 3. Average use of computer time (percentage of leisure time, per age group). (Source: http://wearesocial.net/blog/2010/08/uks-media-consumption-habits/)

a users' desktop. Consequently, developers using different frameworks need to use different technologies for implementing and testing their user applications.

This is not directly perceived by the user, of course, but it has the potential of slowing down the improvement in quality that we could achieve by applying novel, advanced methods for testing, for instance. Specifically, property-based testing is a verification technique that has been gaining attention due to the appearance of tools like QuickCheck [1]. QuickCheck has proven very effective in many case studies [8–12], which is leading to the appearance of many clone implementations [4–7].

In this work, we propose an alternative for developers instead of waiting for a technology-specific clone of QuickCheck being implemented that they can use. Instead, we enable the use of the original QuickCheck for testing desktop applications, more precisely FreeDesktop applications, via a common inter-process communication system, D-Bus. This enables the use a powerful and mature implementation of PBT for testing desktop applications today, regardless of the specific development framework we use to build an application.

2   Example of Typical Desktop Ecosystem Inhabitants: Heterogeneous Components of an Alarm Service

To illustrate our proposal, we borrow an example from [13], in which a simple alarm clock service is used to explain how the D-Bus intercommunication system works. We will discuss the characteristics of this system in the next section, but for now we will focus on the conducting example.

Take a simple functionality consisting in setting up a count-down timer, which needs to raise a visual alarm. To implement this functionality we could

design three separate pieces which need to integrate, but need not be implemented in the same language nor be developed by the same person/group of
people. Of course, we could also implement this functionality as a single component developed in a single technology by one developer alone, but the consideration of different heterogeneous pieces scalates better to larger, more complex
software applications. Figure 4 shows a representation of the heterogeneous scenario, in which the core of the service is developed in a low-level language such as
C, while the other two pieces, the configurator and the alarm GUI are developed
in higher-level languages, namely Python and JavaScript.

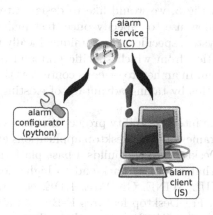

Fig. 4. Heterogeneous components of a simple alarm service.

In a traditional development scenario, after the agreement on the integration APIs amongst the components of the system, each person/group of people
would design, implement and test each component. Usually, the tests for each
component would consist on a set of unitary test scenarios, individually chosen,
written and run by the component developer(s), as shown in Fig. 5. Additionally,
once the components are integrated into the final system, system-level testing
in the form of smoke testing is frequently performed, which in an heterogeneous
case like this requires either setting up a series of coordinated test scripts (at
operating-system level) to run again a set of designed scenarios, or else some
monkey testing performed manually by beta testers or selected users.

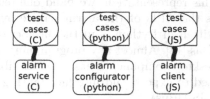

Fig. 5. Traditional unit testing of heterogeneous system components.

As one can easily see, the 'proper' testing of any heterogeneous software system like the one in our example quickly becomes a hassle when system size and complexity grow, constituting an error-prone, hard to maintain, inefficient, and ineffective testing infrastructure. In the next section, we propose an alternative that can help reduce the maintenance effort of unit and system-level tests of such systems, also improving test definition, repeatability, and error debugging.

3 Running QuickCheck-Generated Tests over D-Bus

To improve the situation presented in the previous section, and depicted in our conducting example in Fig. 5, we would like to design a testing strategy which infrastructure would allow use to "specify once, test multiple times". In other words, given that the system specification is unique, ideally we would like to have a unique test specification from which specific unit and integration test levels could be derived and run. In an heterogeneous context as the desktop ecosystem, we propose to achieve this by taking advantage of existing intercommunication facilities.

FreeDesktop [2] is an interoperability project that seeks to ensure that differences in development frameworks for desktop applications are not user-visible. In other words, the FreeDesktop project builds a base platform (both specification and implementation) that serves as back-end to higher-level application APIs such as Qt, GTK+, XUL, WINE, GNOME, KDE, etc. As an example of this interoperability efforts, FreeDesktop features D-Bus [3], a free and open-source inter-process communication (IPC) system, that allows multiple, concurrently-running software applications to communicate with one another.

Our proposal is to use D-Bus to communicate with any FreeDesktop application for testing purposes. In particular, D-Bus can be used as a way to interact with desktop applications within the context of test sequence execution. Given that a desktop application is compliant with the FreeDesktop guidelines, we can test it, and its components, even if they do not use D-Bus for inter-communication purposes. D-Bus functionalities include information sharing, meaning that FreeDesktop applications 'publish' their services (i.e. APIs) via D-Bus, enabling auto-discovery and thus even automatic black-box test generation, which we propose to steer by using a PBT tool like QuickCheck. The use of a test model rather than a set of specific unitary test cases has a number of benefits in terms of quality assurance [14].

Specifically, the application of this idea to our alarm service example is depicted in Fig. 6. In this representation, we build one test model (labelled `QC model`) which exercises the APIs of the alarm service implemented in C, the alarm configuration written in Python, and the JavaScript alarm client, all of them accessible via D-Bus [13]. Almost any programming language that is commonly used to build desktop components has a D-Bus library available, which is programmatically used to expose said interface (cf. Fig. 6, libraries C-DBus, Python-DBus [15] and JS-DBus).

Depending on the test module we write, we can exercise only one component at a time (i.e. unit-testing the C-core of the service alone) or several/all of them

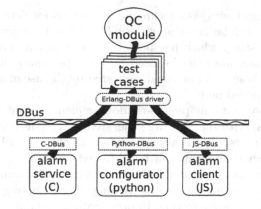

Fig. 6. Integrated PBT testing of the alarm service via D-Bus.

(i.e. their integration testing). The key aspect is, since the test cases would be generated from the QC model, they are technology-agnostic, and can be run against any specific implementation of each and every component thanks to the inter-connection of the generated test case to a given component execution via D-Bus.

The general architecture of the testing infrastructure we propose for these heterogeneous desktop applications is presented in Fig. 7.

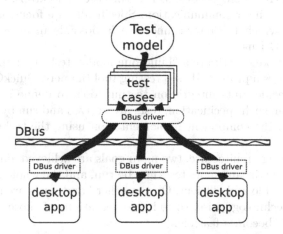

Fig. 7. General PBT testing architecture for heterogeneous components via D-Bus.

4   Discussion

There have been previous attempts to use D-Bus as a vehicle to enable other kinds of black-box, technology-independent testing of applications, specifically fuzz testing [16]. Fuzz testing is a technique well suited for detecting bugs stemming from improper validation of input data, but it is not adequate for functional unit-/integration testing, which has been our focus in this work. Admittedly, many bugs in software are indeed caused by improper validation and handling of input data, but these could be equally covered by the use of a property-based testing tool, as proposed here.

Using a PBT tool, not only pseudo-random sequences of interactions (this is, method invocations) with the SUT are generated to serve as test cases, the data to be used in such interactions is also generated. To this end, while the available interactions for each component can be obtained via D-Bus, the tester needs to manually define *data generators*. These data generators may produce only 'proper data', thus focusing on positive testing, or else may generate 'random data', thus enabling negative testing. In other words, the data-focused negative testing that one can perform using a property-based testing is equivalent to the aforementioned fuzz testing.

On the contrary, the effort required to use a PBT tool is unarguably greater. While the use of a fuzz tool requires no learning from the tester, adopting PBT as testing strategy does, and it should not be disregarded [17].

5 Conclusions

In this paper, we present a novel testing approach to applications or systems which are inherently heterogeneous, as it is the case of desktops, but for which it exists some form of inter-communication. Specifically, we focus on FreeDesktop applications, for which the inter-connection is possible in an end-technology-agnostic way via D-Bus.

In this setting, we contribute a "build one model, test any implementations" approach which uses a property-based testing tool (namely, QuickCheck) instead of technology-specific unit-/integration testing tools to define a high-level test specification. From such specification, tests are derived and run by the PBT tool, and submitted to the component implementation using the technology-specific D-Bus driver.

With this testing architecture, two main goals are achieved: on the one hand, tests are easier to maintain, more tests can be run, and the whole testing process becomes more reliable and efficient. On the other hand, tests are independent of the component technology-wise, so re-implementations of those, or even re-use of the test model, becomes feasible.

References

1. Hughes, J.: QuickCheck testing for fun and profit. In: Hanus, M. (ed.) PADL 2007. LNCS, vol. 4354, pp. 1–32. Springer, Heidelberg (2007)
2. FreeDesktop website. http://www.freedesktop.org/. Accessed October 2014
3. Pennington, H., Carlsson, A., Larsson, A.: D-Bus specification. http://dbus. freedesktop.org/doc/dbus-specification.html. Accessed October 2014

4. Holser, P.: JUnit-QuickCheck: QuickCheck-style parameter suppliers for JUnit Theories. https://github.com/pholser/junit-quickcheck/. Accessed May 2015
5. Nilsson, R.: ScalaCheck: Property-based testing for Scala. http://www.scalacheck.org/. Accessed May 2015
6. Pennebaker, A.: QC: a C port of the QuickCheck unit test framework. https://github.com/mcandre/qc. Accessed May 2015
7. Soldani, C.: QuickCheck++. http://software.legiasoft.com/quickcheck/. Accessed May 2015
8. López, M., Castro, L.M., Cabrero, D.: Feasibility of property-based testing for time-dependent systems. In: Moreno-Díaz, R., Pichler, F., Quesada-Arencibia, A. (eds.) EUROCAST. LNCS, vol. 8112, pp. 527–535. Springer, Heidelberg (2013)
9. Arts, T., Hughes, J., Johansson, J., Wiger, U.: Testing telecoms software with quviq QuickCheck. In: Proceedings of 5th ACM SIGPLAN Workshop on Erlang (2006)
10. Arts, T., Castro, L.M., Hughes, J.: Testing erlang data types with quviq QuickCheck. In: Proceedings of 7th ACM SIGPLAN Workshop on Erlang (2008)
11. Arts, T., Castro, L.M.: Model-based testing of data types with side effects. In: Proceedings of the 10th ACM SIGPLAN Workshop on Erlang (2010)
12. Castro, L.M.: Advanced management of data integrity: property-based testing for business. J. Intell. Inf. Syst. **44**(3), 1–26 (2014)
13. Morgado, A.: Introduction to D-Bus. GNOME ASIA 2014 (2014). https://aleksander.es/data/GNOMEASIA2014%20-%20Introduction%20to%20DBus.pdf. Accessed May 2014
14. Fink, G., Bishop, M.: Property-based testing: a new approach to testing for assurance. ACM SIGSOFT Softw. Eng. Notes **22**(4), 74–80 (1997)
15. McVittie, S.: dbus-python tutorial. http://dbus.freedesktop.org/doc/dbus-python/doc/tutorial.html. Accessed May 2015
16. Marhefka, M., Muller, P.: Dfuzzer: a D-Bus service fuzzing tool. In: Proceedings of 7th IEEE International Conference on Software Testing, Verification and Validation (2014)
17. Nilsson, A., Castro, L.M., Rivas, S., Arts, T.: Assessing the effects of introducing a new software development process: a methodological description. J. Softw. Tools Technol. Transf. **17**(1), 1–17 (2015)

Adaptation Engine for Large-Scale Distributed Systems

Tania Nemes[(✉)]

Christian-Doppler Laboratory for Client-Centric Cloud Computing (CDCC),
Softwarepark 21, 4232 Hagenberg im Mühlkreis, Austria
tania.nemes@cdcc.faw.jku.at
http://www.cdcc.faw.jku.at/

Abstract. One of the primary concerns with the increased complexity of large-scale distributed systems is to ensure efficiency, resilience and reliability of the system under changing contextual circumstances. A poorly handled outage as unavailability of parts of the network or services, performance bottlenecks or core network failure leads to down rated reliability and quality of service and, in extreme cases, lengthy downtime of the system. The current paper proposes a dynamic failure handling adaptation solution for cloud-enabled large-scale distributes systems that is composed (so far) of two phases. The first phase represents identification of a possible solution by means of case-based reasoning. The second one is a modeling phase, where the adaptation strategy is configured and described in terms of adaptation actions.

Keywords: Large-scale distributed systems · Adaptation · Decentralization · Case-based reasoning

1 Introduction

Over the last years, there have been growing recognition and interest gain among enterprises and academia throughout the world regarding the cloud computing paradigm and a new emerging notion, cloud-enabled, large scale, distributed systems (CELDS). Such systems, as a pool of collaborated stand-alone sub-clouds, enhance the performance, availability and reduced cost of the resources by employing usability of each cloud's capability. They come as an answer to the single cloud provider's serving limitation in matters of processing and storage requirements in relation to the continuously growing number of resource and service consumers.

For CELDS, adaptability is a valuable and an almost inevitable process mainly because cloud environments are not static: they evolve, and the parties must respectively adapt to new contexts varying from network traffic fluctuations to unavailability of different system components. In this paper we propose a set of standards for adaptation, that will guarantee that the structure as well as the level of analysis and action are sufficiently detailed and scalable to allow

© Springer International Publishing Switzerland 2015
R. Moreno-Díaz et al. (Eds.): EUROCAST 2015, LNCS 9520, pp. 244–251, 2015.
DOI: 10.1007/978-3-319-27340-2_31

the system to handle accordingly detected failures while supporting evolution of the system over time through higher flexibility and maximized performance. The adaptation component must abide by a balance between preventing violations of established Service Level Agreements (SLAs) and resource consumption while conveying the recovery method that triggers the repair action associated to a particular event and allows the system to be rolled back to a state in which continuation with the new execution plan can be performed [1]. The adaptation engine would be embedded in a larger architecture that envisions CELDS in terms of abstract state machines (ASMs) [2] as a three-layered model handling the service work flow, monitoring and adaptation which are distributed throughout the system [3]. Monitoring components [4] and adaptation components must cohesively work together in order to detect and enforce the correct solutions in case of failures. The adaption component reacts to the data collected and assessed by the monitoring components and employs the repair of the encountered problem under presumably optimal performance. Identification and management of the solution are done through patterns of Case Base Reasoning (CBS) and action workflows described in detail in the following sections.

The reminder of the paper is organized as follows. Section 2 presents case base reasoning and its corresponding components in the current architecture. Section 3 introduces our approach for supporting the adaptation action of multi-cloud systems. Section 4 gives an outlook for further research in this fields. Section 5 analyzes related work. Main conclusions are provided in Sect. 6.

2   Knowledge Management Using Case-Based Reasoning

This section is intended to give a short summary of some key concepts in knowledge management -based systems, and to provide focus on the CBR approach and its applicability within the adaptation model.

2.1   Motivation

One of the most effective methods to assure the cooperation and collaboration in a dynamically changing cloud enabled environment is knowledge sharing among all computing objects. By sharing knowledge and leveraging the existing information resources, intelligent behaviors that target a better coverage, robustness, and efficiency of the system at hand can be built.

Therefore, through reactive and proactive adaptation policies, the adaptation manager exploits the components' properties and registered behavior (average of quality of service (QoS) failures, cloud's violations responsiveness etc.), in building and continuously enhancing a catalog of rules that bind certain events to specific adaptation actions [5]. Thus, at any time point, the knowledge management system receives input measurements and notifications from the monitoring component and outputs a set of actions that are executed within the Adaptation Engine in order to retaliate the reported problems and avoid complete system failure.

Knowledge can be structured by employing one of the well known knowledge management methods like:

- Rule-based system: with rules in the format "IF *Condition* THEN *Action*", it leaves room for concern regarding scenarios of handling contradicting rules, employing a definite decision without hindering the rules' load
- Default logic [6]: used mainly in areas with contradicting information, represents a version of a rule-based system in which the rules are represented as: "IF *Condition* and all statements are consistent with the current system assumptions, THEN *Action*"
- Situation Calculus [7]: data is observed as states, more specific fluents (logic expression that can be true or false) and situations (a finite set of actions). As situations observe fluents, their state is determined by the set of all valid fluents for a given situation.

Although some of these alternatives can be worked out for a substantial part of erroneous conditions, they are either incredibly complex (Situation Calculus), time consuming or not feasible, basing their construction on contradicting information rather than reason oriented (Default Logic). Most critically, they are difficult to extend or maintain and are prone to break-down when faced with complexity specific to large systems like CELDS (Rule-based system).

2.2   Case-Based Reasoning

CBR is defined by identifying, adapting and applying past registered solutions/experiences to similar problems by heavily relying on the quality and amount of the collected data, the background knowledge and the pattern discovery mechanism that determines the similarity between two problems/cases [8].

As the project is in its incipient stage, we assume the knowledge base is filled with some meaningful initial cases, representative for the actions that can be triggered. In cloud management, a case (CB_r) represents a formatted instance of a problem linked (P_r) to a recorded solving experience (S_r):

$$CB_r = P_r + S_r,$$

The problem part of the adaptation case consists of description attributes and features subject to a common pattern recognition mechanism, whereas the solution denotes the set of actions that have to be performed on the retrieved solution. For organizing our case bases in a manageable manner that supports efficient search and retrieval, we use either [9] the flat/linear memory model (all cases are organized in the same level) characterized by maximum accuracy, easy maintenance, and easy but rather slow retention in large case bases; or the footprint memory model (all cases are in hierarchical form) characterized by a fast retrieval at a high cost of care base construction and maintenance.

In general, a typical CBR cycle comprises 4 activities, which adapted to the given context of failure handling in CELDS, work in close relationship with the monitoring components and the adaptation manager, depicted also in Fig. 1:

1. **Retrieve** the case(s) deemed most similar to the new one. Identifying initial matches represents applying domain-specific similarity measures ($Sim(f_i^I, f_i^E)$) between the new case (I) and the existing ones (E), for each of the specified features (f_i) in the case base. For flat memory models, initial and best match are done through a nearest neighbor assessment, based on a weighted (w) sum of all the features :

$$x = \frac{\sum_{i=1}^{n} w_i \times Sim(f_i^I, f_i^E)}{\sum_{i=1}^{n} w_i}$$

The retrieval complexity of this approach is O(n). The footprint model, on the other hand, uses a proprietary method that locates the target's nearest footprint case and then searches for the most similar case among the cases covered by that footprint case.

2. **Reuse** the information in the similar case to perform the needed adaptation. In this phase of the process, through simple operations of copy and adapt, the retrieved case is adapted to the current situation by abstracting away the differences ($D_{t,r}$) between the target problem (P_T) and the retrieved case solution part (S_r):

$$CB_t = P_t + D_{t,r} + S_r$$

The definitory actions for that particular solution are loaded and passed on to the Adaption Manager where they are executed according to the action workflow schema describing them.

3. **Revise** the proposed solution. As the solution is being carried out according to its specification, the monitoring component evaluates the solution's performance, accuracy and output to specific threshold values. If the results

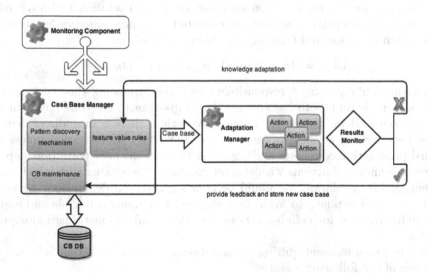

Fig. 1. Proposed case-base manager model

are positive, then the Case Base Manager is notified to classify it as a valid solution and retain the parts of the experience likely to be useful for future problem solving. The Case Base Manager is notified also in case of failures (problems persists or is partially satisfactory) as it needs then to optimize the definition of aggregated features by applying a set of rules to the feature values of the current case, making it a better fit with the new case requirements. And thus the cycle is repeated for the newly refined case.

4. **Retain** the case. The new problem-solving experience (be it a new case or an old case generalized to include the new case as well) is indexed for future retrieval and integrated into the case repository. Existing cases need to have a refined indexing as well as a strengthened or weakened weight of features, based on their correlation of retrieving relevant or irrelevant cases.

3   Adaptation Approach in Terms of Action Management

As indicated in the previous section, a solution for any case r (S_r) represents a set of N actions, all equally necessary to completing the solution:

$$S_r = \{a_0, ..., a_{N-1}\}$$

We do not want to impose any constraint on this set meaning that the order of definition does not necessarily represent the order of execution. Still, in order to support ordered execution for any given set of actions, we need additionally a starting execution action and a set of transitions (t_i) from one action execution to other(s):

$$t_i = s \begin{cases} \{(a_i, a_0), ..., (a_i, a_j)\} & \text{if } 0 \leq j \leq N\text{ - }1 \\ \emptyset, & \text{if } j = i \end{cases}$$

Introducing a new term, an action workflow for a given solution r (AW_{S_r}) indicates that the adaptation actions are executed in a prescribed order starting from an initial action and following the defined transitions.

$$AW_{S_r} = (\{a_0, ..., a_{N-1}\}, \ a_{\text{initial}}, \{t_0, ..., t_{N-1}\})$$

Actions are built on single responsibility principle, meaning that each action denotes a single update to the system. More importantly, they are autonomous and self-aware. If we look at the order of execution, there is an indirect dependency between the actions as one action cannot start its execution unless its needed prior action completes and implicitly triggers the next transition step. If we were to annotate actions with characteristics of the actions with which they are engaged in a relation, we would be creating a strong dependency between all the involved actions. To avoid this, we need to employ a flexible and easily extendable method for defining actions and their underlying transition dependencies.

At any given moment, during the adaptation process, an action is bound to have one of the following 4 states:

$$state : \{a_0, ..., a_{N-1}\} = \{active, passive, failed, run\}$$

Starting with a *passive* state, the action awaits its determining action to complete its update. Once the prior action is completed, the passive action moves to state *run* where the execution process handles the needed update. Depending on the results of the execution, the action can become either *active* or *failed*. An *active* action indicates that its defining update was already performed successfully. If the execution was interrupted due to some detected failures or errors, the running action becomes *failed*.

One way of handling action ordering is by means of notification/signaling. Starting with a fixed set of notifications:

$$signals = \{actionStarted, actionCompleted, actionFailed\}$$

every action would now embody concrete instances of those three notifications. Based on this construction, every action state change would now imply broadcasting the associated notification/signal:

$$\begin{cases} passive_{a_i} \rightarrow run_{a_i}, & broadcastNotification(actionStarted_{a_i}) \\ run_{a_i} \rightarrow active_{a_i}, & broadcastNotification(actionCompleted_{a_i}) \\ run_{a_i} \rightarrow failed_{a_i}, & broadcastNotification(actionFailed_{a_i}) \end{cases}$$

Through this mechanism, the problem is partially solved, as actions still need to be linked to data specific to other actions, in this case associated notifications. Fragmenting the notification mechanism by introducing an intermediate component, Action Controller or Handler (illustrated in Fig. 2), gives us the complete independence between the given actions of an adaptation solution. The Action Controller would therefore intercept all the raised notifications and respond to them based on its established contract. The reaction implies either enacting and executing its corresponding action, or ignoring the notification as it is not of interest in the given solution configuration. Besides pertaining to the independence of the actions, having controllers in place to monitor and handle the interaction between given actions emphasizes new properties of the complete model like: *built-in extensibility and substitution capabilities* by enabling the possibility to add or remove any given number of actions without the need to update the current actions; *reusability capabilities* as actions are not specified in terms of other actions but in terms of needed input, concrete implementation and resulting output; *reverse state capabilities*, offering in case of failures the possibility to revert the system to a stable state through a notification based compensating transaction. All the pertaining notions like actions (with their corresponding properties and notifications), action controllers (with their associated action and notification contract) as well as the starting action are described in the configuration file workflow schema. Each adaptation case has such a schema which, once is passed on to the Action Manager, is compiled and all the relevant data (initial action and all action controllers) are loaded to handle the execution of the adaptation (the actions are loaded once that particular update is requested as a result of one action completing). While an adaptation strategy is acted out in compliance to the established factors, new changes in the environment may require other methods, which, if not treated accordingly, can lead to a continuous adaptation loop, also referred to as oscillation. Depending on the completion time of the actions, the time frequency of the requests and in equal part the components involved, the Action Manger must either interrupt the undergoing update or prioritize the remaining ones.

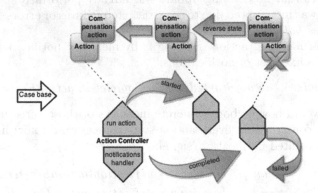

Fig. 2. Proposed action manager model

4   Future Development

Having only one component in charge of the adaptability process is rather risky as faulty situations can occur also at this level. Therefore, redundancy should be considered so that every component is annotated with a subset of rules and actions that allows adaptation enactment at component level in case the adaptation engine is not viable. Before reaching the execution of an adaptation solution, the decision process based on prior experiences needs further refinement: feature and attribute description and classification for an adaptation case and similarity functions definition based on the established parameters. A parallel development would be to model the evolving solution in terms of ASMs which would allow us to verify and validate the models before starting the development of the code.

5   Related Work

Research in software adaptation ranges from the development of generic architectural platforms to specific middleware using component frameworks and reflective technologies for specialized domains. The proposed mechanisms include: dynamic adaptation by generic interceptors [10], which do not modify a component's behavior, but intercept messages between components; dynamic adaptation with aspect-orientation [11]; parametric adaptation [12] or dynamic reconfiguration by means of adjusting or fine-tuning predefined parameters in software entities.

6   Conclusions

This article pertains to identify adaptation approaches of dynamic and scalable distributed systems to facilitate a mapping of current challenges and fault tolerance procedures to CELDS characteristics. The approaches presented herein for identifying and configuring an adaptation solution and its corresponding set of executable actions, represent building blocks in our (on-going) research and development project, focused on analysis, design, specification and formal modeling of an adaptation engine.

References

1. Ferry, N., Rossini, A., Chauvel, F., Morin, B., Solberg, A.: Towards model-driven provisioning, deployment, monitoring, and adaptation of multi-cloud systems. In: IEEE Sixth International Conference on Cloud Computing (2013)
2. Borger, E., Stark, R.F.: Abstract State Machines: A Method for High-Level System Design and Analysis. Springer-Verlag New York Inc., Secaucus (2003)
3. Bósa, K.: A formal model of a cloud service architecture in terms of ambient ASM. Technical report, Christian Doppler Laboratory for Client-Centric Cloud Computing (CDCC), Johannes Kepler University Linz, Hagenberg, Austria (2012)
4. Buga, A.: A scalable monitoring solution for large-scale distributed systems. In: Moreno-Díaz, R., Pichler, F., Quesada-Arencibia, A. (eds.) EUROCAST 2015. LNCS, vol. 9520, pp. 219–227. Springer, Heidelberg (2015)
5. Aamodt, A., Plaza, E.: Case-based reasoning: foundational issues, methodological variations, and system approaches. IOS Press **7**(1), 39–59 (1994)
6. Antoniou, G.: A tutorial on default logics. ACM Comput. Surv. **31**(4), 337–359 (1999)
7. Levesque, H., Pirri, F., Reiter, R: Foundations for the situation calculus. In: Modelling Autonomic Communicatiosn Environments, pp. 120–125 (1998)
8. Althoff, K.-D.: Case-based reasoning. In: Handbook on Software Engineering and Knowledge Engineering, vol. 1, pp. 549–587 (2001)
9. Soltani, S.: Case-based reasoning for diagnosis and planning. Technical report, Queens University, Kingston (2013)
10. Sadjani, S., McKinley, P.: An adaptive CORBA template to support unanticipated adaption. In: International Conference on Distributed Computing Systems, pp. 74–83 (2004)
11. Yang, Z., Cheng, B., Stirewalt, R., Sowell, J., Sadjadi, S., McKinley, P.: An aspect-oriented approach to dynamic adaptation. In: WOSS, pp. 85–92 (2002)
12. Pellegrini, M.-C., Riveill, M.: Component management in a dynamic architecture. J. Supercomputing **24**(2), 151–159 (2003)

Theory and Applications
of Metaheuristic Algorithms

A Multi-stage Approach Aimed at Optimizing the Transshipment of Containers in a Maritime Container Terminal

Eduardo Lalla-Ruiz[✉], Jesica de Armas, Christopher Expósito-Izquierdo,
Belén Melián-Batista, and J. Marcos Moreno-Vega

Department of Computer and Systems Engineering, University of La Laguna,
38271 La Laguna, Spain
{elalla,jdearmas,cexposit,mbmelian,jmmoreno}@ull.es

Abstract. This paper addresses the management of container flows in a maritime container terminal. In this context, we propose a multi-stage approach that allows to provide a complete schedule of the container flows from their arrival within container vessels to their delivery to receiving companies. Our proposed approach is aimed at minimizing the total maximum waiting time of the companies after they have requested containers. The computational results indicate that there are some relations subjected to the involved resources that have to be considered when tackling this problem.

Keywords: Container transshipment · Maritime container terminal · Metaheuritics

1 Introduction

The multi-modal transportation involves the interconnection of several means of transport (*e.g.*, container vessels, trucks, trains, etc.). In this environment, maritime container terminals play a highlighted role. These facilities are open systems dedicated to the exchange of containers in multimodal transportation networks, allowing to move goods from their production sources towards their final destinations. However, the management of a given maritime container terminal is extremely complex due to the high volume of containers to handle, the number and the characteristics of the heterogeneous processes brought together within it, and the increasingly demand of reliable services.

For this reason, the availability of support systems that aid to achieve an efficient management of maritime container terminals is of essential interest in this transportation area. Thus, in order to tackle some of the most challenging issues for obtaining a support system, the main goals of this paper are (*i*) to analyse the main flows of containers in a maritime container terminal between the quay area and external companies that pick up the containers, and (*ii*) to propose a multi-stage approach aimed at modelling the transshipment of containers in a terminal.

© Springer International Publishing Switzerland 2015
R. Moreno-Díaz et al. (Eds.): EUROCAST 2015, LNCS 9520, pp. 255–262, 2015.
DOI: 10.1007/978-3-319-27340-2_32

The remainder of this paper is organized as follows. Section 2 introduces an analysis of the main flows of containers arisen in maritime container terminals. Section 3 overviews the most highlighted papers found in the related literature. Afterwards, Sect. 4 introduces a multi-stage approach aimed at optimizing the transshipment of containers in a given maritime container terminal. Several computational experiments are presented and discussed in Sect. 5. Finally, Sect. 6 draws the main conclusions extracted from the work and proposes several lines for further research.

2   Maritime Container Terminals

The maritime container terminals are huge facilities found within multi-modal transport networks mainly dedicated to exchange containers among different transport modes. The layout of a terminal can be split into the following three different functional areas (Günther and Kim [10]):

- The *quay area* is the part of the port in which the container vessels are berthed in order to load and unload containers to/from them. The main seaside operations in maritime container terminals are studied in [14].
- The *yard area* is aimed at storing the containers until their subsequent retrieval. The main storage yard operations and several directions for further research are analysed in [2].
- The *mainland interface* connects the terminal with the land transport modes. The transport operations in container terminals are reviewed in [3].

The containers in a maritime container terminal arrive by means of container vessels, trucks, or trains. Once a container vessel arrives to the terminal, a suitable berth is assigned to it according to its particular characteristics (*i.e.*, draft, stowage plan, etc.) and all its containers are unloaded by means of the available quay cranes. Simultaneously, some containers can be loaded to be transported by the vessel towards another port in its shipping route. The loading and unloading operations are termed *transshipment operations* and have a great impact on the competitiveness of the terminal due to the fact that they determine the turnaround time of the vessels at the terminal.

Internal transport vehicles found at the terminal are aimed at moving containers from the quay cranes towards their storage locations on the yard, and vice-versa. The containers are stored on the yard of the terminal until their subsequent retrieval, which is determined by their loading time in vessels or the expected arrival time in private companies found outside the terminal.

The containers are moved between the terminal and the existing private companies found outside the terminal by means of external transport vehicles. The containers requested by the external transport vehicles can be picked up from the quay after the quay crane has unloaded them or from their current locations in the yard blocks. Once a container has been picked up by an external transport vehicle can be directly transported towards its destination private company outside the terminal. It is worth mentioning that, due to space and security restrictions, only a maximum number of external transport vehicles can be simultaneously in the terminal.

The optimization objective studied in this paper is the minimization of the waiting times of the private companies requesting containers. This can be formally expressed as follows:

$$\min \sum_{e \in E} wt(e), \tag{1}$$

where E is the set of existing private companies and $wt(\cdot)$ is the maximum waiting time of a company after requesting containers.

3   Related Works

The container transshipment management at maritime container terminals involves, at a first stage, the berthing of container vessels and the storage of their containers on the yard. In this regard, the quay and yard operations play an outstanding role due to their direct impact on the overall management of transshipment flows.

The main logistic problem at the seaside is the so-called Berth Allocation Problem (BAP). Its goals are assigning and scheduling incoming vessels to berthing positions along the quay. As indicated in [12], this problem has a relevant impact on the container terminal performance. The reason is found in that a bottleneck derived from a poor schedule of its resources may be translated into a delay of the remaining logistic operations at the terminal.

Once the vessels have been berthed, their containers are unloaded [7] and moved towards the yard, where they are stored in the yard blocks until their subsequent retrieval [9]. However, the space on the yard is a scarce resource, and therefore suitable stacking strategies are required. This way, a continuous flow of goods in the supply chain is kept. Optimization approaches have been proposed in [11] and [1] among others with the aim of satisfying the container requests of a container terminal.

On the other hand, a relevant problem arises in the land-side, the route planning problem, which can be split into two stages: the design of service networks (tactical), whose goal is to find the best set of services dealing with transport and logistics, and the transport programming or operational planning (operational), which determines the best service under scenarios with available resources and imposed constraints. Most inter-modal problems described in the literature follows the first format (*i.e.*, design and planning of networks and flow), aimed at finding the best combined transport route in an inter-modal transport network. These problems are solved and modelled as a shortest path problem, since their objective is to find the best path given specified starting and ending points, and doing stops at diverse nodes. See the works [4,5], and [15] for further discussion.

4   Optimization Approach

The flow of containers around a maritime container terminal in their way towards receiving companies can be addressed by a multi-stage approach, as discussed

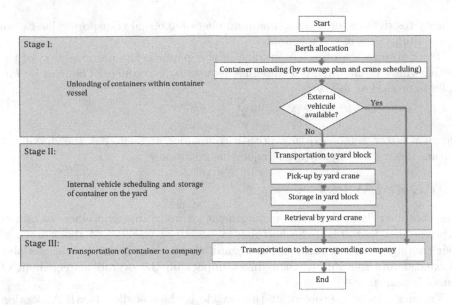

Fig. 1. Diagram of the multi-stage approach

in the following. This is depicted in Fig. 1. Those container vessels arriving to port must be adequately berthed along the quay in order to load and unload their containers while minimizing their waiting times. Thus, at Stage I, the vessels are allocated and the transshipment containers to be loaded and unloaded from/into are scheduled by the quay cranes according to their stowage plans. An efficient Tabu Search algorithm with a Path-Relinking-based restarting strategy (Lalla-Ruiz et al. [13]) is used at this stage.

Moving containers from the terminal to the companies requires to manage a fleet of external transport vehicles. With this goal in mind, a heuristic approach is proposed. This approach allows to assign each container to one of the available external transport vehicles with the aim of minimizing the total transportation times of containers to companies. This way, each container unloaded from a vessel is assigned to a vehicle to be transported to its destination company as shown in Stage III. In those cases in which there is not external transport vehicle, the container must be stored in one of the yard blocks and follow the process shown in Stage II.

As above mentioned, in some cases, containers cannot be delivered immediately to their destination companies, and then they have to be temporarily stored on the yard of the terminal. In this case, each container is moved to the yard by one of the internal vehicles of the terminal and stored in a yard block by means of the stacking cranes. The management of the storage and retrieval operations in blocks is known as Stacking Problem (SP). Its objective is to minimize the number of relocation movements performed by the stacking cranes at the yard. A heuristic algorithm [8] to solve this problem is used. The rationale behind our heuristic is to exploit those time periods in which the stacking cranes are idle in order to arrange the stored containers according to their retrieval orders.

5   Computational Experiments

This section is devoted to assess the performance of the multi-stage approach proposed in this paper. The influence of the different elements of the maritime container terminal in the companies waiting time has been studied, and the correct behaviour of our approach has been checked. The approach has been implemented using the programming language Java Standard Edition 7.0. All the computational experiments have been carried out on a PC equipped with Ubuntu 13.10, a processor Intel Core 2 Duo 3.16 GHz, and 4 GB of RAM.

Some parameters, such as number of containers nC, number of companies nE, number of berths nB, and number of arriving vessels nV, have been taken into account to generate scenarios with different features. These scenarios have been executed changing some other parameters values, such as number of quay cranes of a berth b denoted as $qc(b)$, number of internal vehicles $nKin$, number of external vehicles $nKout$, and maximum number of internal vehicles simultaneously allow inside container terminal.

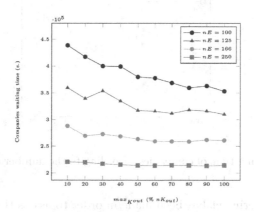

Fig. 2. Average companies waiting time according to a percentage over a maximum number of external vehicles (max_{Kout}).

For the first experiment, we have checked the influence of the number of external vehicles simultaneously allowed inside the terminal (max_{Kout}) over the companies waiting time. Figure 2 shows the behaviour of the companies waiting time when the percentage of external vehicles allowed inside the terminal max_{Kout} increases. Each line corresponds to a different number of companies $nE = \{100, 125, 166, 250\}$, and the number of containers nC has been fixed to 500.

As can be seen in Fig. 2, the rank of the waiting time is different based on the number of companies to which containers belong, going from 4 days to 2 days. It has been possible to verify that the higher the percentage, the smaller the companies have to wait.

Moreover, there is a certain stability in terms of companies waiting time obtained when a percentage is reached. In this regard, this stability is achieved earlier when the number of external vehicles increases, since the percentage of allowed vehicles in the terminal is calculated on the basis of the total number of external vehicles. Hence, the higher the total number of external vehicles, the larger the number of external vehicles allowed inside terminal, and therefore the better the results in terms of the companies waiting time. This way, when the total number of external vehicles is very high there is no difference between allowing 10 % or 100 % of them inside terminal. With this kind of graphic it is possible to determine which is the limit number of external vehicles allowed inside terminal for which no significant improvement occurs in terminal performance according to the particular characteristics of the studied terminal.

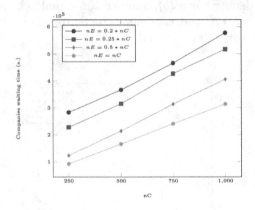

Fig. 3. Average waiting time of companies according to the number of containers (nC)

The second experiment has been made in order to assess the influence of the number of required containers over the companies waiting time. Figure 3 represents the increment of companies waiting time when the number of required containers increases. In the figure, each line corresponds to a number of companies, $nE = \{0.2 * nC, 0.25 * nC, 0.5 * nC, nC\}$, which depends on the workload in terms of the number of containers $nC = \{250, 500, 750, 1000\}$.

As can be checked in the figure, the increment over the companies waiting time increases with the number of containers. This increment is quasi-linear which makes sense taking into account the increase of containers within a terminal with the same characteristics. Moreover, in those cases where the number of companies is small, the companies waiting time is higher and vice-versa. This is agree with real-scenarios since the higher the number of companies, the larger the number of external vehicles hired by them for picking-up the containers.

Furthermore, other important factor in a maritime container terminal is the number of available internal vehicles. For this reason, in the last experiment the effect of this parameter in the waiting time of companies is evaluated. Table 1 report the waiting time of companies regarding the number of internal vehicles. Each column in the table represent the different number of companies considered. As can be seen, the higher the number of vehicles, the lower the waiting time. In this regard, the reduction is more relevant in terms of objective function value when the number of companies increases. That is, when the number of companies is high, the number of external vehicles is also high, so it is more likely that an external transport vehicle may carry a container directly to a company without requiring the use of any internal vehicle.

Table 1. Average waiting time of companies according to the number of internal vehicles (nK_{in}) and number of companies (nE)

nK_{in}	nE			
	100	125	250	500
5	393152.39	324464.09	221071.60	167157.47
10	366842.52	315150.17	214457.18	166005.43
15	361079.06	307337.74	215206.25	165432.28
20	360385.22	304778.57	215020.96	164726.63

6 Conclusions and Further Research

In this work, we analyze the flow of containers in a maritime container terminal from their arrival into container vessels to their delivery to receiving companies. During this complete process, we have recognized three main stages and, hence, proposed a multi-stage approach for providing a complete schedule. The computational experiments carried out suggest that the performance of the proposed multi-stage approach corresponds with expectations while it provides a complete schedule of the resources involved in the management of container flows.

Moreover, through our propose approach terminal managers are also able to analyse the impact that some resources have over the terminal from the viewpoint of the companies. This feature provides them a support when taking strategic decisions such as increasing the number of either internal vehicles or quay cranes, extending the quay to include more berths, etc.

In future works, on the basis of the contributions presented in this paper, we will focus on the introduction of dynamism related to the arrival of the vessels and the movement of containers.

Acknowledgements. This work has been partially funded by the Spanish Ministry of Economy and Competitiveness (project TIN2012-32608). Eduardo Lalla-Ruiz and Christopher Expósito-Izquierdo would like to thank the Government of Canary Island for the financial support they receive through their post-graduate grants. The research by Jesica de Armas is supported by the Canary Islands CIE: Tricontinental Atlantic Campus.

References

1. Bortfeldt, A., Wäscher, G.: Constraints in container loading - a state-of-the-art review. Eur. J. Oper. Res. **229**(1), 1–20 (2013)
2. Carlo, H.J., Vis, I.F.A., Roodbergen, K.J.: Storage yard operations in container terminals: literature overview, trends, and research directions. Eur. J. Oper. Res. **235**(2), 412–430 (2014). Maritime Logistics
3. Carlo, H.J., Vis, I.F.A., Roodbergen, K.J.: Transport operations in container terminals: Literature overview, trends, research directions and classification scheme. Eur. J. Oper. Res. **236**(1), 1–13 (2014)
4. Cho, J., Kim, H., Choi, H.: An intermodal transport network planning algorithm using dynamic programming case study: from Busan to Rotterdam in intermodal freight routing. Appl. Intell. **36**(3), 529–541 (2012)
5. Cho, J.H., Kim, H.S., Choi, H.R., Park, N.K., Kang, M.H.: An intermodal transport network planning algorithm using dynamic programming. In: Okuno, H.G., Ali, M. (eds.) IEA/AIE 2007. LNCS (LNAI), vol. 4570, pp. 1012–1021. Springer, Heidelberg (2007)
6. de Armas, J., Melián-Batista, B., Moreno-Pérez, J.A., Brito, J.: GVNS for a real-world rich vehicle routing problem with time windows. Eng. Appl. Artif. Intell. Rev. **42**, 45–56 (2014)
7. Expósito-Izquierdo, C., González-Velarde, J.L., Melián-Batista, B., Moreno-Vega, J.M.: Hybrid estimation of distribution algorithm for the quay crane scheduling problem. Appl. Soft Comput. **13**(10), 4063–4076 (2013)
8. Expósito-Izquierdo, C., Lalla-Ruiz, E., de Armas, J., Melián-Batista, B., Moreno-Vega, J.M.: A Heuristic algorithm for the stacking problem. Comput. Ind. Eng. Rev. (2014)
9. Expósito-Izquierdo, C., Melián-Batista, B., Moreno-Vega, J.: A domain-specific knowledge-based heuristic for the blocks relocation problem. Adv. Eng. Inform. **28**(4), 327–343 (2014)
10. Günther, H.O., Kim, K.H.: Container terminals and terminal operations. OR Spectrum **28**(4), 437–445 (2006)
11. Kim, K.H., Hong, G.: A heuristic rule for relocating blocks. Comput. Oper. Res. **33**(4), 940–954 (2006)
12. Lalla-Ruiz, E., González-Velarde, J.L., Melián-Batista, B., Moreno-Vega, J.M.: Biased random key genetic algorithm for the tactical berth allocation problem. Appl. Soft Comput. **22**, 60–76 (2014)
13. Lalla-Ruiz, E., Melián-Batista, B., Moreno-Vega, J.M.: Artificial intelligence hybrid heuristic based on tabu search for the dynamic berth allocation problem. Eng. Appl. Artif. Intell. **25**(6), 1132–1141 (2012)
14. Meisel, F.: Seaside Operations Planning in Container Terminals. Contributions to Management Science. Physica-Verlag HD, Heidelberg (2010)
15. Xiong, G., Wang, Y.: Best routes selection in multimodal networks using multi-objective genetic algorithm. J. Comb. Optim. pp. 1–19 (2012)

A Greedy Randomized Adaptive Search Procedure for Solving the Uncapacitated Plant Cycle Problem

Israel López-Plata, Christopher Expósito-Izquierdo[✉], Eduardo Lalla-Ruiz,
Belén Melián-Batista, and J. Marcos Moreno-Vega

Department of Computer and Systems Engineering,
University of La Laguna, 38271 La Laguna, Spain
iloppla@gmail.com, {cexposit,elalla,mbmelian,jmmoreno}@ull.es

Abstract. The Uncapacitated Plant Cycle Problem seeks to select a subset of potential locations in which to open plants dedicated to provide service to customers scattered abroad upon the field. The locations are known and each plant can serve an unlimited number of customers through a vehicle route. The objective of this problem is to (i) determine the number of plants to open, (ii) select the subset of locations in which to open the plants, (iii) assign a non-empty subset of customers to each plant, and (iv) determine a vehicle route dedicated to serve the subset of customers assigned to each plant. With the goal of solving this problem from an approximate point of view, a Greedy Randomized Adaptive Search Procedure is proposed in this paper. The computational experiments disclose the suitable performance of this algorithmic approach, which allows to reach high-quality solutions in reasonable computational times.

Keywords: Greedy randomized adaptive search procedure · Uncapacitated plant cycle problem · Logistics

1 Introduction

Determining the most adequate locations of logistic facilities is a challenging objective in many fields, such as distribution, transportation, infrastructure management, and so forth. This decision is usually subject to conflicting criteria: maximizing the coverage of the customers to serve, minimizing the average transportation times to reach the customers, minimizing the costs derived from opening the infrastructures, etc.

Over the last few decades, an special interest has arisen through the combination of location and routing decisions. Location-routing problems [11] involve the integration of those decisions regarding facility location, at strategic level, and the design of vehicle routes to fulfil the demand of customers geographically dispersed on a two-dimensional area, at tactical level. Addressing these logistic

© Springer International Publishing Switzerland 2015
R. Moreno-Díaz et al. (Eds.): EUROCAST 2015, LNCS 9520, pp. 263–270, 2015.
DOI: 10.1007/978-3-319-27340-2_33

decisions independently gives rise to only sub-optimal results in most of the practical applications [1]. Hence, it is highly advisable to develop new optimization approaches which consider their interdependencies jointly.

The focus of the present paper is put on the Uncapacitated Plant Cycle Problem [8]. It is an optimization problem that seeks to determine a subset of locations with unknown cardinality in which to open plants to provide service to customers scattered abroad upon the field. The customers are assigned to the plants and their service is given by means of vehicle routes. In this problem no capacity constraints are considered, thus each plant can serve an unlimited number of customers.

The main objective of this work is to propose a Greedy Randomized Adaptive Search Procedure to solve the Uncapacitated Plant Cycle Problem from an approximate point of view. The computational results disclose the suitability of this algorithm when addressing the Uncapacitated Plant Cycle in realistic scenarios and open several promising lines for further research.

The remainder of this work is organized as follows. Firstly, Sect. 2 describes the Uncapacitated Plant Cycle Problem. Section 3 presents a Greedy Randomized Adaptive Search Procedure aimed at solving the Uncapacitated Plant Cycle Problem. The computational experiments carried out in the work are presented and discussed in Sect. 4. Finally, Sect. 5 extracts the main conclusions from the work and indicates several lines for further research.

2   Problem Description

In this work, the Uncapacitated Plant Cycle Problem (hereafter termed UPCP) proposed in [8] is addressed. In the UPCP, a set of potential locations is given, $M = \{1, 2, \ldots, m\}$, in which to open plants (*i.e.*, infrastructures, warehouses, etc.), $P = \{1, 2, \ldots, k\}$, with the goal of serving a set of customers, denoted as $N = \{1, 2, \ldots, n\}$. The number of plants to open, k, is positive but unknown in advance. However, opening a plant $p \in P$ in a location produces a certain cost, $o_p > 0$. Moreover, each customer must be assigned to exclusively one of the opened plants. The assignment of a customer $i \in N$ to the plant $p \in P$ involves an assignment cost, $c_{ip} > 0$. Furthermore, the customers assigned to a given plant $p \in P$ must be visited by a vehicle with no capacity constraints. The travel cost between each pair of points, $i, j \in M \cup N$, is $d_{ij} > 0$. It is assumed that all the travel costs satisfy the triangle inequality [5].

The optimization objective of the UPCP is to minimize the sum of the opening costs of the plants, the customer assignment costs, and the vehicle routing costs. This objective can be formally expressed as follows

$$\min \sum_{j \in M} o_j \cdot y_j + \sum_{i \in N} \sum_{j \in M} c_{ij} \cdot z_{ij} + \sum_{i \in M \cup N} \sum_{j \in M \cup N} d_{ij} \cdot x_{ij}, \tag{1}$$

where y_j is a binary variable that takes a value of one if and only if a plant is open at location $j \in M$, z_{ij} is a binary variable that takes a value of one if and only if customer $i \in N$ is assigned to a plant open at location $j \in M$, and x_{ij} is a binary variable that takes a value of one if and only if the distance from the points $i, j \in M \cup N$ is travelled by some vehicle.

According to the previous description of the UPCP, it should be noted that the decisions to take are the following ones:

- Determining the number of plants to open. This is denoted as k.
- Selecting the subset of k locations in which to open the plants.
- Assigning a non-empty subset of customers to each plant.
- Determining a vehicle route dedicated to serve the subset of customers assigned to each plant.

Finally, it is worth mentioning that, the UPCP is an optimization problem that belongs to the $\mathcal{NP}$-hard class of problems by reduction to the well-known Travelling Salesman Problem [6].

3   Algorithm Approach

This work proposes a Greedy Randomized Adaptive Search Procedure (hereafter termed GRASP) for solving the Uncapacitated Plant Cycle Problem (UPCP) introduced in Sect. 2 from an approximate point of view. The GRASP [2,3] is a well-known multi-start or iterative meta-heuristic algorithm developed in the late 1980 s that has been successfully applied to a wide range of optimization problems found in many fields of research. Representative examples of its application can be found in vehicle routing [13], scheduling [10], and web services composition [9]. Outstanding reviews of the GRASP have been published in [4,7,12].

The rationale behind a GRASP is to make up feasible solutions by means of a constructive procedure and then exploit them through the application of an improvement algorithm. This process is iteratively repeated until a given stopping criterion is satisfied. The execution of a GRASP usually starts with an empty solution and, at each step, the constructive procedure includes a promising element in the partial solution obtained so far. The potential elements to be included in the partial solution are conventionally evaluated according to a greedy evaluation function, which determines the increment or decrement caused in the objective function value after including the relevant element. If the solution obtained by means of the constructive procedure is not feasible, a repair procedure must be then applied to recover the feasibility. Once a feasible solution is obtained, a local optimum solution is frequently achieved by applying a local search method.

Specifically, the GRASP proposed in this paper has a threefold purpose. That is, (i) selecting a subset of locations in which to open plants, (ii) assigning each customer to a plant, and (iii) building the route to serve all the customers assigned to each plant. The pseudo-code of the GRASP is depicted in Algorithm 1. In this case, the GRASP iterates until a maximum number of consecutive iterations without improvement in the best found solution have been executed (lines 3–17). This number of iterations is denoted as λ and its value

---

Algorithm 1. Pseudocode of the Greedy Randomized Adaptive Search Procedure for the Uncapacitated Plant Cycle Location Problem

---

Require: λ, maximum number of consecutive iterations without improvement in the best solution found

1: $s_{best} \leftarrow \emptyset$
2: $iterations \leftarrow 0$
3: **while** $(iterations < \lambda)$ **do**
4:     $k \leftarrow 1$
5:     **while** $(k \leq m)$ **do**
6:       $P \leftarrow$ Select k plants randomly from available locations
7:       $s \leftarrow$ Assign customers and determine routes associated with the plants in P
8:       $s_{local} \leftarrow$ Apply local search to s
9:       **if** $(f(s_{local}) < f(s_{best}))$ **then**
10:        $s_{best} \leftarrow s_{local}$
11:        $iterations \leftarrow 0$
12:      **else**
13:        $iterations \leftarrow iterations + 1$
14:      **end if**
15:      $k \leftarrow k + 1$
16:    **end while**
17: **end while**
18: Return s_{best}

---

is pre-defined by the user. In Algorithm 1, *iterations* represents the number of consecutive iterations without improvement of the best found solution. Both, the best solution achieved by the GRASP and *iterations* are initialized to empty and zero, respectively (lines 1–2).

The selection of locations in which to open plants is the first decision to take in the GRASP proposed in this paper. In this regard, $k > 0$ locations are selected at random. With this goal in mind, the value of the parameter k is initialized to one (line 4) and is increased in one unit from one iteration to the next (line 15). This process is carried out until the maximum number of locations, m, is achieved (lines 5–16). Recall that, according to the definition of the UPCP introduced in Sect. 2, the set of locations in which plants are going to be open is denoted as P. This set of locations is selected in line 6.

Once the plants are open, the underlying solution must be completed with the assignment and routing of the customers (line 7). In this regard, successive constructions of a greedy randomized solution for the assignment and routing of the available customers in the problem are carried out. With this goal in mind, the impact of assigning each customer to the previously selected plants and its position in the corresponding route is evaluated. At this step, one of the best $r > 0$ assignments is selected according to the roulette-wheel selection process on the basis of the increment in the objective function value. Each feasible solution is improved through a local search algorithm based upon the reinsertion movement (line 8). Finally, at each step, if the local optimum solution provided by the improvement procedure improves the best solution found during the search process in terms of objective function value, this is updated (lines 9–10). Additionally, the count of iterations without improvement of the best solution found during the search is set to zero again (line 11). Otherwise, the count is increased in one unit.

4   Analysis

In the following, the suitability of the Greedy Randomized Adaptive Search Procedure (GRASP) introduced in Sect. 3 to solve the Uncapacitated Plant Cycle Problem (UPCP) described in Sect. 2 is adequately assessed. Specifically, its performance is evaluated in comparison with those of the Honey Bees Mating Optimization (HBMO) algorithm proposed in [8] and an optimization model for the UPCP developed by the authors of the present paper in a wide range of realistic scenarios. The proposed optimization technique has been been implemented in Java Standard Edition 7 and executed on a computer equipped with an Intel Dual Core 3.16 GHz and 4 GB of RAM.

Table 1. Comparative results obtained by the Honey Bees Mating Optimization algorithm [8] and the Greedy Randomized Adaptive Search Procedure (Sect. 3)

Instance				Optimum	HBMO [8]		GRASP	
n	m	o_p	Index		Gap (%)	t (s.)	Gap (%)	t (s.)
5	2	1	1	4644	0.000	0.272	0.000	0.004
		1	2	4990	0.000	0.297	0.000	0.004
		250	1	3112	0.000	0.278	0.000	0.004
		250	2	3046	1.250	0.256	0.000	0.003
		500	1	5913	0.000	0.309	0.000	0.004
		500	2	3207	0.000	0.281	0.000	0.004
		645	1	5627	0.000	0.241	0.000	0.004
		645	2	4784	0.000	0.313	0.000	0.004
		1000	1	4728	0.000	0.303	0.000	0.004
		1000	2	5865	0.000	0.291	0.000	0.003
10	5	1	1	6545	0.825	0.391	0.199	0.018
		1	2	6615	1.077	0.406	0.000	0.016
		250	1	6074	1.962	0.372	0.000	0.015
		250	2	5215	2.429	0.303	0.000	0.015
		472	1	5126	0.000	0.587	0.000	0.015
		472	2	7015	1.792	0.294	0.000	0.016
		500	1	7105	1.401	0.328	0.000	0.014
		500	2	8044	1.203	0.572	0.000	0.016
		1000	1	6648	1.773	1.119	0.000	0.015
		1000	2	8042	0.000	0.412	0.000	0.014

(Continued)

Table 1. *(Continued)*

Instance				Optimum	HBMO [8]		GRASP	
n	m	o_p	Index		Gap (%)	t (s.)	Gap (%)	t (s.)
10	10	1	1	4779	0.374	0.269	0.000	0.039
		1	2	5028	3.456	0.278	0.000	0.036
		250	1	5417	3.612	0.303	0.000	0.025
		250	2	5004	3.309	0.266	0.000	0.036
		500	1	5348	3.467	0.300	0.000	0.022
		500	2	4450	1.420	0.384	0.000	0.023
		715	1	7466	3.045	0.569	0.000	0.027
		715	2	6479	2.179	0.356	0.000	0.023
		1000	1	8258	1.822	0.384	0.000	0.044
		1000	2	7937	2.565	0.669	0.202	0.039
25	10	1	1	8746	2.009	0.697	0.000	0.121
		1	2	7764	0.836	0.684	0.000	0.122
		250	1	10449	1.348	0.722	0.000	0.191
		250	2	10227	3.352	0.912	0.000	0.261
		500	1	12320	4.771	0.734	1.372	0.313
		500	2	11033	3.398	0.797	2.275	0.170
		508	1	11593	3.958	1.125	0.000	0.213
		508	2	11827	4.161	0.859	0.000	0.318
		1000	1	14153	6.553	1.316	3.519	0.294
		1000	2	12837	0.000	7.212	1.416	0.407
25	25	1	1	6776	1.593	0.491	0.000	0.391
		1	2	5368	1.360	0.494	0.000	0.400
		70	1	7250	1.662	0.500	0.000	0.625
		70	2	8670	4.129	0.509	0.000	0.400
		250	1	8955	7.738	0.487	0.000	0.377
		250	2	10380	6.794	0.559	0.000	0.360
		500	1	9827	15.438	0.747	0.000	0.437
		500	2	9166	11.115	0.522	0.000	0.436
		1000	1	13812	9.977	1.238	4.134	0.348
		1000	2	12603	10.702	1.653	1.992	0.513

Table 1 shows the comparison between the GRASP and the HBMO. The first column (*Instance*) depicts the characteristics of the problem instances to solve. Particularly, the number of customers (n), the number of potential locations (m), the opening costs of the plants (o_p), and the identifier of the instance (*Index*) are respectively shown. The subsequent column (*Optimum*) reports the optimum objective function value obtained by the optimization model developed by the authors of the present paper. Finally, the last columns (*i.e.*, *HBMO* and *GRASP*) show the deviations (*Gap (%)*) and computational times measured in seconds (*t (s.)*) of the HBMO and the GRASP when solving the problem instances under analysis, respectively. It is worth mentioning that, λ takes a value of 100 in all the executions of the GRASP.

The computational results indicate that the performance of the GRASP overcomes that of the previous approach from the related literature. In this regard, the GRASP obtains the optimal or near-optimal solutions in all the scenarios under analysis (below 4.2 %) by means of short computational times, less than one second. Unlike this, the HBMO reports noticeable deviations in terms of objective function value. This fact is specially evidenced in the largest problem instances, where deviations around 15 % have been obtained. Additionally, HBMO requires larger computational times than the GRASP, around 7 s in some cases.

5   Conclusions and Future Work

The Uncapacitated Plant Cycle Problem (UPCP) is a location-routing optimization problem whose objective is to select a subset with unknown cardinality of potential locations in which to open plants dedicated to provide service to customers distributed on the field. The positions of the available locations and customers are known in advance. Additionally, the plants to open can serve an unlimited number of customers. Solving the UPCP involves to take several decisions. These are (i) determining the number of plants to open, (ii) selecting the subset of locations in which to open the plants, (iii) assigning a non-empty subset of customers to each plant, and (iv) determining a vehicle route dedicated to serve the subset of customers assigned to each plant.

In this paper, a Greedy Randomized Adaptive Search Procedure (GRASP) is proposed to solve the UPCP from an approximate point of view. This metaheuristic approach is nested into a restarting strategy, which allows to iteratively select the number of plants to open. The plants are selected at random by taking into account the pre-defined number of plants selected. Afterwards and by means of a constructive procedure, the customers are adequately assigned to the plants open, whereas a route is efficiently built for the subset of customers assigned to each plant. The computational experiments conducted in this paper indicate the suitable performance of the proposed algorithmic approach, which allows to reach high-quality solutions in reasonable computational times. This allows to overcome a previous algorithmic proposal found in the related literature.

Several promising lines are still open for further research. One of them is to tackle dynamic data in the problem. For instance, changes in the assignment costs, travel costs, etc. Additionally, considering multi-route, fuzzy, or capacitated variants of this optimization problem should be also explored in subsequent works.

Acknowledgements. This work has been partially funded by the Spanish Ministry of Economy and Competitiveness (project TIN2012-32608). Christopher Expósito-Izquierdo and Eduardo Lalla-Ruiz would like to thank the Canary Government for the financial support they receive through their post-graduate grants.

References

1. Drexl, M., Schneider, M.: A survey of variants and extensions of the location-routing problem. Eur. J. Oper. Res. **241**(2), 283–308 (2015)
2. Feo, T.A., Resende, M.G.C.: A probabilistic heuristic for a computationally difficult set covering problem. Oper. Res. Lett. **8**(2), 67–71 (1989)
3. Feo, T.A., Resende, M.G.C.: Greedy randomized adaptive search procedures. J. Global Optim. **6**(2), 109–133 (1995)
4. Festa, P., Resende, M.G.C.: Grasp: an annotated bibliography. In: Festa, P., Resende, M.G.C. (eds.) Essays and Surveys in Metaheuristics. Operations Research Computer ScienceInterfaces Series, vol. 15, pp. 325–367. Springer, Heidelberg (2002)
5. Fleming, C.L., Griffis, S.E., Bell, J.E.: The effects of triangle inequality on the vehicle routing problem. Eur. J. Oper. Res. **224**(1), 1–7 (2013)
6. Gutin, G., Punnen, A.P.: The Traveling Salesman Problem and Its Variations, 1st edn. Springer, Heidelberg (2002)
7. Martí, R., Campos, V., Resende, M.G.C., Duarte, A.: Multiobjective grasp with path relinking. Eur. J. Oper. Res. **240**(1), 54–71 (2015)
8. Melián-Batista, B., Moreno-Vega, J.M., Vaswani, N., Yumar, R.: A nature inspired approach for the uncapacitated plant cycle location problem. In: Krasnogor, N., Melián-Batista, M.B., Pérez, J.A.M., Moreno-Vega, J.M., Pelta, D.A. (eds.) NICSO 2008. SCI, vol. 236, pp. 49–60. Springer, Heidelberg (2009)
9. Parejo, J.A., Segura, S., Fernandez, P., Ruiz-Cortés, A.: QOS-aware web services composition using grasp with path relinking. Expert Syst. Appl. **41**(9), 4211–4223 (2014)
10. Park, C., Seo, J.: A grasp approach to transporter scheduling and routing at a shipyard. Comput. Ind. Eng. **63**(2), 390–399 (2012)
11. Prodhon, C., Prins, C.: A survey of recent research on location-routing problems. Eur. J. Oper. Res. **238**(1), 1–17 (2014)
12. Resende, M.G.C., Ribeiro, C.C.: Grasp with path-relinking: recent advances and applications. In: Ibaraki, T., Nonobe, K., Yagiura, M. (eds.) Metaheuristics: Progress as Real Problem Solvers. Operations Research/Computer Science Interfaces Series, vol. 32, pp. 29–63. Springer, US (2005)
13. Villegas, J.G., Prins, C., Prodhon, C., Medaglia, A.L., Velasco, N.: A grasp with evolutionary path relinking for the truck and trailer routing problem. Comput. Oper. Res. **38**(9), 1319–1334 (2011)

On the Comparison of Decoding Strategies for a Memetic Algorithm for the Multi Layer Hierarchical Ring Network Design Problem

Christian Schauer$^{(\boxtimes)}$ and Günther R. Raidl

Institute of Computer Graphics and Algorithms, TU Wien, Vienna, Austria
schauer@ads.tuwien.ac.at, raidl@ac.tuwien.ac.at

Abstract. We address the Multi Layer Hierarchical Ring Network Design Problem, which arises in the design of large telecommunication backbone networks. To ensure reliability for the network the nodes are assigned to different layers and connected using a hierarchy of rings of bounded length. Previously we presented a memetic algorithm that clusters the nodes of each layer into disjoint subsets and then uses a decoding procedure to determine rings connecting all nodes of each cluster. In this paper we compare several decoding procedures based on construction heuristics for the Traveling Salesman Problem and an integer linear programming approach. We observe that a nearest neighbor procedure outperforms the other constructive methods, while the exact approach proves to be to slow for practical use.

1 Introduction

In this paper we analyze several decoding strategies for candidate solutions in a memetic algorithm for the *Multi Layer Hierarchical Ring Network Design* (MLHRND) problem. MLHRND arises in the field of telecommunication network design and finds applications in large, hierarchically structured networks with a strong need of survivability. The problem description originates from a cooperation with an Austrian telecommunication provider.

With the increasing demand of large and fast telecommunication networks, the matter of reliability became more and more important. Hence, it has to be avoided that larger parts of the network become disconnected in case of limited failures of devices or links. In principle, the simplest way to ensure survivability in a network is the use of a ring topology since a node or link failure can be compensated by re-routing the connection in the other direction. For the backbone of wide area networks a single ring would not be efficient anymore. The failure of two nodes or links at the same time could disconnect large parts of the network. Moreover, requirements with respect to bandwidth and maximal delays physically limit the size of a ring. To fulfill physical constraints and ensure a high degree of survivability in larger networks, multiple interconnected rings are frequently used as backbones. Gendreau et al. describe in [1] the *Ring Design Problem*, where nodes are connected via such interconnected rings, and propose

© Springer International Publishing Switzerland 2015
R. Moreno-Díaz et al. (Eds.): EUROCAST 2015, LNCS 9520, pp. 271–278, 2015.
DOI: 10.1007/978-3-319-27340-2_34

an integer programming formulation with a quadratic objective function. Moreover, the authors present three ring construction heuristics based on heuristics for the Traveling Salesman Proplem (TSP) and three destroy and reconstruct approaches for post-optimization to solve large size instances.

To allow scalability this interconnection is often realized in a hierarchical fashion using rings on every layer of the hierarchy. Such a network is hence called a *Hierarchical Ring Network* (HRN). When two rings are connected over a single node (*single homing*) the network can compensate for a link failure but does not stay connected if the concatenation node fails. To additionally cover this situation the rings must be connected over two different nodes on each ring, which is also called *dual homing*. Proestaki and Sinclair present in [2] a variant of HRN with dual homing for matters of survivability, where the node to layer assignment is not given a priori but to determine during the optimization process. The objective function incorporates both the traffic on the rings and the overall ring length. As an exact approach the authors present a binary integer linear programming formulation. Additionally, they discuss a partition, construct, and perturb heuristic that iteratively, for each layer, creates a solution.

The *Multi Layer Hierarchical Ring Network Design* (MLHRND) deals with a hierarchical structure spanning nodes on multiple layers using rings of bounded length and dual homing to ensure fault tolerance in case of single link and node failures. In MLHRND the node to layer assignment is given a priori. In [3], we introduced MLHRND for the three-layer case and described a variable neighborhood search (VNS) and a greedy randomized adaptive search procedure for heuristically solving it. We further argued that MLHRND is NP-hard, even for the three layer case, since the classical *Capacitated Vehicle Routing Problem* can be reduced to MLHRND.

In [4] we generalized the definition to an arbitrary number of layers, i.e., MLHRND, and described a memetic algorithm (MA). The idea of the MA is to divide MLHRND into two depending subproblems, a partitioning problem to determine the nodes belonging to each ring and a ring computation problem for each partition. As a side effect we were able to further improve our VNS during the design of the local search for the MA. In the end the MA outperforms the VNS in 13 out of 30 instances, while in eight instances they perform on par. In [4] we focused on the partitioning problem, in this work we discuss and evaluate six different ring computation strategies.

The rest of the paper is organized as follows. In Sect. 2 we give a formal definition of the problem and present the main principles of the MA in Sect. 3. In Sect. 4 we describe several decoding strategies designed for MLHRND and compare their performance in Sect. 5. We conclude this work in Sect. 6.

2   Multi Layer Hierarchical Ring Network Design

Let $G = (V, E)$ be an undirected graph with vertex set V and edge set E. A weighting function assigns costs $c_{ij} \geq 0$ to each edge $(i, j) \in E$. Moreover, V is partitioned into $K \geq 3$ disjoint subsets $V_1, \ldots, V_K$ representing the layers each node belongs to. Edges exist between all pairs of nodes of the same and the successive layer, i.e., $E = \bigcup_{k=1,\dots,K}(V_k \times V_k) \cup \bigcup_{k=1,\dots,K-1}(V_k \times V_{k+1})$.

A feasible solution to MLHRND is a subgraph $G_L = (V, E_L)$ connecting all nodes in V and satisfying the following conditions; see Fig. 1 for an example.

1. All nodes in V_1 are connected by a single independent ring containing no other node.
2. The remaining layers are connected by $K - 1$ respective sets of paths containing no nodes from other layers. Each node must appear in exactly one path, i.e., the paths are node and edge disjoint to ensure reliability.
3. The end nodes of each path at layer $k \in \{2, \dots, K\}$ are further connected to two different nodes (*hubs*) in layer $k - 1$, i.e., dual homing is realized. We refer to the edges connecting paths to hubs as *uplinks*.
4. The two hub nodes, a path is connected to, must themselves be connected by a simple path at their layer, i.e., the connection to a ring may not be established via more than two layers.
5. The lengths of layer $k \in \{2, \dots, K\}$ paths in terms of the number of edges is bounded below and above by $b_k^l \geq 1$ and $b_k^u \geq b_k^l$, respectively.

The objective is to find a feasible solution with minimum total costs:

$$c(E_L) = \sum_{(i,j) \in E_L} c_{ij}$$

3   A Memetic Algorithm for MLHRND

From condition 1 we can conclude that finding the layer 1 ring resembles the classical TSP. Since there are no further limitations for the layer 1 ring, this subproblem can be solved independently. We use in our experiments the Concorde TSP solver[1] to determine an optimal layer 1 ring.

The MA is intended to solve the structurally more complex further layers. As already mentioned before, the main idea behind the MA is to split MLHRND into two subproblems: the first, to cluster the nodes of each layer into different subsets; the second, to compute Hamiltonian paths through the subsets and determine the uplinks for the paths in order to form together with the upper layer feasible rings. While the MA is used to optimize the clusters, a decoding procedure calculates the paths and rings. For a detailed description about the MA including crossover and mutation operators as well as local improvement methods we refer to [4].

In this paper we solely focus on the path and ring computation problem. A generic decoding procedure is described in Algorithm 1. For each cluster on each layer at first a Hamiltonian path is computed through the cluster (line 5). We also tested the possibility to further improve each path by a local search incorporating a two edge exchange neighborhood structure (line 6). Then the uplinks connecting the end nodes of the current path to the preceding layer are determined (line 7). We discuss an efficient algorithm to determine the uplinks

---

[1] www.math.uwaterloo.ca/tsp/concorde.

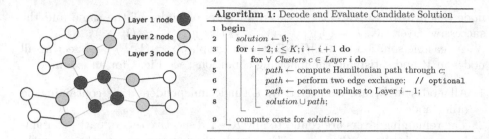

Fig. 1. A schematic representation for $K = 3$ and a generic decoding strategy.

in [4]. Obviously, the crucial part of Algorithm 1 is to compute the Hamiltonian path, which is an NP-complete problem. Since Algorithm 1 is called in every generation of the MA for each cluster in each candidate solution, i.e., thousands of times, the runtime is a crucial factor. Therefore, we need to rely on heuristic methods to solve this problem in reasonable time.

4   Decoding Strategies

In this section we discuss several heuristics to solve line 5 in Algorithm 1, i.e., the computation of a Hamiltonian path, efficiently. We designed our methods based on various construction heuristics for the TSP.

Nearest Neighbor. In our first strategy (**NN1**) we start with the cheapest edge of the cluster as initial path. Then we successively append the path at one end with the cheapest edge available at this end until all nodes of the cluster are connected. Out tests showed that this approach is too naive since the edge connecting the last node can be of arbitrary length. To overcome this problem at least in practice our next approach (**NN2**) is able to append both ends of the path. We again start with the cheapest edge but in the following steps we select the cheapest edge considering both ends and add this edge at the respective end.

Insertion. Our third strategy (**INS**) is based on the insertion heuristic using farthest insertion. This method starts with the most expensive edge in the cluster as initial path. From the set of remaining nodes INS iteratively considers all minimum cost connections to a node on the path and selects the node with the maximum min-costs. This node is then inserted into the path at the best position, i.e., the least increase in path costs. To additionally improve the quality of this approach we also allow to append the path at the begin and end.

Savings. Furthermore, we were interested in an approach that also considers the uplinks during the path calculation. We adapted the savings heuristic for the TSP to meet this demand and designed two strategies, one in favor of quality (**SAV-Q**) and one in favor of speed (**SAV-S**). In the first step we compute the two closest hub nodes for each node on the cluster to form initial subpaths. Then the best saving when connecting two paths is computed and these two paths are merged. This procedure is repeated until all nodes are connected to a single path. For SAV-Q we only consider feasible subpaths regarding the dual homing and the hub path constraints. Therefore, the hub nodes for subpaths must be adapted, when to paths are merged, which induces an enormous overhead in runtime. But is it really necessary to consider these constraints during the path creation? Why not relax them and only consider the hub nodes as an additional indicator? Then all savings could be computed in a preprocessing step at the beginning of the MA. This idea is realized in SAV-S, which follows the same scheme as described before but without updating the hub nodes.

Exact Approach. To optimally decode a candidate solution we calculate a minimum length Hamiltonian path including the uplinks for each cluster with n nodes on layer k. We developed a single commodity flow mixed integer linear programming formulation **MIP** for this task. Due to space restrictions we cannot present the model here but it can easily be determined from the description of the following constraints. For the flow start send a flow of n units from a hub node $z^+ \in V_{k-1}$. At each node in the cluster drop one unit of flow, i.e., flow conservation, and connect to a second hub node $z^- \neq z^+$, i.e., the dual homing and hub path constraints. Additionally, each node in the cluster must have one incoming and one outgoing edge to fulfill the degree constraint.

5 Results

For testing purposes we focus on the $K = 3$ layer scenario and use the same 30 benchmark instances as in [4], which consist of random graphs and graphs from the TSPLIB[2]. By varying the number of nodes on each layer we generated 74 test instances with up to 439 nodes[3]. By using different combinations of upper bounds b_k^u for the path lengths we obtained 380 test cases. For the lower bound b_k^l we always assumed one edge as the minimum length for all paths.

We implemented our approach in Java 1.6 using IBM CPLEX 12.6 for MIP. For each of the test cases we performed 30 runs executed on a single core of an Intel Xeon (Nehalem) Quadcore CPU with 2.53 GHz and 3 GB of RAM. The presented results show the average value over all test runs for each of the 30 benchmark instances. All statistical tests are based on a Wilcoxon rank sum test with an error level of 5 %.

We performed our tests in two steps. In the first step we used each of the three randomized construction heuristics from [4] to generate 30 networks for each test case, which we then evaluated with our different decoding strategies. We used MIP to determine the optimal decoding and considered the quality of a solution as relative deviation from the optimal solution. Moreover, we tested our strategies with and without local search, see Algorithm 1 (line 6). The results of the first step are summarized in Table 1.

Without local search NN1 performed rather poor, while NN2 and INS performed best for 15 instances each. In three cases the differences were significant

---

[2] http://comopt.ifi.uni-heidelberg.de/software/TSPLIB95
[3] All instances are available at www.ac.tuwien.ac.at/research/problem-instances

Table 1. Experimental results for the evaluation of the different decoding strategies without and with local search. The first column lists the instance names including the number of nodes in the graphs. For each heuristic approach the deviation (dev) from the optimal decoding in percent and the runtime (t) in milliseconds is presented. Note the runtime for MIP is given in seconds! Since the deviation of MIP is always 0 this column was omitted. Columns p show a statistical comparison between the best heuristic method (printed bold), once without and once with local search, and each other method, ≈ indicates no significant difference and > that the current method performs significantly worse than the best.

| | without local search | | | | | | | | | | | | | with local search | | | | | | | | | | | | | | MIP |
| | NN1 | | NN2 | | INS | | | SAV-S | | | SAV-Q | | | NN1 | | | NN2 | | | INS | | | SAV-S | | | SAV-Q | | | |
instance	dev [%]	t [ms]	dev [%]	t [ms]	dev [%]	t [ms]	p	dev [%]	t [ms]	p	dev [%]	t [ms]	p	dev [%]	t [ms]	p	dev [%]	t [ms]	p	dev [%]	t [ms]	p	dev [%]	t [ms]	p	dev [%]	t [ms]	p	t [s]
ulysses22	4.6	0.06	**1.6**	0.06	1.5	0.09	≈	9.5	0.08	≈	2.2	0.39	≈	3.7	0.07	>	**1.4**	0.07	≈	1.5	0.11	≈	8.4	0.10	>	1.6	0.40	>	0.62
rand25	7.9	0.06	**1.4**	0.06	1.9	0.10	≈	5.6	0.09	≈	4.4	0.43	≈	7.7	0.07	>	**1.1**	0.07	≈	1.9	0.12	≈	3.3	0.11	>	3.3	0.46	>	0.68
rand30	8.1	0.07	**1.6**	0.07	2.3	0.12	≈	5.6	0.11	≈	3.9	0.51	>	7.0	0.09	>	**1.4**	0.09	≈	2.2	0.14	≈	4.6	0.13	>	3.0	0.54	>	0.85
rand35	8.7	0.09	**2.3**	0.09	2.8	0.14	≈	4.9	0.12	≈	4.1	0.60	>	7.4	0.10	>	**2.0**	0.10	≈	2.5	0.16	≈	4.1	0.14	>	3.3	0.64	>	1.04
rand45	10.0	0.11	**2.5**	0.11	2.6	0.19	≈	7.4	0.16	≈	4.9	0.86	>	8.1	0.14	>	**2.0**	0.14	≈	2.3	0.22	≈	5.0	0.18	>	3.7	0.83	>	1.35
att48	8.6	0.12	**1.6**	0.12	2.1	0.22	≈	5.6	0.16	≈	4.6	0.86	>	7.4	0.15	>	**1.4**	0.15	≈	1.9	0.25	≈	4.3	0.20	>	3.2	0.90	>	1.47
eil51	11.2	0.13	**2.7**	0.13	2.9	0.23	≈	5.6	0.17	≈	5.2	0.92	>	8.8	0.17	>	**2.2**	0.17	≈	2.7	0.28	≈	4.2	0.21	>	3.6	1.01	>	1.60
berlin52	10.2	0.13	**2.8**	0.13	4.1	0.24	>	5.8	0.18	≈	4.9	0.97	>	8.4	0.16	>	**2.5**	0.16	>	4.0	0.27	>	4.6	0.21	>	3.5	0.95	>	1.50
rand55	9.8	0.14	**2.4**	0.14	3.1	0.24	≈	7.1	0.19	≈	4.8	0.98	>	8.2	0.17	>	**2.1**	0.17	>	2.8	0.27	>	5.3	0.37	>	3.8	1.00	>	1.90
rand70	10.9	0.23	**3.4**	0.24	3.7	0.40	≈	7.9	0.30	≈	6.5	1.84	>	8.8	0.29	>	**2.7**	0.30	≈	3.5	0.45	≈	4.8	0.42	>	4.4	1.90	>	2.77
eil76	11.3	0.26	**3.0**	0.28	3.5	0.50	>	6.8	0.32	≈	6.6	2.14	>	8.9	0.35	>	**2.3**	0.37	≈	3.1	0.56	≈	5.4	0.48	>	4.3	2.22	>	3.07
rand85	10.2	0.31	**3.1**	0.34	3.5	0.55	>	7.9	0.38	≈	7.0	2.43	>	8.1	0.40	>	**2.4**	0.42	≈	3.2	0.61	≈	5.0	0.60	>	4.5	2.52	>	4.07
gr96	11.8	0.38	**2.9**	0.41	3.3	0.72	≈	8.3	0.42	≈	5.7	2.96	>	9.5	0.52	>	**2.3**	0.55	≈	2.9	0.85	≈	5.9	0.64	>	3.6	3.14	>	4.49
kroA100	11.0	0.39	**3.1**	0.45	3.5	0.76	≈	9.5	0.46	≈	6.7	3.18	>	9.0	0.56	>	**2.4**	0.59	≈	3.3	0.88	≈	5.8	0.63	>	4.3	3.35	>	4.72
kroB100	12.1	0.39	**3.3**	0.44	3.5	0.77	≈	8.6	0.45	≈	7.0	3.18	>	9.9	0.55	>	**2.7**	0.58	>	3.2	0.88	>	5.4	1.20	>	4.4	3.33	>	4.68
bier127	12.2	0.70	**4.4**	0.80	4.4	1.47	≈	7.9	0.72	≈	7.5	6.82	>	8.7	1.14	>	**3.2**	1.15	≈	3.9	1.74	≈	5.6	1.64	>	4.7	7.20	>	7.99
ch150	13.5	0.93	**4.1**	1.09	4.4	2.05	≈	10.9	0.91	≈	9.9	9.21	>	10.1	1.53	>	**2.8**	1.58	≈	3.9	2.45	≈	6.3	1.97	>	5.6	10.01	>	9.96
rand175	14.3	1.18	**4.6**	1.39	4.6	2.46	≈	11.6	1.11	≈	10.3	11.73	>	10.8	1.84	>	**3.2**	1.94	≈	4.2	2.89	≈	5.8	2.83	>	5.8	12.46	>	12.39
kroA200	13.8	1.58	**4.3**	1.90	4.3	3.70	≈	12.0	1.37	≈	10.3	15.80	>	10.3	2.76	>	**3.0**	2.90	≈	3.9	4.43	≈	6.4	2.87	>	5.7	16.93	>	15.11
kroB200	13.9	1.55	**4.3**	1.85	4.2	3.64	≈	12.4	1.35	≈	10.3	15.54	>	10.3	2.75	>	**3.0**	2.90	≈	3.8	4.49	≈	6.8	2.87	>	6.1	17.14	>	14.81
gr229	12.6	2.77	**3.9**	3.11	3.1	6.16	≈	11.2	2.36	≈	9.0	31.17	>	8.1	5.16	>	**2.3**	5.08	≈	2.8	7.50	≈	6.9	5.46	>	5.1	34.12	>	23.21
rand250	15.0	3.27	**5.6**	3.82	5.1	7.07	≈	12.8	2.85	≈	12.5	37.00	>	10.4	5.48	>	**3.5**	5.60	>	4.6	8.29	>	6.5	7.04	>	6.3	40.11	>	30.87
rand275	15.4	4.25	**5.3**	4.96	4.9	8.96	≈	13.2	3.61	≈	12.8	47.70	>	10.8	7.02	>	**3.3**	7.17	>	4.3	10.42	>	6.7	9.91	>	6.4	50.63	>	36.19
pr299	15.7	4.98	**4.7**	5.70	4.2	10.92	>	13.1	3.90	≈	11.3	54.32	>	11.0	9.32	>	**2.9**	9.41	>	3.7	13.61	>	6.2	10.98	>	6.1	61.60	>	36.31
lin318	15.5	5.75	**5.5**	6.50	4.7	12.59	>	13.0	4.59	≈	11.2	59.79	>	10.5	10.62	>	**3.5**	10.77	>	4.2	15.56	>	6.5	12.75	>	5.8	66.00	>	39.22
rand350	15.8	7.26	**5.8**	8.65	5.2	15.87	≈	14.9	5.68	≈	13.2	81.04	>	10.8	12.49	>	**3.8**	12.85	≈	4.7	18.69	≈	7.3	15.25	>	6.6	88.31	>	47.61
rand375	15.6	9.13	**5.6**	10.83	5.1	18.85	≈	14.4	7.41	≈	13.0	99.00	>	11.1	14.91	>	**3.6**	15.58	≈	4.6	22.26	≈	6.9	17.51	>	6.6	107.97	>	53.63
rand400	16.0	10.59	**5.8**	12.61	5.2	22.34	≈	15.0	8.35	≈	13.6	117.59	>	11.1	17.28	>	**3.7**	18.07	≈	4.6	25.80	≈	6.6	25.80	>	6.8	125.89	>	58.66
gr431	13.9	12.16	**4.8**	13.79	3.9	27.48	≈	10.4	9.23	≈	9.6	133.33	>	8.9	24.02	>	**3.0**	23.59	>	3.5	34.20	>	5.4	24.51	>	5.0	148.76	>	58.06
pr439	15.4	12.99	**5.2**	14.75	4.7	28.49	>	13.7	9.85	≈	11.1	142.14	>	10.6	24.34	>	**3.3**	24.36	>	4.2	35.04	>	6.8	24.64	>	5.8	151.65	>	57.73

Table 2. Experimental results for the MA using 1PX or UX as crossover operators and NN2 or INS as decoding strategies with the respective results (score) and standard deviations (dev). The first column lists the instance names including the number of nodes in the graphs. Columns p show a statistical comparison between the best (printed bold) and each other approach. As before ≈ indicates no significant difference and > that the current approach performs significantly worse than the best.

instance	NN2 with local search 1PX			UX			INS without local search 1PX			UX		
	score	dev	p	score	dev	p	score	dev	p	score	dev	p
ulysses22	123.31	0.28	>	**123.20**	0.24	≈	123.33	0.36	>	123.23	0.29	>
rand25	**71255.47**	221.34	≈	**71255.47**	221.34	≈	72115.70	791.21	>	72034.08	842.77	≈
rand30	88484.53	3542.46	≈	**88365.69**	3422.10	≈	88373.45	3417.27	≈	88520.03	3517.76	≈
rand35	89182.22	2888.34	≈	**89167.36**	2874.31	≈	89207.88	2905.87	≈	89219.38	2921.30	≈
rand45	99145.13	2039.62	≈	**99126.84**	1992.77	≈	99257.84	1879.57	≈	99197.98	1899.85	≈
att48	59663.81	632.16	≈	**59596.17**	681.46	≈	59665.21	670.47	≈	59597.99	617.41	≈
eil51	743.72	15.56	≈	743.02	15.63	≈	**742.34**	16.68	≈	742.41	16.62	≈
berlin52	13370.03	201.04	≈	**13364.96**	197.50	≈	13415.79	187.50	≈	13442.45	208.13	>
rand55	**111846.88**	2971.71	≈	111882.44	2878.37	≈	112080.33	3092.02	≈	112034.15	3078.47	≈
rand70	126402.60	2322.23	>	**125926.40**	2264.60	≈	126444.95	2410.38	>	126350.88	2460.84	>
eil76	902.71	21.82	≈	**902.03**	23.09	≈	903.92	22.30	≈	902.58	21.50	≈
rand85	136312.04	3237.14	≈	**136050.13**	3227.32	≈	136356.85	3247.76	≈	136371.92	3188.22	≈
gr96	**925.80**	21.40	≈	926.07	22.21	≈	927.05	22.25	≈	926.81	22.50	≈
kroB100	**40759.91**	1068.90	≈	40780.24	1122.37	≈	40785.50	1048.49	≈	40836.23	1052.94	≈
kroA100	40043.51	1132.73	≈	**39992.35**	1151.43	≈	40045.00	1071.77	≈	40073.78	1127.82	≈
bier127	202817.43	2601.11	≈	**202674.00**	2836.98	≈	202840.11	2636.28	≈	203059.76	2891.91	≈
ch150	11719.20	236.62	≈	**11715.27**	246.43	≈	11745.00	246.83	≈	11743.80	249.00	>
rand175	**184434.64**	4073.46	≈	184749.36	4161.79	≈	184827.76	4163.57	≈	184575.13	4062.15	≈
kroA200	**53045.74**	986.66	≈	53183.41	1089.88	≈	53130.83	1027.43	≈	53124.99	972.16	≈
kroB200	**53148.67**	1024.49	≈	53229.85	1023.96	≈	53233.90	1093.49	≈	53225.21	1097.12	≈
gr229	2840.61	66.71	≈	2842.48	65.43	≈	2840.89	68.60	≈	**2839.64**	68.63	≈
rand250	**214841.28**	2983.39	≈	215245.46	3347.49	≈	215298.52	2823.12	>	215748.21	3095.64	>
rand275	**219517.82**	4488.71	≈	220505.76	4672.04	>	219986.49	4072.93	>	219977.24	4066.65	>
pr299	**88667.95**	1264.57	≈	88920.18	1383.50	>	89039.56	1229.15	>	89023.79	1248.33	>
lin318	**77173.81**	1718.17	≈	77612.38	1835.81	>	77413.53	1695.41	>	77369.73	1616.14	>
rand350	**248766.28**	5152.62	≈	250009.87	5706.74	>	249898.38	4995.30	>	249620.92	4888.68	>
rand375	**259471.79**	5313.26	≈	261068.47	6000.87	>	259663.98	5009.27	≈	259802.65	4989.60	>
rand400	**269699.91**	5854.83	≈	271924.26	6542.30	>	270367.61	5656.84	>	270318.90	5640.60	≈
gr431	**3373.65**	57.92	≈	3401.35	63.94	>	3383.81	59.06	>	3384.23	57.47	>
pr439	**201790.51**	6992.98	≈	204776.11	7414.42	>	202670.12	6514.25	>	202878.68	6508.17	>

for NN2 and in eight for INS. Nevertheless, the runtime of NN2 is only half of INS for the larger instances. To our surprise the savings approaches are not competitive in terms of solution quality. While SAV-S is the overall fastest method for the larger instances SAV-Q is by far the slowest. Therefore, we conclude that considering the uplinks during the decoding process is more misleading than helpful. The local search was able to improve all five methods. The generally weaker approaches benefit more form the local search, which goes along with a certain increase in runtime. In the end NN1, NN2, and SAV-S show the same runtime behavior. Nevertheless, with local search NN2 performs best in all instances and in 21 cases significantly. Unluckily, MIP performs too slow to be used within the MA on a regular base.

In the second step we incorporated the two most promising approaches within the MA and compared their performance. We decided to use the NN2 approach with and the INS approach without local search, since both show a comparable runtime behavior and performed best in their specific category. We applied MIP only to the best solution found by the MA to finally guarantee an optimal decoding. The MA settings are exactly the same as in [4] only varying the decoding strategy for it. The results are summarized in Table 2.

Used within the MA the NN2 approach performs best with 1PX for 15 instances (six times significantly) and with UX for 12 instances (twice significantly). INS only performs best once for 1PX and UX each but not significantly. A special case is the rand25 instance. Here NN2 found the optimal solution for all test runs with both crossover operators while INS did not! Therefore, we conclude that NN2 is our decoding method of choice and for larger instances especially in combination with the 1PX crossover operator.

6   Conclusions and Future Work

We presented several decoding strategies for an MA to solve the Multi Layer Hierarchical Ring Network Design problem. The basic concept is to use the MA to cluster the nodes of each layer into disjoint subsets and then use a decoding procedure to compute a Hamiltonian path through each cluster and find appropriate uplinks. We designed and compared five different procedures based on construction heuristics for the TSP and an exact approach. In the end a nearest neighbor method combined with a local search performed best. The exact approach proved to be to slow to be used frequently. In the future we want to focus on a faster exact approach that can better be incorporated in the MA to evaluate promising candidate solutions on a regular base.

References

1. Gendreau, M., Labbé, M., Laporte, G.: Efficient heuristics for the design of ring networks. Telecommun. Syst. **4**(1), 177–188 (1995)
2. Proestaki, A., Sinclair, M.: Design and dimensioning of dual-homing hierarchical multi-ring networks. IEE Proc.Commun. **147**(2), 96–104 (2000)
3. Schauer, C., Raidl, G.R.: Variable neighborhood search and GRASP for three-layer hierarchical ring network design. In: Coello, C.A.C., Cutello, V., Deb, K., Forrest, S., Nicosia, G., Pavone, M. (eds.) PPSN 2012, Part I. LNCS, vol. 7491, pp. 458–467. Springer, Heidelberg (2012)
4. Schauer, C., Raidl, G.R.: A memetic algorithm for multi layer hierarchical ring network design. In: Bartz-Beielstein, T., Branke, J., Filipič, B., Smith, J. (eds.) PPSN 2014. LNCS, vol. 8672, pp. 832–841. Springer, Heidelberg (2014)

Metaheuristics and Cloud Computing: A Case Study on the Probabilistic Traveling Salesman Problem with Deadlines

Dennis Weyland[1,2]([✉])

[1] Universitá Della Svizzera Italiana, Lugano, Switzerland
[2] Department of Economics and Management, University of Brescia, Brescia, Italy
dennisweyland@gmail.com

Abstract. In this work we study the potential of cloud computing in the context of optimization. For this purpose we perform a case study on the Probabilistic Traveling Salesman Problem with Deadlines, an extremely difficult stochastic combinatorial optimization problem. By using a large amount of computational resources in parallel, it is possible to obtain significantly better solutions for the Probabilistic Traveling Salesman Problem with Deadlines in the same amount of time. For many different applications this advantage clearly outweighs the requirement for additional computational resources, in particular considering the convenience of modern cloud infrastructures.

Keywords: Stochastic combinatorial optimization · Cloud computing · Probabilistic traveling salesman problem with deadlines

1 Introduction

In recent years cloud computing has evolved towards a hot topic in computer science and related fields. Based on technical improvements of the last decades, in particular the availability of broadband internet and mobile internet, the usage of cloud services and resources has become increasingly convenient. The huge amount of resources provided by cloud computing is of extreme interest in the field of optimization and operations research. The majority of research in these fields has focused on algorithms using only a single computer or a very small network. It has been argued, that this allows for fair comparisons in a realistic environment, since the access to computer clusters and high performance computing systems is assumed to be limited. This assumption is no longer valid and a paradigm shift is necessary. Instead of using a single computer and measuring computational time and memory consumption for this system, it can be assumed that a large number of computers with different specifications is available. The development of algorithms that exploit this huge amount of resources is of great

D. Weyland—This work has been supported by the *Swiss National Science Foundation* as part of the *Early Postdoc.Mobility* grant 152293.

R. Moreno-Díaz et al. (Eds.): EUROCAST 2015, LNCS 9520, pp. 279–285, 2015.
DOI: 10.1007/978-3-319-27340-2_35

importance. Of course, computational time (of the whole system) and memory consumption (of the whole system and its parts) are still crucial indicators, but additionally the costs for using the cloud resources should be taken into account.

In this work we study the potential of cloud computing using the PROBABILISTIC TRAVELING SALESMAN PROBLEM WITH DEADLINES (PTSPD, [1,2]) as a case study. The PROBABILISTIC TRAVELING SALESMAN PROBLEM WITH DEADLINES is an extremely difficult stochastic combinatorial optimization problem. In fact, it has been shown that even the evaluation of the objective function is #P-hard [7]. The design of good heuristics for the PTSPD is a very challenging task. The current state-of-the-art algorithm for the PTSPD [8] is exploiting the computational power of graphics processing units (GPUs), and we further modify this algorithm such that it can be applied in parallel on any number of computers and GPUs. The main goal of our research is to investigate in which way the quality of the final solution is influenced by the number of computers and GPUs and to estimate the potential benefits that could be obtained by using cloud computing.

The remainder of this paper is organized as follows. In Sect. 2 we introduce the PTSPD and give a formal definition for this problem. After that, we present the computational studies and their results in Sect. 3. Finally, we conclude the paper with a brief discussion of our findings in Sect. 4.

2   The Probabilistic Traveling Salesman Problem with Deadlines

In this section we give a formal definition of the PROBABILISTIC TRAVELING SALESMAN PROBLEM WITH DEADLINES (PTSPD). We then discuss related literature and give an overview about known facts and algorithms for the PTSPD.

The PTSPD is an a-priori stochastic vehicle routing problem [5] in which the presence of the customers are modeled in a stochastic way and additionally time constraints in terms of deadlines are imposed. It is a generalization of the well-known PROBABILISTIC TRAVELING SALESMAN PROBLEM (PTSP, [4]) which is itself a generalization of the famous TRAVELING SALESMAN PROBLEM (TSP, [6]). The task is to find a so-called a-priori tour starting at the depot, visiting all the customers exactly once, and returning to the depot, such that the expected costs of the a-posteriori tour is minimized. For a given realization of the random events (the presence of the customers) the a-posteriori tour is derived from a given a-priori tour in the following way. The vehicle starts at the depot and visits the customers which are present in the order defined by the given a-priori tour. The customers which do not require to be visited are just skipped. The costs of such an a-posteriori tour are then the travel costs plus penalties for missed deadlines.

More formally, the PTSPD is defined as follows. We have given a set of locations $V = \{v_0, v_1, \ldots, v_n\}$. Here v_0 is the depot and the set $V' = V \setminus \{v_0\}$ is the set of customers. Additionally, we have given a function $d : V \times V \to \mathbb{R}^+$ representing travel times between the different locations, a function $p : V' \to [0, 1]$

representing the presence probabilities of the customers, a function $t : V' \rightarrow \mathbb{R}^+$ representing the deadlines of the customers and a function $h : V' \rightarrow \mathbb{R}^+$ representing the penalties for deadlines violations for the customers. The task is to find a so-called a-priori tour starting at the depot and visiting all the customers exactly once, such that the expected costs over the a posteriori tours (with respect to the given probabilities) is minimized. For a given realization of the customers' presence an a-posteriori tour is derived by visiting the present customers in the order defined by the a priori tour while skipping the other customers. The costs for such an a posteriori tour is the sum of the travel times plus the penalties for violated deadlines. Figure 1 illustrates the relation between a-priori and a-posteriori tours for a specific input instance. A more detailed definition of this problem, including a thorough motivation, is given in [1].

The PTSPD has been introduced in 2008 [1]. Some fundamental properties of the four different models of this problem are discussed in [1,2]. In [7,9] the computational complexity of the PTSPD has been examined. Here it has been shown that several computational tasks related to the PTSPD are #P-hard (which implies NP-hardness and is a much stronger statement): the evaluation of the objective function, determining the probability with which a deadline is violated, the decision variant of the problem and the optimization variant of the problem. Therefore, heuristics are of great importance for this problem. In particular, methods which are based on an approximation of the objective function. Such methods have been introduced in [2,8,10]. The method in [8] is currently the state-of-the-art approach for the PTSPD. Here the evaluation of solutions is performed in parallel on the graphics processing unit (GPU) using an approximation based on Monte Carlo sampling.

3   Computational Studies

For the computational studies conducted in this section we use an adaptation of the state-of-the-art algorithm [8] of the PROBABILISTIC TRAVELING SALESMAN PROBLEM WITH DEADLINES which can be executed in a proper cloud environment. The resulting algorithm is a first improvement local search algorithm which can be executed in parallel on a given number of computational devices in the cloud which provide a GPU supporting the CUDA framework. The objective function is approximated using Monte Carlo sampling. The neighborhood used for the local search is the famous 3-opt neighborhood [6]. Statistical tests are used to avoid the evaluation of too many samples. Additionally, the massive computational power of modern GPUs is exploited. Each local search is performed independent and at the end the best solution over all the final solutions computed by the local search algorithms is returned. The computational time is the maximum computational time of the different local search algorithms.

3.1   Benchmark Instances

For our experiments we use common benchmark instances for the PTSPD. These benchmark instances were introduced in [1] and are derived from instances for

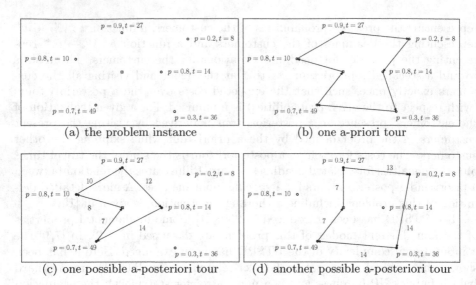

(a) the problem instance

(b) one a-priori tour

(c) one possible a-posteriori tour

(d) another possible a-posteriori tour

Fig. 1. Example of how a-posteriori tours are derived from a given a-priori tour for the PTSPD. Part (a) shows the given PTSPD instance and (b) shows the given a-priori tour. Parts (c) and (d) represent two particular realizations of the random events. Here the filled circles represent the customers that require a visit. These customers are visited in the order specified by the a-priori tour, while the other customers are just skipped. Note that penalties for missed deadlines are not visualized here.

the TRAVELING SALESMAN PROBLEM WITH TIME WINDOWS (TSPTW, [3]). More in detail, the instances for the PTSPD are derived from the TSPTW instances with time window lengths of 20 and instance sizes of 40, 60 and 100 in the following way. There are five TSPTW instances available for every instance size of 40, 60 and 100. For each of those instances four different types of customer probabilities are added. The first one uses probabilities taken uniformly at random from $[0, 1]$ and is referred to as *range*. Then two types with homogeneous probabilities of 0.1 and 0.9 are used. The last type is referred to as *mixed*, here customer probabilities are taken uniformly at random from the two values $\{0.1, 1.0\}$. Moreover, in those instances the penalty values are the same for all customers. We distinguish between two different values for the penalties, 5 and 50, and between two different types of deadlines. The first deadline type is called *early* and uses the starting times of the time windows for the original TSPTW instances as deadlines. The second one is called *late* and uses the finishing times of the time windows as deadlines. In total we have 48 different instance classes (3 different instance sizes, 4 probability types, 2 penalty values, 2 deadline types) consisting of 5 instances each.

3.2   Experimental Setup

We run our newly developed algorithm on each of these instance classes. The number of computational devices (and therefore also the number of parallel local searches) is set to 1, 2, 3, 5, 10, 20, 50 or 100. For each setting we perform 20 repetitions of the experiment (only 5 for the latter two settings). We then measure the average solution quality obtained by the algorithm as well as the average computational time of the algorithm, which is the maximum computational time over the independent local search algorithms.

3.3 Results

First of all, the overall running time of the parallel approach differs only slightly from the computational time required by a single local search algorithm. Therefore, we will focus here on the quality of the final solution, which is the more interesting indicator in this setting. Of course, we are able to compare multiple runs against a single run, since this was also included in our experiments. But additionally, we will also compare our results to the state-of-the-art results reported in [8].

Figures 2 and 3 show representative results for two instances. In Fig. 2 the costs of the final solution obtained by the different approaches for an instance with 100 customers, early deadlines, probabilities of 0.9 and a penalty value of 50 are shown. Figure 3 visualizes the same results for an instance with 100 customers, late deadlines, probabilities of 0.1 and a penalty value of 5.

The results of our computational studies clearly reveal the potential benefits of cloud computing in optimization. For the PTSPD better solutions could be obtained in the same amount of computational time. This implies a trade-off between the costs of the final solution and the costs of the computational resources that are used. Depending on the actual operational costs, a rather small investment for computational resources might result in huge overall savings.

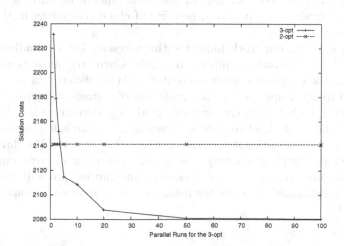

Fig. 2. A plot of the solution quality obtained by the different approaches for an instance with 100 customers, early deadlines, probabilities of 0.9 and a penalty value of 50.

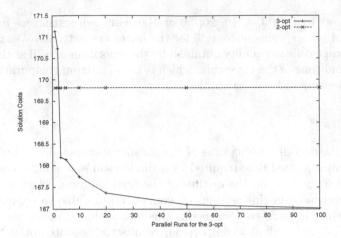

Fig. 3. A plot of the solution quality obtained by the different approaches for an instance with 100 customers, late deadlines, probabilities of 0.1 and a penalty value of 5.

4 Discussion and Conclusions

In this work we have studied the potential of cloud computing in the context of optimization. For this purpose we adapted and improved the state-of-the-art algorithm for the PROBABILISTIC TRAVELING SALESMAN PROBLEM WITH DEADLINES such that it can be easily used in a cloud environment. We then performed a series of experiments on common benchmark instances for the PTSPD. We could clearly demonstrate that by using cloud computing we are able to obtain significantly better solutions in the same amount of running time. Our results definitely show the potential benefits of cloud computing in the field of optimization.

Apart from that, our work indicates the necessity for a paradigm shift in the field of heuristics and operations research. Currently, most heuristics are developed for the usage on a single computer and the efficiency of such methods is compared to other approaches that make use of a single computer. We think that this view is highly restrictive and outdated, in particular with respect to the general availability of cloud resources. Nowadays, we can safely assume that a large number of computational devices is available to everyone. The development of algorithms that exploit this huge amount of resources is of great importance. Of course, computational time and memory consumption are still crucial indicators, but additionally the costs for using the cloud resources should be taken into account.

References

1. Campbell, A.M., Thomas, B.W.: Probabilistic traveling salesman problem with deadlines. Transp. Sci. **42**(1), 1–21 (2008)
2. Campbell, A.M., Thomas, B.W.: Runtime reduction techniques for the probabilistic traveling salesman problem with deadlines. Comput. Oper. Res. **36**(4), 1231–1248 (2009)
3. Dumas, Y., Desrosiers, J., Gelinas, E., Solomon, M.M.: An optimal algorithm for the traveling salesman problem with time windows. Oper. Res. **43**(2), 367–371 (1995)
4. Jaillet, P.: Probabilistic traveling salesman problems. PhD thesis, MIT, Department of Civil Engineering (1985)
5. Jaillet, P.: A priori solution of a traveling salesman problem in which a random subset of the customers are visited. Oper. Res. **36**(6), 929–936 (1988)
6. Johnson, D.S., McGeoch, L.A.: The traveling salesman problem: a case study in local optimization. Local Search Comb. Optim. **1**, 215–310 (1997)
7. Weyland, D.: On the computational complexity of the probabilistic traveling salesman problem with deadlines. Theor. Comput. Sci. **540**, 156–168 (2014)
8. Weyland, D., Montemanni, R., Gambardella, L.M.: A metaheuristic framework for stochastic combinatorial optimization problems based on GPGPU with a case study on the probabilistic traveling salesman problem with deadlines. J. Parallel Distrib. Comput. **73**, 74–85 (2012)
9. Weyland, D., Montemanni, R., Gambardella, L.M.: Hardness results for the probabilistic traveling salesman problem with deadlines. In: Mahjoub, A.R., Markakis, V., Milis, I., Paschos, V.T. (eds.) ISCO 2012. LNCS, vol. 7422, pp. 392–403. Springer, Heidelberg (2012)
10. Weyland, D., Montemanni, R., Gambardella, L.M.: Heuristics for the probabilistic traveling salesman problem with deadlines based on quasi-parallel monte carlo sampling. Comput. Oper. Res. **40**(7), 1661–1670 (2013)

Optimizing Set-Up Times Using the HeuristicLab Optimization Environment

Johannes Karder[1]([⊠]), Andreas Scheibenpflug[1,2], Stefan Wagner[1], and Michael Affenzeller[1,2]

[1] Heuristic and Evolutionary Algorithms Laboratory School of Informatics, Communications and Media, University of Applied Sciences Upper Austria, Campus Hagenberg, Softwarepark 11, 4232 Hagenberg, Austria
{jkarder,ascheibe,swagner,maffenze}@heuristiclab.com
[2] Institute for Formal Models and Verification, Johannes Kepler University Linz, Altenbergerstraße 69, 4040 Linz, Austria

Abstract. This publication shows the application of set-up time optimization to machinery that requires some components to be preloaded from a component storage to the work zone before jobs can be processed. Component loading and unloading, which is normally done by the machine operators, should be done automatically. The machine has access to a component storage consisting of multiple racks. Components can be moved by using different strategies. These strategies also affect the storage layout over time. Applying simulation-based optimization to the set-up process yields good machine configuration parameters (i.e. initial storage layout, sequence of jobs and used strategies) for a given job sequence. A simulator which models the machinery is used to evaluate different strategies and machine parameters. For all optimization aspects, HeuristicLab is used as the underlying software environment in combination with a new specific problem type that can be solved with evolutionary algorithms such as genetic algorithms or evolution strategies.

1 Introduction

Rapid changes in production cycles lead to time windows that do not generate added value. The minimization of set-up times can increase the net product, because a certain percentage of time formerly used to prepare machinery can be converted to time used for actual production. In the studied environment, machines have to be loaded manually with certain components by the operators for each job. The components vary in size and weight. Lifting components is demanding for the operator, especially if lots of components have to be changed in short intervals. Therefore, this set-up process should be done automatically by the machine itself.

Within this publication, set-up times of machines that automatically fetch the necessary machine components for specific jobs from a component storage

R. Moreno-Díaz et al. (Eds.): EUROCAST 2015, LNCS 9520, pp. 286–293, 2015.
DOI: 10.1007/978-3-319-27340-2_36

are optimized using simulation-based optimization with HeuristicLab (HL)[1] [1]. In the specific case, implementing an according machine simulator requires a static, deterministic and discrete model of the real system. This model is then used to analyze and evaluate different loading and unloading cycles as well as different strategies, which helps in the implementation of a robust optimization technique for set-up time minimization.

Three different optimization aspects, i.e. the storage organization, the job sequence order and the component movement strategies, are presented. The initial storage layout and the way the storage is managed over time plays an important role in the machine's readiness. Five different movement strategies were implemented and can be used by the simulation to unload components back to the storage. These strategies also affect the storage layout, because components are moved back according to specific rules. Job sequence ordering can only be done if more than one job is known.

The simulation was incorporated into a new HL problem type that provides the necessary operators to be optimized with evolutionary algorithms such as genetic algorithms or evolution strategies. Different parameters of the simulation were analyzed and tuned by applying parametric optimization using a genetic algorithm with offspring selection [2]. The parameters include all three optimization aspects. Three different optimization approaches were executed, starting from a naive approach and ending with a well optimized technique. The main focus of the study lies in analyzing and optimizing the storage layout, i.e. how components should be positioned inside the storage area.

Another approach for set-up time minimization has been shown in [3]. Sequence dependent set-up costs were reduced by applying automatically generated dispatching and scheduling rules to artificial and real world production scenarios. This approach used several similarity measures instead of a simulation model within the objective function.

2 Set-Up Time Optimization

2.1 Concept

Set-up time minimization requires analysis of different loading and unloading cycles of the machine in use. Many strategies exist and often it is not clear which one works well under which conditions. Although creating an objective function for simulation models can often be a difficult task [4], it is easy to measure the fitness in this particular case by the time the machine needs to prepare itself for one or more jobs.

Implementing an according machine simulator requires a static, deterministic, discrete model of the real system. The architecture of the specific machinery is depicted in Fig. 1. Components can be stored in 20 different storage racks. The racks' contents can be manipulated by the changers, which are able to slide components in and out of the right side of each rack. From the changers, components can be slid to the rack zero and the work zone using the movers.

---

[1] http://dev.heuristiclab.com/.

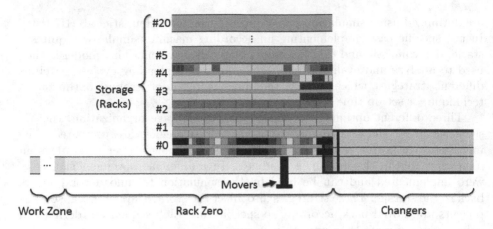

Fig. 1. Simplified machine architecture

All actions (i.e. movements) that are executed by the simulator can be represented atomically by phases and consume a certain part of the total time that is used to load and unload the machine.

2.2   Strategies

There are three key aspects that can be optimized. First of all, the organization of the component storage can be improved. Depending on how components are stored and managed over time, set-up times can be reduced. The second optimization potential can be found in changing the order of the jobs being processed. The last aspect that can lead to performance improvements is the strategy used to move components. On-the-fly switching between sliding and other types of transportation can speed up the loading and unloading cycles. The following sections contain more detailed information about all optimization aspects

Storage Organization. The way the component storage is managed over time plays an important role in the machine's readiness. Unloading components to their original position seems to be a good strategy, keeping in mind that components are often sorted in a logical and reasonable way by the machine operators. A tidy storage should be quickly accessible and each job will start with the original storage layout. In Fig. 2, the upper left image shows the storage layout after applying the `DownloadToOriginalPosition` strategy. The layout equals the initial storage layout. Using a chaotic storage, it is possible to slide the components back to their original racks, but not to their original position. The upper right image in Fig. 2 shows the storage layout after unloading using the `DownloadToOriginalRack` strategy. Another strategy to unload components is to always fill up the first available rack when moving down the storage area from rack zero. The result of applying this so called

DownloadToFirstFillableRack strategy can be seen in the lower left image of Fig. 2. Unloading components to the least filled rack is also an option. By applying the DownloadToLeastFilledRack strategy, component for component is moved to the rack with the most free space. This strategy's outcome is displayed in the lower right image in Fig. 2.

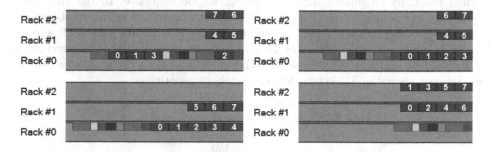

Fig. 2. Results of the different component movement strategies

The last strategy, namely UnloadGroupsWithMaximumLength, has nothing to do with where components are unloaded to, but rather how many components are unloaded at once. The machine is able to unload connected components (i.e. component groups) one at a time or as many components as physically possible.

Job Sequence Order. Once all jobs are in the queue, job sequence order optimization can be applied. Depending on the subset of components that are shared by multiple jobs, the order of execution can be optimized. If two jobs use many different components (i.e. the subset of components used in both jobs is small or empty), many movements are necessary to switch from one job configuration to another. Thus the set-up time increases. Chaining jobs with similar configurations decreases these movements and leads to quicker set-up times. Using the simulation, the theoretically best execution order in combination with a certain set of applied strategies can be found.

Component Movement. There is also optimization potential in the component movement method itself. Sliding is a pretty fast way to move bulks of components. Another method is to pick and place components between different locations. Picking and placing can be used to remove or exchange some components in a component group and leave other components for further use. Here, both the combination of sliding as well as picking and placing and especially the decision when to use one and only one strategy are key. Since the picking and placing features are not implemented in the simulator, this optimization aspect will be excluded from this study.

3   Experiments

The test series starts with a naive approach that uses a manually configured storage layout and no active optimization. The order of the jobs and the chosen strategies are then optimized for the manual storage layout using HL. The layout is then optimized autonomously with HL. The best layout configuration is finally tuned manually to further optimize the whole job sequence. In the end, the resulting best solution – i.e. job sequence, layout configuration and strategies – is applied to each job separately to analyze the specific quality gain of all parts.

HL's implementation of the OSGA produced the best results (compared to a standard GA and a RAPGA) and was therefore used with the manually tuned parameters shown in Table 1 for all tests with 10 repetitions.

Table 1. Parameters for the OSGA experiment

Name	Value
Elites	1
MaximumGenerations	100
MaximumSelectionPressure	100
MutationProbability	25 %
PopulationSize	200
Selector	ProportionalSelector
SuccessRatio	1

3.1   Naive Approach

In the naive approach the jobs are executed in random order and components are unloaded to their original positions. The manually configured storage layout that is used is depicted in Fig. 3. Rack #0 to #2 contain all components that are used in the first four jobs, whereas rack #3 and #4 store all other components. The set-up time required in the naive approach is 22 min 4.181 s.

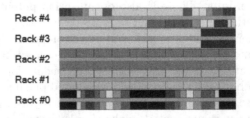

Fig. 3. The manually configured storage layout

3.2   Optimized Approach I

The first optimized approach tries to find a good execution order for the jobs as well as a good set of strategies that should be used with that order. Storage layout optimization is omitted. All best solutions of each OSGA run had equal quality and only differed in the proposed job sequence. Compared to the naive approach, the set-up time was reduced by approximately 17.11 % to 18 min 17.573 s by using one of the proposed job sequences and the UnloadGroupsWithMaximumLength strategy.

3.3   Optimized Approach II

In the second optimized approach, storage layout optimization is enabled and mutation probability is reduced from 25 % to 10 %. With storage layout optimization enabled, the solution space explodes. The number of solutions can be computed by multiplying the number of different job sequences (10!) with the number of different strategy settings (8) and the number of different rack configurations. This leads to a greater variance in solution qualities. Compared to the naive approach, the set-up time was reduced by approximately 18.74 % to 17 min 56.07 s by applying the DownloadToFirstFillableRack and UnloadGroupsWithMaximum Length strategies. Components in the resulting storage layout were fractionated all over the storage which seems to be a good strategy due to the fact that some component movements that are needed to access components inside highly populated racks are eliminated. These component movements are more time consuming than moving the changers along the storage.

3.4   Optimized Approach III

In the last optimized approach the best storage layout configuration found by the second optimized approach is manually tuned. Components are placed so that they are quickly accessible. This was not done for all components due to the fact that sometimes components are carried to other storage racks and unloaded there. Transposing these components would lead to inefficiencies later on. Compared to the naive approach, the set-up time was reduced by approximately 20.21 % to 17 min 36.511 s using the same job sequence and strategies proposed by the second optimized approach.

3.5   Overall Performance

Nearly every job gets executed faster with the third optimized approach, as can be seen in Table 2. The set-up time becomes even less when all jobs are executed in an optimized sequence as shown in Table 3, since the component movements of each job change the storage structure and the OSGA optimizes the storage layout exactly for this sequence.

Table 2. Single job comparison

Job	Set-up time (mm:ss.fff)		
	Naive	Opt. III	Delta
Job 1	02:31.851	02:15.443	−00:16.408
Job 2	03:29.314	03:30.670	+00:01.356
Job 3	04:18.186	03:42.467	−00:35.719
Job 4	03:27.401	03:17.892	−00:09.509
Job 5	01:26.121	01:12.725	−00:13.396
Job 6	01:25.083	01:14.090	−00:10.993
Job 7	01:15.088	01:10.913	−00:04.175
Job 8	01:28.845	01:05.990	−00:22.855
Job 9	01:31.596	01:18.956	−00:12.640
Job 10	01:10.696	01:09.122	−00:01.574
		$\sum$	−02:05.913

Table 3. Job sequence comparison

Set-up time (mm:ss.fff)		
Naive	Opt. III	Delta
22:04.181	17:36.511	−04:27.670

4   Conclusion

Creating a sorted storage as it was done in the first approach seems to be natural but inefficient. Many racks are empty and not used at all, whereas the remaining racks are completely filled with components. This leads to many sliding operations that are needed to access certain components inside the racks. Dividing components inside the storage can reduce these sliding operations. Operating in more racks leads to more changer movements, but moving changers along the storage does not take as much time as the sliding operations.

Compared to the first (naive) approach, set-up times were reduced by approximately 20.21 % (267.67 s). Using more powerful and likewise more time consuming algorithm parameter settings, set-up times could be reduced even more by approximately 21.24 % (281.217 s), but empirical tests with a sufficient number of repetitions have not been conducted because of the long runtime of each repetition. Concerning the problem implementation, instead of using a permutation encoding for the storage layout, a special layout encoding and appropriate crossover and mutation operators could yield even better results.

When manually improving the storage, two things have to be kept in mind. Firstly the storage should not be modified so that the component groups needed for each job are already present. Probably this would not even be possible since multiple components might be needed in more than one job, but nevertheless building such a "perfect" rack configuration is not the goal of this study. Secondly one has to be careful not to optimize "too much". Components should be made quickly accessible by the changers, but not all component transpositions improve performance.

There is still much optimization potential in the set-up process. A factor that can be improved further is the component selection, i.e. which components to chose from which rack. Some optimization is done inside the simulation, but this selection process can be extended with priority rules that propose the next steps depending on the current storage layout. Furthermore, the component movement strategies can be improved and new ones can be added. Picking and placing features simultaneously extend and increase the complexity of strategic options.

Rack configurations and strategies turned out to be (in-)efficient and including the job sequences, first distinctions between good and bad settings could be made. Valuable information was gathered which can be used in the development of a more profound optimization module for the machinery.

Acknowledgments. The work described in this paper was conducted within the NPS (Sustainable Production Steering) project and funded by the Austrian Research Promotion Agency (FFG).

References

1. Wagner, S., Kronberger, G., Beham, A., Kommenda, M., Scheibenpflug, A., Pitzer, E., Vonolfen, S., Kofler, M., Winkler, S., Dorfer, V., Affenzeller, M.: Architecture and design of the HeuristicLab optimization environment. In: Klempous, R., Nikodem, J., Jacak, W., Chaczko, Z. (eds.) Advanced Methods and Applications in Computational Intelligence. TIEI, vol. 6, pp. 193–258. Springer, Heidelberg (2013)
2. Affenzeller, M., Wagner, S.: Offspring selection: a new self-adaptive selection scheme for genetic algorithms. In: Ribeiro, B., Albrecht, R.F., Dobnikar, A., Pearson, D.W., Steele, N.C. (eds.) Adaptive and Natural Computing Algorithms. Springer Computer Series, pp. 218–221. Springer, Vienna (2005)
3. Kofler, M., Wagner, S., Beham, A., Kronberger, G., Affenzeller, M.: Priority rule generation with a genetic algorithm to minimize sequence dependent setup costs. In: Moreno-Díaz, R., Pichler, F., Quesada-Arencibia, A. (eds.) EUROCAST 2009. LNCS, vol. 5717, pp. 817–824. Springer, Heidelberg (2009)
4. Law, A.M., Kelton, D.W.: Simulation Modelling and Analysis. McGraw-Hill Education, Europe (2000)

The Bike Request Scheduling Problem

Kenneth Sörensen and Nicholas Vergeylen[✉]

University of Antwerp Operations Research Group ANT/OR, Antwerp, Belgium
{kenneth.sorensen,nicholas.vergeylen}@uantwerpen.be
http://antor.uantwerpen.be

Abstract. In this paper we introduce the *bike request scheduling problem*, a new approach to city bike repositioning problems. The rationale behind this approach is explained, and a mixed-integer programming formulation is given. We prove that the bike request scheduling problem is NP-hard and formulate recommendations for future research.

1 Introduction: The Bike Request Scheduling Problem

Bicycle sharing systems (BSSs) are popping up in cities all over the world. These initiatives allow individuals to rent a bike from an automated rental station, use it for a short period of time, and return it to any other rental station in the city. A 2011 report of the Commission on Sustainable Development of the United Nations Department of Economic and Social Affairs (Midgley 2011) put the number of BSSs at 375, using around 236,000 bikes, and there is very little doubt that these numbers have only increased since. Clearly, "bikesharing" has evolved from an interesting experiment to a viable addition to the modal mix of public passenger transport, even in large cities. For a historical perspective on BSSs, as well as some future trends we refer to DeMaio (2009).

Demand and supply at specific rental stations are rarely balanced, and fluctuations in supply and demand in the long or the short term might cause stations to fill up or deplete, preventing users from collecting or returning bikes. BSSs therefore typically use a fleet of light vehicles to transfer bikes between stations, attempting to rebalance the system. The vehicles are in constant contact with the dispatching station, where the current inventory of each station is monitored, and from where the repositioning activities are directed.

In the literature, several contributions have tackled the problem of determining the optimal routing of the repositioning vehicles. The family of related optimization problems solved in these papers is generally referred to as the *bike repositioning problem* (BRP). The *static* BRP (SBRP) is applicable when use of the BSS is negligible (i.e., at night). Examples of papers that tackle this problem are Benchimol et al. (2011), Chemla et al. (2012), Erdoğan et al. (2013), Raviv et al. (2012), Rainer-Harbach et al. (2014). Other authors, like Contardo et al. (2012), Kloimüllner et al. (2014), focus on the *dynamic* BRP (DBRP), in which demand and supply at each station during the day is taken into account. Their objective is to minimize the total unmet demand (which is expressed as

© Springer International Publishing Switzerland 2015
R. Moreno-Díaz et al. (Eds.): EUROCAST 2015, LNCS 9520, pp. 294–301, 2015.
DOI: 10.1007/978-3-319-27340-2_37

the number of users who tried to collect bikes from empty stations or to bring back bikes to full stations).

A large majority of approaches in the literature combine two distinct problems into one single optimization problem: (1) deciding how many bikes to load or unload at the different stations throughout the day, and (2) the vehicle routing problem of the repositioning vehicles. This forces them to either model user demand and supply of bikes at the various stations as zero (the static BRP) or as a highly simplified process (the dynamic BRP). In reality, however, determining the expected demand and supply of bikes at each station and deriving from this information the number of bikes to load or unload at the different stations, as well as the best moment to do so, is a difficult problem that deserves attention in its own right. Ignoring the stochastic nature of this problem may lead to solutions that are not implementable. Moreover, it is unlikely that the process of determining the number of bikes to load and unload can and should be always fully automated: the complexity of the real-life situation will most likely call for some human interaction in the planning process. For these reasons, we propose an alternative modelling approach, which we call the *bike request scheduling problem* (BRSP) is a better alternative.

The remainder of this article is organized as follows. Our methodology for tackling repositioning problems is explained in Sect. 2. A mathematical model of the BRSP is presented in Sect. 3. In Sect. 4 a proof is given that the BRSP is NP-hard. Finally, conclusions and recommendations for further work are given in Sect. 5.

2   Methodology

We propose a novel approach that tackles the bicycle repositioning problem by decomposing it into two distinct subproblems: (1) the generation of loading or unloading *requests* (essentially an order to pick up or drop off a certain number of bikes at a certain station within a certain time window), and (2) the (dynamic) assignment of these requests to vehicles and the scheduling of requests within each vehicle. In this contribution we focus on the latter problem, which has been called the *bike request scheduling problem* (BRSP). This approach differs from the traditional approaches (using the BRP) in that it explicitly separates the process of determining the demand and supply of bikes at the different stations from the problem of routing the repositioning vehicles. The objective of the BRSP is to determine the assignment and sequencing of requests to vehicles that minimizes the priority-weighted number of unscheduled requests, subject to the time windows of the requests, as well as the capacities of the replenishment vehicles.

Decomposing the problem of request generation and the problem of scheduling those requests into two distinct subproblems requires that an information exchange protocol is established between both subproblems. At the core of the boundary are the so-called *requests*. They encapsulate the necessary information for the scheduling algorithm to create a set of vehicle routes such that preferably all requests are handled. The attributes of a request are defined in Table 1.

Table 1. Attributes of a request

Name	Explanation
Issue time	The time at which the request is issued
Type	Pick-up (load) or deliver (unload)
Quantity	Number of bikes to load or unload
Station	Identity of the station at which to load or unload bikes
Priority	A weight that indicates the relative importance of the request
Earliest time	Start of the time window during which the request can be fulfilled
Latest time	Expiration time of the request
Drop time	Time required to execute the request

All common taxonomies of vehicle routing problems distinguish between static and dynamic vehicle routing problems (Pillac et al. 2013), which differ in the availability of all information at the start of the planning period (static problems) or not (dynamic problems). Both static and dynamic variants of the BRSP can be defined through the issue time of the requests. The static BRSP will be agnostic of future requests, which is equivalent to all requests having an issue time of zero (assuming that the planning period starts at time zero or after). The dynamic BRSP can introduce positive issue times that fall within the interval defined by the start and end of the planning period. The rest of this paper will discuss the static BRSP, although dynamic variants of the BRSP will be investigated in future research.

3 Problem Definition and Mathematical Model

Given a set of requests, the objective of the (static) BRSP is to minimize the priority-weighted number of unscheduled requests. To this end, requests can be scheduled on a (given) set of vehicles, each having identical capacity. Executing a request requires a vehicle to visit the station where this request occurs. Travel times between stations are assumed to be known. Each request has a time window (earliest and latest time), and the request can only be executed during this time. Executing a request takes a certain amount of time, which needs to be spent before the vehicle can start traveling towards the station at which its next request occurs. Vehicles are allowed to wait before starting service if they arrive before the earliest time of the request. It is assumed that a vehicle can always start executing their first request at its earliest time and return to the depot after the latest time of their last request. This makes it unnecessary to model a depot in the mathematical model. Each request requires a number of bikes to be either picked up or dropped off. The number of bikes on a vehicle after each pick-up or drop-off can never fall below zero or exceed the vehicle's capacity. Each request has a priority, and the priority of all requests that have not been assigned to a vehicle, are added to the objective function.

Table 2. Parameters of the static BRSP

I	Set of requests
N	Set of positions within a vehicle tour
K	Set of vehicles
b_i	Number of bikes picked up or delivered at request i ($> 0 \rightarrow$ delivery, $< 0 \rightarrow$ pick-up)
w_i	Weight of request i
o_i	Working time at request i
a_i^e	Earliest arrival time at request i
a_i^l	Latest arrival time at request i
t_{ij}	Travel time from request i to request j
C	Capacity of the vehicles

Table 3. Decision variables of the static BRSP

x_{in}^k	1 if request i is served as the n-th request of vehicle k, 0 otherwise
y_i	1 if request i is not served, 0 otherwise
a_i	Arrival time at request i
z_{ij}	1 if request j is visited immediately after request i by the same vehicle

In this section a mixed-integer programming model is developed for the (static) BRSP. The parameters used in the model are shown in Table 2. The decision variables can be found in Table 3.

Using this notation, the problem can be written as follows.

$$\min \sum_i y_i w_i \tag{1}$$

s.t.

$$\sum_k \sum_n x_{in}^k + y_i = 1 \qquad\qquad \forall i \in I \tag{2}$$

$$z_{ij} \geq x_{jn+1}^k + x_{in}^k - 1 \qquad \forall i,j \in I, k \in K, n \in N \tag{3}$$

$$\sum_i x_{i(n+1)}^k \leq \sum_i x_{in}^k \qquad\qquad \forall k \in K, n \in N \tag{4}$$

$$\sum_i x_{in}^k \leq 1 \qquad\qquad \forall n \in N, k \in K \tag{5}$$

$$\sum_i \sum_{n' \leq n} x_{in'}^k b_i \leq C \qquad\qquad \forall n \in N, k \in K \tag{6}$$

$$\sum_i \sum_{n' \leq n} x_{in'}^k b_i \geq 0 \qquad\qquad \forall n \in N, k \in K \tag{7}$$

$$a_j \geq a_i + o_i + t_{ij} - (1 - z_{ij})M \qquad\qquad \forall i,j \in I \tag{8}$$

$$a_i^e \le a_i \le a_i^l \qquad\qquad\qquad \forall i \in I \qquad (9)$$

$$x_{in}^k, z_{ij}, y_i \in (0,1) \qquad\qquad \forall i \in I, k \in K, n \in N \qquad (10)$$

$$a_i \ge 0 \qquad\qquad\qquad\qquad \forall i \in I \qquad (11)$$

The objective function (1) minimizes the total weight of all unscheduled requests. Constraints (2) ensure that each request is not served more than once. Constraints (3) link the decision variables z_{ij} and x_{in}^k so that z_{ij} is forced to be equal to 1 if a vehicle serves request j immediately after request i. Constraints (4) ensure that a contiguous set of adjacent positions in the vehicle is used, starting from the first position. Constraints (5) force each position in the vehicle to be used only once. For a vehicle moving between requests i and j, constraints (8) ensure that the vehicle can only serve request j after its arrival time at i plus its drop time at i plus the time it takes to travel between i and j. Constraints (6) and (7) ensure that the number of bikes on a vehicle never exceed the vehicles' capacity or goes below zero respectively. Constraints (9) force the arrival time at request i to be between its earliest and latest arrival time. Finally, constraints (10) to (11) define the domains of the decision variables.

4   NP Hardness of the BRSP

In this section we show that the BRSP is NP-hard by demonstrating that a subset of BRSP instances are knapsack problems which are studied in Martello and Toth (1990) and Dasgupta et al. (2008). A subset of BRSP instances can be transformed to 0-1 knapsack problems and any 0-1 knapsack problem can be transformed into a BRSP instance. Solving the BRSP implies solving the knapsack problem. Therefore the BRSP is at least as hard as the knapsack problem, or, in other words, the BRSP is NP-hard.

Instances of the BRSP that can be modeled as knapsack problems are those where (1) only one vehicle is used, (2) every request has a positive quantity of bicycles, and (3) time windows are non-constraining. The latter will be the case when all early time limits are zero and all late time limits are at least as late as the length of the longest vehicle trip, which we denote T_m. This means the time windows, as enforced by constraints (3) and (8)–(9) are always satisfied. To see this, notice the arrival time for any request in any instance will necessarily be between these bounds:

$$a_i^e = 0 \le a_i < T_m = a_i^l, \forall i \in I \qquad (12)$$

This means we can leave those constraints explicitly out of consideration when solving the subproblem.

All b_i are positive. This means we can drop constraints (7) explicitly as well. It also means that vehicle load will increase monotonously with the request sequence in constraints (6):

$$\sum_i \sum_n x_{in} b_i = \sum_i \sum_{w=1}^{n'} x_{iw} b_i + \sum_i \sum_{w=n'+1}^{n} x_{in} b_i \le C, \quad \forall n \in N, 1 \le n' < n$$

So

$$\sum_i \sum_n x_{in} b_i \leq C \Rightarrow \sum_i \sum_{w=1}^{n'} x_{iw} b_i \leq C, \qquad \forall n \in N, 1 \leq n' < n$$

This means we can only consider the constraint where n is the position of the last scheduled request. For a certain schedule, we can permute the requests without changing the left hand side of the constraint. This means the order of the schedule becomes irrelevant in terms of the capacity constraints and the time window constraints. It was already irrelevant in terms of the objective function. Therefore we can now remove order information from the model together with constraints (4) and (5) as they become redundant.

The remaining model minimizes the priority-weighted number of unscheduled requests. The decision variables x_i are the complement of the y_i variables: $x_i + y_i = 1, \forall i \in I$. This means we can further simplify the model by removing y_i and expressing the model only in terms of x_i. This removes the need to express constraints (2) explicitly, but changes the sense of the objective function. The resulting model after applying the simplifications is given by:

$$\max \quad P_i \cdot x_i \tag{13}$$

s.t.

$$\sum_i x_i b_i \leq C \tag{14}$$

$$x_i \in \{0, 1\} \qquad \forall i \tag{15}$$

This is exactly the formulation of the *0-1 knapsack problem* with profits P_i and weigths b_i. We can therefore conclude that the highly restricted case of the BRSP we consider here is identical to the knapsack problem.

On the other hand, every knapsack problem can be transformed to a special case of the BRSP. This can be done as follows. Given a set I of items, each with a profit P'_i and a weight b'_i, a request is created with the following attributes:

- $b_i = b'_i, \forall i \in I$
- $w_i = P'_i, \forall i \in I$

Further, a set of stations should exists, to which requests may be assigned in any possible way. Travel times between stations are irrelevant, as are working times for each requests. Further, a single vehicle is defined with the same capacity as the knapsack. Time windows for each request are set to zero for the earliest time and an arbitrarily large number of the latest time. The optimal solution of the BRSP with these characteristics is the same as the optimal solution of the original knapsack problem.

We set up experiments to verify how the model scales when implemented in a general purpose solver (Gurobi). Without going into much detail, we report that the presented model is prone to combinatorial explosion, even for small instances. When enforcing a time limit of 3600 s, we see that the number of time constraint violations increases exponentially ranging from 3 for 9 requests to 189 for 12 requests. Notice that an instance of 12 requests is extremely small when looking at real life situations where we have more than 100 stations in networks of medium size.

5   Conclusion

In this contribution we have described the problem of bicycle repositioning and highlighted the problems of the approaches that exist today. We have proposed a new approach to tackle this problem, that separates the process of determining the number of bikes and the time window within which to pick them up or deliver them at each station, and the vehicle routing of the repositioning vehicles. The concept of a *request* was introduced as the core communication between both subproblems. We have proven that the static version of the bike repositioning problem is NP-hard and developed a mixed-integer programming model.

One possible avenue for future research is an improvement of the exact model, including strategies to reduce computational effort such as introducing problem-specific cutting planes, an intelligent column generation strategy, or the use of lazy constraints. The aim of this line of research would be to solve realistic instances in a more acceptable time limit. The empirical analysis presented in this contribution could then be extended to these cases, yielding results of more practical significance.

Another path for further research will focus on the development of heuristic solution algorithms to obtain a better ratio of resource consumption to objective value. In practice, for example, the unpredictable calculation time of the exact model will be unacceptable, especially in a dynamic situations where the changing list of requests requires a constant re-evaluation of the current solution. Heuristics are the only alternative in this case. This research path could also focus on matheuristics, trying to combine the best from the exact models and heuristics.

Future research also will consider the request generation algorithm. Requests should be generated to reflect patterns found in user behavior. Modeling usage behavior could be of great value for the research on the BRSP as well, as it will allow to generate more realistic test cases compared to the extended Solomon cases used in this research.

References

Benchimol, M., Benchimol, P., Chappert, B., Taille, A.D.L., Laroche, F., Meunier, F., Robinet, L.: Balancing the stations of a self service bike hire system. RAIRO Oper. Res. **45**(1), 37–61 (2011)

Chemla, D., Meunier, F., Calvo, R.W.: Bike sharing system: solving the static rebalancing problem. Discrete Optim. **10**, 120–146 (2012). (Accepted for publication in Discrete Optimization)

Contardo, C., Morency, C., Rousseau, L.-M.: Balancing a dynamic public bike-sharing system. Centre Interuniversitaire de Recherche sur les Réseaux d'entreprise, la Logistique et le Transport (2012)

Dasgupta, S., Papadimitriou, C.H., Vazirani, U.: Algorithms, 1st edn. McGraw-Hill Inc, New York (2008)

DeMaio, P.: Bike-sharing: History, impacts, models of provision, and future. J. Public Transp. 12(4), 41–56 (2009)

Erdoğan, G., Laporte, G., Calvo, R.W.: The one-commodity pickup and delivery traveling salesman problem with demand intervals. Submitted for publication to Transportation Science (2013)

Kloimüllner, C., Papazek, P., Hu, B., Raidl, G.R.: Balancing bicycle sharing systems: an approach for the dynamic case. In: Blum, C., Ochoa, G. (eds.) EvoCOP 2014. LNCS, vol. 8600, pp. 73–84. Springer, Heidelberg (2014)

Martello, S., Toth, P.: Knapsack Problems: Algorithms and Computer Implementations. Wiley, New York (1990)

Midgley, P.: Bicycle sharing schemes: enhancing sustainable mobility in urban areas. Background paper CSD19/2011/BP 8, United Nations Department of Economic and Social Affairs, Commission on Sustainable Development (2011)

Pillac, V., Gendreau, M., Guret, C., Medaglia, A.L.: A review of dynamic vehicle routing problems. Eur. J. Oper. Res. 255(1), 1–11 (2013)

Rainer-Harbach, M., Papazek, P., Raidl, G.R., Hu, B., Kloimllner, C.: PILOT, GRASP, and VNS approaches for the static balancing of bicycle sharing systems. J. Glob. Optim. 63, 1–33 (2014)

Raviv, T., Tzur, M., Forma, I.A.: Static repositioning in a bike-sharing system: models and solution approaches. EURO J. Transp. Logistics 2, 1–43 (2012)

Classification of the States of Human Adaptive Immune Systems by Analyzing Immunoglobulin and T Cell Receptors Using ImmunExplorer

Susanne Schaller[1]([✉]), Johannes Weinberger[2], Raúl Jiménez-Heredia[2],
Martin Danzer[3], and Stephan M. Winkler[1]

[1] Bioinformatics Research Group, University of Applied Sciences Upper Austria,
Hagenberg Campus Softwarepark 11, 4232 Hagenberg, Austria
{susanne.schaller,stephan.winkler}@fh-hagenberg.at
[2] Experimental and Clinical Traumatology, Ludwig Boltzmann Institute,
Garnisonstrasse 21, 4020 Linz, Austria
johannes.weinberger@o.roteskreuz.at
[3] Red Cross Blood Transfusion Service of Upper Austria,
Krankenhausstrasse 7, 4020 Linz, Austria
martin.danzer@o.roteskreuz.at

Abstract. The behavior and actions of the human adaptive immune system and its key players, namely B and T cells, are often hard to understand in their entirety. We here present a workflow for modelling the states of adaptive immune systems by analyzing B and T cell receptor repertoires using next-generation sequencing data. For our workflow, we have blood and kidney tissues from diseased patients, who suffered from different kidney diseases (e.g., renal carcinoma), and healthy proband. A set of features based on clonal expansion and diversity of immunoglobulins and T cell receptor next-generation sequencing data, isolated from patients, are calculated. Using different machine learning methods such as support vector machines, random forests, artificial neural networks and genetic programming in HeuristicLab, we are able to classify and distinguish between healthy and diseased individuals up to 80 % accuracy using ImmunExplorer.

Keywords: IG and TR immune repertoire · Clonality and diversity feature extraction · ImmunExplorer · Machine learning · HeuristicLab

1 Introduction: The Adaptive Immune System and Its Receptors

Today's research and investigation in the field of immunology demands for a deep understanding of the clonal expansion, diversity, and the overall behavior of the immunoglobulins (IG) or antibodies and T cell receptors (TR) of the

The work performed in this paper was done within *ImmuneProfiler*, a research project funded by the basic research funding program of the University of Applied Sciences Upper Austria.

© Springer International Publishing Switzerland 2015
R. Moreno-Díaz et al. (Eds.): EUROCAST 2015, LNCS 9520, pp. 302–309, 2015.
DOI: 10.1007/978-3-319-27340-2_38

human adaptive immune system. The immune system is composed of various cells that usually are able to prevent pathogen growth, to generate responses for eliminating pathogens, and to develop an immunological memory. Especially, the B and T cells are major players in the immune system, characterized by special proteins on the cell membrane, the so-called immune IG and TR. Modern high-throughput next-generation sequencing (NGS) technologies [1] are nowadays the method of choice when it comes to analyzing IG and TR in the human adaptive immune system. NGS enables researchers to read the bases of DNA derived from samples (e.g., blood, tissue) of different species. Due to the high-throughput, scalability, and speed, NGS machines are able to produce billions of short sequences (reads) per run, which needs algorithms to analyze this huge amount of generated data.

Our research goal is to use these preprocessed NGS-based IG and TR data as input to calculate and determine the clonality and diversity of the antigen immune repertoire and therefore, to extract features to differentiate the states of human adaptive immune systems using machine learning algorithms (see Fig. 1). This immunological modelling approach shall be used to distinguish states of immune systems between patients having immunological reactions (e.g., allergies) or diseases (e.g., autoimmune disorders, HIV), and states of healthy proband using blood and tissue samples.

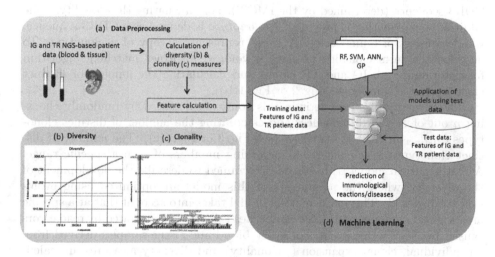

Fig. 1. Schematic workflow of the modelling approach for the prediction of the health status of the human adaptive immune system.

2   Methods

Only blood or blood and tissue (kidney) samples have been obtained from healthy proband and every diseased patient, respectively. B and T cells were isolated and preprocessed for NGS experiments. Diseased patients had any kind of kidney disease e.g., cirrhosis of the kidney, sacculated kidney, or renal carcinoma. By using NGS we are able to determine bases of DNA from all samples, and furthermore the NGS sequences are analyzed using the ImmunoGeneTics information system (IMGT) [2,3]. The IMGT enables a broaden nucleotide analysis of IG and TR V-(D)-J repertoires, polymorphisms, and mutations of different species (e.g., homo sapiens, mus musculus). IG and TR contain different gene segments, including the V-(D)-J gene repertoire, which is also known as somatic recombination. The expressed IG and TR repertoires represent a potential of 10^{12} IG and 10^{12} TR per individual. This huge diversity occurs from mechanisms that happened during the IG and TR molecular synthesis [4,5]. These mechanisms include the combinatorial rearrangements of the variable (V), diverse (D), and joining (J) gene segments. The IMGT enables the alignment and assignment of these V-(D)-J genes on the basis of DNA sequences determined by NGS. The output files derived from the IMGT information system are used as input for further analyses implemented in the tool ImmunExplorer (IMEX)[1]. IMEX contains descriptive statistics, clonality and diversity algorithms, primer efficiency methods, various visualization options and comparison analysis. Moreover, IMEX is a freely available tool, currently available for Windows and with Linux/Unix support planned for future releases.

Algorithms have been implemented (integrated in IMEX) for calculating the clonality and diversity based on the most variable part in IG and TR [6], the CDR3 sequence (determined by the IMGT). For calculating the clonality, some additional explanation is provided: A *clonotype* is defined as a CDR3 sequence, which consists of amino acids. A *clone* represents a copy of a clonotype. To describe the term clonality we have developed an exact matching algorithm for determining all IG and TR clones and calculating the number of distinct clonotypes of a sample (see Fig. 2 or Fig. 1(b)).

The diversity of a sample is in this context calculated by randomly choosing n out of N CDR3 sequences and calculating the number of distinct clonotypes $c_{distinct}$ in these n sequences (see Fig. 3 or Fig. 1(c)). The number of distinct clonotypes is calculated for increasing numbers of n in a specific range. A mathematical model [7] has been determined to describe the development of the diversity, where the parameters of this model are optimized using evolution strategies [8]. This mathematical model takes into account that at a specific area a certain amount of distinct clonotypes is identified generated by read errors caused by NGS technologies. For every blood and tissue samples derived from an individual, clonal expansion (=clonality) and diversity measures are calculated using IMEX. The next two figures illustated clonality (Fig. 2) and diversity (Fig. 3) frequency plots obtained using IMEX. For each sample (blood and kidney) of each patient and proband those measures are calculated to determine features for the classification of the states of adaptive immune systems.

To compare and analyze data samples concerning clonality and diversity we have defined features that characterize the sequences of the distinct clonotypes and the diversity of IG and TR derived from blood and kidney tissue samples:

---

[1] http://bioinformatics.fh-hagenberg.at/immunexplorer/.

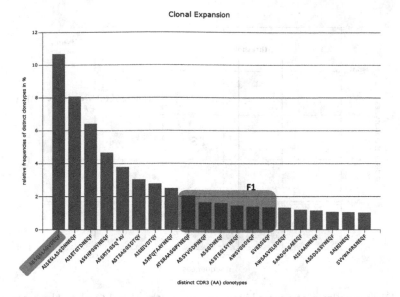

Fig. 2. In this particular example the top 20 CDR3 (AA) clonotypes are calculated of a kidney sample from a patient. The most frequent clonotype (ASSQSLAGVDEQF) can be found 8583 (10.65 %) times. The total number of identified clonotypes is 1939 and the total number of genes are 84145.

Clonality features [2]:

- ratio between the highest frequent clonotype and the average frequency of the top $[n_1;n_2]$ clonotypes (F1)
- mean and standard deviation of the frequencies of the top n distinct clonotypes (F2, F3)
- area under the clonality curve of the top n clonotypes (F4)
- number of the distinct clonotypes that cover t % of the area under the clonality curve (F5)

Diversity features [3]:

- area under the diversity (F6)
- area under the frequencies of the top n distinct clonotypes (F7)
- area under specific parts of the diversity (F8)
- relative frequencies of distinct clonotypes without read errors (F9)

3   Empirical Study

In the empirical section we evaluated data of 7 diseased patients and 4 healthy proband with respect to clonality and diversity of IG and TR on CDR3 (AA) sequence level. We had approximately 30 blood and kidney samples of those 11

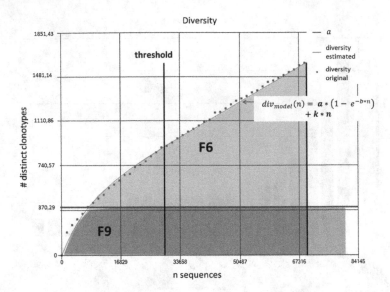

Fig. 3. Diversity plot of the same kidney sample as the clonality plot. The green points show the original calculated diversity by randomly choosing 1500 out of 84145 CDR3 sequences. The orange line shows the estimated diversity using the mathematical model and performing parameter optimization using an evolution strategy. Two diversity features (F6 and F9) are included in the diversity curve for better illustration (Color figure online).

patients/probands due to different primer settings: for IG, we used three different primer sets (which are redundant), while for TR, we used only two different primer sets (which are additive). The following machine learning methods were used: random forests (RF) [9], artificial neural networks (ANN) [10], and genetic programming (GP) [11] were performed using the framework HeuristicLab[2] [12] to predict the states of patient's adaptive immune systems. HeuristicLab is as well integrated in IMEX and will be available online soon. All approaches were performed using a five-fold crossvalidation and each fold were evaluated using ten repetitions and for each receptor repertoire separately. Three different analyses were performed:

– from each patient only blood samples,
– blood and kidney samples depending whether the patient is healthy or diseased have been considered. If the patient is healthy only blood samples were used, for diseased patients we have blood and kidney samples,
– and for healthy patients blood and for diseased patients the blood and kidney primer set feature values were averaged.

---

[2] http://dev.heuristiclab.com/.

Table 1. Accuracy, sensitivity and specificity for blood, blood and kidney, and blood and kidney tissue averaged analyzing the **TR repertoire** using all eleven patients. It is illustrated that the test accuracies for blood and kidney enable a distinction between healthy and ill patients due to kidney diseases. It can also be seen that the test sensitivity and specificity for the TR repertoire show better results using only blood but as well as the averaged primer sets of blood and kidney values.

	Blood	Blood and Kidney	Blood and Kidney Averaged
		Acccuracy	
RF	53.84	86.66	83.30
ANN	53.85	86.60	75.00
GP	53.84	83.33	81.25
		Sensitivity	
RF	0.45	0.79	0.60
ANN	0.67	0.79	0.79
GP	0.55	0.60	0.67
		Specificity	
RF	0.63	1.0	1.0
ANN	0.50	0.92	0.72
GP	0.75	0.88	0.79

Table 2. Accuracy, sensitivity and specificity for blood, blood and kidney, and blood and kidney tissue averaged analyzing the **IG or antibody repertoire** using all eleven patients. Interestingly, the test accuracies are much higher using only blood instead of blood and kidney compared to the TR repertoire analysis. Sensitivities and specificities show better results using blood or blood and kidney values averaged more promising results.

	Blood	Blood and Kidney	Blood and Kidney Averaged
		Acccuracy	
RF	84.27	97.45	95.22
ANN	92.67	94.87	88.88
GP	92.56	96.65	94.44
		Sensitivity	
RF	0.88	1.00	1.00
ANN	0.95	1.00	1.00
GP	1.00	0.88	1.00
		Specificity	
RF	0.75	0.94	0.88
ANN	0.89	0.91	0.77
GP	0.75	1.00	0.88

Tables 1 and 2 represent test accuracies, specificities and sensitivities of all analyses and for IG and TR repertoire, respectively. Specificity and sensitivity are defined as:

$$specificity = \frac{true_{negative}}{true_{negative} + false_{positive}} \tag{1}$$

$$sensitivity = \frac{true_{positive}}{true_{positive} + false_{negative}} \tag{2}$$

4   Conclusion and Outlook

A workflow for analyzing the health states of human adaptive immune systems using NGS generated IG and TR repertoire data, derived from blood and kidney tissue samples from healthy proband and diseased patients, which are pre-processed using the IMGT information system have been designed and developed. The outputs are used as input for our freely available and designed software IMEX for performing clonality, diversity, descriptive statistics, comparing and visualization analyses. Clonality and diversity features have been calculated and machine learning methods have been applied on IG and TR repertoire data. The first results of the here proposed workflow show promising results, including best classification accuracies up to 80 % by using information of blood and kidney samples from a patient. In future the workflow needs to be tested and evaluated with more collected data from patients and the application of this approach shall be extended to other immunological disease e.g., allergies or other tissue samples. In conclusion the medical goal would be to track the adaptive immune response to specific diseases which could lead to a better understanding of the evolution of the disease and also to a better focused treatment depending on each individual immune response.

References

1. Reis-Filho, J.S., others: Next-generation sequencing. 11 (2009) S12
2. Alamyar, E., Giudicelli, V., Li, S., Duroux, P., Lefranc, M.P.: IMGT/HighV-QUEST: the IMGT web portal for immunoglobulin (IG) or antibody and t cell receptor (TR) analysis from NGS high throughput and deep sequencing. Immunome research **8**, 26 (2012)
3. Li, S., Lefranc, M.P., Miles, J.J., Alamyar, E., Giudicelli, V., Duroux, P., Freeman, J.D., Corbin, V.D.A., Scheerlinck, J.P., Frohman, M.A., Cameron, P.U., Plebanski, M., Loveland, B., Burrows, S.R., Papenfuss, A.T., Gowans, E.J.: IMGT/HighV QUEST paradigm for t cell receptor IMGT clonotype diversity and next generation repertoire immunoprofiling. Nature Communications **4**, 2333 (2013)
4. Alamyar, E., Duroux, P., Lefranc, M.P., Giudicelli, V.: IMGT() tools for the nucleotide analysis of immunoglobulin (IG) and t cell receptor (TR) v-(d)-j repertoires, polymorphisms, and IG mutations: IMGT/v-QUEST and IMGT/HighV-QUEST for NGS. In: Christiansen, F.T., Tait, B.D. (eds.) Immunogenetics. Methods in Molecular Biology (Clifton, N.J.), vol. 882, pp. 569–604. Springer, Heidelberg (2012)

5. Giudicelli, V., Chaume, D., Lefranc, M.P.: IMGT/GENE-DB: a comprehensive database for human and mouse immunoglobulin and t cell receptor genes. Nucleic Acids Research (33) D256–D261

6. Diss, T.C., Liu, H.X., Du, M.Q., Isaacson, P.G.: Improvements to b cell clonality analysis using PCR amplification of immunoglobulin light chain genes. Molecular Pathology **55**, 98–101 (2002)

7. Schaller, S., Weinberger, J., Danzer, M., Gabriel, C., Oberbauer, R., Winkler, S.M.: Mathematical modeling of the diversity in human b- and t-cell receptors using machine learning. In: Proceedings of the 26th European Modeling and Simulation Symposium. (2014)

8. Schwefel, H.P.: Evolution strategies: A family of non-linear optimization techniques based on imitating some principles of organic evolution. Annals of Operations Research **1**, 165–167 (1984)

9. Breiman, L.: Random forests. Machine Learning **45**, 5–32 (2001)

10. Haykin, S.: Neural Networks. A Comprehensive Foundation. Prentice-Hall, Upper Saddle River NJ (1999)

11. Koza, J.R.: Genetic Programming: On the Programming of Computers by Means of Natural Selection. The MIT Press (1992)

12. Wagner, S., Kronberger, G., Beham, A., Kommenda, M., Scheibenpflug, A., Pitzer, E., Vonolfen, S., Kofler, M., Winkler, S., Dorfer, V., Affenzeller, M.: Architecture and Design of the HeuristicLab Optimization Environment. In: Klempous, R., Nikodem, J., Jacak, W., Chaczko, Z. (eds.) Advanced Methods and Applications in Computational Intelligence. TIEI, vol. 6, pp. 193–258. Springer, Heidelberg (2013)

Classifying Human Blood Samples Using Characteristics of Single Molecules and Cell Structures on Microscopy Images

Daniela Borgmann[1]([✉]), Sandra Mayr[2], Helene Polin[3], Lisa Obritzberger[1], Susanne Schaller[1], Viktoria Dorfer[1], Jaroslaw Jacak[2], and Stephan Winkler[1]

[1] Bioinformatics Research Group, University of Applied Sciences Upper Austria, Hagenberg Campus, Softwarepark 13, 4232 Hagenberg, Austria
{daniela.borgmann,lisa.obritzberger,susanne.schaller, viktoria.dorfer,stephan.winkler}@fh-hagenberg.at
[2] Department of Medical Engineering, University of Applied Sciences Upper Austria, Linz Campus, Garnisonstrasse 21, 4020 Linz, Austria
{sandra.mayr,jaroslaw.jacak}@fh-linz.at
[3] Red Cross Blood Transfusion Service of Upper Austria, Krankenhausstrasse 7, 4017 Linz, Austria
helene.polin@o.roteskreuz.at

Abstract. In this paper we present a method for the definition of characteristics of single molecules as well as of cell structures on fluorescence microscopy images for classifying human disease states. Fluorescence microscopy is one of the most emerging fields in modern laboratory diagnostics and is used in various research areas, for instance in studies of protein-protein interactions, analyses of cell interactions, diagnostics, or drug distribution studies. We have developed a new combinatory workflow comprising image processing and machine learning techniques to define characteristics out of given fluorescence microscopy images and to classify given images of blood samples according to their level of protein expression (high or low), i.e. according to their disease state. This combinatory workflow is not adapted to a specific illness but is usable for all kinds of diseases that can be characterized using single molecule fluorescence microscopy.

Keywords: Fluorescence microscopy · Bioinformatics · Image analysis · Machine learning

The work described in this paper has been done within the FFG FIT-IT project *NanoDetect: A Bioinformatics Image Processing Framework for Automated Analysis of Cellular Macro and Nano Structures (project number 835918)* sponsored by the Austrian Research Promotion Agency.

R. Moreno-Díaz et al. (Eds.): EUROCAST 2015, LNCS 9520, pp. 310–317, 2015.
DOI: 10.1007/978-3-319-27340-2_39

1   Introduction

Recent developments in the field of highly sensitive microscopy have changed the way of thinking of cell biologists and medical experts. Since it became more and more important to study the structural origin of cellular functions or cellular interactions, special focus is set on the required instruments, their improvements, and of course, also on the applied software frameworks and algorithms. A specific field of highly sensitive microscopy, namely fluorescence microscopy, already reached all-time sensitivity by resolving the signal of a single, fluorescence-labeled biomolecule within a living cell. The principles of this microscopy technique can be quickly explained in the following: Cell components on the cell surfaces are fluorescently labeled using antibodies targeting the specific cell component to be analysed; small molecules, named fluorophores, are attached to those antibodies and emit light signals upon light excitation. Those light signals are detected as fluorescence intensity values and can thereby help to localize and quantify the abundance and the expression level of proteins in cell membranes on acquired images. Exemplary generated fluorescence microscopy images and labeled blood cell compounds are depicted in Fig. 1.

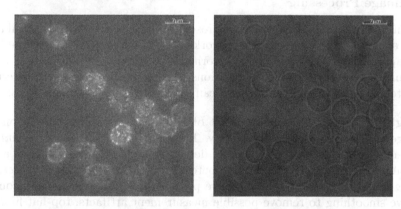

Fig. 1. Exemplary fluorescence microscopy image: (left) blood cell compounds labeled using primary antibodies, (right) corresponding white-light image showing red blood cells.

Using this information it is possible to study living specimens in their native environment in a non-invasive and non-destructive way [1]. Moreover, detected fluorescence intensities can provide further information about conformation and movement of cell compounds as well as about their surroundings, i.e. other molecules, viscosity, oxygen concentration, or pH characteristics [2].

Research topics addressed using by this techniques are spread among various application areas: For example, single molecule studies on protein expression and clustering within the cell membranes have been shown to play a significant role in signal transduction in T-cells, as stated in [3]. Further research was done concerning the statistical analysis of the relationship between fluorescence signal signatures and structures in microscopy images of brain tissue (further described

in [4]) or in the context of PNH research as the definition of motion characteristics of single molecules enables the classification of PNH affected cells [5].
We here present a combinatory workflow consisting of fluorescence microscopy,
image processing techniques, and machine learning approaches for the automatic
identification of characteristics at single molecule level, followed by a classification in critical and non-critical disease states based on human blood sample data,
which is highly important in the context of modern laboratory diagnostics, as
further medications or treatments are based on those classification results.

2   An Automatic Detection and Feature Extraction Algorithm for Classifying Human Disease States

The proposed workflow for the identification of single molecules and cell structures and the associated disease state classification can be divided into three
main steps: image processing, feature extraction, and machine learning. In the
following sections all workflow steps will be explained in detail.

2.1   Image Processing

As mentioned in Sect. 1 fluorescence microscopy images form the basis for all integrated analyses in the here presented workflow. Therefore, it is indispensable to
apply appropriate image processing algorithms to extract all information about
single molecule occurrences, their positions, their intensities, and cell structures
accurately. The image processing task can be divided into two main steps:

- **Single Molecule Detection:** First of all, single molecules present on the
  images have to be detected correctly. This step is crucial, as all results are
  dependent on the correct number of detected single molecules and on a low
  amount of false-positives. In this context, images are further preprocessed
  using a combination of various image processing techniques, namely conservative smoothing to remove possible measurement artifacts, top-hat filtering
  using a ring formed structure element to further emphasize small, bright, and
  round signals on the images, binary thresholding to extract all areas of interest, and region growing to separate all existing signals and to exclude regions
  smaller as a given size threshold. Each extracted region is finally analyzed and
  its maximum intensity value and its x-y coordinates in nano-scale precision
  are considered as a detected molecule. More detailed information about the
  used image processing techniques can be found in [6].
- **Cell Detection:** As information about the location and intensity of each
  molecule is not enough to state a hypothesis of a sample's disease state, it is
  indispensable to detect all cell structures on each white-light image accurately
  and to connect the single molecule information with the corresponding cell
  information. The cell detection is performed using a white-light image of each
  measured area of the sample, which shows all cell structures and its boundaries
  more clearly compared to the fluorescence signal images, as depicted in Fig. 1.
  First, a binary image showing all edges is created using a canny edge detector

[7] and thresholding operations. As a result, regions containing cells with a high probability are marked. In the second step, those highlighted regions are extracted and converted into a first guess cell using a convolution operation parameterized with a fixed ring-structured kernel. With the help of this kernel it is possible to find the approximate center of each cell, which is then further optimized using an evolution strategy. Finally, the resulting cells and their boundaries are further optimized using an active contour method that automatically adjusts all cell features for each cell independently. As a consequence, all cells, regardless of which shape or size, are detected automatically without any user interactions. Furthermore, the algorithm discards incomplete or malformed cells, which results in an even more robust statistic result.

2.2 Feature Extraction

Using the correct location of all cells, it is possible to assign all single molecules to the corresponding cell. Single molecules not belonging to any cell are discarded. Further statistical analyses on image level as well as on cell level are performed to extract features that shall help to differentiate between samples of critical and non-critical disease states. In detail the following features are extracted:

- **Average cell intensity:** average intensity of all detected molecules on cell level
- **Standard deviation of average cell intensities:** variability between average intensities of all detected molecules on cell level
- **Average molecule density:** average number of detected molecules per cell area
- **Average complete distance:** average distance between all molecules on cell level
- **Average neighboring distance:** average distance between all nearest neighboring molecules on cell level
- **Average intensity ratio:** average intensity ratio between cell and background areas

All features are further used as input for the here applied machine learning approaches as described in the next section.

2.3 Machine Learning

In the final step of our analysis workflow, various machine learning approaches are applied on extracted image features to assign the corresponding disease state to images of a given blood sample. For this purpose we applied the following machine learning approaches, using the implementation in HeuristicLab[1] [8]:

- **Random forest (RF):** RFs are ensembles of decision trees, each depending on randomly chosen samples and features. Every tree votes for a certain label and the final prediction for the given sample is the mode vote of all trees [9].

---

[1] http://dev.heuristiclab.com/.

- **Genetic Programming (GP):** Genetic programming is an algorithmic concept that works on populations of solution candidates and is based on selection (and offspring selection), recombination, and mutation [10, 11].
- **k-nearest neighbor algorithm (kNN):** k-nearest neighbor approaches work without creating and using any explicit model; a sample is classified using k training samples showing the smallest distance from the sample [12].
- **Artificial neural network (ANN):** Artificial neural networks are inspired by the structure of biological neural networks and have been frequently used in the context of pattern recognition and image analysis [13].

All analysed samples consist of multiple imaged areas (that are used in the classification tasks independently) to cover the possible heterogeneity of human blood samples; as a consequence, we introduce a majority voting step to be able to provide a clear statement about the classified disease state of each sample. This majority vote is performed in the following manner:

Whether a sample is classified as class 1 or class 0 is decided using the number of images ($im(sample) : imageset$) that are classified as class 1. If the number of images that are classified as class 1 is higher or equal than a declared threshold θ of the total number of images, the sample is classified as class 1; if the number is lower than θ the sample is classified as class 0.

$$classification(sample) = \begin{cases} 0 & \frac{|im(sample)_i \, : \, class(im(sample)_i)=1|}{|im(sample)|} < \theta \\ 1 & else \end{cases} \qquad (1)$$

The used threshold value θ for the majority voting can be set for each classification task independently; disease states that comprise highly significant differences may need a higher θ, datasets comprising low or subtle differences should be analysed using a lower θ.

3 Empirical Study: Classifying Blood Samples of Patients at Critical and Non-Critical Disease States

In order to prove the functionality and reliability of the here presented methods, we tested our workflow using an exemplary dataset composed of human blood samples of critical and non-critical patients. The dataset consists of 55 samples, comprising 8 critical and 47 non-critical blood samples; in total approximately 800 acquired images are analysed and involved in the classification tasks. All preliminary results of all image processing algorithms were reviewed and manually corrected to eliminate the possibility of biased data. In Fig. 2 we exemplarily show processed images and the detected single molecules as well as detected cell structures.

3.1 Majority Vote Thresholding

As mentioned in Sect. 2.3 the determination of the appropriate threshold θ used for the majority vote process is of great significance, as this parameter determines

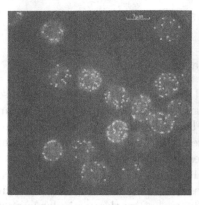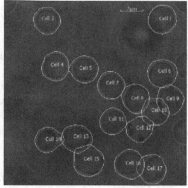

Fig. 2. Exemplary image processing result: (left) detected single molecules, (right) detected cell structures.

the stringency of the performed classification. In Table 1 the achieved accuracies using different values for θ are listed. It can be seen that a constant decrease of θ leads to a steady increase with regard to classification sensitivities and accuracies. As a result, an optimal value θ of 5 % was determined for the here used dataset. It can therefore be concluded, that the here used dataset is composed of classes characterized through minor differences to each other that can be balanced and classified correctly by using a low θ value.

Table 1. Summary of tested θ values used for majority voting: Each algorithm was repeated 10 times; all sensitivity and accuracy values represent majority vote test results.

		θ						
		50 %	33 %	25 %	20 %	15 %	10 %	5 %
RF	Sensitivity	95.75 %	100.00 %	100.00 %	100.00 %	100.00 %	100.00 %	100.00 %
	Accuracy	88.91 %	99.82 %	98.55 %	98.91 %	99.82 %	99.82 %	100.00 %
GP	Sensitivity	52.50 %	78.75 %	86.25 %	91.25 %	92.50 %	100.00 %	100.00 %
	Accuracy	89.45 %	94.73 %	97.82 %	98.73 %	98.91 %	100.00 %	100.00 %
kNN	Sensitivity	50.00 %	62.50 %	62.50 %	100.00 %	100.00 %	100.00 %	100.00 %
	Accuracy	90.91 %	92.73 %	94.55 %	100.00 %	100.00 %	100.00 %	100.00 %
ANN	Sensitivity	50.00 %	75.00 %	76.25 %	87.50 %	100.00 %	100.00 %	100.00 %
	Accuracy	89.09 %	94.55 %	96.55 %	98.18 %	100.00 %	100.00 %	100.00 %

3.2   Classification Results

All classification algorithms were repeated 10 times using 10-fold cross validation. The used machine learning algorithms were applied using the implementation in HeuristicLab and parameterized as follows:

- **Random forests**: number of trees = 50
- **Genetic programming**: generations = 1000, population size = 100
- **k-nearest neighbor algorithm**: k = 3
- **Artificial neural network**: hidden layers = 1

Altogether six features, as described previously in Sect. 2.2, were used as input for machine learning; the target variable was defined as 1 (critical sample) and 0 (non-critical sample). In Table 1 the achieved test classification results are also depicted in detail: It can be seen that all applied machine learning approaches yielded at highly satisfying results, with a constant sensitivity value of 100 % and classification accuracies of 100 % for a θ value of 5 %.

Summed up, all critical blood samples were classified correctly without any false-negative predictions. This fact highly emphasizes the particular importance of our workflow and the robustness of the defined and extracted characteristics regarding single molecules and cell structures, as in modern diagnostics sensitive and reliable results are indispensable.

4   Conclusion and Outlook

In this paper we presented an innovative and highly promising combinatory approach for the definition of characteristics of single molecules and cell structures on fluorescence microscopy images. This new approach combines three different application areas, namely fluorescence microscopy, image processing techniques, and machine learning to enable a new analysis possibility for human disease states based on imaged human blood samples. Single molecules and cell structures were identified using various image processing techniques, namely smoothing, thresholding, edge detection, active contour methods, and convolution. All classification tasks were performed using multiple machine learning approaches to ensure and validate the quality of the here presented results.

In the empirical part of our work, we tested the proposed workflow by using critical and non-critical human blood samples. All image processing techniques performed well and could be applied on various diverse images without any configuration changes. All classification results were highly satisfying, as accuracies of 100 % and a constant sensitivity value of 100 % were achieved.

Those high sensitivity values and the high robustness of the here presented methods are of great significance regarding modern laboratory diagnostic routines, as reliable and sensitive results are extremely important key factors for diagnostics, further treatments, or medication settings.

References

1. Stephens, D., Allan, V.: Light microscopy techniques for live cell imaging. Science **300**, 82–86 (2003)
2. Lakowicz, J.: Principles of Fluorescence Spectroscopy. Springer, New York (2006)

3. Douglass, A.D., Vale, R.D.: Single-molecule microscopy reveals plasma membrane microdomains created by protein-protein networks that exclude or trap signaling molecules in T Cells. Cell **121**, 937–950 (2005)
4. Schaller, S., Jacak, J., Silye, R., Winkler, S.M.: Statistical analysis of the relationship between spots and structures in microscopy images. In: Moreno-Díaz, R., Pichler, F., Quesada-Arencibia, A. (eds.) EUROCAST 2013. LNCS, vol. 8111, pp. 211–218. Springer, Heidelberg (2013)
5. Schaller, S., Jacak, J., Gschwandtner, D., Bettelheim, P., Winkler, S.: Identification of PNH affected cells by classifying motion characteristics of single molecules. In: Proceedings of the International Workshop on Innovative Simulation for Health Care (IWISH), Athen, Greece (2013)
6. Burger, W., Burge, M.J.: Principles of Digital Image Processing: Fundamental Techniques. Springer, London (2011)
7. Canny, J.: A computational approach to edge detection. IEEE Trans. Pattern Anal. Mach. Intell. **8**, 679–698 (1986)
8. Wagner, S., Kronberger, G., Beham, A., Kommenda, M., Scheibenpflug, A., Pitzer, E., Vonolfen, S., Kofler, M., Winkler, S., Dorfer, V., Affenzeller, M.: Architecture and design of the HeuristicLab optimization environment. In: Klempous, R., Nikodem, J., Jacak, W., Chaczko, Z. (eds.) Advanced Methods and Applications in Computational Intelligence. TIEI, vol. 6, pp. 197–261. Springer, Heidelberg (2013)
9. Breiman, L.: Random forests. Mach. Learn. **45**, 5–32 (2001)
10. Koza, J.R.: Genetic Programming: On the Programming of Computers by Means of Natural Selection. The MIT Press, Cambridge (1992)
11. Affenzeller, M., Winkler, S., Wagner, S., Beham, A.: Genetic Algorithms and Genetic Programming - Modern Concepts and Practical Applications. Chapman & Hall/CRC, London (2009)
12. Dasarathy, B.: Nearest Neighbor (NN) Norms: NN Pattern Classification Techniques. IEEE Computer Society Press, Silver Spring (1991)
13. Haykin, S.: Neural Networks. A Comprehensive Foundation. Prentice-Hall, Upper Saddle River (1999)

Prediction of Stem Cell Differentiation in Human Amniotic Membrane Images Using Machine Learning

Lisa Obritzberger[1]([✉]), Daniela Borgmann[1], Susanne Schaller[1],
Viktoria Dorfer[1], Andrea Lindenmair[2,3], Susanne Wolbank[2,3],
Simone Hennerbichler[4], Heinz Redl[2,3], and Stephan Winkler[1]

[1] Bioinformatics Research Group, University of Applied Sciences Upper Austria,
Softwarepark 13, 4232 Hagenberg, Austria
{lisa.obritzberger,daniela.borgmann,susanne.schaller,viktoria.dorfer,
stephan.winkler}@fh-hagenberg.at
[2] Ludwig Boltzmann Institute for Experimental and Clinical Traumatology,
AUVA Research Center, Donaueschingenstraße 13, 1200 Vienna, Austria
{andrea.lindenmair,susanne.wolbank,heinz.redl}@trauma.lbg.ac.at
[3] Trauma Care Consult, Traumatologische Forschung Gemeinnützige GmbH,
Gonzagagasse 11/25, 1010 Vienna, Austria
office@traumacareconsult.com
[4] Red Cross Blood Transfusion Service for Upper Austria, Austrian Cluster
for Tissue Regeneration, Krankenhausstraße 9, 4020 Linz, Austria
simone.hennerbichler@o.roteskreuz.at

Abstract. It has been shown that it is possible to differentiate viable amniotic membrane towards osteogenic lineage, i.e. bony tissue. This process of mineralization may take several weeks and can show different manifestations per sample. The tissue can only be used, when the mineralization process is advanced in a certain degree. Therefore, a forecast of the development of mineralization would be helpful to save time and resources. This paper shows how a prediction on the development of mineralization can be made by using several image processing techniques, machine learning methods, and hybrid ensembles of machine learning algorithms.

Keywords: Osteogenic tissue engineering · Hybride machine learning ensembles · Image processing

1 Research Goal

The human amniotic membrane is the thin, highly flexible innermost of the fetal membranes and a part of the placenta. For regenerative medicine, the membrane has shown great potential as it is bacteriostatic, reduces pain, suppresses

The work described in this paper was done within the FIT-IT project number 835918 *NanoDetect* sponsored by the Austrian Research Promotion Agency (FFG).

© Springer International Publishing Switzerland 2015
R. Moreno-Díaz et al. (Eds.): EUROCAST 2015, LNCS 9520, pp. 318–325, 2015.
DOI: 10.1007/978-3-319-27340-2_40

inflammation, inhibits scarring, and promotes wound healing [1,2] and epithelialization [3].

In addition, the amniotic membrane is used for tissue engineering, as it is possible to differentiate viable amniotic membrane towards osteogenic tissue (i.e., bone cells). [4] During this process amniotic cells mineralize to osteogenic tissue, which can be used for medical purposes. A tissue can only be used for medical purposes if the degree of its mineralization is high. Unfortunately, the mineralization is not distributed homogeneously among the tissue but shows patches of positive areas which is depicted in Fig. 1.

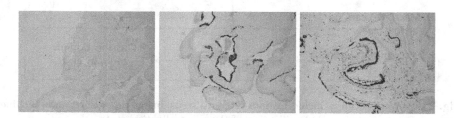

Fig. 1. Differentiation of amniotic membrane to bone tissue over time (day 0, 14 and 28); dark areas represent the mineralization. (Figure taken from [4])

As the mineralization process takes several weeks in the laboratory, it would be of great advantage to be able to predict the degree of mineralization already after some days. It is assumed that the positioning of the cell nuclei inside of the tissue supplies information about the progress of mineralization after a few days. In order to verify this theory we have developed an algorithm that is able to automatically process the images of the tissues and can be used to predict the degree of mineralization during the first days using image processing and machine learning techniques.

2   Methods

The analysis techniques performed to classify the mineralization degree can be divided into three major steps shown in Fig. 2.

Microscopy images from differentiated amnion membranes were taken weekly to document the tissues development.

In order to identify the structures of the tissue we use image processing techniques that include dilation, erosion, and edge detection. Reference [5] Further image processing is needed to identify the positions of the cell nuclei, which are determined through thresholding. The generated images are used to calculate several features which are used to train the following machine learning techniques: genetic programming, random forests, support vector machines, artificial neural networks, and linear regression. These algorithms shall help to predict the progression of mineralization of amnion membrane.

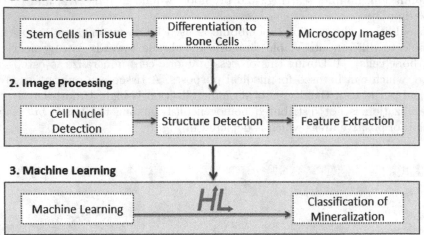

Fig. 2. Detailed workflow including data retrieval steps, image processing, and machine learning for the automated classification of the mineralization state.

2.1 Image Processing

To extract features used as input for machine learning methods, several image processing steps have been performed. These steps are intended to detect the structure in the image and identify all cell nuclei that are contained in the structure. All image processing steps used in this approach will be explained in this section.

Tissue Structure Identification: All tissue images showed heterogenous intensity values, therefore we split the images into several parts and calculated an individual threshold for each part. As threshold we used the average of the intensities in each image part. All image parts were merged back together which can be seen in Fig. 3(a). Further image processing techniques were applied that including sobel edge detection, dilatation, erosion and thresholding to identify pixels belonging to the structure. [5]

To identify all pixels that form the structure a floodfill algorithm was performed to detect continuous areas. To detect those areas that belong to the tissue, regions with a minimum number of pixels that exceed a certain threshold were selected as part of the tissue. In order to fill remaining gaps in the structure, dilatation and erosion was applied which lead to results shown in Fig. 3(b).

Cell Nuclei Detection: Identifying the location of cell nuclei was achieved quite easily as the cell nuclei have different intensity values as the structure and the background of the image. To emphasize the cell nuclei we used sobel edge detection and subsequently, a thresholding operation, where pixels that exceed

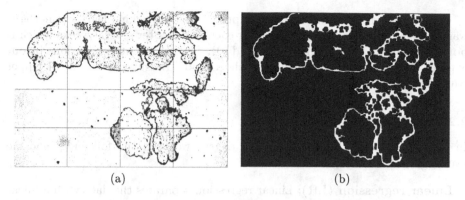

(a)   (b)

Fig. 3. (a): Merged image after applying thresholding on each image part. (b): The final identified structure used as input for machine learning methods.

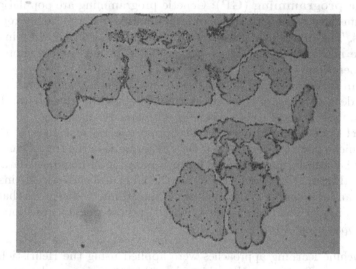

Fig. 4. Cell nuclei identified using thresholding operations.

the defined threshold value are identified as part of the image and are marked as green dots as demonstrated in Fig. 4.

Feature Extraction: The preprocessed images were further used to extract the following features:

- number of epithelial cells (cells in the outer area of the tissue)
- number of mesenchymal cells (cells in the inner area of the tissue)
- average distance between cells and outer surface of the tissue
- median distance between cells and outer surface of the tissue
- number of distances in different distance intervals ($[0px - 5px[$, $[5px - 10px[$, $[10px - 15px[$, $[15px - 20px[$, $> 20px$)

The target variable that had to be predicted by machine learning methods was the quality of the mineralization for each image after several weeks which is binary classified in either good (1) or bad (0). The classification was done by our experts of Trauma Care Consult and the Blood Transfusion Service of Upper Austria.

2.2   Machine Learning Methods

In order to predict the mineralization degree we used the following machine learning methods:

- **Linear regression (LR):** Linear regression separates the data with a linear function. It is hereby attempted to minimize the distances between a straight line and the data points [6].
- **Genetic programming (GP):** Genetic programming are population based algorithms that work with a pool of individuals which are usually represented by trees. The individuals are selected, recombined, and mutated in order to generate new individuals. Those with the best fitness are promoted to the next generation [7].
- **Random forests (RF):** Random forests use a combination of multiple uncorrelated decision trees of those every tree classifies the given data. The class with the most votes is chosen as the result class [8].
- **Support vector machines (SVM):** Support vector machines use the kernel trick, which allows the algorithm to fit a hyperplane in the transformed feature space. The transformation allows linear separation of nonlinear data [9].
- **Artificial neural networks (NN):** Artificial neural networks are inspired by the human brain and present a network of interconnected neurons that process the given input. The neurons are weighted and the weights are adopted using back propagation [10].

All machine learning approaches were applied using the HeuristicLab[1] [11] implementation. To improve the achieved machine learning results, we additionally used a hybrid ensemble of machine learning algorithms that combined the results of the individually applied methods as described in 3.1.

3   Results

3.1   Ensemble Modeling Approach

Each of the above described machine learning techniques were applied on image parts to train a model. These trained models were used for a hybrid ensemble approach where each model classifies the image.

The predictions of the different models are used to estimate the class of an image via majority voting. [12] This allows an estimation of the confidence calculated by the agreement of the classifications which is demonstrated in Table 1.

---

[1] HeuristicLab: http://dev.heuristiclab.com/.

Table 1. Combining several machine learning methods (GP, RF, ANN, SVM, LR) allows a majority vote that selects the class with the majority of the votes as the final class for the image.

ID	GP	RF	ANN	SVM	LR	Final classification	Confidence
1	0	0	0	1	0	0	80 %
2	1	1	1	1	1	1	100 %
3	1	0	1	0	0	0	60 %
4	0	0	0	1	0	0	80 %
5	0	0	0	0	0	0	100 %

3.2   Results for Image Parts

Each image is split into 15×15 parts, as explained in [13] and the model majority vote is applied for each of the image parts. Based on the intermediate results for each image part a calculation is made determining the number of votes for each class. The class with the majority of the votes was chosen as the final class for a whole image.

We used 41 images for the classification process and split them into parts. As we only used relevant parts that contain amniotic structure and cells we received 2032 that could be used for classification. Using the hybrid ensemble approach we achieved 70.08 % correctly classified image parts, which is shown in Table 2.

3.3   Results for Merged Image Parts

To identify the class of one merged image the majority of the votes for a class is calculated and determined as the final class of the merged image.

The hybrid ensemble approach of the image parts allowed to include only those parts of the images in the vote for the final classification that exceed a minimum confidence value. This should increase the accuracy of the classification of the merged images.

Only those image parts where the hybrid ensemble approach got a confidence of at least 80 % were included in the final classification. Therefore, it was possible that only a few image parts were allowed to vote and it could occur that no image part was included in the final classification process. This decreases the coverage

Table 2. The confusion matrix shows how many image parts were estimated correctly; using a confidence of 60 % a coverage of 100 % of all image parts could be achieved.

Estimated target	0	1	
0	721	283	
1	325	703	
			1424 (70.08 %)

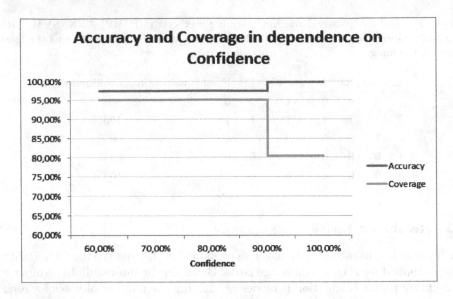

Fig. 5. Higher confidence values lead to an improvement of the accuracy and to a lower coverage rate.

of the merged images that are classified: Using a confidence value of at least 80 % resulted in a coverage of 95.12 % with 97.44 % correctly classified images. With minimum confidence of 90 % all images were classified correctly and a coverage of 80.49 % could be achieved which is depicted in 5.

4   Conclusion

The mineralization process of amniotic membrane towards bone tissue takes several weeks in the laboratory and can only be used for medical treatments if the degree of mineralization has advanced sufficiently. In this paper we showed that it is possible to predict the degree of mineralization already after some days: The classification could predict the mineralization degree with an accuracy of 97.44 %. By increasing the confidence rate to 90 % it was even possible to classify all images correctly. This shows that it is possible to predict the degree of mineralization already after several days which is of great advantage for reasearchers as it saves a lot of time and resources.

References

1. Faulk, W., Matthews, R., Stevens, P., Bennett, J., Burgos, H., Hsi, B.: Human amnion as an adjunct in wound healing. Lancet **1**, 1156–1158 (1980)
2. Gruss, J., Jirsch, D.: Human amniotic membrane: a versatile wound dressing. Can. Med. Assoc. J. **118**, 1237–1246 (1978)
3. Ganatra, M.: Amniotic membrane in surgery. J. Pak. Med. Assoc. **53**, 29–32 (2003)

4. Lindenmair, A., Wolbank, S., Stadler, G., Meinl, A., Peterbauer-Scherb, A., Eibl, J., Polin, H., Gabriel, C., van Griensven, M., Redl, H.: Osteogenic differentiation of intact human amniotic membrane. Biomaterials **31**, 8659–8665 (2010)
5. Burger, W., Burge, M.: Principles of Digital Image Processing: Fundamental Techniques. Springer, London (2011)
6. Ljung, L.: System Identification - Theory For the User, 2nd edn. PTR Prentice-Hall, Upper Saddle River, NJ (1999)
7. Koza, J.R.: Genetic Programming: On the Programming of Computers by Means of Natural Selection. The MIT Press, Cambridge (1992)
8. Breiman, L.: Random forests. Mach. Learn. **45**, 5–32 (2001)
9. Vapnik, V.: Statistical Learning Theory. Wiley, New York (1998)
10. Haykin, S.: Neural Networks. A Comprehensive Foundation. PTR Prentice-Hall, Upper Saddle River, NJ (1999)
11. Wagner, S., Kronberger, G., Beham, A., Kommenda, M., Scheibenpflug, A., Pitzer, E., Vonolfen, S., Kofler, M., Winkler, S., Dorfer, V., Affenzeller, M.: Architecture and design of the HeuristicLab optimization environment. In: Klempous, R., Nikodem, J., Jacak, W., Chaczko, Z. (eds.) Advanced Methods and Applications in Computational Intelligence. TIEI, vol. 6, pp. 193–258. Springer, Heidelberg (2013)
12. Winkler, S., Schaller, S., Dorfer, V., Affenzeller, M., Petz, G., Karpowicz, M.: Data-based prediction of sentiments using heterogeneous model ensembles. Soft Comput. **18**, 1–12 (2014)
13. Obritzberger, L., Borgmann, D., Schaller, S., Dorfer, V., Lindenmair, A., Wolbank, S., Redl, H., Winkler, S.: Prediction of mineralization degree in human amniotic membrane using image processing techniques and machine learning. To be published in Proceedings of the XI Metaheuristics International Conference (MIC2015) (2014)

Dynamics of Predictability and Variable Influences Identified in Financial Data Using Sliding Window Machine Learning

Stephan M. Winkler[1,3]([✉]), Gabriel Kronberger[1], Michael Kommenda[1,3],
Stefan Fink[2], and Michael Affenzeller[1,3]

[1] Hagenberg Campus Heuristic and Evolutionary Algorithms Laboratory,
University of Applied Sciences Upper Austria,
Softwarepark 11, 4232 Hagenberg, Austria
{stephan.winkler,gabriel.kronberger,michael.kommenda,
michael.affenzeller}@fh-hagenberg.at
[2] Department of Economics, Johannes Kepler University Linz,
Altenberger Straße 69, 4040 Linz, Austria
stefan.fink@jku.at
[3] Institute for Formal Models and Verification, Johannes Kepler University Linz,
Altenberger Straße 69, 4040 Linz, Austria

Abstract. In this paper we analyze the dynamics of the predictability and variable interactions in financial data of the years 2007–2014. Using a sliding window approach, we have generated mathematical prediction models for various financial parameters using other available parameters in this data set. For each variable we identify the relevance of other variables with respect to prediction modeling. By applying sliding window machine learning we observe that changes of the predictability of financial variables as well as of influence factors can be identified by comparing modeling results generated for different periods of the last 8 years. We see changes of relationships and the predictability of financial variables over the last years, which corresponds to the fact that relationships and dynamics in the financial sector have changed significantly over the last decade. Still, our results show that the predictability has not decreased for all financial variables, indeed in numerous cases the prediction quality has even improved.

1 Research Goal

The goal of the research presented in this paper is to describe the predictability and impact factors in financial data of the years 2007–2014. Using a sliding window approach, we have generated prediction models for various financial parameters using other available parameters in this data set. For each variable we identify in how far other features are relevant for modeling it; the relevance of a variable can in this context be defined via the decrease in modeling quality after removing it from the data set.

© Springer International Publishing Switzerland 2015
R. Moreno-Díaz et al. (Eds.): EUROCAST 2015, LNCS 9520, pp. 326–333, 2015.
DOI: 10.1007/978-3-319-27340-2_41

Keeping in mind that relationships and dynamics in the financial sector have changed significantly over the last decade, we expect to see changes of relationships and the predictability of financial variables. By applying sliding window machine learning we see that changes of the relationships as well as of the predictability of financial variables can be identified by comparing modeling results generated for different periods of the last 8 years.

Figure 1 schematically shows this approach:

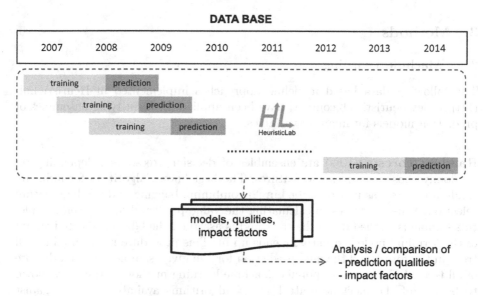

Fig. 1. Data based identification of regression models and variable impacts in financial data using sliding window machine learning.

2   Data and Data Preprocessing

For the here presented empirical tests we have used various financial variables measured daily between April 2007 and August 2014. The here used data base includes 24 variables, namely currency exchange rates, several stock indices, nominal yields of treasury bonds, Euribor and Libor, CDS spreads, gold price, key interest rates, and financial indices.

For each variable x we train classifiers for the following targets:

- $c(x_{d+1})$: Trend (positive, neutral, or negative) for x at day $d + 1$ relative to the value of x at day d
- $c(x_{d+5})$: Trend (positive, neutral, or negative) for x at day $d + 5$ relative to the value of x at day d
- $c(x_{d+10})$: Trend (positive, neutral, or negative) for x at day $d + 10$ relative to the value of x at day d

A trend is classified positive if the difference is at least $+1\%$ and negative if the difference is at least -1%.

For each variable x we additionally calculate the following features that are used as input for training classifiers:

- x_{d-1}: x at day $d-1$ relative to the value of x at day d
- x_{d-5}: x at day $d-5$ relative to the value of x at day d
- x_{d-10}: x at day $d-10$ relative to the value of x at day d

3   Methods

3.1   Machine Learning

The following data based modeling approaches implemented in HeuristicLab (http://dev.heuristiclab.com) [1] have been applied for identifying ensembles of prediction models for financial variables:

Random Forests (RFs) are ensembles of decision trees, each depending on randomly chosen samples and features. The best known algorithm for inducing random forests was first described in [2] combining bagging and random feature selection. When it comes to calculating the value predicted for a given sample, this sample is pushed down the trees and is assigned the label (predicted value) of the terminal node it eventually ends up in. This procedure is executed for all trees in the forest and the final prediction for the given sample is the mode vote of all trees. RFs are a very popular machine learning method as they are known to be one of the most accurate learning algorithms available, robust against overfitting, and a very efficient learning method.

Genetic Programming: We have also applied a symbolic regression algorithm based on genetic programming (GP) [3] using a structure identification framework described in [4] and [5], in combination with strict offspring selection; this GP approach has been implemented in HeuristicLab [6]. We have used the following parameter settings for our GP test series: The mutation rate was set to 20%, a combination of random and roulette parent selection was applied as well as strict offspring selection [5] (OS) with success ratio as well as comparison factor set to 1.0. The functions set described in [4] (including arithmetic as well as logical ones) was used for building composite function expressions.

In addition to splitting the given data into training and test data, the GP based training algorithm implemented in HeuristicLab has been designed in such a way that a part of the given training data is not used for training models and serves as validation set; in the end, when it comes to returning classifiers, the algorithm returns those models that perform best on validation data. This approach has been chosen because it is assumed to help to cope with over-fitting; it is also applied in other GP based machine learning algorithms as for example described in [7].

3.2   Accuracy and Confidence of Model Ensembles

All so created models are then applied on test partitions as indicated in Fig. 1; the final classification for each sample is calculated in the following way (as described in detail in ([8]):

For each sample s various models are trained; models are here referred to as m_i where i represents the current model index. Subsequently, a voting over all models for each sample s is performed:

$$vote(c, s, m) = |m_i : m_i(s) = c| \tag{1}$$

where c represents an arbitrary, but fix class c. The final classification fc for a sample s is calculated by using a majority voting of votes $vote(c, s, m)$. Finally, we define the confidence of classification c for a sample s on the basis of a set of models m:

$$fc(s, m) = \operatorname*{argmax}_{c}(vote(c, s, m)) \tag{2}$$

$$conf(c, s, m) = \frac{|m_i : m_i(s) = c|}{|m|} \tag{3}$$

As we are here facing ternary classification tasks, the classification confidence for any final classification fc (that is a majority vote winner and thus must have more than $1/3$ of the votes) will always be in the interval $[1/3, 1]$.

In the empirical tests documented in the following sections we use a confidence threshold $\theta \in [0 \ldots 1]$. If the confidence for a sample's classification is smaller than this threshold, then there is no estimation statement for this sample. As a consequence, the ratio of samples for which a classification statement is given will be below 100%; we expect this samples coverage ratio to decrease for increasing values of θ.

3.3   Calculation of the Relevance of Variables

There are several methods for calculating the relevance of variables as described, for instance, in [9], [10], and [11]. The following approach is used in the context of this research work: We estimate the relevance of variables with respect to algorithm performance by removing them from the list of available inputs and repeating the modeling process. We use $r(Data_v)$ as the available data collection with variable v replaced or removed for calculating the relevance of variable v; we define the relevance of variable v with respect to a modeling method mm, a replacement method r and a fitness function ff as

$$impact_{alg}(v, mm) = 1 - \frac{ff(eval(mm, r(Data_v)))}{ff(eval(mm, Data))}. \tag{4}$$

As fitness function we calculate the accuracy of prediction models. For example, this means the following: If using the full data base leads to models that explain validation samples with 90% accuracy and models not using a variable y show 80% accuracy, then the impact of y is $1 - 0.8/0.9 = 0.111 = 11.1\%$.

4 Modeling Results

Using sliding window modeling with RFs and GP as described in Sects. 1 and 3 we trained sets of models for varying training and test data partitions. Each modeling method was executed with varying configurations, and for each data partition the 10 best models (with respect to performance on training data) were selected and applied on test data. The results achieved using this approach are summarized in this section.

4.1 Dynamics of Accuracies and Classification Confidence over Time

This sliding window modeling approach was executed for each target variable and partitions of training and test samples as given in Table 1. This table shows exemplary test results for prediction models for the next day's trend of the exchange rate of US dollar and Euro. As we see, in most cases the prediction accuracy rises by increasing the confidence threshold θ, which on the other hand also decreases the samples coverage. Furthermore, the accuracies and coverages vary for the analyzed partitions.

This analysis was done for all available target variables, and comparing results for the first partition (2009/2010) with those calculated for the last partition (2013/2014) and $\theta = 0$ we observe the following results:

- For 42 % of the target variables, the accuracy of the next day's trend increased by at least 10 %, while it decreased by at least 10 % for 38 % of the variables.
- For 45 % of the target variables, the accuracy of the next week's trend increased by at least 10 %, while it decreased by at least 10 % for 32 % of the variables.
- For 42 % of the target variables, the accuracy of the next two weeks's trend increased by at least 10 %, while it decreased by at least 10 % for 33 % of the variables.

These results are graphically displayed in Fig. 3 where we show the relative progress of classification accuracies (with $\theta = 0$) as well as of classification confidences for all analyzed test partitions.

4.2 Dynamics of Variable Impacts over Time

For each target variable we also calculated impact factors of all input variables with respect to prediction modeling with one day, 5 days, and 10 days offset. Figure 2 graphically shows impact factors for selected target values calculated using Formula 4 evaluated on test samples. We see that the impact of variables varies significantly; for 38 % of the analyzed potential input variables the impact changed by at least 10 % over the analyzed period, and for 11 % it changed by at least 20 %. Interestingly, there are phases in which no variables show significant impact, which can be seen as white horizontal lines.

Table 1. Accuracy and coverage of ensemble models predicting the trend of the exchange rate between US dollar and Euro for varying confidence thresholds (θ).

Training samples	Test samples	Accuracy						
		$\theta = 0$	$\theta = 0.5$	$\theta = 0.6$	$\theta = 0.7$	$\theta = 0.8$	$\theta = 0.9$	$\theta = 1.0$
0–400	400–500	32 %	33 %	33 %	42 %	35 %	36 %	36 %
100–500	500–600	47 %	44 %	48 %	49 %	54 %	50 %	50 %
200–600	600–700	36 %	38 %	39 %	41 %	42 %	32 %	32 %
300–700	700–800	35 %	33 %	31 %	40 %	41 %	42 %	42 %
400–800	800–900	28 %	28 %	27 %	29 %	37 %	54 %	54 %
500–900	900–1000	37 %	36 %	34 %	28 %	30 %	30 %	30 %
600–1000	1000–1100	38 %	40 %	41 %	41 %	44 %	44 %	44 %
700–1100	1100–1200	39 %	42 %	48 %	44 %	50 %	67 %	67 %
800–1200	1200–1300	61 %	62 %	61 %	60 %	56 %	58 %	58 %
Training samples	Test samples	Coverage						
		$\theta = 0$	$\theta = 0.5$	$\theta = 0.6$	$\theta = 0.7$	$\theta = 0.8$	$\theta = 0.9$	$\theta = 1.0$
0–400	400–500	100 %	85 %	58 %	33 %	23 %	11 %	11 %
100–500	500–600	100 %	90 %	71 %	51 %	24 %	8 %	8 %
200–600	600–700	100 %	90 %	66 %	51 %	43 %	25 %	25 %
300–700	700–800	100 %	88 %	64 %	42 %	29 %	12 %	12 %
400–800	800–900	100 %	89 %	73 %	58 %	35 %	13 %	13 %
500–900	900–1000	100 %	76 %	47 %	32 %	20 %	10 %	10 %
600–1000	1000–1100	100 %	92 %	73 %	46 %	27 %	9 %	9 %
700–1100	1100–1200	100 %	89 %	60 %	41 %	18 %	6 %	6 %
800–1200	1200–1300	100 %	99 %	95 %	87 %	72 %	50 %	50 %

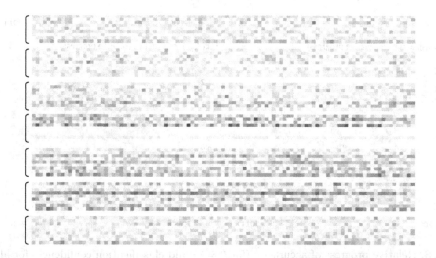

Fig. 2. Graphical representation of impacts of variables for 7 randomly chosen target variables. For each target variable, 9 training and test data partitions were used (as given in Table 1) and each horizontal row shows graphical representations of the impacts calculated on the respective test data; light squares represent low impacts, dark squares high impacts.

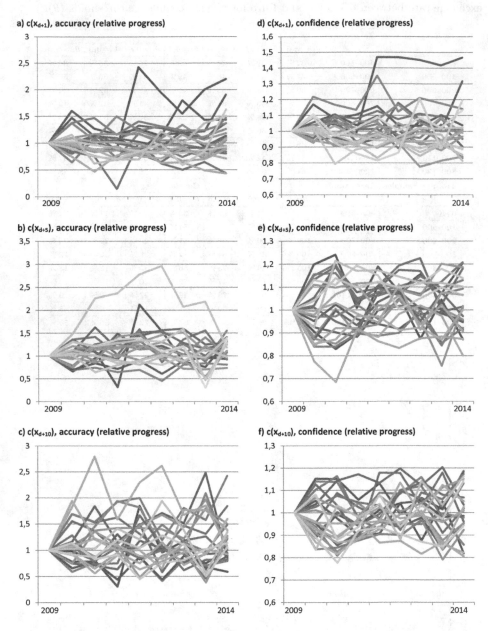

Fig. 3. Relative progress of accuracies (for $\theta = 0$) and classification confidences for all target variables and 9 partitions of training and test data (as given in Table 1). For each target variable and partition we give classification accuracy and confidence relative to the respective values calculated for the first partition.

5   Conclusion

We have seen that the identification of prediction model ensembles for financial values reveals dynamics and changes over time of classification accuracies and confidences. Still, by far not for all financial indicators the predictability has decreased over the last years – indeed, classification accuracy and also classification confidence have increased for several indicators. Impact values also vary significantly: In some cases, there are no variables for which significant impacts are calculated, which can be interpreted as situations in which no variable is identified as connected to the prediction of the target variable; this makes predictions less trustworthy than in situations in which significantly relevant variables can be identified.

References

1. Wagner, S., Kronberger, G., Beham, A., Kommenda, M., Scheibenpflug, A., Pitzer, E., Vonolfen, S., Kofler, M., Winkler, S., Dorfer, V., Affenzeller, M.: Architecture and design of the HeuristicLab optimization environment. In: Klempous, R., Nikodem, J., Jacak, W., Chaczko, Z. (eds.) Advanced Methods and Applications in Computational Intelligence. TIEI, vol. 6, pp. 193–258. Springer, Heidelberg (2013)
2. Breiman, L.: Random forests. Mach. Learn. **45**, 5–32 (2001)
3. Koza, J.R.: Genetic Programming: On the Programming of Computers by Means of Natural Selection. The MIT Press, Cambridge (1992)
4. Winkler, S.: Evolutionary System Identification: Modern Concepts and Practical Applications. Schriften der Johannes Kepler Universität Linz, Universitätsverlag Rudolf Trauner (2009)
5. Affenzeller, M., Winkler, S., Wagner, S., Beham, A.: Genetic Algorithms and Genetic Programming - Modern Concepts and Practical Applications. Chapman & Hall CRC, Boca Raton (2009)
6. Kommenda, M., Kronberger, G., Wagner, S., Winkler, S., Affenzeller, M.: On the architecture and implementation of tree-based genetic programming in heuristiclab. In: Proceedings of the 14th Annual Conference Companion on Genetic and Evolutionary Computation, GECCO 2012, pp. 101–108. ACM, New York, NY, USA (2012)
7. Banzhaf, W., Lasarczyk, C.: Genetic programming of an algorithmic chemistry. In: O'Reilly, U., Yu, T., Riolo, R., Worzel, B. (eds.) Genetic Programming Theory and Practice II, pp. 175–190. Springer, New York (2004). Ann Arbor
8. Winkler, S., Schaller, S., Dorfer, V., Affenzeller, M., Petz, G., Karpowicz, M.: Data-based prediction of sentiments using heterogeneous model ensembles. Soft Comput. (2014)
9. Kronberger, G.: Symbolic Regression for Knowledge Discovery. Schriften der Johannes Kepler Universität Linz, Universitätsverlag Rudolf Trauner (2011)
10. Pearl, J.: Causality: Models, Reasoning and Inference, 2nd edn. Cambridge University Press, New York (2009)
11. Winkler, S.M., Kronberger, G., Affenzeller, M., Stekel, H.: Variable interaction networks in medical data. Int. J. Priv. Health Inf. Manage. **1**, 1–16 (2013)

Modeling a Lot-Aware Slab Stack Shuffling Problem

Judith Fechter[1,2]([✉]), Andreas Beham[1,2], Stefan Wagner[1],
and Michael Affenzeller[1,2]

[1] Heuristic and Evolutionary Algorithms Laboratory School of Informatics,
Communications and Media, University of Applied Sciences Upper Austria,
Hagenberg Campus, Softwarepark 11, 4232 Hagenberg, Austria
{judith.fechter,andreas.beham,stefan.wagner,
michael.affenzeller}@fh-hagenberg.at
[2] Institute for Formal Models and Verification, Johannes Kepler University Linz,
Altenbergerstr. 69, 4040 Linz, Austria

Abstract. Stacking and shuffling problems are key logistics problems
in various areas such as container shipping or steel industry. The aim of
this paper is motivated by a real world instance arised in steel production. Slabs, continously but randomly casted, need to be arranged for
transport while having a certain number of buffer stacks available. The
optimization problem arising is assigning transport lotnumbers, regarding properties of slabs, as well as minimizing shuffling movements while
arranging the slabs, regarding the implicitly given transport order. For
that purpose, a combined optimization problem, being composed of two
sub-problems is developed. Further computational studies are conducted
in order to investigate the complexity of the problem. A combined solution approach is developed solving the problem in a sequential way using
customized algorithms in order to make advantage of specialised algorithms.

1 Introduction

The problem of stacking and restacking plays an important role in production and logistics, arising in various areas such as container terminals and
steel production. The former addresses the shuffling of containers within a yard
where containers are stacked temporarily. [5] developed a simulated annealing
(SA) algorithm for finding stacking strategies. Results show that the number of
shuffling movements is reduced compared to a strategy grouping same-weight-
containers. In an earlier work [2] considered two stacking strategies. One aims
to keep all stacks at an equal height. The other one locates containers according
to their arrival time. The results show that the measures of a bay most influence the expected number of shuffling movements. In [9] a comprehensive literature review of operations, space allocation, yard layout and stacking logistics is
provided.

Another approach for optimal stacking is the pre-marshalling problem. It
considers the optimal shuffling of blocks that are assumed to be of the same size.

© Springer International Publishing Switzerland 2015
R. Moreno-Díaz et al. (Eds.): EUROCAST 2015, LNCS 9520, pp. 334–341, 2015.
DOI: 10.1007/978-3-319-27340-2_42

The delivery order is assumed to be known. [6] propose a method for finding an optimal strategy for shuffling containers by decomposing the problem into two stages and three subproblems. They use dynamic programming and the transportation problem technique, which overall take a considerable computational time. In [8] a mathematical model is proposed for the shuffling while considering a given loading sequence as well as a given yard layout. They present an integer programming model based on a multi commodity flow problem. A simple heuristic is proposed in order to solve problems close to real-world size.

Considering steel industry, most research work has been done on the Slab Stack Shuffling (SSS) problem which aims to choose appropriate slabs for the rolling schedule out of ponderous stacks of slabs while minimizing the shuffling movements needed. [11] propose an integer programming model for the SSS problem and developed a two-phase heuristic algorithm. In [12] a genetic algorithm using specially designed operators is presented. For the SSS problem considered in [10], an improved parallel genetic algorithm is proposed in [12]. Two operators are developed, namely a modified crossover operator and a kin selection operator. [10–12] consider that a lifted slab is moved back immediately after the required slab is taken out. [13] takes into account that lifted slabs can be placed on other stacks. [3] propose a linearization of the SSS problem solved by using a linear binary integer programming (BIP) model.

1.1   Motivation

Considering the hot storage area, slabs are continuously casted and then lifted to buffer stacks to allow for an arranging process, while the number of stacking locations is limited. Subsequently the slabs are lifted to a delivery point to be picked up by transportation facilities. As there is only a limited number of vehicles, it is essential that slabs are carried to the delivery point in assorted lots. The slabs should be arranged according to measurements and properties.

[7] propose an exact method for solving a stacking problem allowing moves from and to a buffer stack and to a target stack with the aim of minimizing shuffling movements. They use ideas from dynamic programming and discrete optimization and obtain a solution quality of 25 % off optimum. Closely related to this problem is the blocks relocation problem (BRP). [1] provide a formal analysis of the problem and developed a heuristic based upon a set of relocation rules.

In contrast to the above mentioned research work, we consider the delivery order not as predefined but as flexible. We developed a combined optimization problem composed of two subproblems: a lot-building problem which provides the transport lots and implicitly the delivery order and a stacking problem which provides the optimal stacking in order to minimize shuffling movements. Further experimental studies are performed and a combined solution approach is proposed. In Sect. 2 a description and formulation of both problems is provided. In Sect. 3 results on complexity and performance and a sequential solution approach are presented.

2   Problem Description

The lot-aware slab stack shuffling problem is composed of a lot-building problem and a stacking problem. This section provides a formulation of both problems as well as of the interrelation on each other. The lot-building problem shall provide the transport lot number as input for the stacking problem (see Eq. 8).

2.1   Lot-Building Problem

Input. A set of slabs with properties (weight, measures, type, production time).

Objective. The aim is to minimize the number of lots used.

Constraints. A lot may only has a maximum weight and minimum number of slabs. Further, one lot may only contains one type of slab and only slabs with certain measurements limits.

$\Omega = \{j\}_{j=1}^{N}$	Set of cast slabs
$\mathcal{L} = \{i\}_{i=1}^{L}$	Set of lots
w_j, t_j, b_j	Weight, production time, measures (width) of slab j
W, T, B	Maximum values of weight, difference of production time and measures per lot

$$\min \sum_{i=1}^{L} y_i \tag{1}$$

$$s.t. \quad x_{ij} \le y_i, \qquad\qquad \forall i \in L, j \in N \tag{2}$$

$$\sum_{i=1}^{L} x_{ij} = 1, \qquad\qquad \forall j \in N \tag{3}$$

$$\sum_{j=1}^{N} x_{ij} \ge 2y_i, \quad \sum_{j=1}^{N} x_{ij} w_j \le W y_i \qquad\qquad \forall i \in L \tag{4}$$

$$(t_j - t_l)x_{ij}x_{il} \le T, \quad (b_j - b_l)x_{ij}x_{il} \le B \qquad \forall i \in L, j, l \in N \tag{5}$$

$$x_{ij} \in \{0,1\}, y_i \in \{0,1\} \qquad\qquad \forall i \in L, j \in N \tag{6}$$

Decision variable x_{ij} takes 1 if slab j is assigned to lot i, otherwise 0. Decision variable y_i takes 1 if lot i is used, otherwise 0. Cosntraints (2) and (3) ensure that each slab is assigned to a lot, but only if the lot exists. (4) state the minimum number of slabs and a maximum weight per lot. (5) ensure that a maximum difference of production time and measures are not exceeded.

The fitness function of the heuristic approach is the sum of the number of lots used and a penalty for each constraint violation.

2.2   Stacking Problem

Input. A set of slabs is produced that arrive on parallel inputs over time. Each slab is assigned to an article depending on its characteristics, as well to a lot. A lot contains only one type of slab.

Objective. The aim is to arrange all slabs on buffer stacks in order to minimize the number of shuffling movements when lifting slabs to the delivery point every time a lot is completely produced.

Stacking Constraints. Due to reasons of stability, slabs must be arranged according to their measures. Predefined stacking constraints determine which slab type is allowed to be placed on another one.

Stacks and Moves. We have a set of buffer stacks and delivery stacks. A buffer stack has a maximum stack height. The initial buffer stacks are assumed to be empty. The delivery stack is assumed to be of infinite capacity. Only moves from the input to a buffer stack are considered as each slab must go to a target stack.

$$
\begin{array}{ll}
\Omega = \{\omega_j\}_{j=1}^{N} & \text{Set of cast slabs} \\
\mathcal{A} = \{a_i\}_{i=1}^{A} & \text{Set of articles} \\
\mathcal{L} = \{l_i\}_{i=1}^{L} & \text{Set of built lots} \\
\mathcal{K} = \{B_k\}_{k=1}^{K} & \text{Set of buffer stacks}
\end{array}
$$

The input may contain the following mappings. Equation (7) assigns one type of article to each slab. Equation (8) assigns a lot to each slab. Equation (9) denotes the last cast slab of one lot. $e(\omega_j)$ takes 1, if ω_j is the last slab of a lot. Based on the input, α (see (10)) takes 1 if two slabs are in the same lot.

$$
\begin{aligned}
f &: \Omega \to \mathcal{A} : f(\omega_j) = a_i & \forall j \in N, i \in A && (7) \\
g &: \Omega \to \mathcal{L} : g(\omega_j) = l_i & \forall j \in N, i \in L && (8) \\
e &: \Omega \to \{0,1\} & && (9) \\
\alpha &: \Omega \times \Omega \to \{0,1\} & && (10)
\end{aligned}
$$

Equations (11) and (12) depend on the decision variable z. β denotes the index of the first cast slab assigned to lot l_i and put on stack B_k. γ denotes whether any of the slabs, belonging to the same lot as ω_j, is put on stack B_k.

$$
\beta : \Omega \times \mathcal{K} \to \Omega : \beta_{ik} = \left\{ \begin{array}{l} \min\{j | \alpha_{ij} z_{kj} = 1\} \\ i, \quad \text{otherwise} \end{array} \right\} \qquad \forall i, j \in N, k \in K \qquad (11)
$$

$$
\gamma : \Omega \times \mathcal{K} \to \{0,1\} \qquad\qquad\qquad\qquad \forall j \in N, k \in K \qquad (12)
$$

Objective Function. Every time a lot l_i is completely produced, given by mapping (9), the shuffling movements are evaluated. The number of shuffling movements has to be minimized and is given in Eq. (13).

$$
\min \sum_{j=1}^{N} \sum_{k=1}^{K} \left((h_{\omega_j}(B_k) + \gamma_{jk} - h'_{\omega_j}(B_k) - n_{\omega_j}(B_k)) * e(\omega_j) \right) \qquad (13)
$$

The objective function is composed of the following parts.

$$h_{\omega_j}(B_k) = \sum_{l=1}^{\omega_j} z_{kl} - \sum_{i=1}^{\omega_j-1} \left(e(\omega_i) \sum_{n=1}^{i} \alpha_{in} z_{kn} \right) \tag{14}$$

$$h'_{\omega_j}(B_k) = h_{\omega_{\beta_{jk}}}(B_k) - \sum_{i=\beta_{jk}}^{\omega_j-1} \left(e(\omega_i) \sum_{n=1}^{\beta_{jk}} \alpha_{in} z_{kn} \right) \tag{15}$$

$$n_{\omega_j}(B_k) = \sum_{l=\beta_{jk}}^{j} \alpha_{jl} z_{kl} \tag{16}$$

Equation (14) denotes the height of buffer stack B_k when slab ω_j is produced. That is the sum of slabs placed on B_k reduced by the sum of slabs moved away. Equation (15) denotes the position of the slab in buffer stack B_k with index β at the time that slab ω_j is cast. Equation (16) denotes the number of slabs of the same lot in buffer stack B_k. Decision variable z determines whether slab ω_j is placed on buffer stack B_k.

$$s.t. \qquad \sum_{k=1}^{K} z_{kj} = 1 \qquad\qquad \forall j \in N \tag{17}$$

$$h_{\omega j}(B_k) \leq H \qquad\qquad \forall j \in N, k \in K \tag{18}$$

$$z_{kj} \in \{0,1\} \qquad\qquad \forall j \in N, k \in K \tag{19}$$

Stacking constraints (20) state whether an article, characterized by its measurements, is allowed to be placed on another one. The constraints are based on a matrix of dimension $C : A \times A : (a_i, a_j) \mapsto \{0,1\}$, being 1 if a_i is allowed to be placed on a_j. Summed up over all stacks and all slabs, Eq. (20) ensures that a constraint is only violated by slabs which are already moved away.

$$\sum_{l=1}^{j} \left((z_{kl})(z_{kj})(1 - C_{a_j a_l}) \right) = \sum_{i=1}^{j-1} \left(e(\omega_i) \sum_{n=1}^{i} \left(\alpha_{in}(z_{kn})(z_{kj})(1 - C_{a_j a_n}) \right) \right) \tag{20}$$

2.3 Interdependency

Due to the fact that slabs are moved to a target as soon as their lot is completely produced, the delivery order is implicitly determined by the assigned lotnumber. Hence, it is reasonable that the assignment of lots has a significant impact on the efficiency of the stacking problem. Thus, an exchange of the solution qualities is worthwhile in order to achieve a best possible combined solution. In empirical studies we focused on the complexity of the problem as well as on a combined solution approach.

3   Empirical Studies

Empircial studies are conducted on problem instances differing in the number of slabs and buffer stacks, indicated by the naming (X-Y stands for X slabs, Y buffer stacks). Instances are solved by using CPLEX [4] and variable neighbourhood search (VNS) in order to show the complexity of the problem by investigating the runtime, solution quality and number of feasible solutions. Instances of higher dimensions are solved by using a multi-objective algorithm namely NSGA II and by using a combined method using VNS. A neighbour is defined as a swap of two assigned stacks/lots as well as the assignment of a random stack/lot to a slab. Studies using heuristic methods are performed by HeuristicLab [14,15]. All tests were calculated on a laptop with a Intel(R) Core(TM) i7-4600U CPU 2.10 GHz 2.70 GHz processor.

Complexity. Results of runtime and number of feasible solutions show that the lot-aware slab stack shuffling problem is of high complexity. CPLEX could solve the problem up to 20 slabs to optimality. Only instances up to 68 slabs could be solved before running out of memory. The runtime of CPLEX shows exponential behaviour. The VNS performs with a rather constant runtime. Table 1 allows a comparison of CPLEX and VNS regarding the best found solutions and runtime. For this study we dissociated the lot-building problem from the stacking problem. Presented results are of the stacking problem only.

Table 1. Results on complexity

Instance	Runtime (sec)		Best solution		Feasible (%)
	CPLEX	VNS	CPLEX	VNS	VNS
30-3	26.73	41.72	**9**	9	79
50-6	213.97	**108.80**	32	**31**	76
60-6	16313.41	**258.12**	41	**40**	79
68-7	7706.96	**339.54**	31	**31**	50
100-8	x	**244.39**	x	**74**	83

We can derive that even for heuristic methods the problem is hard to solve. For solving real world instances of more than 200 slabs only heuristic approaches work. Due to the number of feasible solutions the algorithm may be adapted by developing specialized operators. Worth to mention is that the best found qualities of VNS are at least as good as obtained by CPLEX.

Sequential Solution Approach. In order to exploit the property of inter-relation we consider a sequential solution approach. Using VNS, the developed method solves the lot-building several times and gives each solution as input to the stacking problem. The best found combined solution is returned. An advantage of this approach is that also sub-optimal solutions of the lot-building problem are considered in order to find the best possible solution for the combined problem. Results are compared to a multi-objective algorithm, NSGA II.

Table 2. Results of combined solving

Instance	Quality	
	NSGA II	Sequ. method
20-5	17	17
50-6	44	**33**
100-8	114	**72**

Table 2 show that the sequential approach achieves good solutions compared to a standard NSGA II. A sequential approach is reasonable in case specialised algorithms for the sub-problems exist since a separate application of both algorithms is allowed.

4 Conclusion and Future Work

In this research work an optimization problem composed of two autonomous but related problems has been developed. Experimental results show that the modelled problem is very hard to solve. Further work will consider customized heuristic algorithms in order to allow the solving of real world instances in reasonable time. Research work will also be done on linking autonomous but related optimization problems. A method for solving several optimization problems in an interrelated way shall be developed. With that purpose an approach for exchanging solution qualities and deduced parameters shall be researched in order to reach a combined sequential solution approach.

Acknowledgments. The work described in this paper was done within the COMET Project Heuristic Optimization in Production and Logistics (HOPL), #843532 funded by the Austrian Research Promotion Agency (FFG).

References

1. Caserta, M., Schwarze, S., Voß, S.: A mathematical formulation and complexity considerations for the blocks relocation problem. Eur. J. Oper. Res. **219**(1), 96–104 (2012)
2. De Castillo, B., Daganzo, C.F.: Handling strategies for import containers at marine terminals. Transp. Res. Part B: Methodol. **27**(2), 151–166 (1993)
3. Fernandes, E.F.A., Freire, L., Passos, A.C., Street, A.: Solving the non-linear slab stack shuffling problem using linear binary integer programming. In: EngOpt 2012–3rd International Conference on Engineering Optimization (2012)
4. IBM, C. IBM Software. Retrieved from CPLEX Optimizer. http://www-01.ibm.com/software/commerce/optimization/cplex-optimizer/, 30 April 2015
5. Kang, J., Ryu, K.R., Kim, K.H.: Deriving stacking strategies for export containers with uncertain weight information. J. Intell. Manuf. **17**, 399–410 (2006)

6. Kim, K.H., Bae, J.W.: Re-marshalling export containers in port container terminals. Comput. Ind. Eng. **35**, 655–658 (1998)
7. König, F.G., Lübbecke, M., Möhring, R.H., Schäfer, G., Spenke, I.: Solutions to real-world instances of PSPACE-complete stacking. In: Arge, L., Hoffmann, M., Welzl, E. (eds.) ESA 2007. LNCS, vol. 4698, pp. 729–740. Springer, Heidelberg (2007)
8. Lee, Y., Hsu, N.Y.: An optimization model for the container pre-marshalling problem. Comput. Oper. Res. **34**, 3295–3313 (2007)
9. Luo, J., Wu, Y., Halldorsson, A., Song, X.: Storage and stacking logistics problems in container terminals. OR Insight **24**, 256–275 (2011)
10. Singh, K.A., Srinivas, Tiwari, M.K.: Modelling the slab stack shuffling problem in developing steel rolling schedules and its solution using improved Parallel Genetic Algorithms. Int. J. Prod. Econ. **91**, 135–147 (2004)
11. Tang, L.X., Liu, J.Y., Rong, A.Y., Yang, Z.H.: An effective heuristic algorithm to minimise stack shuffle in selecting steel slabs from the slab yard for heating and rolling. J. Oper. Res. Soc. **52**, 1091–1097 (2001)
12. Tang, L.X., Liu, J.Y., Rong, A.Y., Yang, Z.H.: Modelling and a genetic algorithm solution for the slab stack shuffling problem when implementing steel rolling schedules. Int. J. Prod. Res. **40**(7), 1083–1095 (2002)
13. Tang, L., Ren, H.: Modelling and a segmented dynamic programming-based heuristic approach for the slab stack shuffling problem. Comput. Oper. Res. **37**, 368–375 (2010)
14. Wagner, S., Kronberger, G., Beham, A., Kommenda, M., Scheibenpflug, A., Pitzer, E., Vonolfen, S., Kofler, M., Winkler, S., Dorfer, V., Affenzeller, M.: Architecture and design of the HeuristicLab optimization environment. Top. Intell. Eng. Inf. **6**, 197–261 (2014)
15. Wagner, S.: Heuristic optimization software systems - modeling of heuristic optimization algorithms in the HeuristicLab software environment. Ph.D. Thesis, Johannes Kepler University Linz (2009)

Heuristic Approaches for the Probabilistic Traveling Salesman Problem

Christoph Weiler[1], Benjamin Biesinger[1(✉)], Bin Hu[2], and Günther R. Raidl[1]

[1] Institute of Computer Graphics and Algorithms, TU Wien,
Favoritenstraße 9-11/1861, 1040 Vienna, Austria
e1029175@student.tuwien.ac.at, {biesinger,raidl}@ac.tuwien.ac.at
[2] Mobility Department - Dynamic Transportation Systems,
AIT Austrian Institute of Technology, Giefinggasse 2, 1210 Vienna, Austria
bin.hu@ait.ac.at

Abstract. The Probabilistic Traveling Salesman Problem (PTSP) is a variant of the classical Traveling Salesman Problem (TSP) where each city has a given probability requiring a visit. We aim for an a-priori tour including every city that minimizes the expected length over all realizations. In this paper we consider different heuristic approaches for the PTSP. First we analyze various popular construction heuristics for the classical TSP applied on the PTSP: nearest neighbor, farthest insertion, nearest insertion, radial sorting and space filling curve. Then we investigate their extensions to the PTSP: almost nearest neighbor, probabilistic farthest insertion, probabilistic nearest insertion. To improve the constructed solutions we use existing 2-opt and 1-shift neighborhood structures for which exact delta evaluation formulations exist. These are embedded within a Variable Neighborhood Descent framework into a Variable Neighborhood Search. Computational results indicate that this approach is competitive to already existing heuristic algorithms and able to find good solutions in low runtime.

Keywords: Probabilistic traveling salesman problem · Variable neighborhood search · Construction heuristics

1 Introduction

The Probabilistic Traveling Salesman Problem (PTSP) is an NP-hard problem [6] introduced by Jaillet [10]. It is a variant of the Traveling Salesman Problem (TSP), where each city has an assigned probability of requiring a visit. We search for an a-priori tour through all cities that minimizes the expected length of the real tour, where some cities might not have to be visited. The real tour, also called realization of the a-priori tour, then follows this a-priori tour and skips cities which do not have to be visited. A real world application for the PTSP would be, e.g., a postman who delivers mails on a fixed assigned route every day. From historical data the probability of each address requiring a visit is known. After each delivery he checks which address he has to visit next and proceeds accordingly.

© Springer International Publishing Switzerland 2015
R. Moreno-Díaz et al. (Eds.): EUROCAST 2015, LNCS 9520, pp. 342–349, 2015.
DOI: 10.1007/978-3-319-27340-2_43

Formally we are given a complete graph $G = \langle V, E \rangle$ with V being a vertex set containing n nodes and E being an edge set containing m edges. Each edge $(i, j) \in E$ is assigned a cost d_{ij} and each node $v \in V$ has a probability p_v of requiring a visit. If the probabilities p_v are equal for every node, the problem is called homogeneous and otherwise it is heterogeneous [9]. A solution $T = \langle v_1, \ldots, v_n \rangle$ is an a-priori tour, represented by a permutation of the n nodes, where the first and last nodes are implicitly assumed to be connected. In this paper we concentrate on the homogeneous PTSP with symmetric distances due to comparability with other papers.

The expected costs of a tour T are defined as

$$c(T) = \sum_{i=1}^{2^n} p(R_i) L(R_i) \tag{1}$$

where R_i is a possible realization, i.e., one possible a-posteriori tour, $p(R_i)$ its occurrence probability, and $L(R_i)$ the resulting length of the tour. Since there are $O(2^n)$ different realizations, it is not convenient to compute the objective value in such a way. Therefore Jaillet [10] showed that the expected length can be calculated in $O(n^2)$ time using the following closed form expression:

$$\begin{aligned} c(T) = \sum_{i=1}^{n} \sum_{j=i+1}^{n} d_{v_i v_j} p_{v_i} p_{v_j} \prod_{k=i+1}^{j-1} (1 - p_{v_k}) \\ + \sum_{j=1}^{n} \sum_{i=1}^{j-1} d_{v_j v_i} p_{v_i} p_{v_j} \prod_{k=j+1}^{n} (1 - p_{v_k}) \prod_{k=1}^{i-1} (1 - p_{v_k}) \end{aligned} \tag{2}$$

This formula represents the most general form for heterogeneous PTSPs. As we concentrate on the homogeneous problem, we will use the following, simplified objective function:

$$c(T) = p^2 \sum_{r=1}^{n-1} (1 - p)^{r-1} \sum_{i=1}^{n} d_{v_i v_{i+r}} \tag{3}$$

The PTSP is a well studied problem in the literature. Bertsimas et al. [4,6] contributed theoretical properties of the PTSP such as bounds and asymptotic analyses. Bianchi et al. [7,8] proposed metaheuristic approaches based on ant colony optimization and local search with exact delta evaluation. Balaprakash et al. [1,2] analyzed sampling and estimation-based approaches. Weyland et al. [14,15] considered new sampling and ad-hoc approximation methods for local search and ant colony system. Marinakis and Marinaki [11] proposed a hybrid swarm optimization approach. The most promising results were obtained by using not the exact objective function as stated in Eq. 3, but either a restricted depth approximation or a sampling approach. In contrast, our approach is based on an efficient exact evaluation.

In Sect. 2 we apply several TSP construction heuristics to the PTSP, consider Jaillet's Almost Nearest Neighbor Heuristic [10], and introduce two new construction heuristics derived for the PTSP: Probabilistic Farthest Insertion and

Probabilistic Nearest Insertion. In Sect. 3 we propose a Variable Neighborhood Descent Framework embedded in a Variable Neighborhood Search to improve constructed solutions. Section 4 presents experimental results and Sect. 5 concludes this work.

2   Construction Heuristics

For generating an initial solution for the subsequent VND/VNS we consider several different construction heuristics. First we investigate construction heuristics having already been used for the TSP and then we improve upon them by taking also the probabilities into account.

2.1   TSP Construction Heuristics on PTSP

To construct a reasonable tour for PTSP we first investigate how well TSP construction heuristics perform. We evaluate the following construction heuristics:

Nearest Neighbor (NN): Starting from a first node $v_0 \in V$, we iteratively append an unvisited node that is nearest to the previously inserted one. The resulting computational complexity is in $O(n^2)$.

Nearest Insertion (NI): Starting with a simple tour T containing only one node $v_0 \in V$, we insert the nearest node to the previously inserted one at the best fitting position. Let v_j be the node to be inserted next, then we calculate the best fitting position by determining

$$\min_{v_i, v_{i+1} \in T} (d_{v_i v_j} + d_{v_j v_{i+1}} - d_{v_i v_{i+1}}) \tag{4}$$

The computational complexity is in $O(n^2)$.

Farthest Insertion (FI): This heuristic is similar to NI. The only difference is that we choose the farthest node to the previously inserted one is chosen for insertion instead of the nearest one.

Space Filling Curve (SFC): SFC was introduced by Bartholdi et al. [3]. The heuristic constructs a Sierpiński curve over all cities and visits them as they appear on this curve. The computational complexity is in $O(n \log n)$.

Radial Sorting (RS): We construct a new virtual city which can be seen as the center of mass of all cities. The cities are then sorted and visited by their angle relative to this center. For TSP this heuristic usually yields poor results, but for stochastic vehicle routing problems with low probabilities it can perform really well [5]. The computational complexity is dominated by the sorting, and thus, is in $O(n \log n)$.

2.2   Construction Heuristics for PTSP Using Probabilities

To take probabilities into account we adapt the first three heuristics from Sect. 2.1.

Almost Nearest Neighbor Heuristic (ANN): ANN was mentioned by Jaillet [10] in his dissertation, but it did not gain much attention until now. It appends the city with the lowest change of expected length from the last inserted city to the tour. The cost of inserting city v_j can be computed the following way for heterogeneous problems:

$$\min_{v_j \in (V-T)} \left(\sum_{i=1}^{|T|} p_{v_i} p_{v_j} d_{v_i v_j} \prod_{k=i+1}^{|T|} (1 - p_{v_k}) \right) \tag{5}$$

For the homogeneous problem we can simplify the formula:

$$\min_{v_j \in (V-T)} \left(\sum_{i=1}^{|T|} d_{v_i v_j} (1-p)^{(|T|-i)} \right) \tag{6}$$

Note that we omitted the p^2 in the homogeneous formula because we try to find a minimum and therefore scaling by p^2 does not matter. The resulting computational complexity is in $O(n^3)$ because we insert each city in the tour and evaluate Eq. 6 on each position in the tour.

Probabilistic Nearest Insertion (PNI): PNI is a new heuristic derived from NI where we insert the node nearest to the last inserted node into the tour and evaluate the objective function on each possible position. This naive approach results in a computational complexity of $O(n^4)$. We use Bianchi et al.'s delta 1-shift [8] local search procedure to solve this heuristic more efficiently: Bianchi showed that 1-shift local search is possible in time $O(n^2)$ using delta evaluation. Therefore we insert the node at the first position in the tour and then perform one iteration of the delta 1-shift procedure. Therefore we are able to reduce the complexity to $O(n^3)$.

Probabilistic Farthest Insertion (PFI): PFI is a new heuristic similar to PNI. The only difference is that the farthest node to the previously inserted one is chosen for insertion instead of the nearest one.

3   Variable Neighborhood Search

Variable Neighborhood Descent (VND) and Variable Neighborhood Search (VNS) were introduced by Mladenović and Hansen in 1997 [12]. VND uses the fact that if a solution is at a local optimum in some neighborhood it is not necessarily locally

Table 1. Results of construction heuristics.

Instance	p	RS	t[s]	SFC	t[s]	NN	t[s]	ANN	t[s]	FI	t[s]	PFI	t[s]	NI	t[s]	PNI	t[s]
eil101	0.1	199.3	<1	206.5	<1	243.9	<1	243.4	<1	202.7	<1	**197.4**	<1	235.3	<1	197.6	<1
	0.2	301.8	<1	301.8	<1	372.7	<1	367.3	<1	296.6	<1	286.9	<1	353.0	<1	**285.2**	<1
	0.3	406.7	<1	377.3	<1	465.4	<1	447.1	<1	373.8	<1	358.3	<1	435.1	<1	**350.6**	<1
	0.4	515.8	<1	442.2	<1	539.7	<1	506.6	<1	439.6	<1	**413.4**	<1	500.6	<1	417.1	<1
	0.5	627.6	<1	500.8	<1	602.4	<1	610.3	<1	496.9	<1	493.8	<1	556.4	<1	**471.6**	<1
d198	0.1	8580.7	<1	7971.6	<1	9010.2	<1	9128.4	<1	7677.0	<1	**7438.9**	3	8011.3	<1	7554.6	3
	0.2	12958.4	<1	10202.3	<1	11523.3	<1	10899.6	<1	9793.1	<1	**9503.8**	3	10259.2	<1	9637.6	3
	0.3	17238.0	<1	11805.9	<1	13037.9	<1	12784.2	<1	11191.6	<1	**10658.1**	3	11731.5	<1	11142.8	3
	0.4	21559.6	<1	13186.4	<1	14190.4	<1	13987.1	<1	12304.8	<1	12069.9	3	12902.4	<1	**12009.5**	3
	0.5	25900.2	<1	14424.3	<1	15141.8	<1	15372.7	<1	13252.8	<1	13001.1	2	13896.9	<1	**12875.3**	3
att532	0.1	54706.7	<1	42508.3	<1	51691.4	<1	45218.4	3	39271.3	<1	**33795.7**	66	43611.1	<1	33933.0	65
	0.2	99168.2	<1	56731.6	<1	67732.8	<1	58060.9	3	53879.0	<1	47245.8	64	59269.2	<1	**46913.2**	53
	0.3	143491.0	<1	67947.3	<1	77856.9	<1	68591.5	2	64473.3	<1	**56196.2**	60	69679.5	<1	57738.6	62
	0.4	187206.0	<1	77640.2	<1	85264.5	<1	80507.1	2	72778.1	<1	**65339.4**	60	77609.6	<1	66619.8	60
	0.5	230028.0	<1	86270.7	<1	91162.4	<1	83988.9	2	79606.1	<1	76768.1	47	84149.3	<1	**72540.6**	59
rat783	0.1	5844.9	<1	3521.5	<1	5038.8	<1	4628.9	9	4174.4	<1	**3339.5**	224	4424.9	<1	3561.6	219
	0.2	11380.1	<1	4978.1	<1	6571.1	<1	5921.0	9	5939.2	<1	**4816.7**	216	6027.2	<1	4985.6	205
	0.3	17005.6	<1	6123.0	<1	7577.0	<1	7294.5	8	7117.3	<1	6381.3	160	7092.5	<1	**6101.9**	206
	0.4	22648.4	<1	7103.9	<1	8360.0	<1	8227.8	8	8008.2	<1	**6782.0**	196	7903.5	<1	6973.7	187
	0.5	28283.8	<1	7978.2	<1	9010.7	<1	8789.8	8	8729.4	<1	**7736.5**	192	8572.2	<1	7795.2	134

optimal in another neighborhood. We use delta 2-opt and delta 1-shift neighborhood structures by Bianchi et al. [8] to combine them within a VND framework because they showed that it is possible to exactly evaluate them using delta evaluation formulations. Therefore, we compute a solution that is locally optimal with respect to both neighborhoods.

Via a general VNS we repetitively randomize the tour by applying shaking, and locally improving it again with VND. In the i-th shaking neighborhood we perform $2i$ random shift moves. Our VNS terminates after 20 iterations without improvement.

4   Computational Results

The algorithms were implemented in C++99 and compiled with GNU GCC 4.6.4. As test environment we used an Intel Xeon E5649, 2.53 GHz Quad Core, running on Ubuntu 12.04.5 LTS (Precise Pangolin). For a comparison with the literature we use test instances from the TSPLIB [13]. Homogeneous visiting probabilities were assumed to be $p \in \{0.1, 0.2, \ldots, 0.5\}$.

Table 1 summarizes our evaluation of the construction heuristics. Generally the probabilistic versions generate better results than their deterministic counterparts but at the price of much higher runtimes. From the deterministic ones, FI performs best, but also SFC performs well. Overall, PFI performs best but PNI is close.

Table 2 shows our Variable Neighborhood Search results compared to results from the literature. Weyland et al. [15] only published results of their EACS for

Table 2. Variable neighborhood descent/search comparison.

Instances	pACS [7]		HPSO [11]		EACS [15]		FI+VND		FI+VNS			PFI+VNS	
p	obj*	t[s]	obj*	t[s]	$\overline{obj}$	t[s]	obj	t[s]	obj*	$\overline{obj}$	$\tilde{t}[s]$	$\overline{obj}$	$\tilde{t}[s]$
eil101													
0.1	199.7	102	200.0	2	213.8	<1	197.4	<1	197.3	**197.3**	<1	**197.3**	<1
0.2	286.7	102	284.9	2	288.8	8	285.3	<1	283.6	**283.6**	8	**283.6**	13
0.3	353.5	102	**283.7**	2	358.7	5	352.0	<1	349.2	349.7	5	350.8	4
0.4	410.9	102	405.4	2	413.1	12	409.2	<1	404.7	405.6	12	**404.7**	1
0.5	470.7	102	455.7	2	462.9	14	459.9	<1	455.5	**456.2**	14	458.8	13
d198													
0.1	7556.1	1011	7504.9	5	8026.1	5	7438.2	1	7436.9	**7436.9**	5	**7436.9**	34
0.2	9489.2	1011	9415.1	5	9372.7	89	9357.8	2	9312.1	**9312.1**	89	9313.1	78
0.3	10951.9	1011	N/M		10635.4	74	10651.8	2	10531.3	**10538.9**	74	10540.3	52
0.4	12047.9	1011	N/M		11621.3	126	11665.0	2	11538.7	11586.6	126	**11555.7**	95
0.5	12745.5	1011	12527.6	5	12556.1	90	12617.9	1	12426.5	**12489.1**	90	12507.9	11
att532													
0.1	35179.7	2830	N/M		**33663.2**	3600	34533.5	50	33665.0	33685.8	2263	33683.0	2426
0.2	47531.4	2830	N/M		**44653.4**	3600	45867.9	47	45011.0	45179.0	2184	45148.6	2426
0.3	55865.3	2830	N/M		54008.2	2330	56150.4	49	53943.9	54111.1	2330	**53846.0**	2567
0.4	63308.0	2830	N/M		61455.6	1790	63973.5	38	61145.7	61500.9	1790	**61175.8**	1777
0.5	69671.2	2830	N/M		**67538.2**	1954	70431.3	33	67600.9	68285.0	1954	68298.6	3000
rat783													
0.1	3368.9	6131	3616.4	70	**3235.6**	3600	3292.4	281	3243.1	3259.7	4752	3255.1	10043
0.2	4781.2	6131	4775.1	63	**4534.0**	3600	4694.4	197	4583.3	4595.5	4627	4590.4	8712
0.3	5794.0	6131	N/M		5591.1	4537	5770.1	169	5574.0	5596.2	4537	**5579.4**	6712
0.4	6643.6	6131	N/M		**6336.3**	4119	6611.1	153	6369.7	6402.7	4119	6352.3	5303
0.5	7334.1	6131	7094.9	64	**6941.2**	4130	7282.4	137	7022.2	7073.5	4130	7007.5	4944

N/M ... not mentioned

instances att532 and rat783 with $p = 0.1$ and $p = 0.2$, and therefore, we performed additional tests using their code and published parameters for the other instances. For the VNS we apply FI and PFI as construction heuristic because FI offers the best tradeoff between efficiency and runtime and PFI performs best. Therefore we only include FI+VND, FI+VNS, and PFI+VNS in our results. In many cases our VND yields good solutions in short time, but VND alone cannot keep up with Weyland et al.'s EACS [15] or Marinakis' HybPSO [11]. However, our VNS is able to achieve new best solutions in 11 cases. We further observe that EACS performs excellent especially on the larger instances but the VNS is typically better on smaller instances. When comparing FI and PFI in combination with the VNS we see that they find solutions of similar quality but for larger instances the runtime of PFI+VNS increases more than the runtime of FI+VNS.

5   Conclusions and Future Work

In this paper the PTSP was discussed and the most important properties were shown. We focused on five TSP construction heuristics to generate an initial solution, namely Radial Sorting, Farthest Insertion, Nearest Insertion, Space Filling Curve, Nearest Neighbor, and compared them on several TSPLIB instances.

C. Weiler et al.

Overall, Farthest Insertion performed best, followed by Space Filling Curve. Then we derived new construction heuristics to take probabilities into account: Almost Nearest Neighbor, Probabilistic Nearest Insertion and Probabilistic Farthest Insertion. They all significantly improve on their deterministic counterparts but are much more time-consuming. To improve these solutions we introduced a VNS framework with embedded VND based on 1-shift and 2-opt neighborhood structures and exact delta evaluation. Results show that FI+VNS and PFI+VNS typically yield the best solutions out of our tested configurations and they are even able to find new best-known solutions for 11 instances.

The major reason why our VNS performs so well is the usage of efficient, exact delta evaluation approaches for 1-shift and 2-opt originally proposed by Bianchi et al. [8]. Future work should consider further neighborhood structures for the PTSP for which exact delta evaluations are possible. In particular we are currently considering Or-opt.

Acknowledgments. The authors thank Dennis Weyland for providing the source code of his EACS for better comparison.

References

1. Balaprakash, P., Birattari, M., Stützle, T., Dorigo, M.: Adaptive sample size and importance sampling in estimation-based local search for the probabilistic traveling salesman problem. Eur. J. Oper. Res. **199**(1), 98–110 (2009)
2. Balaprakash, P., Birattari, M., Stützle, T., Yuan, Z., Dorigo, M.: Estimation-based ant colony optimization and local search for the probabilistic traveling salesman problem. Swarm Intel. **3**(3), 223–242 (2009)
3. Bartholdi III, J.J., Platzman, L.K.: An $O(n \log n)$ planar travelling salesman heuristic based on spacefilling curves. Oper. Res. Lett. **1**(4), 121–125 (1982)
4. Bertsimas, D., Howell, L.H.: Further results on the probabilistic traveling salesman problem. Eur. J. Oper. Res. **65**(1), 68–95 (1993)
5. Bertsimas, D.J., Chervi, P., Peterson, M.: Computational approaches to stochastic vehicle routing problems. Transp. Sci. **29**(4), 342–352 (1995)
6. Bertsimas, D.J., Jaillet, P., Odoni, A.R.: A priori optimization. Oper. Res. **38**(6), 1019–1033 (1991)
7. Bianchi, L., Gambardella, L.M., Dorigo, M.: An ant colony optimization approach to the probabilistic traveling salesman problem. In: Guervós, J.J.M., Adamidis, P.A., Beyer, H.-G., Fernández-Villacañas, J.-L., Schwefel, H.-P. (eds.) PPSN 2002. LNCS, vol. 2439, pp. 883–892. Springer, Heidelberg (2002)
8. Bianchi, L., Knowles, J., Bowler, N.: Local search for the probabilistic traveling salesman problem: correction to the 2-p-opt and 1-shift algorithms. Eur. J. Oper. Res. **162**(1), 206–219 (2005)
9. Chervi, P.: A computational approach to probabilistic vehicle routing problems. Master's thesis, Massachusetts Institute of Technology, Department of Electrical Engineering and Computer Science (1988)
10. Jaillet, P.: Probabilistic traveling salesman problems. Ph.D. thesis, Massachusetts Institute of Technology (1985)

11. Marinakis, Y., Marinaki, M.: A hybrid multi-swarm particle swarm optimization algorithm for the probabilistic traveling salesman problem. Comput. Oper. Res. **37**(3), 432–442 (2010)
12. Mladenović, N., Hansen, P.: Variable neighborhood search. Comput. Oper. Res. **24**(11), 1097–1100 (1997)
13. Reinelt, G.: TSPLIB. http://www.iwr.uni-heidelberg.de/groups/comopt/software/ TSPLIB95/. Accessed 7 May 2015
14. Weyland, D., Bianchi, L., Gambardella, L.M.: New approximation-based local search algorithms for the probabilistic traveling salesman problem. In: Moreno-Díaz, R., Pichler, F., Quesada-Arencibia, A. (eds.) EUROCAST 2009. LNCS, vol. 5717, pp. 681–688. Springer, Heidelberg (2009)
15. Weyland, D., Montemanni, R., Gambardella, L.M.: An enhanced ant colony system for the probabilistic traveling salesman problem. In: Di Caro, G.A., Theraulaz, G. (eds.) BIONETICS 2012. LNICST, vol. 134, pp. 237–249. Springer, Heidelberg (2014)

Increasing the Sensitivity of Cancer Predictors Using Confidence Based Ensemble Modeling

Michael Affenzeller[1]([✉]), Karin Zölzer[1], Stephan M. Winkler[1], Erwin Hopf[1], Herbert Stekel[2], Rupert Frechinger[2], and Stefan Wagner[1]

[1] Heuristic and Evolutionary Algorithms Laboratory School of Informatics, Communications and Media, University of Applied Sciences Upper Austria, Hagenberg Campus, Softwarepark 11, 4232 Hagenberg, Austria
{michael.affenzeller,karin.zoelzer,stephan.winkler,erwin.hopf, stefan.wagner}@fh-hagenberg.at
[2] General Hospital of Linz, Central Laboratory, Krankenhausstraße 9, 4021 Linz, Austria
{herbert.stekel,rupert.frechinger}@akh.linz.at

Abstract. This paper discusses the use of symbolic regression based ensemble modeling for obtaining more sensitive cancer predictors. The ensemble models are generated on the basis of blood parameters acting as model inputs which have been coupled with diagnosis data in order to predict breast cancer. In addition to previous works this contribution focuses on the use of ensemble predictors in order to achieve more sensitive models. For achieving this goal the best models in terms of accuracy, sensitivity and in terms of a combined measure are selected based on training data in order to analyze to which extent the more sensitive model behavior is also reflected on test data. In addition to the a-posteriori selection of ensemble models with certain properties first results are shown that have been achieved with a new evaluation function which favors more sensitive predictors and guides the search towards more sensitive models already in the model generation phase.

1 Introduction

In the last decades various machine learning techniques have been applied in the field of medical data mining [1]. Many contributions in this field, for example [2], use benchmark data sets such as those offered by the UCI machine learning repository [3].

The data sets used for the research described in this paper have been collected and pre-processed by the authors in cooperation with researchers at the General Hospital of Linz. In order to learn models for cancer prediction, blood parameters recorded at the central laboratory have been combined with the hospital's information about diagnoses (recorded according to the ICD-10 standard for the classification of diseases). The data preprocessing steps required in order to prepare data sets for the prediction of the several cancer types are explained in the authors' previous research work like e.g. in [4] or [5]. In [6] the data preprocessing steps are also reflected; however, the main focus of this contribution

© Springer International Publishing Switzerland 2015
R. Moreno-Díaz et al. (Eds.): EUROCAST 2015, LNCS 9520, pp. 350–358, 2015.
DOI: 10.1007/978-3-319-27340-2_44

is on the integration of ensemble modeling into genetic programming based classification. In this work concepts are presented how to use specific features based on ensemble congruence for achieving new confidence indicators that estimate the trustworthiness of predictions. Based on this work, an analysis of confidence based ensemble estimators for the prediction of several types of cancer was presented in [7].

Especially the approaches using ensembles of symbolic classification models as well as hybrid ensembles coupled with confidence measures based on ensemble congruence are able to achieve convincing results in terms of prediction accuracy for those data samples which are considered trustworthy w.r.t. ensemble confidence. As for example detailed in [7], the best single training model for the prediction of respiratory system cancer could achieve an accuracy of 85.15 % on the test data; the accuracy could be increased to 87.17 % using standard ensemble interpretation based on majority voting. The introduction of ensemble confidence measures based on ensemble congruence lead to an increase of the test accuracy to 96 % while still explaining 60 % of the data. For the remaining 40 % of the data samples, the ensemble congruence was not clear enough; the results for these samples are therefore considered as too uncertain in order to state a confident prediction. The goal of this approach is to present a classification statement only if the congruence of the several hundred ensemble predictors is high enough for stating a decision. This approach denotes a compromise between prediction accuracy and data coverage and seems especially suited for medical data mining.

However, even if the above mentioned approach already leads to satisfying results, there is no differentiation between false positive and false negative predictions, even though this is an important aspect in the field of medical data mining. Especially in the context of data-based pre-screening for cancer prediction, the number of false negative results should be minimized. The main research question stated in this paper is to which extent an ensemble based interpretation of symbolic classification models coupled with confidence analysis is suited to further minimize the ratio of false negative predictions and therefore increase sensitivity. Even more concretely, the research question is, whether or not model ensembles with higher sensitivity on the training data will remain this property when being applied on the test data. Beside this a-posteriori ensemble model selection strategy a new combined evaluation operator is introduced which is based on the normalized mean squared error, but additionally considers sensitivity, in order to guide the hypothesis search already towards more sensitive models already in the model generation phase.

2 Ensemble Modeling

In contrast to the generation of single models for the prediction of a certain output parameter, within ensemble modeling numerous stochastically independent predictors are generated in order to reduce error caused by variance. For classification problems the result of an ensemble prediction is usually stated by a majority decision. Basically, the concept of ensemble modeling can be combined with any machine learning technique that may be used for supervised learning. Figure 1 shows the basic workflow of ensemble model based cancer prediction using blood parameters as inputs. Like in [7] also in this contribution symbolic classification models are used, where the aim of generating stochastically more independent models is supported by using different functional bases (FB1, FB2, and FB3 as stated in Table 2) and different model complexities as stated in Table 1. Table 1 also shows the parameter settings for the offspring selection genetic programming algorithm [8] which has been used for generating the symbolic classification ensemble models.

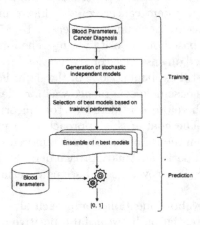

Fig. 1. Basic workflow of ensemble model based cancer prediction.

Like in [6,7] a confidence measure cm has been used based on the clearness of prediction. The confidence measure is based on ensemble clearness where a confidence value of 0.0 indicates that the number of votes for the positive class is equal to the number of votes for the negative class whereas a confidence value of 1.0 indicates that all ensemble members vote for the same class. By claiming a confidence threshold which defines the level of confidence that has to be reached in order to consider a prediction result trustable, the original two-class classification problem is transformed into a three-class interpretation introducing a third class – samples for which the confidence threshold is not reached are considered *uncertain*. The coverage which is reported in the experiments indicates the ratio of samples that can be interpreted as the ensemble clearness exceeds the given confidence threshold.

$$cm := 2 \cdot \left(\frac{|votes(winnerclass)|}{|votes|} - 0.5 \right) \in [0, 1] \tag{1}$$

In addition to the previous works which aimed to use confidence based ensemble interpretation for increasing the accuracy of prediction, the focus of this work

Table 1. Genetic programming parameter configuration

Algorithm	Offspring Selection Genetic Programming
Runs	100 per tree size (with three different tree sizes)
Symbols	+, -, *, /, sin, cos, tan, exp, log, IfThenElse, <, >, and, or, not
TreeCreator	Probabilistic Tree Creator
Fitness function	MSE (mean squared error)
Selector	GenederSpecific (Random, Proportional)
Mutator	ChangeNodeTypeManipulation, FullTreeShaker, One-PointTreeShaker, ReplaceBranchManipulation
Crossover	SubtreeCrossover
Elites	1
Population Size	700
Mutation Rate	20 %
Maximal Generations	1000
Maximal Selection Pressure	100
Cross Validation Folds	5
Tree size (Length/Depth)	20/7
	35/8
	50/10

Table 2. Function symbols

FB1 (original)	+, -, *, /, sin, cos, tan, exp, log, IfThenElse, <, >, and, or, not
FB2	+, -, *, /, IfThenElse (Init = 3), <, >, and, or, not
FB3	IfThenElse, <, >, and, or, not

is to use this approach to increase not only the accuracy but also the sensitivity of the ensemble interpretation. This shall be achieved by selecting the best models not only on the basis of accuracy on training data but also on the basis of a combined measure (accuracy and sensitivity) or just based on sensitivity. The combined measure is implemented as a ranking-based selection of the best models based on the combined measure *accuracy + sensitivity*.

In order to empirically validate or invalidate this assumption, we analyze the behavior of ensemble configurations for the test data.

The empirical discussion for the prediction of breast cancer shows the results achieved on test data based on applying the best 75 models out of the 900 (3 * 3 * 100) models generated by the combination of the 3 different functional bases and the 3 different model complexities. The reported results on the test data have been achieved with 5-fold cross-validation.

Table 3 shows the results that have been achieved by selecting the best 75 models based on training quality for the quality measures accuracy, sensitivity and the combined measure. As can be seen in Table 3 the respective selection criteria on the training data are reflected in the test qualities.

Table 3. Breast cancer ensemble results on the basis of the best 75 out of 900 ensemble models based on training quality.

Criteria	Training			Test		
	Accuracy	Sensitivity	Specificity	Accuracy	Sensitivity	Specificity
Best accuracy	81.87 %	89.79 %	72.53 %	74.36 %	84.29 %	62.65 %
Best sensitivity	76.63 %	95.29 %	54.63 %	74.08 %	92.67 %	52.16 %
Best of both	77.05 %	95.55 %	55.25 %	74.36 %	91.88 %	53.70 %

Table 4. Breast cancer confidence (75 best models from 900 by accuracy)

Confidence	Accuracy	Sensitivity	Specificity	Coverage
0	0.7436261	0.8429319	0.6265432	1
0.1	0.7559524	0.8630137	0.6286645	0.9518414
0.3	0.7834395	0.8786127	0.6666667	0.8895184
0.5	0.8200371	0.8976898	0.720339	0.7634561
0.7	0.8633257	0.9007937	0.8128342	0.621813
0.9	0.9107807	0.9337748	0.8813559	0.3810198
0.95	0.9197861	0.9439252	0.8875	0.2648725
1	0.9333333	0.974026	0.8604651	0.1699717

Tables 4, 5 and 6 show the test results achieved by combining the model selection strategies based on accuracy, sensitivity and the combined measure in combination with confidence interpretation. Also in this more sophisticated analysis it can be seen that the tendency of the model selection strategies based on training results is reflected in the correspondingly reported test qualities. However, as accuracy and sensitivity are basically complementary objectives, the improvements go hand in hand. The first column (confidence) in the corresponding tables states the confidence threshold which has to be surpassed in order to use the result for classification; the last column (coverage) reports the ratio of samples that can still be explained when using the corresponding threshold. Of course the ratio of predictable samples (coverage) decreases while the confidence threshold is increased.

3   Ensemble with Weighted Performance Measures

In contrast to the approach described in Sect. 2, this approach already guides the hypothesis search towards models with a good overall sensitivity. For this

Table 5. Breast cancer confidence (75 best models from 900 by sensitivity)

Confidence	Accuracy	Sensitivity	Specificity	Coverage
0	0.7407932	0.9267016	0.5216049	1
0.1	0.7421203	0.9261214	0.523511	0.9886686
0.3	0.7444279	0.9245283	0.5231788	0.9532578
0.5	0.75	0.9281609	0.5285714	0.8895184
0.7	0.7690909	0.9419355	0.5458333	0.7790368
0.9	0.8387097	0.9598214	0.6068376	0.4830028
0.95	0.9086758	0.9803922	0.7424242	0.3101983
1	0.9347826	0.9705882	0.8333333	0.1954674

Table 6. Breast cancer confidence (75 best models from 900 by accuracy and sensitivity)

Confidence	Accuracy	Sensitivity	Specificity	Coverage
0	0.7436261	0.9188482	0.537037	1
0.1	0.7460545	0.9253333	0.5372671	0.9872521
0.3	0.7530488	0.9220056	0.5488215	0.9291785
0.5	0.7594728	0.9255952	0.5535055	0.8597734
0.7	0.8088803	0.9331104	0.6392694	0.733711
0.9	0.8791209	0.96	0.7346939	0.3866856
0.95	0.9105263	0.969697	0.7758621	0.2691218
1	0.9126214	0.9726027	0.7666667	0.1458924

purpose the Weighted Performance Measure Evaluator – a special genetic programming fitness evaluator was implemented. Besides considering a normalized mean squared error, this evaluator also takes the false negative and false positive rate of the symbolic classification model into account. To each of the 3 measures a weight needs to be assigned. The model fitness is calculated as followed:

$$fitness := NMSE * weight_{NMSE} + FNR * weight_{FNR} + FPR * weight_{FPR}$$

In order to increase the sensitivity, the false negative rate needs to be minimized. Table 7 shows the ensemble results achieved by applying this method on 300 models with 3 different complexities using functional basis 1 with the following weights:

- NMSE: 1
- FNR: 0.2
- FPR: 0

Table 7. Breast cancer ensemble results on the basis of the best 75 out of 300 ensemble models based on training quality of the weighted performance measure.

Criteria	Training			Test		
	Accuracy	Sensitivity	Specificity	Accuracy	Sensitivity	Specificity
Best accuracy	76.91 %	73.51 %	96.34 %	92.67 %	54.01 %	50.93
Best sensitivity	76.06 %	72.38 %	98.17 %	94.76 %	50 %	45.99
Best of both	77.05 %	73.23 %	97.38 %	93.72 %	53.09 %	49.07

Table 8. Breast cancer confidence with weighted performance measures (75 best models from 300 by accuracy)

Confidence	Accuracy	Sensitivity	Specificity	Coverage
0	0.7351275	0.9267016	0.5092593	1
0.1	0.7357143	0.9267016	0.5062893	0.9915014
0.3	0.743025	0.9413333	0.5	0.9645892
0.5	0.7461774	0.9430894	0.4912281	0.9263456
0.7	0.7562189	0.9602273	0.4701195	0.8541076
0.9	0.7472767	0.9829352	0.3313253	0.6501416
0.95	0.7690058	0.9873418	0.2761905	0.4844193
1	0.8024194	0.9945946	0.2380952	0.3512748

Table 9. Breast cancer confidence with weighted performance measures (75 best models from 300 by sensitivity)

Confidence	Accuracy	Sensitivity	Specificity	Coverage
0	0.723796	0.947644	0.4598765	1
0.1	0.7202899	0.9472296	0.4437299	0.9773371
0.3	0.7250384	0.9569892	0.4157706	0.9220963
0.5	0.720268	0.967033	0.3347639	0.8456091
0.7	0.7226415	0.9884726	0.2185792	0.7507082
0.9	0.7116279	1	0.05343511	0.6090652
0.95	0.7245179	1	0	0.5141643
1	0.7537313	1	0	0.3796034

For the ensemble the best 75 models have been selected based on their training performance regarding accuracy and sensitivity. Tables 8, 9 and 10 show the test performance using confidence thresholds. The accuracy and sensitivity could be further improved at the expense of specificity and coverage.

Table 10. Breast cancer confidence with weighted performance measures (75 best models from 300 by accuracy and sensitivity)

Confidence	Accuracy	Sensitivity	Specificity	Coverage
0	0.7322946	0.9371728	0.4907407	1
0.1	0.7339056	0.939314	0.490625	0.990085
0.3	0.7385524	0.944	0.4834437	0.9589235
0.5	0.7407407	0.9538043	0.4607143	0.917847
0.7	0.7487002	0.977208	0.3938053	0.8172805
0.9	0.7342342	0.9869281	0.173913	0.6288952
0.95	0.7472222	0.992278	0.1188119	0.509915
1	0.8047809	1	0.09259259	0.3555241

4   Conclusion and Future Perspectives

In this contribution new ensemble techniques based on symbolic classification have been introduced in order to increase the sensitivity of diagnosis prediction for breast cancer. In order to increase sensitivity two approaches have been considered: The first approach selects more sensitive models based on training sensitivity and analyzes the properties on the test data. However, the training models have been learned using normalized mean squared error evaluation which basically supports accuracy. The second approach introduces a new combined evaluator which aims to lead the hypothesis search towards more sensitive models. The results indicate that both strategies are capable to find more sensitive predictors. The results further show the properties of the described strategies for breast cancer; preliminary results which have recently been generated also for respiratory system cancer and melanoma show very similar behavior and shall be further considered in future studies and publications.

References

1. Lavrač, N.: Machine learning for data mining in medicine. In: Horn, W., Shahar, Y., Lindberg, G., Andreassen, S., Wyatt, J.C. (eds.) AIMDM 1999. LNCS (LNAI), vol. 1620, pp. 47–62. Springer, Heidelberg (1999)
2. Winkler, S., Affenzeller, M., Wagner, S.: Using enhanced genetic programming techniques for evolving classifiers in the context of medical diagnosis - an empirical study. Genet. Program. Evolvable Mach. **10**(2), 111–140 (2009)
3. Bache, K., Lichman, M.: UCI machine learning repository. http://archive.ics.uci.edu/ml (2013)
4. Winkler, S., Affenzeller, M., Stekel, H.: Evolutionary identification of cancer predictors using clustered data: a case study for breast cancer, melanoma, and cancer in the respiratory system. In: Proceedings of the GECCO 2009 Workshop on Medical Applications of Genetic and Evolutionary Computation (MedGEC 2006), pp. 1463–1470. Association for Computing Machinery (ACM) (2009)

5. Winkler, S., Jacak, M.A.W., Stekel, H.: Identification of cancer diagnosis estimation models using evolutionary algorithms - a case study for breast cancer, melanoma, and cancer in the respiratory system. In: Proceedings of the Genetic and Evolutionary Computation Conference GECCO 2010 (2011)
6. Affenzeller, M., Winkler, S.M., Forstenlechner, S., Kronberger, G., Kommenda, M., Wagner, S., Stekel, H.: Enhanced confidence interpretations of GP based ensemble modeling results. In: Jimenez, E., Sokolov, B. (eds.) The 24th European Modeling and Simulation Symposium, EMSS 2012, Vienna, Austria, 19–21 September 2012, pp. 340–345 (2012)
7. Affenzeller, M., Winkler, S.M., Stekel, H., Forstenlechner, S., Wagner, S.: Improving the accuracy of cancer prediction by ensemble confidence evaluation. In: Moreno-Díaz, R., Pichler, F., Quesada-Arencibia, A. (eds.) EUROCAST. LNCS, vol. 8111, pp. 316–323. Springer, Heidelberg (2013)
8. Affenzeller, M., Wagner, S.: Offspring selection: a new self-adaptive selection scheme for genetic algorithms. In: Ribeiro, B., Albrecht, R.F., Dobnikar, A., Pearson, D.W., Steele, N.C. (eds.) Adaptive and Natural Computing Algorithms, pp. 218–221. Springer, Vienna (2005)

Optimization Strategies for Integrated Knapsack and Traveling Salesman Problems

Andreas Beham[1,2]([✉]), Judith Fechter[1,2], Michael Kommenda[1,2],
Stefan Wagner[1], Stephan M. Winkler[1], and Michael Affenzeller[1,2]

[1] Heuristic and Evolutionary Algorithms Laboratory School of Informatics,
Communications and Media, University of Applied Sciences Upper Austria,
Hagenberg Campus, Softwarepark 11, 4232 Hagenberg, Austria
{andreas.beham,judith.fechter,michael.kommenda,stefan.wagner,
stephan.winkler,michael.affenzeller}@fh-hagenberg.at
[2] Institute for Formal Models and Verification, Johannes Kepler University Linz,
Altenberger Straße 69, 4040 Linz, Austria

Abstract. In the optimization of real-world activities the effects of solutions on related activities need to be considered. The use of isolated problem models that do not adequately consider related processes does not allow addressing system-wide consequences. However, sometimes the complexity of the real-world model and its interplay with related activities can be described by a combination of simple, existing, problems. In this work we aim to discuss strategies to combine existing algorithms for simple problems in order to solve a more complex master problem. New challenges arise in such an integrated optimization approach.

1 Introduction and Literature Review

The orienteering problem (OP) can be seen as a combination between the knapsack problem (KP) and the travelling salesperson problem (TSP) [1]. The traveling thief problem (TTP) is a similar combination of the TSP and the KP, but interleaves the two sub-problems to a higher degree [2]. Another problem is the knapsack constrained profitable tour problem (KCPTP) [3] that also combines a KP and a TSP.

In contrast to solving these problems with specialized algorithms or solution manipulation operators it is worthwhile to consider combining existing algorithms and studying the necessary interaction patterns that lead to good solutions in short time. Instead of solving the master, also denoted as integrated problem, several solvers are employed to obtain solutions to sub-problems. These solutions are called partial or sub-solutions to the master or integrated solution.

Past approaches that have to be mentioned include cooperative co-evolution [4] where the partitioning of problems has been used as a major tool. However, the problems in co-evolution are still tightly coupled within the variation loop of a genetic algorithm. The interaction between more specialized solvers for the sub-problems is not considered.

© Springer International Publishing Switzerland 2015
R. Moreno-Díaz et al. (Eds.): EUROCAST 2015, LNCS 9520, pp. 359–366, 2015.
DOI: 10.1007/978-3-319-27340-2_45

From a mathematical programming point, top-down approaches such as problem decomposition have to be mentioned. The application of Lagrangian decomposition on a mathematical formulation of the integrated problem allows splitting it into two sub-problems [3,5]. Such a closed form mathematical formulation is not always possible however. We will perform a Lagrangian decomposition of the KCPTP next in order to derive an idea for a more general methodology.

1.1 Lagrange Decomposition

A description of the KCPTP model is given in Eqs. (1) to (5).

$$\text{KCPTP: } \max \sum_{i=1}^{n} y_i * p_i - t * \sum_{j=i+1}^{n} x_{ij} * d_{ij} \tag{1}$$

$$\sum_{i=1}^{n} y_i * w_i \leq K \tag{2}$$

$$\sum_{i=1}^{n} x_{ij} + \sum_{k=1}^{n} x_{jk} = 2 * y_j \quad \forall_j \in [1..n] \tag{3}$$

$$x \text{ has exactly one subtour} \tag{4}$$

$$y_1 = 1, y_i, x_{ij} \in 0, 1 \tag{5}$$

Constraint (2) is the knapsack constraint that limits the number of visited cities. By applying Langrangian decomposition y_i in Eq. (2) is substituted with a new decision variable z_i and a new equality constraint is added $y_i = z_i$ which is then again relaxed using Lagrangian multipliers λ. By rearranging the sums the objective function may be split with λ being a shared variable. The decomposed sub-problems are given in Eqs. (6) to (12).

$$\text{KCPTP-LD-PTP}(\lambda): \quad \max \sum_{i=1}^{n} y_i * (p_i - \lambda_i) - t * \sum_{j=i+1}^{n} x_{ij} * d_{ij} \tag{6}$$

$$\sum_{i=1}^{n} x_{ij} + \sum_{k=1}^{n} x_{jk} = 2 * y_j \quad \forall_j \in [1..n] \tag{7}$$

$$x \quad \text{has exactly one subtour} \tag{8}$$

$$y_1 = 1, y_i, x_{ij} \in 0, 1 \tag{9}$$

$$\text{KCPTP-LD-KP}(\lambda): \quad \max \sum_{i=1}^{n} \lambda_i z_i \tag{10}$$

$$\sum_{i=1}^{n} z_i * w_i \leq K \tag{11}$$

$$z_1 = 1, z_i \in 0, 1 \tag{12}$$

The master problem in form of the Lagrange dual problem given in Eqs. (13) to (14) then is to optimize λ such that the sum of the optimal solutions which is given by function ν to these two problems becomes minimal. This problem is piecewise linear and can be solved using a sub-gradient approach [5].

$$\text{KCPTP-LD:} \quad \min \quad \nu(\text{KCPTP-LD-KP}(\lambda)) + \nu(\text{KCPTP-LD-PTP}(\lambda)) \qquad (13)$$

$$\lambda_i \in \mathbb{R}^+ \qquad (14)$$

2   A General Integrated Optimization Methodology

While Lagrange decomposition is a very useful concept, it becomes apparent that we cannot achieve a reduction to the TSP as we intended, but still have to solve the rather complex PTP, albeit without knapsack constraint. Furthermore, in Lagrangian decomposition the requirement is to solve sub-problems optimally in order to calculate the objective of the Lagrange dual problem. Combining this decomposition with heuristic approaches seems difficult or even impossible to achieve.

Still, we can use the hint that λ can be seen as a control parameter that adjusts the profits in the individual sub-problems. Generalizing this rather strict approach it seems feasible to assume that we may alter inputs such as profits so as to obtain solutions that are "good" with respect to the sub-problems *and* with respect to the master problem. In defining a rather general variegation strategy for sub-problem inputs we can come to a general methodology for solving integrated problems. Two slightly different approaches shall be presented first.

Sequential Approach: In the sequential approach sub-problems can be ordered such that the solution of one sub-problem describes restrictions to another problem. For example, in the KCPTP solutions to the KP limit the problem space of the TSP as only those customers need to be routed which have been selected. The integration between master and subordinate solver can be *tight* in that for every solution to the master problem a sub-problem needs to be solved or *loose* in that the master problem is solved and only for the best solution the problem reduction is performed and the subordinate solver is launched (Fig. 1).

Cooperative Approach: In the cooperative approach, both problems are optimized concurrently, but the solvers are collaborating with each other. Collaboration could be *tight*, in that solvers exchange solutions during their search or *loose* in that the final results of solvers are used to parameterize the problems for a new optimization run. In the KCPTP, for example the solver for the KP can use a tour through all customers as a frame to evaluate the tour length on the subset of customers actually picked (Fig. 2).

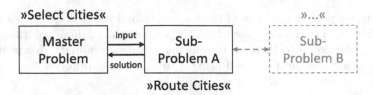

Fig. 1. Sequential approach

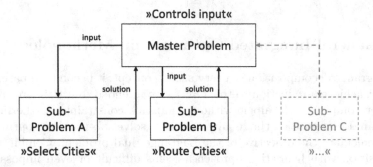

Fig. 2. Cooperative approach

2.1   Orchestration of Solvers

As mentioned before for this approach to work well, it is required to control the subordinate solvers. For simple problems usually a number of methods are available such as problem-specific heuristics, metaheuristics, or exact approaches. But not in all cases is it useful to employ exact approaches or complex metaheuristics. It is not guaranteed that an optimal solution to a certain sub-problem instance can be integrated well into a solution to the master problem. The difficult part is to tune the sub-problem instances such that good solutions thereof align with good integrated solutions. Such a tuning can be thought of as an orchestration of solvers where two decisions have to be made.

(A) *Solution Effort* - The effort with which the sub-problems are to be solved. For example, sub-problems that do not show to have a large impact on the master objective should be solved with less computational effort compared to sub-problems that have a very high impact.

(B) *Sub-problem Variegation* - When the sub-problem landscape shows optima that are very bad for the integrated problem, the instance of the sub-problem needs to be altered in order to obtain solutions that are suitable for both master and sub-problem.

In this work we will not yet treat the first topic of deciding solution effort and use simple local search techniques to solve the sub-problems. But the second topic of variegating the sub-problem instances will be discussed in the following sections.

2.2   Sub-problem Input Variegation

The adjustment of the sub-problems' inputs can be seen as a change of the fitness landscapes with the goal to align it with the landscape of the master problem. Figure 3 attempts to sketch this idea schematically. A simple example shall further elaborate this idea: A remote, but profitable customer with low weight in a KCPTP is naturally attractive to be included in a knapsack solution. But on the other hand, servicing that customer requires to perform a larger detour. In a situation where travel costs are higher than the value of the detour an adjustment of this customer's profit will direct the knapsack solver to visit different customers.

The alignment between fitness landscapes can be seen as an optimization problem and has to be solved by a coordinating agent. In the case of Lagrangian decomposition such an "agent" would be the sub-gradient approach. However, in general for integrated problems sub-gradients are not available. Hence, a different measurement of the quality of such an input configuration is necessary.

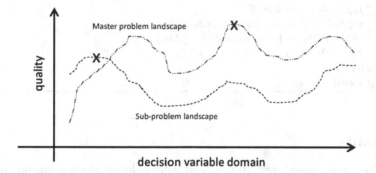

Fig. 3. A simplified schematic drawing of the sub-problem landscape given the master problem's objective function with all other partial solutions fixed compared to the sub-problem's landscape. The example should illustrate that some local optima are well aligned, but the global optimum still leads to inferior solutions for the master problem.

The evaluation of some candidate input can be performed by applying a subordinate solver to the sub-problem and evaluate the obtained partial solution using the master problem's objective function (in combination with other partial solutions). This can then be seen as a fitness for the sub-problem's inputs. But while this approach is simple, the downside is that only the resulting solution, e.g. a local optimum, is used and the shapes of the landscapes are ignored. Another approach would be to compare a range of solutions obtained during the search from worse ones to better ones and calculate a correlation coefficient such as Spearman's rank correlation between sub-problem and master problem objective. The correlation coefficient can then be used as a measurement between the alignment of the two landscapes and therefore as a fitness for the actual sub-problem's inputs.

2.3   Algorithms

Algorithm 1 describes a loosely coupled sequential approach that includes the above mentioned input variegation. The coordinating agent requires four methods that *Reduce a problem* based on a solution as input, *Expand a solution* of a reduced problem to the original inputs, that *Evaluate* the master objective given the partial solutions and that *Variegate* the inputs of. Both reduction, expansion and variegation are only concerned with the type of the sub-problems and may be independent of whether the KCPTP, the OP, or the TTP is solved. *Evaluate* however is specific to the concrete master problem and contains the implementation of the master objective.

Algorithm 1. Pseudocode of a sequential integrated solver

1: **procedure** SOLVE($KpSolver, TspSolver$)
2:      $kp, kp' \leftarrow$ InitializeKp()
3:      **for** $iter = 0$ To $MaxIter$ **do**
4:          $kpSol \leftarrow KpSolver$.Solve($kp'$)
5:          $tsp \leftarrow$ Reduce($kpSol$)
6:          $tspSol \leftarrow Expand(TspSolver$.Solve($tsp$))
7:          $masterObj \leftarrow$ Evaluate($kpSol, tspSol$)
8:          $kp' \leftarrow$ Variegate($kp, masterObj$)
9:      **end for**
10: **end procedure**

---

3   Results

All results are averaged over 10 runs and were calculated on a laptop equipped with a 3rd generation Intel Core i7 running at 2.6 Ghz. Only a single core was used in all tests. Results are computed for some instances of the KCPTP, OP, and the TTP. For the KCPTP we used benchmark instances for orienteering problems that originally only specified a profit per location [6,7]. The weights for the knapsack were generated to be correlated to the profits using Eq. (15) where $U(0,1)$ returns a random number in the interval $[0,1)$. The maximum size of the knapsack has been calculated using Eq. (16). The transport cost factor for each instance has been scaled in a geometric progression between minimum and maximum profit to distance ratio for a total of 6 different variants per instance and results have been averaged. For the TTP, we relaxed the constraints of having to visit all locations and visit only the locations where something is actually stolen.

$$w_i = T_{max} * (0.1 + U(0,1) * 0.8 * \frac{p_i - \min(p)}{\max(p) - \min(p)}) \tag{15}$$

$$K = (0.2 + U(0,1) * 0.6) * \sum_i^n w_i \tag{16}$$

Table 1. Results of the sequential approach applied to several instances of the KCPTP and TTP problems.

KCPTP instances	With variegation			Without variegation		
	Avg	StdDev	[sec]	Avg	StdDev	[sec]
chao64.set_64_1_25	**701.1**	9.7	1.3	698.7	7.2	0.7
chao64.set_64_1_50	**856.2**	9.2	1.5	849.5	6.3	1.0
chao64.set_64_1_80	**801.7**	6.9	1.5	799.1	5.2	0.9
tsi1.budget_15	**11.2**	5.1	0.4	8.6	4.2	0.1
tsi1.budget_30	**16.2**	5.1	0.4	11.5	4.1	0.1
tsi1.budget_60	**39.3**	4.4	0.5	30.6	3.1	0.3
OP instances	Avg	StdDev	[sec]	Avg	StdDev	[sec]
chao64.set_64_1_25	**109.2**	22.9	5.0	-	-	0.5
chao64.set_64_1_50	382.2	37.4	0.2	**445.2**	10.9	0.2
chao64.set_64_1_80	**501.6**	11.4	0.4	492.6	9.6	0.3
tsi1.budget_15	-	-	1.1	-	-	0.2
tsi1.budget_30	**57.0**	11.8	0.7	-	-	0.2
tsi1.budget_60	141.5	21.4	0.1	**175.5**	2.8	0.2
TTP instances berlin52_n51	Avg	StdDev	[sec]	Avg	StdDev	[sec]
bounded-strongly-corr_01-10	**15269.5**	529.7	1.0	14246.9	505.3	0.6
uncorr-similar-weights_01-10	**7934.2**	269.6	1.0	5476.9	329.7	0.5
uncorr_01-10	**8777.0**	405.3	1.0	5559.1	422.5	0.5

The results in Table 1 show that the variegation of input is beneficial for the search when using the same algorithm. For the OP, also the knapsack weights were variegated in order to achieve more feasible solutions. Still, constraint variegation still needs to be improved as the results indicate. The difference in runtime can be explained by the variegation strategy that employed a CMA-ES algorithm to modify the profit vector. Both times the same number of iterations were given. While the results for the KCPTP do not convince as much, the results for the TTP show that input variegation actually makes a significant difference and that an adjustment of the sub-problem's fitness landscapes is necessary to deliver better results for the master problem.

4   Conclusions and Future Work

In this work we discussed a general methodology for solving integrated problems. We showed that complex problems that consist of simpler sub-problems can be decomposed using Lagrange decomposition. We also discussed the disadvantage of these techniques in the requirement of exact solution approaches and went on to present a more general methodology for solving integrated problems. Thoughts have been presented on how a variegation of the sub-problem's inputs is able to shift the sub-problem's fitness landscape so that it aligns with the fitness landscape of the master problem. This more general methodology may be applied between arbitrary combinations of sub-problems and is not limited to closed-form mathematical descriptions. First results have shown that the variegation is indeed beneficial for the search. The acceptance of this approach will certainly depend on the simplicity of its use. But to be successful, it must be considerably simpler than the development of a new algorithm for solving a new complex problem while still achieving competitive results.

Acknowledgments. The work described in this paper was done within the COMET Project Heuristic Optimization in Production and Logistics (HOPL), #843532 funded by the Austrian Research Promotion Agency (FFG).

References

1. Vansteenwegen, P., Souffriau, W., Oudheusden, D.V.: The orienteering problem: a survey. Eur. J. Oper. Res. **209**, 1–10 (2011)
2. Polyakovskiy, S., Bonyadi, M.R., Wagner, M., Michalewicz, Z., Neumann, F.: A comprehensive benchmark set and heuristics for the traveling thief problem. In: Genetic and Evolutionary Computation Conference, GECCO 2014, Vancouver, BC, Canada, pp. 477–484 (2014)
3. Feillet, D., Dejax, P., Gendreau, M.: Traveling salesman problems with profits: an overview. Transp. Sci. **39**, 188–205 (2001)
4. Potter, M.A., De Jong, K.A.: A cooperative coevolutionary approach to function optimization. In: Davidor, Y., Männer, R., Schwefel, H.-P. (eds.) PPSN 1994. LNCS, vol. 866, pp. 249–257. Springer, Heidelberg (1994)
5. Pirkwieser, S., Raidl, G.R., Puchinger, J.: Combining lagrangian decomposition with an evolutionary algorithm for the knapsack constrained maximum spanning tree problem. In: Cotta, C., van Hemert, J. (eds.) EvoCOP 2007. LNCS, vol. 4446, pp. 176–187. Springer, Heidelberg (2007)
6. Chao, I.M., Golden, B.L., Wasil, E.A.: A fast and effective heuristic for the orienteering problem. Eur. J. Oper. Res. **88**, 475–489 (1996)
7. Tsiligirides, T.: Heuristic methods applied to orienteering. J. Oper. Res. Soc. **35**, 797–809 (1984)

On the Effectiveness of Genetic Operations in Symbolic Regression

Bogdan Burlacu[1,2]([✉]), Michael Affenzeller[1,2], and Michael Kommenda[1,2]

[1] Heuristic and Evolutionary Algorithms Laboratory School of Informatics,
Communications and Media, University of Applied Sciences Upper Austria,
Softwarepark 11, 4232 Hagenberg, Austria
{bogdan.burlacu,michael.affenzeller,michael.kommenda}@fh-hagenberg.at
[2] Institute for Formal Models and Verification, Johannes Kepler University Linz,
Altenbergerstr. 69, 4040 Linz, Austria

Abstract. This paper describes a methodology for analyzing the evolutionary dynamics of genetic programming (GP) using genealogical information, diversity measures and information about the fitness variation from parent to offspring. We introduce a new subtree tracing approach for identifying the origins of genes in the structure of individuals, and we show that only a small fraction of ancestor individuals are responsible for the evolvement of the best solutions in the population.

Keywords: Genetic programming · Evolutionary dynamics · Algorithm analysis · Symbolic regression

1 Introduction

Empirical analysis in the context of different benchmark problems and tentative algorithmic improvements (such as various selection schemes or fitness assignment techniques) has a limited ability of explaining genetic programming (GP) behavior and dynamics. Results usually confirm our intuitions about the relationship between selection pressure, diversity, fitness landscapes and genetic operators, but they prove difficult to extend to more general theories about the internal functioning of GP.

This work is motivated by the necessity for a different approach to study the GP evolutionary process. Instead of looking for correlations between different selection or fitness assignment mechanisms and solution quality or diversity, we focus on the reproduction process itself and the effectiveness of the variation-producing operators in transferring genetic material.

Achieving good solutions depends on the efficient use of the available gene pool given its inherent stochasticity (random initialization, random crossover, random mutation). Under the effects of selection pressure, many suboptimal exchanges of genetic information will cause a decrease in the amount of genetic material available to the evolutionary engine. Measures to mitigate this phenomenon usually use various heuristics for guiding either selection or the crossover operator towards more promising regions of the search space [1,2].

© Springer International Publishing Switzerland 2015
R. Moreno-Díaz et al. (Eds.): EUROCAST 2015, LNCS 9520, pp. 367–374, 2015.
DOI: 10.1007/978-3-319-27340-2_46

Diversity is an important aspect of GP, considered to be a key factor in its performance. Multiple studies dedicated to GP diversity analyze diversity measures (based on various distance metrics, for example [3]) in correlation with the effects of genetic operators [4–6]. Genotype operations – crossover in particular – often have a negative (or at most, neutral) effect on individuals, leading to diversity loss in the population following each selection step. This effect is due to the interplay between crossover and selection which leads to an increase in average program size [7] (when sampling larger programs, crossover has a higher chance of having a neutral effect).

2   Methodology

In this paper we introduce a new methodology for the exact identification ("tracing") of any structural change an individual is subjected to during evolution. We use this methodology in combination with population diversity and genealogy analysis methods to investigate the effects of the genetic operators in terms of how often they lead to a fitness improvement, how often they overlap (for example when the same area inside the tree is repeatedly targeted by crossover), and how often they cancel each other out.

2.1   Tracing of Genotype Fragments

This method is based on previous work on population genealogies [8,9]. During the algorithm run, every new generation is added to the genealogy graph with arcs connecting child vertices to their parents. When crossover is followed by mutation, both the results of crossover and mutation are saved in the graph (Fig. 1).

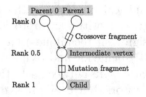

We define an individual's *trace graph* as a collection of vertices representing its ancestors from which the various parts of its genotype originated, connected by a collection of arcs representing the different genotype operations that gradually assembled those parts.

The tracing procedure uses a set of simple arithmetic rules to navigate genealogies and identify the relevant subtrees, based on the indices of the subtree to be traced and the index of the received fragment

Fig. 1. Saving intermediate results in the genealogy graph

(Fig. 2). The nodes in each tree are numbered according to their preorder index i such that, given two subtrees A and B, $B \subset A$ if $i_A < i_B < i_A + l_A$, where i_A, i_B are their respective preorder indices and l_A, l_B are their lengths.

Since some individuals within the ancestry of the traced individual may have contributed parts of their genotype to multiple offspring, there may exist multiple evolutionary trajectories in the trace graph passing through the same vertex or sequence of vertices, reflected in the graph by multiple arcs between the same two vertices, each arc representing the transmission of different genes or building blocks.

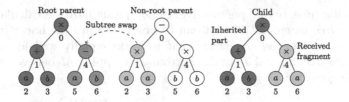

Fig. 2. Preorder arithmetics for subtree inclusion

2.2 Analysis of Population Dynamics

The various measurements used to quantify the behavioral aspects of GP are described in more detail within the following paragraphs.

Genetic Operator Effectiveness. Operator effectiveness is calculated as the difference in fitness between the child and its root parent.

Average Fitness Improvement. Let N be the total number of individuals in the population, t_i one individual and p_i its parent:

$$\bar{q} = \frac{1}{N} \cdot \sum_{i=1}^{N} \left(Fitness(t_i) - Fitness(p_i) \right)$$

Best Fitness Improvement. Return the difference between the fitness values of the best individual t_{best} and its parent p_{best}

$$q_{best} = Fitness(t_{best}) - Fitness(p_{best})$$

The average and best fitness improvements are calculated individually for crossover and mutation operations.

Average Relative Overlap. We define the relative overlap between two sets A_1 and A_2 using the Sørensen-Dice coefficient[1] which can also be seen as a similarity measure between sets:

$$s(A_1, A_2) = \frac{2 \cdot |A_1 \cap A_2|}{|A_1| + |A_2|}$$

The reason for using this measure is to see how much overlap exists between the trace graphs and root lineages of the individuals in the population. A high relative overlap would mean that diversity is exhausted as all the individuals have the same parents or ancestors.

Genotype and Phenotype Similarity. These similarity measures provide information about the evolution of diversity from both a structural (genotype)

---

[1] It was also possible to use the *Jaccard index* $J(A_1, A_2) = \frac{|A_1 \cap A_2|}{|A_1 \cup A_2|}$ as it is very similar to the Sørensen-Dice coefficient. However this choice makes no practical difference for the results presented in this publication.

and a semantic (phenotype) perspective. Genotype similarity is calculated using a *bottom-up tree mapping* [10] that can be computed in time linear in the size of the trees and has the advantage that it works equally well for unordered trees. For two trees T_1 and T_2 and a bottom-up mapping M between them, the similarity is given by:

$$GenotypeSimilarity(T_1, T_2) = \frac{2 \cdot |M|}{|T_1| + |T_2|}$$

Phenotype similarity between two trees is calculated as the Pearson R^2 correlation coefficient between their respective output values on the training data.

Contribution Ratio. While it is clear that under the influence of random evolutionary forces (such as genetic drift or hitchhiking) each of an individual's ancestors plays an equally important role in the events leading to its creation, the trace graph represents a powerful tool for analyzing the origin of genes and the way solutions are assembled by the genetic algorithm.

The size of the trace graph relative to the size of the complete ancestry can be used as a measure of the effort spent by the algorithm to achieve useful adaptation. For example, a small trace graph means that a small number of an individual's ancestors contributed to the assembly of its genotype, via an equally small number of genetic operations (crossover and mutation). The effort, seen as the ratio of effective genetic operations over the total number of genetic operations, can give an indication of how easy new and better solutions can be assembled by the algorithm.

The contribution ratio r is given by the percentage of individuals from the best solution ancestry that had an actual contribution to its structure:

$$r = \frac{|Trace(\text{bestSolution})|}{|Ancestry(\text{bestSolution})|}$$

3   Experiments

For the experimental part, we use GP to solve two symbolic regression benchmark problems:

Vladislavleva-8

$$F_8(x_1, x_2) = \frac{(x_1 - 3)^4 + (x_2 - 3)^3 - (x_2 - 3)}{(x_2 - 2)^4 + 10}$$

Poly-10

$$F(\mathbf{x}) = x_1 x_2 + x_3 x_4 + x_5 x_6 + x_1 x_7 x_9 + x_3 x_6 x_{10}$$

The Vladislavleva-8 problem was solved using the standard GP algorithm (SGP) with a population size of 500 individuals and 50 generations (in order to be able to compute the trace graphs of each individual in the population in feasible time). For the Poly-10 problem the offspring selection GP (OSGP) [11]

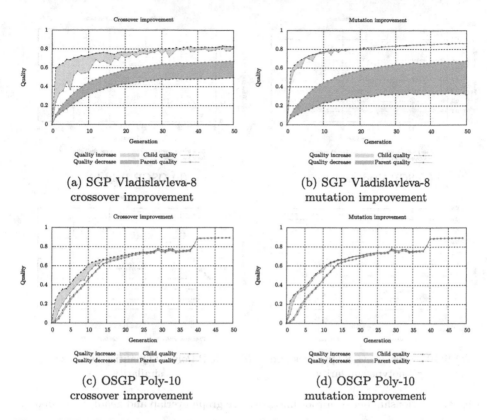

Fig. 3. SGP Vladislavleva-8 and Poly-10 best (above) and average (below) operator improvement

was also tested with a population size of 300 individuals and gender-specific selection.

We analyzed the algorithm dynamics using the genealogy graph, the ancestry of the best solution and the trace history of its genotype. Other additional measurements such as diversity, size and quality distributions were included for a more complete picture. All the results were averaged on a collection of 20 algorithmic runs for each problem and algorithm configuration.

In the case of SGP, we see in Fig. 3 that the genetic operators produce negative improvement on average, meaning that in most cases the fitness of the child is worse than the fitness of the parent. The light-colored curves filled with green in Fig. 3 represent the best improvement while the dark-colored once filled with red represent the average improvement. As average fitness improvement produced by genetic operators tends to be negative, the increase in average population fitness can be attributed to the interplay between recombination operators and selection. OSGP operator improvement is always small but positive due to the requirement that offspring are better than their parents.

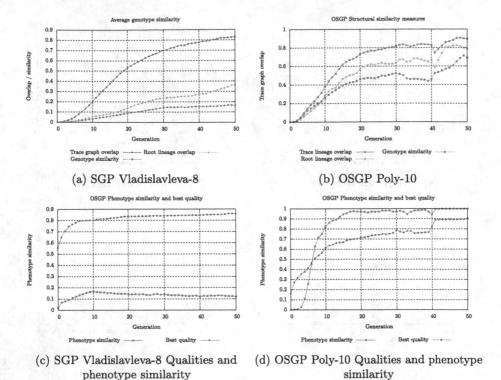

(a) SGP Vladislavleva-8

(b) OSGP Poly-10

(c) SGP Vladislavleva-8 Qualities and phenotype similarity

(d) OSGP Poly-10 Qualities and phenotype similarity

Fig. 4. Relationship between root lineage/trace graph overlap and genotype similarity

The ability to produce useful genetic variation (leading to fitness improvements) is directly related to the structural diversity of the population which cannot be controlled through fitness-based selection. Results in Fig. 4a and b reveal the relationship mediated by the selection mechanism between the structural similarity between two trees and the degree to which their root lineages and their trace graphs overlap. The high correlation (calculated as the Pearson R^2 coefficient) between the three curves corresponds intuitively to the fact that similar individuals come from similar (partially overlapping) lineages, with the important difference that trace graphs do not represent lineages in the strictest sense, as they only include those ancestors whose genes survived in the structure of the traced individual. In Fig. 4c and d we show the correlation between semantic similarity and quality of the best solution. We see that SGP does not suffer from loss of semantic diversity. With offspring selection, as children are required to outperform their parents, the semantic similarity increases rapidly to a value close to 1.

Another aspect of GP search is illustrated in Fig. 5a, where we can observe the exploratory behavior of the OSGP algorithm in the beginning of the run, when the building blocks representing the terms of the formula are gradually discovered, and the exploitative behavior towards the end, when no big jumps in

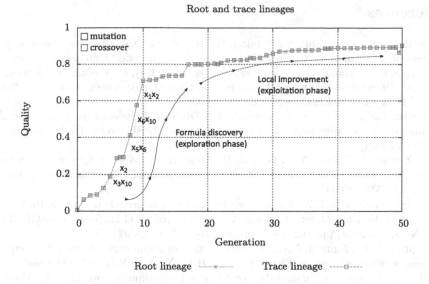

Fig. 5. (a) OSGP Poly-10 best solution (the term x_3x_4 was already present in the initial formula)

quality are produced, but the solution is incrementally improved through small changes of the tree constants and variable weighting factors.

Finally, the contribution ratio for SGP and OSGP was calculated at 13 % and 4 %, respectively, showing a high degree of interrelatedness between individuals which leads to low genetic operator efficiency. Fit individuals contribute multiple times, but selection pressure exceeds their variability potential. Offspring selection improves efficiency by adapting selection pressure.

4 Conclusion and Outlook

Our results show that in most cases GP operators do not lead to fitness improvement. The tracing of the best solution indicates that a few critical operations when the algorithm is able to assemble high fitness solution elements out of pre-existing, disparate genes are responsible for the performance of the entire run. A significantly small fraction (around 13 % for SGP and 4 % for OSGP) of all ancestors of the best individual have an actual contribution to its final structure.

The tracing methodology can reveal interesting and previously unexplored aspects of GP evolution regarding genetic operators and their effects on population dynamics. In contrast to other methods and techniques, our approach provides a more accurate and complete description of the evolutionary process.

Acknowledgments. The work described in this paper was done within the COMET Project Heuristic Optimization in Production and Logistics (HOPL), #843532 funded by the Austrian Research Promotion Agency (FFG).

References

1. Burke, E.K., Gustafson, S., Kendall, G., Krasnogor, N.: Is increased diversity in genetic programming beneficial? An analysis of the effects on performance. In: Sarker, R., Reynolds, R., Abbass, H., Tan, K.C., McKay, B., Essam, D., Gedeon, T. (eds.) Proceedings of the 2003 Congress on Evolutionary Computation CEC2003, pp. 1398–1405. IEEE Press, Canberra (2003)
2. Burke, E.K., Gustafson, S., Kendall, G.: Diversity in genetic programming: An analysis of measures and correlation with fitness. IEEE Trans. Evol. Comput. **8**, 47–62 (2004)
3. Mattiussi, C., Waibel, M., Floreano, D.: Measures of diversity for populations and distances between individuals with highly reorganizable genomes. Evol. Comput. **12**, 495–515 (2004)
4. Ekárt, A., Németh, S.Z.: Maintaining the diversity of genetic programs. In: Foster, J.A., Lutton, E., Miller, J., Ryan, C., Tettamanzi, A.G.B. (eds.) EuroGP 2002. LNCS, vol. 2278, pp. 162–171. Springer, Heidelberg (2002)
5. Nguyen, T.H., Nguyen, X.H.: A brief overview of population diversity measures in genetic programming. In: Pham, T.L., Le, H.K., Nguyen, X.H. (eds.) Proceedings of the Third Asian-Pacific workshop on Genetic Programming, pp. 128–139. Military Technical Academy, Hanoi, VietNam (2006)
6. Jackson, D.: Phenotypic diversity in initial genetic programming populations. In: Esparcia-Alcázar, A.I., Ekárt, A., Silva, S., Dignum, S., Uyar, A.Ş. (eds.) EuroGP 2010. LNCS, vol. 6021, pp. 98–109. Springer, Heidelberg (2010)
7. Dignum, S., Poli, R.: Crossover, sampling, bloat and the harmful effects of size limits. In: O'Neill, M., Vanneschi, L., Gustafson, S., Esparcia Alcázar, A.I., De Falco, I., Della Cioppa, A., Tarantino, E. (eds.) EuroGP 2008. LNCS, vol. 4971, pp. 158–169. Springer, Heidelberg (2008)
8. Burlacu, B., Affenzeller, M., Kommenda, M., Winkler, S.M., Kronberger, G.: Evolution tracking in genetic programming. In: Jimenez, E., Sokolov, B. (eds.) The 24th European Modeling and Simulation Symposium, EMSS 2012, Austria, Vienna (2012)
9. Burlacu, B., Affenzeller, M., Kommenda, M., Winkler, S., Kronberger, G.: Visualization of genetic lineages and inheritance information in genetic programming. In: GECCO 2013 Companion: Proceeding of the Fifteenth Annual Conference Companion on Genetic and Evolutionary Computation Conference Companion, pp. 1351–1358. ACM, Amsterdam (2013)
10. Valiente, G.: An efficient bottom-up distance between trees. In: Proceedings of the 8th International Symposium of String Processing and Information Retrieval, pp. 212–219. Press (2001)
11. Affenzeller, M., Winkler, S., Wagner, S., Beham, A.: Genetic Algorithms and Genetic Programming: Modern Concepts and Practical Applications. Numerical Insights. CRC Press, Singapore (2009)

Smooth Symbolic Regression: Transformation of Symbolic Regression into a Real-Valued Optimization Problem

Erik Pitzer[(✉)] and Gabriel Kronberger

Heuristic and Evolutionary Algorithms Laboratory, School of Informatics,
Communications and Media, University of Applied Sciences Upper Austria,
Franz-Fritsch Strasse 11, 4600 Wels, Austria
{erik.pitzer,gabriel.kronberger}@fh-hagenberg.at
http://heal.heuristiclab.com

Abstract. The typical methods for symbolic regression produce rather abrupt changes in solution candidates. In this work, we have tried to transform symbolic regression from an optimization problem, with a landscape that is so rugged that typical analysis methods do not produce meaningful results, to one that can be compared to typical and very smooth real-valued problems. While the ruggedness might not interfere with the performance of optimization, it restricts the possibilities of analysis. Here, we have explored different aspects of a transformation and propose a simple procedure to create real-valued optimization problems from symbolic regression problems.

1 Introduction

When analyzing complex data sets not only to predict a variable from others but also trying to gain insights into the relationships between variables, symbolic regression is a very valuable tool. It can often produce human-interpretable explanations for relationships between variables. The considered formulas are explored by substituting variables or re-organizing the syntax tree. This results in rather abrupt changes in the behavior of these formulas.

Genetic programming (GP) [12] is a technique that uses an evolutionary algorithm to evolve computer programs that solve a given problem when executed. These programs are often represented as symbolic expression trees, and operations such as crossover and mutation are performed on sub-trees. One particular problem that can be solved by GP is symbolic regression [12], where the goal is to find a function, mapping the known values of input variables to the value of a target variable with minimal error.

Several specialized and improved variants of GP for symbolic regression have already been described in the literature e.g. [9–11,20] and it has been shown that other techniques are also viable for solving symbolic regression problems such as FFX [14] or dynamic programming [23].

While GP – or other (quasi-)combinatorial methods – typically work well in identifying formulas that describe relations between variables and, therefore, do

© Springer International Publishing Switzerland 2015
R. Moreno-Díaz et al. (Eds.): EUROCAST 2015, LNCS 9520, pp. 375–383, 2015.
DOI: 10.1007/978-3-319-27340-2_47

not create a black-box function but an opaque and often human-interpretable description of these relations, the process for obtaining these formulas is complicated and large effort is necessary to grasp their progression.

During the optimization, the symbolic expression tree can vary wildly between individuals and between generations. In other words, when a GP fitness landscape is analyzed it appears extremely rugged. A typical measure for ruggedness, the autocorrelation [22] between two "neighboring" solution candidates, is usually very close to zero.

This makes it very hard to derive any meaningful conclusions of GP fitness landscapes as typical "neighbors" are too dissimilar to each other, even more so, when crossover operators are employed which creates even more drastic changes, let alone the difficulties of crossover landscapes themselves [18].

In this paper, we present the idea of creating a smoother fitness landscape for symbolic regression problems by borrowing ideas from neural networks and combining them with typical tree formulations found in genetic programming. The intent is to have a smooth transition from one syntax tree to another. At the same time, we want to ensure that the final output settles for and determines one of the available operators at each node.

1.1   Symbolic Regression

In a regression problem the task is to find a mapping from a set of input variables to on or more output variables so that using only the input values, the output can be accurately predicted. This task can be tackled with two fundamentally different approaches. On the one hand, so-called black-box models focus on providing predictions with maximum quality sacrificing "understanding" of the model for exampling when employing neural networks [16] and deep learning [4] or Support Vector Machines [3]. On the other hand, white box models try not only to give good quality explanations but also try to provide some insight into how the relationship between the variables. Examples are most prominently linear regression [5] and generalized linear regression [15].

As an extension to these methods, symbolic regression provides great freedom in the formulation of a regression formula. By allowing an arbitrary syntax tree as the formulation for the relationship between the variables. This freedom, however, comes with the price of a much large solution space and, hence, much more possibilities for a goo solution. Therefore, powerful methods have to be used to control the complexity of this approach.

Genetic Programming (GP) [12] is a method that is able to conquer these problems and create white-box models with good quality and often understandable models that can give new insights into the relationships between the variables in addition to the provided predictions.

In Genetic Programming, syntax trees are usually modified using two different methods both drawing the solution candidates from a pool called the current generation. The most important form of modification is achieved via crossover, where two trees are recombined into a new tree that has some features from both predecessors. The second form of modification is mutation that randomly introduces or changes some features of the syntax tree, such as replacing operators or changing constants.

Overall, genetic programming provides powerful means of evolving symbolic trees and has proven its effectiveness and efficiency in providing good quality white box models of difficult regression problems. On the downside, however, the changes introduced during the evolution of syntax trees are quite drastic and the process, how genetic programming arrives at these solutions is very difficult to follow through, and its analysis is complicated.

1.2   Fitness Landscape Analysis

Every optimization problem implies a so-called fitness landscape that describes the relationship of solution candidates and their associated fitness. Formally, a fitness landscape can be defined as the triple $\mathcal{F} := \{\mathcal{S}, f, \mathcal{X}\}$, where $\mathcal{S}$ is an arbitrary set of solution candidates for the optimization problems at hand. The function $f : \mathcal{S} \rightarrow \mathbb{R}$ is the actual fitness function that assigns a value of desirability to every solution candidate and is often the most expensive part in the optimization of a problem. Finally, $\mathcal{X}$ describes how solution candidates relate to each other: A very simple case would be to define $\mathcal{X} \subseteq \mathcal{S} \times \mathcal{S}$ a relation of neighboring solution candidates or alternatively as distance function $\mathcal{X} : \mathcal{S} \times \mathcal{S} \rightarrow \mathbb{R}$. The important observation is that this definition of a fitness landscape can be made for any optimization problem and, therefore, provides the foundation for very general and portable problem analysis techniques.

Based on this formulation several different analysis methods have been proposed. Many of which require a sample of the solution space, i.e. so called walkable landscapes [7]. This sample often comes in the form of a trajectory inside the solution space, following the neighborhood relation or distance function.

Based on these trajectories, different measures can be defined that characterize the fitness landscape. Examples are auto correlation [22] that measures the average decay of correlation of fitness values as the trajectory moves away from a point. Typically, it is only defined for the very first step but can be continued to an arbitrary distance. The distance at which the correlation is not statistically significant anymore is called the correlation length also defined in [22].

Other techniques include the information analysis proposed in [19] where several measure are defined that try to capture information theoretic characteristics of these trajectories. One particularly simple but interesting property is the information stability which simply captures the maximum fitness difference between neighboring solution candidates and has proven to be a very characteristic property of a problem instance.

Besides these trajectory-based analysis methods several other methods have been proposed such as analytical decomposition into elementary landscapes [2, 17] or fitness distance correlation [8].

2   Transformation

As described in the previous sections most landscape analysis methods as well as trajectory-based optimization algorithms rely on a relatively smooth landscape or, in other words, high correlation between neighboring solution candidates. Conversely, typical modifications in genetic programming are very large and previous attempts of applying classic fitness landscape analysis (FLA) have failed.

Figure 1 summarizes the basic ideas for this transformation: To overcome the drastic fitness changes induced by changes in the tree structure, the first simple ideas is to fix the tree structure (Fig. 1a) to a full (e.g. binary) tree. This is comparable to the limited tree depth or tree size that can often be found in genetic programming. This limits the maximum change to the replacement of an operator in the tree. However, directly switching from e.g. an addition to a multiplication can still have quite a large impact on the behavior of the formula. Therefore, the second idea is to make this transition smooth too, as illustrated in Fig. 1b. A very simple way to achieve this smooth transition is to simply use a weighted average over all possible operators as shown in Eq. 1, where the $op_i(x, y)$ are the possible operators and $op(x, y)$ is the overall operation result. In the simplest case, when only two operators are available, i.e. addition and multiplication, only a single factor needs to be tuned, i.e. $op(x, y) := \alpha \cdot (x + y) + (1 - \alpha) \cdot (x \cdot y)$.

$$op(x, y) := \sum_{i}^{2^d - 1} \alpha_i \cdot op_i(x, y) \tag{1}$$

(a) fixed structure   (b) operation average

Fig. 1. Basic ideas

So far, this yields a smooth optimization problem for the operator choices where only real values have to be adjusted. However, this simply replaces every operator with a weighted average of other operators and make the formula much more complicated. Therefore, another simple addition is necessary: The overall fitness function is augmented with a penalty for undecided operator choices. In the simplest possible case where two possible operators are chosen an inverted quadratic function that peaks at 0.5 and intersects with the abscissa at zero and one can be used. When more than two operations are available a different penalty function is required. In this case the least penalty should occur when exactly one operator is chosen and it should increase progressively the more weight other operators are receiving. Therefore, the simple formula shown in Eq. 2 can been used to steer the optimization towards a unique operator choice.

$$p_{\text{op}}(\alpha) := \left(\sum_i^{2^d-1} \alpha_i - \max_i \alpha_i \right) / (2^d - 2) \tag{2}$$

Now that the structure and the operators of the tree can be selected using only real values, the last remaining aspect is how to make a smooth choices between variables. This task is a litte more complicated as the variables should also have a weight attached. However, another simple solution can be applied as shown in Eq. 3 where the operation in the leaf node is selected in addition to the variables, and n is the number of input variables in X. Please note that one additional weight $\beta_{i,n+1}$ is included to allow a constant to be selected which gives the ability to "mute" parts of the tree by selecting for example a multiplication with one or an addition with zero for some subtree.

$$\text{op}(X) := \sum_i^{2^d-1} \alpha_i \cdot \text{op}(\beta_{i,1} \cdot X_1, \dots, \beta_{i,n} \cdot X_n, \beta_{i,n+1}) \tag{3}$$

This yields quite a large number of variable weights. As the number of leaf nodes increases exponentially with the tree depth and is further multiplied with the number of input variables. For example a smooth symbolic regression problem with ten variables and a tree depth of five has only 31 operator weights but 176 variable weights.

In Fig. 2 several alternative ideas are shown for variable selection schemes with fewer resulting variables. However, they have not been very promising in preliminary tests. Therefore, we can only recommend to use the variable selection scheme with more variables, given the complexity of the variable selection problem per se. The first idea was to use only a single angle and take the two closest variables weighted by distance, as shown in Fig. 2a, however, this blinds the algorithm by completely hiding other choices. This might still be a good option for other algorithms where diversity of the population is kept very high. Another idea was to use multidimensional scaling [1] to project the variables according to their correlation onto e.g. a two dimensional plane and use only two coordinates to choose between all variables. Figure 2b shows the selection of the two nearest neighbors, which has similar problems as the angular selection as it completely hides other variable choices. The second alternative is to use again a weighted average, however, using the distance to the coordinates as the weights.

It has to be noted, that also for the variable selection the optimization has to be guided towards limiting the number of variables. This can be achieved similarly to the operator choice, only that this time two or more non-zero weights are acceptable and their weights can be subtracted from the penalty.

In summary, the new encoding transforms a problem with $2^d - 1$ tree nodes, where d is the depth of the tree, k possible operations at each node and n input

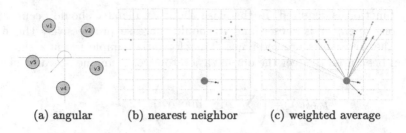

(a) angular   (b) nearest neighbor   (c) weighted average

Fig. 2. Alternative variable selection strategies

variables into a problem with $(2^d - 1) \cdot (k - 1)$ operator weights α and $(2^{d-1}) \cdot n$ variable weights β. So, for example, for a depth of five, with two operations and ten variables we get a $31 + 176 = 207$ dimensional real-valued problem instead of a combinatorial problem with $6 \cdot 10^{20}$ possible choices. Obviously this does not make the problem less complex, i.e. dimensions compared with choices, however it makes the fitness landscape much smoother. One could think of discrete points in space in the combinatorial formulation and filling the volume between them in the smooth approach.

3 Experimental Results

We have tested this new implementation only on comparatively simple problems most notably the Poly-10 Problem [13] using custom operators in HeuristicLab [21] with a CMA Evolution Strategy [6]. One very interesting aspect is shown in Fig. 3 where the penalties for operators and variable weights have been successively turned on. It can be seen that the correlation of the formula slightly decreases as the optimization tries to lower the operator penalty but quickly recovers with very low operator penalties, indicating a crisp operator choice. This choice is also achieved rather quickly indicating that it might not be so difficult to make this crisp operator choice. When turning on the variable selection penalty a distinct knee and steeper slope can be seen in the variable selection penalty curve, however, it is much harder to decrease as many more weights are involved.

Finally, we have used the new formulation to calculate some fitness landscape analysis measures. For the first time, traditional techniques can be applied to symbolic regression problems and reasonable results can be obtained as shown in Table 1, where the fitness landscape of the Poly-10 Problem was analyzed using different neighborhoods: In particular polynomial one position or all position manipulators where used with contiguity of 15 or only 2 as well as a uniform one position manipulator. Both random and up-down walks [8] where performed to get a first impression of the landscape's characteristics.

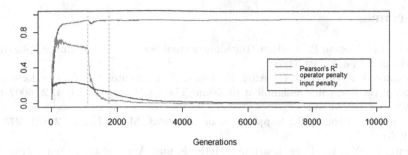

Fig. 3. Results

Table 1. Fitness Landscape Analysis of Symbolic Regression Problem

	Poly-1-15	Poly-All-15	Poly-1-2	Poly-All-2	Uni-1
Auto correlation	0.999	0.910	0.998	0.547	0.991
Corr. length	2245	57	1246	11	290
Density basin information	0.628	0.619	0.626	0.593	0.628
Information content	0.546	0.394	0.686	0.403	0.399
Information stability	0.058	0.141	0.058	0.255	0.037
Partial inf. content	0.476	0.532	0.457	0.586	0.506
Up walk length	328.063	124.872	14.321	5.179	83.433
Up walk len. variance	46668.196	5405.852	35.814	3.176	870.758
Down walk length	296.563	123.400	12.140	4.878	83.100
Down walk len. variance	27152.263	4627.477	26.232	2.713	832.024

4 Conclusions

While there is certainly still a lot of work needed to fine tune the optimization process and play with different variants of variable selection and penalty schemes, this transformation principle opens the door for classical fitness landscape analysis applied to symbolic regression problems. The focus of future work should therefore not be the tuning of algorithm performance but rather the interpretation and utilization of FLA results generated for the class of symbolic regression problems.

Acknowledgments. The work described in this paper was done within the COMET Project Heuristic Optimization in Production and Logistics (HOPL), #843532 funded by the Austrian Research Promotion Agency (FFG).

References

1. Borg, I., Groenen, P.: Modern Multidimensional Scaling: Theory and Applications. Springer, New York (2005)
2. Chicano, F., Whitley, L.D., Alba, E., Luna, F.: Elementary landscape decomposition of the frequency assignment problem. Theoret. Comput. Sci. **412**, 6002–6019 (2011)
3. Cortes, C., Vapnik, V.: Support-vector networks. Mach. Learn. **20**(3), 273–297 (1995)
4. Deng, L., Yu, D.: Deep Learning: Methods and Applications, Foundations and Trens in Signal Processing, vol. 7. Now Publishers Inc., Hanover (2013)
5. Freedman, D.A.: Statistical Models: Theory and Practice. Cambridge University Press, Cambridge (2009)
6. Hansen, N.: The CMA evolution strategy: a comparing review (chap.). In: Lozano, J.A., Larrañaga, P., Inza, I., Bengoetxea, E. (eds.) Towards a New Evolutionary Computation: Advances on Estimation of Distribution Algorithms. STUDFUZZ, vol. 192, pp. 75–102. Springer, Berlin (2006)
7. Hordijk, W.: A measure of landscapes. Evol. Comput. **4**(4), 335–360 (1996)
8. Jones, T.: Evolutionary algorithms, fitness landscapes and search. Ph.D. thesis, University of New Mexico, Albuquerque, New Mexico (1995)
9. Keijzer, M.: Improving symbolic regression with interval arithmetic and linear scaling. In: Ryan, C., Soule, T., Keijzer, M., Tsang, E.P.K., Poli, R., Costa, E. (eds.) EuroGP 2003. LNCS, vol. 2610, pp. 70–82. Springer, Heidelberg (2003)
10. Kommenda, M., Kronberger, G., Winkler, S., Affenzeller, M., Wagner, S.: Effects of constant optimization by nonlinear least squares minimization in symbolic regression. In: GECCO 2013 Companion: Proceeding of the Fifteenth Annual Conference Companion on Genetic and Evolutionary Computation Conference Companion, pp. 1121–1128. ACM, Amsterdam, The Netherlands (2013)
11. Kotanchek, M., Smits, G., Vladislavleva, E.: Trustable symbolic regression models: using ensembles, interval arithmetic and pareto fronts to develop robust and trust-aware models (Chap. 12). In: Riolo, R.L., Soule, T., Worzel, B. (eds.) Genetic Programming Theory and Practice V, pp. 201–220. Genetic and Evolutionary Computation, Springer (2007)
12. Koza, J.R.: Genetic Programming: On the Programming of Computers by Means of Natural Selection. MIT Press, Cambridge (1992)
13. Langdon, W.B., Banzhaf, W.: Repeated patterns in genetic programming. Nat. Comput. **7**(4), 589–613 (2008)
14. McConaghy, T.: FFX: fast, scalable, deterministic symbolic regression technology. In: Riolo, R., Vladislavleva, E., Moore, J.H. (eds.) Genetic Programming Theory and Practice IX, pp. 235–260. Springer, New York (2011)
15. Nelder, J., Wedderburn, R.: Generalized linear models. J. Roy. Stat. Soc. Ser. A (General) **135**(3), 370–384 (1972)
16. Rosenblatt, F.: The perceptron: a probabilistic model for information storage and organization in the brain. Psychol. Rev. **65**(6), 386–408 (1958)
17. Stadler, P.F.: Linear operators on correlated landscapes. J. Phys. I France **4**, 681–696 (1994)
18. Stadler, P., Wagner, G.: The algebraic theory of recombination spaces. Evol. Comp. **5**, 241–275 (1998)
19. Vassilev, V.K., Fogarty, T.C., Miller, J.F.: Information characteristics and the structure of landscapes. Evol. Comput. **8**(1), 31–60 (2000)

20. Vladislavleva, E.J., Smits, G.F., Hertog, D.D.: Order of nonlinearity as a complexity measure for models generated by symbolic regression via pareto genetic programming. IEEE Trans. Evol. Comput. **13**(2), 333–349 (2009)
21. Wagner, S.: Heuristic optimization software systems - modeling of heuristic optimization algorithms in the heuristicLab software environment. Ph.D. thesis, Johannes Kepler University, Linz, Austria (2009)
22. Weinberger, E.: Correlated and uncorrelated fitness landscapes and how to tell the difference. Biol. Cybern. **63**(5), 325–336 (1990)
23. Worm, T., Chiu, K.: Prioritized grammar enumeration: symbolic regression by dynamic programming. In: GECCO, pp. 1021–1028 (2013)

A Scalable Approach for the K-Staged Two-Dimensional Cutting Stock Problem with Variable Sheet Size

Frederico Dusberger$^{(\boxtimes)}$ and Günther R. Raidl

Institute of Computer Graphics and Algorithms, TU Wien, Vienna, Austria
{dusberger,raidl}@ac.tuwien.ac.at

Abstract. We present a new scalable approach for the K-staged two-dimensional cutting stock problem with variable sheet size, particularly aiming to solve large-scale instances from industry. A construction heuristic exploiting the congruency of subpatterns efficiently computes sheet patterns of high quality. This heuristic is embedded in a beam-search framework to allow for a meaningful selection from the available sheet types. Computational experiments on benchmark instances show the effectiveness of our approach and demonstrate its scalability.

1 Introduction

The two-dimensional cutting stock problem occurs in many industrial applications, such as glass, paper or steel cutting, container loading, and VLSI [7]. It is particularly relevant in the manufacturing industry, where large amounts of material are processed and significant commercial benefits can be achieved by minimizing the used material.

Formally, we consider in this work the *K-staged two-dimensional cutting stock problem with variable sheet size* (K2CSV) in which we are given a set of n_E rectangular *element types* $E = \{1, \dots, n_E\}$, each $i \in E$ specified by a height $h_i \in \mathbb{N}^+$, a width $w_i \in \mathbb{N}^+$, and a demand $d_i \in \mathbb{N}^+$. Furthermore, we have a set of n_T *stock sheet types* $T = \{1, \dots, n_T\}$, each $t \in T$ specified by a height $H_t \in \mathbb{N}^+$, a width $W_t \in \mathbb{N}^+$, an available quantity $q_t \in \mathbb{N}^+$, and a cost factor $c_t \in \mathbb{N}^+$. Both elements and sheets can be rotated by 90°. A feasible solution is a set of *cutting patterns* $\mathcal{P} = \{P_1, \dots, P_n\}$, i.e. an arrangement of the elements specified by E on the available stock sheets specified by T without overlap and using guillotine cuts up to depth K only. Each pattern P_j, $j = 1, \dots, n$, has an associated stock sheet type t_j and a quantity a_j specifying how often the pattern is to be applied, i.e. how many sheets of type t_j are cut following pattern P_j. More precisely, a cutting pattern is represented by a tree structure that is detailed in Sect. 1.1.

In particular, we are considering here large-scale instances from industry, where the number of different element and sheet types is moderate but the demands of the element types are rather high. Reasonable solutions need to be

---

We thank LodeStar Technology for their support and collaboration in this project.

R. Moreno-Díaz et al. (Eds.): EUROCAST 2015, LNCS 9520, pp. 384–392, 2015.
DOI: 10.1007/978-3-319-27340-2_48

found within moderate runtimes. The objective is to find a feasible set of cutting patterns $\mathcal{P}$ minimizing the weighted number of used sheets $c(\mathcal{P})$.

$$\min \ c(\mathcal{P}) = \sum_{t \in T} c_t \sigma_t(\mathcal{P}) \tag{1}$$

where $\sigma_t(\mathcal{P})$ is the number of used sheets of type $t \in T$ in the set $\mathcal{P}$.

1.1 Cutting Tree

Each cutting pattern $P_j \in \mathcal{P}$ is represented by a (cutting) tree structure. Its leaf nodes correspond to individual elements (possibly in their rotated variants) and its internal nodes are either *horizontal* or *vertical compounds* containing at least one subpattern. Vertical compounds always only appear at odd stages (levels), starting from stage 1, and represent parts separated by horizontal cuts of the respective stage. Horizontal compounds always only appear at even stages and represent parts separated by vertical cuts. Each node thus corresponds to a rectangle of a certain size (h, w), which is in case of compound nodes the bounding box of the respectively aligned subpatterns. A pattern's root node always has a size that is not larger than the respective sheet size, i.e. $h \leq H_{t_j}$, $w \leq W_{t_j}$. Recall that a_j represents the quantity of sheets cut according to pattern P_j. Similarly, compound nodes store congruent subpatterns only by one subtree and maintain an additional quantity. Compounds with only one successor are required in cases where a cut is necessary to cut off a waste rectangle, otherwise they are avoided. In this tree structure, residual (waste) rectangles are never explicitly stored, but can be derived considering a compound node's embedding in its parent compound or sheet.

Each pattern $P_j \in \mathcal{P}$ can be transformed into *normal form* having equal objective value, hence it is sufficient to consider patterns in normal form only. In normal form, subpatterns of vertical (horizontal) compounds are arranged from top to bottom (left to right), ordered by nonincreasing width (height), and aligned at their left (top) edges, i.e. in case the subpatterns have different widths (heights), remaining space appears to their right (at their bottom). Figure 1 shows a 3-staged cutting pattern and the cutting tree representing it.

2 Related Work

A classical solution approach to the K2CSV has been proposed by Gilmore and Gomory [4] who employ column generation, solving the pricing problem by dynamic programming. Although more recently, both column generation and dynamic programming still have been successfully used in approaches to the K2CSV [2,11], the high computational effort prohibits an efficient application to large-scale instances. More reasonable approaches in terms of runtime are fast construction heuristics. In their survey on solution approaches to two-dimensional cutting stock problems, Lodi et al. [8] compare the most well-known

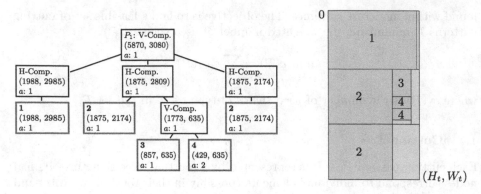

Fig. 1. A three-staged cutting tree (left) and the corresponding cutting pattern (right). The leaves represent actual elements of types $1, \ldots, 4$ obtained after at most K stages of guillotine cuts. Note that the two elements of type 4 belong to the same vertical compound and are thus only stored once.

ones, such as First-Fit Decreasing Height or Hybrid First-Fit. Being rather simple in their nature, a major drawback of these heuristics is their inflexibility. Recently, Fleszar [3] proposed three more involved construction heuristics for the $K2CSV$ with only a single sheet type achieving excellent results in short time. A solution is constructed element by element using a sophisticated enumeration of the possible ways of adding the current element to it.

The literature on heuristic approaches for the $K2CSV$ specifically (i.e. when multiple sheet types are given) is rather scarce. Only recently, Hong et al. [5] embedded fast construction heuristics in a backtracking framework to address the problem of a meaningful sheet type selection. Several solutions are computed in a sheet by sheet manner and the best one is returned. Backtracking is applied to choose a different sheet type, if a choice leads to a poor solution. Another promising technique, generally applicable to problems where solutions can be computed in terms of sequences, is beam-search, which was first applied in speech recognition [9]. Beam-search is a heuristic breadth-first tree-search algorithm that only further explores a most promising restricted-size subset of nodes at each level.

3 A Congruency-Aware Construction Heuristic

In the following, we describe our heuristic for computing a pattern for a given sheet. One of the major drawbacks of conventional construction heuristics is their lack of scalability. A solution is usually constructed element by element leading to rather high runtimes for large-scale instances with high demands. To overcome this problem, we exploit congruent subpatterns during the solution construction using the following principle: The heuristic operates not on single elements but on element types. When considering a certain element type $i \in E$ for insertion into a compound c, we attempt to simultaneously insert multiple instances of i. This is realized by inserting a completely filled grid of $a_i^{\text{vert}} \times a_i^{\text{hor}}$ instances of i in c and doing the same for the compounds congruent to c. The congruent compounds can be determined by considering the quantities along the path from the current node representing c to the root of the cutting tree. Let accum_a be the accumulated quantity over these congruent compounds and let d_i^r be the *residual demand* of element type i. We can then, in total, insert

$$\min\left\{a_i^{\text{vert}} \cdot a_i^{\text{hor}} \cdot \text{accum}_a, \left\lfloor \frac{d_i^r}{a_i^{\text{vert}} \cdot a_i^{\text{hor}}} \right\rfloor \cdot a_i^{\text{vert}} \cdot a_i^{\text{hor}}\right\} \tag{2}$$

instances of i at once. Figure 2 demonstrates this principle on a simple example.

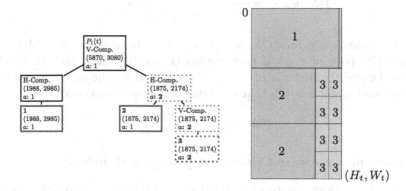

Fig. 2. Congruency-aware pattern insertion: considering the insertion of element type 3, eight instances can be added at once by exploiting the quantities in the cutting tree.

Another drawback of conventional construction heuristics we aim to avoid is their inflexibility w.r.t. already placed elements. In particular, the sizes of the (sub-)patterns currently in the pattern tree, as well as its general structure, are usually fixed. Towards a more flexible construction heuristic, we therefore extend the concept of Fleszar [3] as follows:

For a pattern p, let $h_p^{\max}$ ($w_p^{\max}$) denote the maximum height (width) of p. The *maximum rectangle* of p is the largest rectangle to which the size of p can be extended such that it remains feasible. Let further $\tilde{h}_p$ ($\tilde{w}_p$) denote the *vertical (horizontal) slack* of p, which is the difference between p's maximum height (width) and its current height (width). The maximum rectangles and the slack values allow us to determine how much space there is left in a given compound – considering a possible resizing of it – for the insertion of a new subpattern.

A further increase of flexibility is achieved by considering not only insertions as a subpattern of a given compound, but also so-called *in-parallel* insertions. For a given compound c and a subsequence S of c's subpatterns, the $a_i^{\text{vert}} \times a_i^{\text{hor}}$ grid is joined in parallel to S, which allows restructuring the pattern. For further details we refer to [3].

When an element type $i \in E$ is considered for insertion, two basic questions need to be addressed: Where should the insertion be made and how many instances of i should be added, i.e. what is the best size of the grid? To answer these questions, we define the fitness of an insertion in a certain compound c as follows: Let $\tilde{h}_c$ and $\tilde{w}_c$ be the vertical and horizontal slacks of the compound after the insertion of $a_i \leq d_i^r$ instances of i, arranged in a completely filled $a_i^{\text{vert}} \times a_i^{\text{hor}}$ grid, i.e. $a_i = a_i^{\text{vert}} \cdot a_i^{\text{hor}}$. Furthermore, let η be the absolute difference between the total height (width) of the inserted grid and the height (width) of the grid's neighbor in c's normal form, given that c is a horizontal (vertical) compound. This neighbor is either the predecessor or the successor, whichever yields the smaller difference. The fitness function is then defined as

$$f(\tilde{h}_c, \tilde{w}_c, \eta) = \frac{1}{(\tilde{h}_c + 1) \cdot (\tilde{w}_c + 1) \cdot (\eta + 1)}. \tag{3}$$

As an exception we define $f(\tilde{h}_c, \tilde{w}_c, \eta) = -1$ if the size of the grid exceeds the available space in c, i.e. if no insertion is possible. To determine the best compound c and the best size of the $a_i^{\text{vert}} \times a_i^{\text{hor}}$ grid for the insertion, we select the compound and quantities that maximize the fitness function (3), i.e.

$$\operatorname*{argmax}_{c, a_i^{\text{vert}}, a_i^{\text{hor}}} f(\tilde{h}_c, \tilde{w}_c, \eta) \tag{4}$$

3.1 Congruency-Aware Critical-Fit Insertion Heuristic

Based on these ideas, we propose the *congruency-aware critical-fit insertion heuristic* (CCF) extending the approach by Fleszar [3], which works as follows:

1. Order the element types in E by nonincreasing area and let further $D = \langle d_1^r, \ldots, d_{n_E}^r \rangle$ be the vector of residual demands, for all $i \in E$.
2. While $D \neq \mathbf{0}$ repeat steps 3 to 5.
3. An element type $i \in E$ *dominates* another type $j \in E$ if $w_i \geq w_j$ and $h_i \geq h_j$. Let U be the set of undominated element types considering only those types for which $d_i^r > 0$.
4. For each $i \in U$, determine the number of sheets in which i fits. Let the *critical element type* i^* be the one that fits in the least number of sheets.
5. Perform the insertion of i^* that has the highest fitness value. If no insertion of i^* is possible, a new sheet is started. Afterwards, decrease $d_{i^*}^r$ accordingly.

4 Sheet Type Selection by Beam-Search

A crucial aspect of solving the $K2CSV$ is a meaningful selection of the sheet types on which the patterns are computed. To address this issue, we employ a beam-search strategy that generates a solution sheet by sheet. Each node in the search tree corresponds to a (partial) solution, starting with the empty solution at the root. A branch from a node reflects the decision for one of the sheet types from T, including the possibly rotated variants. At each level, all the nodes on that level are evaluated and all but the BW best ones are pruned, where BW is the chosen beam-width. Note that some nodes might also be pruned earlier, e.g. if there is no more sheet available of a certain type. This procedure continues until all residual demands are zero. Figure 3 shows an example for BW $= 2$.

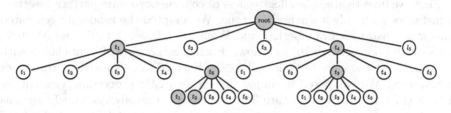

Fig. 3. Beam-search example for BW $= 2$. At each level, each node is evaluated by computing a pattern on the sheet type corresponding to it. The search is continued only for the two best (highlighted) nodes from that level, the remaining ones are pruned.

We compute the pattern for a single sheet using the following variant of the CCF heuristic (cf. Sect. 3.1): As there is only one sheet to fill, the critical element type is simply the one having the highest fitness. If there is no $i \in U$ that fits, consider all $i \in E$. Finally, if no type $i \in E$ fits, the pattern is considered finished. Exploiting congruency, the pattern resulting from the evaluation of a certain sheet type is considered to be used as often as possible. Let $\text{elems}_i(P_j)$ be the number of elements of type $i \in E$ contained in the computed pattern P_j, let t_j be the type of the sheet P_j is defined on and let d_i^r be the residual demand of i before the computation of P_j. The usable quantity for pattern P_j is then

$$\min \left\{ \min_{i \in E} \left\lfloor \frac{\text{elems}_i(P_j)}{d_i^r} \right\rfloor, q_{t_j} \right\} \tag{5}$$

4.1 Node Evaluation

To evaluate the tree nodes the following criterion is applied: Let $\mathcal{P}$ be the set of patterns in the current partial solution, i.e. the patterns selected when following the path in the search tree from the root down to the current node. Furthermore, $\text{wr}(P_j)$ denotes the waste ratio of pattern P_j, i.e. the unused area on the sheet, c_{t_j} is the cost factor of the sheet type used for pattern P_j and a_j is the quantity of P_j. We prefer (partial) solutions for which the average waste ratio over $\mathcal{P}$, weighted by the respective cost factors is comparatively smaller. Formally, this ratio is defined by:

$$\frac{\sum_{P_j \in \mathcal{P}} \text{wr}(P_j) \cdot c_{t_j} \cdot a_j}{\sum_{P_j \in \mathcal{P}} c_{t_j} \cdot a_j}. \tag{6}$$

5 Computational Results

Our algorithms have been implemented in C++, compiled with GCC version
4.8.2 and executed on a single core of a 3.40 GHz Intel Core i7-3770. For all
experiments, the stage limit was set to $K = 10$.

First, we investigated the effectiveness of congruency-aware pattern insertion
on instances with only a single sheet type. We adapted the randomly generated
benchmark instances from Berkey and Wang [1] (classes 1 to 6) and Martello
and Vigo [10] (classes 7 to 10) as follows: Each class consists of 5 subclasses with
$|E| = 4, \ldots, 20$ and $d_i = 1000$, for all $i \in E$. Each of these subclasses comprises
10 instances. We compared a simple first-fit heuristic proceeding element by
element (FF), a congruency-aware first-fit heuristic that always naively adds as
many instances of an element type as possible at once (CFF), and the CCF
heuristic. For each subclass, the average objective values $\overline{c(\mathcal{P})}$ and runtimes
$\overline{t}$ were computed. In Table 1 we give the results for classes $5, 6, 7$ and 8. As
expected, for CFF we observe a significant speed-up over FF, but also an overall
worse solution quality. Remarkably, the much more involved CCF heuristic has
runtimes in the same order of magnitude and additionally yields significantly
better solutions for each subclass. The same holds for the remaining classes.

Second, we tested our beam-search approach on the benchmark set by
Hopper and Turton [6]. The set comprises 3 categories of increasing complex-
ity. Each category consists of 5 randomly generated instances with $|T| = 6$,
$2 \leq q_t \leq 4$ for all $t \in T$ and $d_i = 1$ for all $i \in E$. We compared our beam-
search approach (BS) with the HHA algorithm by Hong et al. [5] as it yields
– to the best of our knowledge – the so far best results on these instances in
the literature and due to its relatedness to our approach. We experimented with
several values for BW and chose BW = 150 and BW = 500 as the best com-
promises for runtime and solution quality, respectively. In Table 2 we report for
each category the average percentage of the used area on the sheets $\overline{a(\mathcal{P})}$ and the
average runtime $\overline{t}$ to be comparable with the results reported in [5]. Although
we cannot exploit congruency, as no element type is needed more than once,

Table 1. Experimental results for classes 5 and 6 from [1] and classes 7 and 8
from [10].The best objective value for each subclass is printed in bold.

		FF		CFF		CCF			FF		CFF		CCF	
	$|E|$	$c(\mathcal{P})$	$t[s]$	$c(\mathcal{P})$	$t[s]$	$c(\mathcal{P})$	$t[s]$	$|E|$	$c(\mathcal{P})$	$t[s]$	$c(\mathcal{P})$	$t[s]$	$c(\mathcal{P})$	$t[s]$
Class 5	4	1442.3	0.2	1450	< 0.1	**1417.4**	< 0.1	4	1091.7	0.1	1099.9	< 0.1	**1087.9**	< 0.1
	8	2285.6	0.5	2318.4	< 0.1	**2190.7**	< 0.1	8	2016	0.4	2030.3	< 0.1	**1949.3**	< 0.1
	12	4197.6	1.4	4213.4	< 0.1	**4071.9**	< 0.1	12	2870	0.9	2885	< 0.1	**2748.1**	< 0.1
	16	4983.6	2.2	5015.2	< 0.1	**4857.3**	< 0.1	16	4533.8	1.9	4541.4	< 0.1	**4401.4**	< 0.1
	20	6344.8	3.5	6366	< 0.1	**6212.8**	< 0.1	20	5442.8	2.9	5466.5	< 0.1	**5215.2**	< 0.1
Class 6	4	126.6	< 0.1	128.6	< 0.1	**124.5**	< 0.1	4	1162.7	0.1	1167.3	< 0.1	**1136.2**	< 0.1
	8	199.3	0.1	200.7	< 0.1	**194.5**	< 0.1	8	1989.3	0.4	1988.3	< 0.1	**1887.3**	< 0.1
	12	375.5	0.2	377.4	< 0.1	**371.4**	< 0.1	12	3052.8	1.0	3063.7	< 0.1	**2949.5**	< 0.1
	16	447.2	0.3	447.5	< 0.1	**440.6**	0.1	16	4241.8	1.9	4248.4	< 0.1	**4059.8**	< 0.1
	20	582.7	0.4	583.4	< 0.1	**573.7**	0.1	20	5273.3	2.9	5297.1	< 0.1	**5178.2**	< 0.1

Note: In the right half of the table, classes are Class 7 (first five rows) and Class 8 (last five rows).

Table 2. Comparison of area utilization for the three instance categories M1 to M3

Instance category	$|E|$	$|T|$	HHA		BS (BW = 150)		BS (BW = 500)	
			$a(\mathcal{P})$	$t[s]$	$a(\mathcal{P})$	$t[s]$	$a(\mathcal{P})$	$t[s]$
M1	100	6	98.4	60	98.4	1.36	98.4	4.10
M2	100	6	95.6	60	95.7	1.18	96.3	3.56
M3	150	6	97.4	60	96.5	3.51	96.5	10.70

our runtimes are significantly lower for all categories, compared to HHA, which always runs for $60s$. Nonetheless, our approach is competitive to HHA, achieving the same solution quality for category M1, surpassing it for category M2, and falling slightly behind for category M3. This even holds for BW = 150. Despite better runtimes, the solution quality only declines for M2, still surpassing the result from HHA.

6   Conclusions and Future Work

We presented a scalable approach for the K2CSV based on the exploitation of congruency during solution construction. The underlying construction heuristic scales, in principle, to arbitrarily high element type demands generating very reasonable results within a few milliseconds. In the light of multiple sheet types, beam-search has been shown to be an effective approach for a meaningful selection of the types to use, even though the underlying construction heuristic could not use its full potential.

Our congruency-aware construction heuristic poses a solid basis for the subsequent application of metaheuristics such as variable neighborhood search, where the heuristic is called very often. In future work, we thus plan to extend our approach by a respective improvement heuristic that is applied to the initially constructed solution.

References

1. Berkey, J.O., Wang, P.Y.: Two-dimensional finite bin-packing algorithms. J. Oper. Res. Soc. **38**(5), 423–429 (1987)
2. Cintra, G., Miyazawa, F., Wakabayashi, Y., Xavier, E.: Algorithms for two-dimensional cutting stock and strip packing problems using dynamic programming and column generation. Eur. J. Oper. Res. **191**(1), 61–85 (2008)
3. Fleszar, K.: Three insertion heuristics and a justification improvement heuristic for two-dimensional bin packing with guillotine cuts. Comput. Oper. Res. **40**(1), 463–474 (2013)
4. Gilmore, P.C., Gomory, R.E.: Multistage cutting stock problems of two and more dimensions. Oper. Res. **13**(1), 94–120 (1965)
5. Hong, S., Zhang, D., Lau, H.C., Zeng, X., Si, Y.: A hybrid heuristic algorithm for the 2D variable-sized bin packing problem. Eur. J. Oper. Res. **238**(1), 95–103 (2014)

6. Hopper, E., Turton, B.C.H.: An empirical study of meta-heuristics applied to 2D rectangular bin packing - Part I. Stud. Informatica Univers. **2**(1), 77–92 (2002)

7. Lodi, A., Martello, S., Monaci, M.: Two-dimensional packing problems: a survey. Eur. J. Oper. Res. **141**(2), 241–252 (2002)

8. Lodi, A., Martello, S., Vigo, D.: Recent advances on two-dimensional bin packing problems. Discrete Appl. Math. **123**(13), 379–396 (2002)

9. Lowerre, B.T.: The harpy speech recognition system. Ph.D. thesis, Carnegie Mellon University, Pittsburgh, PA, USA (1976)

10. Martello, S., Vigo, D.: Exact solution of the two-dimensional finite bin packing problem. Manage. Sci. **44**(3), 388–399 (1998)

11. Pisinger, D., Sigurd, M.: The two-dimensional bin packing problem with variable bin sizes and costs. Discrete Optim. **2**(2), 154–167 (2005)

Diversity-Based Offspring Selection Criteria for Genetic Algorithms

Andreas Scheibenpflug[1,2]([✉]), Stefan Wagner[1], and Michael Affenzeller[1,2]

[1] Heuristic and Evolutionary Algorithms Laboratory, School of Informatics,
Communications and Media University of Applied Sciences Upper Austria,
Campus Hagenberg, Softwarepark 11, 4232 Hagenberg, Austria
{ascheibe,swagner,maffenze}@heuristiclab.com
[2] Institute for Formal Models and Verification, Johannes Kepler University Linz,
Altenberger Straße 69, 4040 Linz, Austria

Abstract. Genetic algorithms can be affected by an early loss of diversity in their populations called premature convergence. To address this problem, this paper presents two extensions for the offspring selection genetic algorithm. Both extensions are based on diversity maintenance mechanisms applied when selecting offspring for the next generation. The first approach focuses on producing solutions that feature a predefined quality improvement as well as an appropriate structural distance from their parents. The second approach monitors the average diversity of the population and selects more diverse offspring if the population does not meet a predefined diversity. We show that these algorithms allow to control diversity and are useful methods for influencing the development of the population independent of the algorithms other parameters.

1 Introduction

The performance of a genetic algorithm (GA) is strongly influenced by the ratio between diversification and intensification [1–4]. Ideally, a GA starts with exploration using a diverse population to identify promising regions in the solution space. As similarity between solutions increases, the population converges towards such an area where the GA then exhibits full intensification. While this behavior is essential for the success of the GA, premature convergence can occur if the algorithm is not able to further improve solution quality.

To overcome this problem, the parameters of GAs can be adjusted, e.g., the mutation rate, population size or operators can be tuned. The danger of high mutation rates and large population sizes is that they may counteract directed search. Furthermore, tuning parameters is a cumbersome trial and error task because there is no parameter that explicitly controls the diversity of the population. Therefore, several parameters have to be adapted to generate the desired behavior, though it is often not clear how these should be changed due to their relations with each other.

For this reason we argue for a diversity control mechanism that is not strongly based on operators or parameters. There is numerous research literature available

© Springer International Publishing Switzerland 2015
R. Moreno-Díaz et al. (Eds.): EUROCAST 2015, LNCS 9520, pp. 393–400, 2015.
DOI: 10.1007/978-3-319-27340-2_49

[5] that describes measures for preventing premature convergence. These works often do not consider diversity at all or try to keep the population diverse by injecting random sampled solutions or restarts. We argue that these mechanisms fail because they do not consider both, quality and diversity. When injecting low quality, high diverse solutions, the selection operator may not even select those solutions for reproduction because of the high quality difference to the rest of the population. Having already improved the population to a certain level, adding new solutions possibly slows down the evolutionary process as they may introduce low-quality genes that first need to be improved before being useful. Furthermore, when controlling diversity, it has been shown that it is important to guarantee "useful diversity" [6], e.g., diversity that *"in some way helps cause (or has helped cause) good strings"* [7]. In our view, a GA should therefore produce solutions that have a certain quality and diversity.

A GA-variant that mainly accepts solutions with a certain quality is the offspring selection genetic algorithm (OSGA) [8]. We extend this approach by adding diversity criteria to offspring selection so that the ratio between diversification and quality improvement can be controlled. The offspring is generated solely from the previous generation and therefore supports and not distracts the search process.

The following sections present two diversity-based extensions to the offspring selection genetic algorithm. Empirical results are shown for comparing the behavior of the algorithms as well as their performance on different instances of the traveling salesman problem.

2   The Offspring Selection Genetic Algorithm

The offspring selection genetic algorithm extends the standard genetic algorithm by a selection step after reproduction (a schematic overview of the OSGA can be found in Affenzeller et al. [9]). While in the genetic algorithm every produced individual takes part in the next generation, OSGA compares the quality of the offspring to its parents. If it surpasses the quality of the parents, it is part of the next generation. If the offspring does not meet this criterion, it is put into a pool of mediocre solutions. The next population is composed of a number of successful individuals determined by the success ratio multiplied with the population size and individuals from the pool. The criterion for determining if an individual is better than the parents may change over the course of algorithm execution. It is often configured to require individuals to be better than the worse parent in the beginning and increases to eventually requiring individuals to surpass the quality of the better parent. Individuals that do not surpass the offspring criterion are counted. The ratio of this count compared to the population size is the selection pressure. It is limited by an algorithm parameter to prevent further execution if it is not possible to make quality improvements anymore.

In the next section the concept of selecting offspring based on a certain criterion is used to create algorithms that assemble new generations not only based on quality of the individuals but also on their diversity.

3   New Offspring Selection Approaches

3.1   Parent Diversity Offspring Selection Criterion

The parent diversity offspring selection criterion (PDC) extends the standard off-spring selection criterion with a diversity component. An offspring is selected for the next generation if its quality surpasses the parents quality and, in addition, if it features a certain, configurable dissimilarity (diversity comparison factor) compared to its parents. An offspring in PDC therefore has to satisfy two criteria which results in higher selection pressures as more individuals have to be created to be able to fill up the next population.

3.2   Population Diversity Preservative Offspring Selection

While PDC considers the difference in diversity of the offspring to their parents, population diversity preservative offspring selection (PDP) uses the standard quality-based rating system. The offspring selection step is extended by calculating the average similarity of the offspring population and checking whether it is below a configurable upper border (diversity comparison factor). If the similarity of the population is lower, execution is continued normally as in the OSGA. Otherwise, the offspring selector calculates the similarity of the offspring to the already accepted next-generation population. It discards new offspring that is beyond the upper border until the desired average population diversity is reached. PDP uses average population diversity to trigger diversity control of the population and therefore does not work on single individuals but on a population level. Compared to PDC, new solutions have to fulfill only one criteria, though this can vary between a quality-based and diversity-based criterion. As a consequence, the success ratio may not be met anymore as quality-based success is neglected when selecting solutions for creating the desired average population diversity.

4   Experiments

In this section the setup of the experiments is first detailed and then a description of the observed behavior of the algorithms and their performance is given.

The parameter configurations in this paper are based on the tests presented in [10,11]. These settings are used as a guideline for configuring the algorithms and are adapted to fit the new variants. The algorithms are applied to selected problem instances from the TSPLIB[1] and are executed in the optimization environment HeuristicLab[2] [12]. Table 1 shows the parameter configurations and variations for each algorithm.

In all experiments proportional selection with multi-crossovers and multi-mutators are used because they lead to good results across different problem

---

[1] http://www.iwr.uni-heidelberg.de/groups/comopt/software/TSPLIB95/.
[2] http://dev.heuristiclab.com.

Table 1. Parameter variations for experiments (dash means no change in parameters compared to OSGA).

Parameter	OSGA	PDC	PDP
Selector	Proportional selection	-	-
Mutation probability	0.1/0.05/0.15	-	-
Maximum generations (thousands)	2.5/5/7	0.5/1/2	0.5/1/1.5/3/5/10
Success ratio	0.7/0.8/0.9	-	-
Population size	250/500	-	-
Max. selection pressure	300	3000	1000
Mutator	Multi: Inversion,Translocation	-	-
Crossover	Multi: MPX,OX,ERX	-	-
Comparison factor u/l bound	0.0–1.0	0.0–1.0	0.5–1.0
Diversity comparison factor u/l bound	-	0.7–1.0	0.35–0.97

instances [10,11]. Mutation probability, success ratio and population size are varied equally for each algorithm. Differences between algorithms are made for the maximum number of generations. PDC has a smaller number of maximum generations because it was not able to reach higher generations (the selection pressure would exceed the maximum very early in algorithm execution because of high constraints). For PDP a higher maximum generation was chosen to allow observing the effect of slow diversity adaption on algorithm performance. Comparison factor bounds have been kept to the standard value except for PDP because it allows violation of the success ratio. The diversity comparison factor lower bound for PDC was chosen higher than for PDP as the selection pressure would otherwise reach the maximum very early. Diversity comparison factor for the PDP is configured to guide the populations diversity linear from high diversity to a nearly collapsed population. Maximum selection pressure is generally configured with high values to allow longer algorithm executions. Especially, the value for PDC was set to a higher value to prevent the algorithm from stopping early.

4.1 Empirical Study

Figure 1 shows sample diversity charts from the experiments for the OSGA and PDC with the same parameter configuration except for PDC which has an additional lower and upper bound in the range of 0.3–1.0 for diversity adaption. It shows that loss of diversity is controlled and slowed down but also that the number of generations is smaller than in OSGA. The reason is that creating individuals that have a certain quality improvement and additionally a certain diversity requires more effort. This can be seen in Fig. 2 which shows that PDC has a higher selection pressure than the OSGA. PDC creates solutions that may have a good quality or a satisfying diversity, but only very little solutions feature both properties. Generating a large number of solutions that are not used because of high diversity constraints is time consuming and has no positive effect on solution quality. This is the reason why a high lower bound for diversity (0.7) was used in the experiments to give a good balance between preventing premature convergence and keeping runtime low.

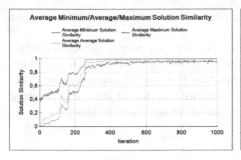 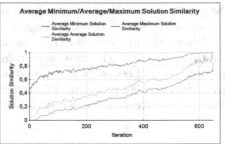

Fig. 1. OSGA (left image) and PDC (right image) sample diversity charts.

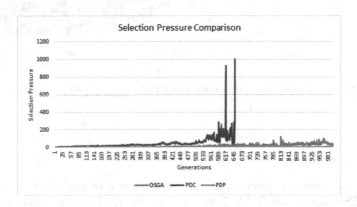

Fig. 2. Selection pressure comparison between OSGA, PDC and PDP.

PDP, compared to PDC and OSGA, exhibits lower selection pressure leading to less evaluated solutions. Figure 3 shows the diversity chart of a sample PDP run with the same parameters used for OSGA and PDC before. It shows that throughout the first few generations, the population quickly looses diversity, as the diversity bound of the offspring selection criteria has not yet been hit. The spike in the line before generation 200 indicates that the border is reached and the standard offspring selection criteria is overridden. The algorithm then starts selecting diverse solutions in favor of high-quality solutions to keep the average population similarity smaller than the diversity comparison factor. This results in a controlled, linear incline in similarity up to the last generation. The switch between OSGA and PDP selection can also be seen on the right chart in Fig. 3. It shows the success ratio, which is the amount of successful offspring relative to the population size that should be included in the next generation. In the beginning the configured value of 0.8 is reached but when the algorithm switches to PDP, this value is not reached anymore as diverse solutions are preferred. In the end, when the diversity comparison factor is near its final value of 0.97 and the population is collapsed, the algorithm again focuses on solution improvement and the success ratio is reached again.

A beneficial property of PDP is its easier, more robust way of diversity control compared to PDC. This can be seen from the diversity chart and the selection pressure curve: Less effort is required to produce the desired average population diversity with high precision. PDP offers therefore an efficient way of preventing premature convergence at a low cost in terms of quality and runtime.

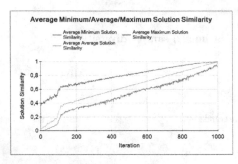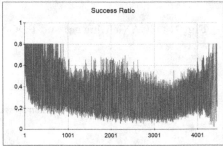

Fig. 3. PDP (left image) diversity chart and PDP success ratio chart (right image).

4.2 Comparison

The following gives an overview of the performance of the algorithms on four different TSP instances. Table 2 shows achieved qualities and the number of

Table 2. Qualities and evaluated solutions (ES) for the experiments.

Algorithm	Problem	Average	Best	Std. dev.	ES average	ES best
OSGA	berlin52	7715.41	7542	86.03	29 187 468.75	4 773 500
	ch130	6 285.67	6 132	65.39	35 962 099.26	2 393 250
	kroA200	30 656.83	29 873	383.39	30 716 573.86	17 449 000
	fl417	15 606.65	12 334	3834.63	7 884 671.05	23 262 250
PDC	berlin52	7 623.19	7 542	112.19	8 229 670.73	938 500
	ch130	6 382.00	6 167	164.77	10 588 479.16	2 711 000
	kroA200	33 080.72	30 302	2640.78	10 313 587.96	9 064 750
	fl417	20 795.77	12 476	6718.55	5 617 263.89	40 226 500
PDP	berlin52	7 680.51	7 542	100.81	6 172 705.56	992 000
	ch130	7 267.05	6 157	525.97	8 024 200.00	17 250 500
	kroA200	33 515.43	29 808	3 214.05	11 542 349.51	48 532 750
	fl417	20 365.42	12 684	7 516.31	9 178 200.00	25 031 250

evaluated solutions, both for the best result and on average with standard deviation for each algorithm and problem instance. The experiments were performed with the parameters from Table 1. It shows that PDC and PDP are not able to outperform OSGA with the used configurations in general. Both variants often evaluated less solutions to reach qualities that are close to the results that OSGA was able to achieve. For berlin52, PDC and PDP outperformed OSGA slightly, reaching better qualities on average and requiring less evaluated solutions compared to OSGA for doing so. In the other cases, OSGA found better solutions and, on average, reached better qualities. One reason for this may be the higher number of evaluated solutions that OSGA often exhibits.

5   Conclusion and Future Work

In this paper two different approaches for diversity maintenance were presented. The first approach (PDC) attempts to create offspring with good quality and useful diversity. This leads to high amounts of individuals that have to be generated to match the desired criteria. The second approach relaxes the high selection pressure observed with PDC by switching between diversity and quality producing phases depending on the average population similarity and by softening the success ratio parameter.

Both PDC and PDP allow to directly control the diversity of the population and prevent premature convergence. They enable better control over the algorithm and make them more predictable. While this is a helpful property of the extensions, it did not result in producing useful diversity and superior quality compared to OSGA in the scope of the presented experiments.

The reason for this may be that linear adaption of the diversity upper bound was performed which leads to short or missing exploitation phases of collapsed populations which OSGA did heavily as configured in the experiments. Future work will therefore include performing tests with different adaptation strategies for the diversity upper bound.

References

1. Hansheng, L., Lishan, K.: Balance between exploration and exploitation in genetic search. Wuhan Univ. J. Nat. Sci. **4**, 28–32 (1999)
2. Leung, Y., Gao, Y., Xu, Z.B.: Degree of population diversity - a perspective on premature convergence in genetic algorithms and its markov chain analysis. IEEE Trans. Neural Netw. **8**, 1165–1176 (1997)
3. Črepinšek, M., Liu, S.H., Mernik, M.: Exploration and exploitation in evolutionary algorithms: a survey. ACM Comput. Surv. **45**, 1–33 (2013)
4. Scheibenpflug, A., Wagner, S.: An analysis of the intensification and diversification behavior of different operators for genetic algorithms. In: Moreno-Díaz, R., Pichler, F., Quesada-Arencibia, A. (eds.) EUROCAST. LNCS, vol. 8111, pp. 364–371. Springer, Heidelberg (2013)
5. Pandey, H.M., Choudhary, A., Mehrotra, D.: A comparative review of approaches to prevent premature convergence in GA. Appl. Soft Comput. **24**, 1047–1077 (2014)

6. Mahfoud, S.W.: Niching methods for genetic algorithms. Ph.D. thesis, University of Illinois at Urbana-Champaign (1995)
7. Goldberg, D.E., Richardson, J.: Genetic algorithms with sharing for multimodal function optimization. In: Proceedings of the Second International Conference on Genetic Algorithms on Genetic Algorithms and Their Application, pp. 41–49, L. Erlbaum Associates Inc. (1987)
8. Affenzeller, M., Wagner, S.: Offspring selection: a new self-adaptive selection scheme for genetic algorithms. In: Ribeiro, B., Albrecht, R.F., Dobnikar, A., Pearson, D.W., Steele, N.C. (eds.) Adaptive and Natural Computing Algorithms. Springer Computer Series, pp. 218–221. Springer, Heidelberg (2005)
9. Affenzeller, M., Wagner, S.: SASEGASA: an evolutionary algorithm for retarding premature convergence by self-adaptive selection pressure steering. In: Mira, J., Alvarez, J.R. (eds.) IWANN 2003. LNCS, vol. 2686, pp. 438–445. Springer, Heidelberg (2003)
10. Affenzeller, M., Wagner, S.: Reconsidering the selection concept of genetic algorithms from a population genetics inspired point of view. In: Trappl, R. (ed.) Cybernetics and Systems 2004, vol. 2, pp. 701–706. Austrian Society for Cybernetic Studies, Vienna (2004)
11. Affenzeller, M., Wagner, S., Winkler, S.: Goal-oriented preservation of essential genetic information by offspring selection. In: Proceedings of the Genetic and Evolutionary Computation Conference (GECCO 2005), vol. 2, pp. 1595–1596. Association for Computing Machinery (ACM) (2005)
12. Wagner, S., Kronberger, G., Beham, A., Kommenda, M., Scheibenpflug, A., Pitzer, E., Vonolfen, S., Kofler, M., Winkler, S., Dorfer, V., Affenzeller, M.: Architecture and design of the heuristiclab optimization environment. In: Klempous, R., Nikodem, J., Jacak, W., Chaczko, Z. (eds.) Advanced Methods and Applications in Computational Intelligence. TIEI, vol. 6, pp. 193–258. Springer, Heidelberg (2013)

CPU Versus GPU Parallelization of an Ant Colony Optimization for the Longest Common Subsequence Problem

David Markvica[✉], Christian Schauer, and Günther R. Raidl

Institute of Computer Graphics and Algorithms, TU Wien, Vienna, Austria
david.markvica@student.tuwien.ac.at,
schauer@ads.tuwien.ac.at, raidl@ac.tuwien.ac.at

Abstract. We analyze the runtime behavior of an ant colony optimization approach for the longest common subsequence problem executed on a many-core GPU and a multi-core CPU. Our approach is a parallelized variant of a previously published algorithm. Moreover, we are able to significantly improve the results of the original one by adapting the heuristic function of the ant colony algorithm. Our results show that despite its many more cores the GPU has no significant advantages over the CPU-based approach.

1 Introduction

Over the last years a paradigm shift in the design of processing units led from single-core to multi-core architectures. Modern central processing units (CPUs) typically contain two to four cores, high-end CPUs even more. As a consequence a rethinking from sequential to parallel algorithms became necessary to efficiently utilize the computational power of modern hardware. Especially graphics processing units (GPUs) used on graphics cards feature hundreds of cores since operations like texture mapping, polygon rendering, and vertex processing are inherently parallel. Nowadays, the peak performance of GPUs is theoretically an order of magnitude larger than that of CPUs. As a consequence the usage of GPUs in the context of scientific computing steadily increased over the last years. Typical application areas (apart from classical graphics and image processing) include, e.g., physics simulations, image processing applications, and statistical modeling.

In the field of computational intelligence population based metaheuristics provide a good basis for parallelization. In recent years many attempts were made on GPUs to accelerate metaheuristics like genetic algorithms or ant colony optimization because they are naturally comprised of parallel components. In this context several articles, e.g., [1,7], report massive speedups for algorithms executed partly or mainly on the GPU compared to the CPU. Taking a closer look these comparisons do not always seem fair. In many cases the programming languages used for the implementations on the GPU and the CPU differ. Usually the runtime of an algorithm executed in parallel on the GPU is compared to the

© Springer International Publishing Switzerland 2015
R. Moreno-Díaz et al. (Eds.): EUROCAST 2015, LNCS 9520, pp. 401–408, 2015.
DOI: 10.1007/978-3-319-27340-2_50

single core runtime of the CPU and not all cores. Often the same parameter settings are used for both architectures but are chosen in favor of the GPU with its many but slower cores. Lee et al. [5] present a detailed critique about this practice.

To form our own opinion we were interested whether we can confirm or soften this critique in the context of a specific problem and metaheuristic. We analyze here the runtime behavior of an *ant colony optimization* (ACO) for the *longest common subsequence* (LCS) problem on a many-core GPU in comparison to a multi-core CPU. The LCS is one of the classical problems in string processing and seeks the longest string that is a subsequence of every string in a set of strings. LCS finds applications in computational biology, data compression, and file comparison. The ACO itself was implemented in OpenCL, which supports parallel execution of the same program on CPU and GPU, allowing a relatively fair side-by-side comparison of the algorithm on both architectures. Our analysis shows that for all instances a fine-tuned approach for the CPU outperforms a fine-tuned approach for the GPU in terms of runtime.

The rest of the paper is organized as follows. We discuss related work for the LCS in Sect. 2 and present a formal definition in Sect. 3. In Sect. 4 we describe our ACO and its parallelization. A comparison between CPU and GPU performance based on computational results is presented in Sect. 5. We conclude this paper in Sect. 6.

2   Related Work

In case of two strings and an alphabet of fixed size, the LCS problem can be solved exactly in polynomial time using dynamic programming, an approach already applied on the GPU by Yang et al. [10]. The complexity changes, when an arbitrary number of strings is considered. Then the LCS problem becomes NP-complete, even with binary alphabet, as shown by Maier [6].

Shyu and Tsai [8] proposed an ACO for the LCS in 2009, which at that time became the state-of-the-art heuristic. Their approach is also the main basis for our ACO and will be described in more detail in Sect. 4.

In 2010 Blum [3] presented a hybrid algorithm that combines *beam search* (BS) with ACO. The so called *beam-ACO* uses BS for the heuristic function of the ACO and provides better solutions than BS alone, especially for DNA sequences. For DNA sequences beam-ACO performs slower than BS alone but for protein sequences it is faster.

The current state-of-the-art heuristic [9] is a *hyper heuristic* proposed by Tabataba and Mousavi. Basically their hyper heuristic uses a BS comprised of two different heuristic functions. Since neither of the heuristic functions alone showed an advantage over the other during their experiments, the hyper heuristic simply uses both. In a preprocessing step both heuristic functions are applied with a small beam size to determine the better function for the particular instance. In a second step the favored heuristic is executed again but this time with the full beam width.

Algorithm 1.1. ACO Algorithm

1 $c^* \leftarrow \lvert LCS2(S_x, S_y) \rvert$	**// CPU**
2 copy strings to execution device memory	**// CPU**
3 initialize pheromone trails & ant memory	
4 $totalBest \leftarrow \emptyset$	
5 **while** *termination condition not met* **do**	
6 **foreach** *ant* **do**	
7 construct *ant* solution	
8 $currentBest \leftarrow$ best solution of this iteration	
9 update pheromone trail	
10 **if** $currentBest$ *is better than* $totalBest$ **then**	
11 $totalBest \leftarrow currentBest$	
12 copy $totalBest$ to main memory	**// CPU**

3   Longest Common Subsequence Problem

Let $A = [a_1, \ldots, a_l]$ be a sequence of l elements (i.e., a string), where each element is chosen from a finite alphabet Σ, $a_i \in \Sigma, \forall i \in \{1, \ldots, l\}$.

A sequence $B = [b_1, \ldots, b_k]$ is called a *subsequence* of A ($B \prec A$), if there exists a strictly increasing sequence of indexes $[i_1, \ldots, i_k]$ such that $A[i_j] = B[j]$, $j \in \{1, \ldots, k\}$ and $k \leq l$ holds. Furthermore, let $S = \{S_1, \ldots, S_n\}$ be a finite set of n strings, then C is a called *common subsequence*, iff $C \prec S_i, \forall i \in \{1, \ldots, n\}$.

As a consequence the *longest common subsequence* (LCS) of S is the common subsequence of maximum length. Note that the LCS need not be unique, i.e., there can be more than one common subsequence with maximum length.

4   An Ant Colony Optimization for LCS

Algorithm 1.1 shows the main loop of the ACO. Apart from the initialization (line 1) and data transfer from and to the execution device (lines 2, 12), the entire program can be run on the GPU or the CPU. Our implementation uses PyOpenCL [4], which allows us to implement the execution device independent parts (lines 3–11) as OpenCL kernels. At runtime each OpenCL kernel is compiled into specialized and optimized machine code for the particular execution device.

The algorithm starts by calculating the optimal LCS c^* of two randomly selected strings (line 1) to determine an upper bound for the length of the expected solution. Since this is not a performance critical part of the algorithm, it can be executed on the CPU using any LCS2 algorithm, e.g., one mentioned by Bergroth et al. [2].

The construction of the ant solutions is done in parallel for each *ant* (lines 6–7). A detailed description of this step is given in Algorithm 1.2 in Sect. 4.1. The ACO tracks the best solution found by an ant during each iteration and stores it in

Algorithm 1.2. Construct Ant Solution

```
1   solution ← ∅
2   randomly choose string S_r,   1 ≤ r ≤ n
3   u_i ← 0,   ∀i : 1 ≤ i ≤ n
4   while u_r ≤ |S_r| do
5       Cand ← [u_r + 1, u_r + 2, ..., max(u_r + d, |S_r|)]
6       foreach c ∈ Cand do
7           char ← character at position c in S_r
8           v_c ← calculate next occurrences of character char in all strings
9           pf_c ← calculate probabilistic transition factor pf(c)
10      q ← random number ∈ [0, 1)
11      choose c from Cand by probabilistic function p(v, pf, q)
12      char ← character at position c in S_r
13      solution ← solution ∪ char
14      for i ← 1 to n do
15          u_i ← v_i
```

currentBest (line 8). During the pheromone update (line 9) the pheromone evaporation is computed and the best solution of the current iteration *currentBest* and the overall best solution *totalBest* deposit new pheromones. If a new best solution is found in the current iteration, it is stored in *totalBest* (lines 10–11). When the specified termination condition, e.g., a time or iteration limit, is met (line 5) the algorithm exits the main loop and copies the best solution found from the execution device into the main memory (line 12).

4.1 Construct Ant Solution

Intuitively, the construction process of a solution can be visualized as an ant walking along a randomly assigned string, looking for "good" characters and incrementally constructing a solution. In Algorithm 1.2 this process is formalized.

The solution construction algorithm is executed by each ant in the main loop of Algorithm 1.1 (line 7). At the beginning a random string S_r is selected for the ant "to walk on" (line 2). An array u is used to track the current position of the ant in all strings (line 3). In the while loop the ant walks along S_r (lines 4–15) from left to right until it reaches the end of the string S_r.

At first a set of candidate positions is selected (line 5). One of the characters at these candidate positions is the next character to be added to the solution. From the current position of the ant u_r, the next d characters to the right are considered as candidate positions *Cand*.

Then for each character *char* at a candidate position, the next occurrence $v_i, 1 \leq i \leq n$, is calculated for all strings n (lines 7–8). The probabilistic transition factor $pf(c)$ (line 9) determines the attractiveness of adding character *char* to the solution, see Eq. (1). It is calculated based on previous experiences in form of pheromones τ and the heuristic factor $\eta \in \{\eta_1, \eta_2\}$ by:

Table 1. The average length of the solutions found by the two heuristic functions η_1 and η_2 on DNA and protein datasets with varying number of strings (n).

n		10	15	20	25	40	60	80	100	150	200
DNA	η_1	181.2	164.2	149.5	150.9	139.2	132.1	121.7	120.8	108.8	104.7
	η_2	183.8	167.8	155.6	154.4	141.0	134.1	124.8	124.2	114.0	107.2
Protein	η_1	66.5	56.5	54.0	50.9	46.5	43.7	42.5	41.8	41.5	40.6
	η_2	68.0	59.0	55.6	52.6	47.0	44.4	43.0	42.0	42.0	41.4

$$pf(c) = \frac{[\tau_{r,c}]^\alpha \cdot [\eta_{r,c}]^\beta}{\sum_{z \in Cand}[\tau_{r,z}]^\alpha \cdot [\eta_{r,z}]^\beta} \tag{1}$$

The heuristic function η is based on greedy local decisions and described below. Shyu and Tsai based their η_1 solely on the number of characters that would have to be skipped, if v_r were added to the solution, i.e., non-chosen characters in all strings are simply summed up.

We apply a slightly different heuristic function η_2. Like η_1 it tries to skip as few characters as possible. But in η_2 the relation between the skipped characters and the remaining characters in each string is considered. As shown in Table 1, the modified heuristic function η_2 consistently yields better average results than η_1.

$$\eta_1 = \frac{1}{\sum_{1 \le i \le n}(v_i - u_i)} \qquad \eta_2 = \frac{1}{\sum_{1 \le i \le n}\frac{(v_i - u_i)}{(|S_i| - u_i)}} \tag{2}$$

Finally, at most one candidate position c is determined by function $p(v, pf, q)$ and the character $char$ at position c is added to the ant solution (lines 10–13). A random number q is used to control exploitation, biased exploration and exclusion. In the exploitation case, the candidate with the best probabilistic transition factor is chosen, regardless of all others. When following the exclusion strategy, none of the candidates is chosen, effectively skipping all the candidates in $Cand$. For biased exploitation the probability of selecting a candidate character is proportional to its probabilistic transition factor. In the end the array tracking the current ant position is updated (lines 14–15).

5   Results

Our implementation was tested on a subset of the dataset proposed by Shyu and Tsai in [8]. All runtimes reported are wall-clock times elapsed from the pheromone initialization, to end of the last iteration of the ACO (Algorithm 1.1, lines 3–11).

The CPU runs were performed on an Intel i7-2820QM, a quad-core processor with Hyper-Threading technology, appearing as 8 virtual cores and running at 2300 MHz. For the corresponding GPU runs we used an NVIDIA GeForce GTX 560 Ti graphics card employing 384 CUDA cores running at 1645 MHz. Both systems were running a pre-release version of PyOpenCL 2013.1.

Table 2. The runtime of the program, in seconds, with varying number of ants using the "DNA rat" dataset.

ants	1	2	4	8	16	32	64	128	256	512	1024	2048
CPU time	0.20	0.21	0.22	0.24	0.32	0.50	0.85	1.52	2.86	5.48	10.54	20.45
GPU time	1.54	1.80	2.18	2.72	3.52	4.94	5.03	5.34	5.82	7.16	12.49	12.70

5.1 Parallel Execution

When only a single core is used (i.e., the number of ants is one), execution on the CPU is 7.9 times faster than on the GPU, as shown in Fig. 2. The GPU has a lower clock speed and is not designed and optimized for this kind of workload. On the CPU, the execution time stays almost the same, when the number of ants is increased from one until it exceeds the number of virtual processor cores (in this case eight). After that point the runtime increases linearly, when the number of ants is doubled, the execution time doubles.

On the GPU the execution time appears to rise in a stepwise pattern. The execution times of the configurations between 32 and 256 ants are very similar (4.94 to 5.82 s). This pattern can again be observed when the number of ants is doubled from 1024 to 2048. The runtime remains almost unchanged, increasing only by less than 2 %, from 12.49 to 12.70 s.

In terms of wall-clock execution time, the GPU is able to outperform the CPU only after about 1300 ants or more working in parallel. If the CPU is restricted to single core execution, the GPU would be faster with 85 ants or more.

5.2 Architecture Specific Parameter Tuning

Based on a series of micro benchmarks, two sets of parameters were chosen and their performance was tested on the CPU and GPU. The first parameter set is called *setCPU* and is a conservative setting using 32 ants and 2000 iterations. As the name implies, it is designed to perform well on the CPU. The second set of parameters (*setGPU*) is optimized for execution on the GPU and uses a high number of ants (1500 – 3000 depending on the instance size due to memory limitations) and a lower number of iterations (200). We tested both parameters sets on both architectures an compared the runtimes. The results are presented in Table 3.

Running the program with the same parameters on the CPU and the GPU gives almost the same solution quality. This is to be expected because exactly the same program is run on both devices.

Also, both parameter sets, *setCPU* and *setGPU*, produce solutions of similar quality, the difference of the LCS is less than 2 characters on average. The solution quality of the ACO alone is comparable to the results reported by Shyu and Tsai in [8] for their ACO plus local search hybrid. On DNA sequences the

Table 3. Comparison of the parameter sets for CPU and GPU executed on both architectures. The first column shows the dataset "DNA rat" and "Protein virus" and the varying number of strings n is printed in the second column. For each parameter set the average length of the LCS in characters and the average runtime in seconds together with the respective standard deviations in parentheses is presented.

| | | CPU | | | | GPU | | | |
| | | setGPU | | setCPU | | setGPU | | setCPU | |
	n	LCS	time [s]	LCS	time [s]	LCS	time [s]	LCS	time [s]
DNA rat	10	184.5(0.6)	43.6(0.5)	183.7(0.7)	6.9(0.5)	185.3(1.0)	25.9(0.0)	183.8(0.6)	99.1(0.0)
	15	169.5(0.9)	52.8(0.5)	167.7(0.6)	9.0(0.3)	168.7(0.6)	42.3(0.0)	169.8(1.7)	141.8(0.0)
	20	155.2(0.4)	164.2(4.8)	155.4(0.5)	21.2(0.5)	155.6(0.7)	75.7(0.1)	155.1(0.2)	448.8(0.2)
	25	155.4(0.9)	214.5(5.9)	154.5(1.1)	27.0(0.9)	155.6(0.6)	107.0(0.1)	154.1(0.2)	588.3(0.1)
	40	142.7(0.5)	316.7(9.0)	141.0(0.3)	37.8(1.3)	142.3(0.7)	169.9(0.2)	141.2(0.8)	877.9(1.1)
	60	135.4(0.6)	502.1(52.2)	134.1(0.9)	53.5(1.9)	135.3(0.8)	251.6(0.6)	133.8(0.5)	1280.9(0.4)
	80	127.2(0.8)	984.9(90.0)	124.8(0.9)	103.7(2.5)	127.5(0.9)	420.6(1.2)	126.7(1.3)	2433.6(1.3)
	100	125.4(0.7)	777.7(77.8)	124.0(0.6)	78.8(3.4)	125.6(0.8)	382.5(1.4)	124.8(0.5)	1983.7(2.3)
	150	115.3(0.8)	1634.0(176.2)	114.0(0.9)	258.6(15.6)	115.1(1.0)	1056.5(1.1)	113.2(0.4)	5959.9(3.3)
	200	108.4(1.0)	684.5(74.8)	106.8(1.0)	132.0(8.9)	108.8(1.1)	477.6(3.1)	107.9(1.0)	3193.0(2.4)
Protein virus	10	69.0(0.4)	89.8(1.7)	68.0(0.0)	11.7(1.0)	68.9(0.3)	48.0(0.1)	68.0(0.0)	295.3(0.2)
	15	59.7(0.5)	102.7(3.7)	59.0(0.0)	13.4(0.4)	60.0(0.5)	63.7(0.3)	59.0(0.0)	370.5(0.2)
	20	55.8(0.4)	126.3(3.4)	55.6(0.5)	16.6(0.6)	55.1(0.4)	85.5(0.2)	55.5(0.5)	467.2(0.4)
	25	52.8(0.4)	149.6(8.8)	52.6(0.5)	19.3(0.7)	52.2(0.4)	110.9(0.2)	51.8(0.4)	577.3(0.5)
	40	47.8(0.4)	220.0(10.0)	47.0(0.0)	26.1(1.7)	47.2(0.4)	177.3(0.2)	47.0(0.0)	837.0(0.9)
	60	44.3(0.5)	316.7(7.7)	44.4(0.5)	37.2(3.0)	44.3(0.5)	250.8(0.8)	44.0(0.0)	1163.8(1.6)
	80	43.0(0.2)	480.2(56.6)	43.0(0.2)	52.0(2.4)	43.0(0.0)	320.4(0.6)	42.2(0.4)	1488.6(1.0)
	100	43.0(0.0)	588.4(98.7)	42.0(0.0)	64.5(3.1)	43.0(0.2)	401.9(2.4)	42.1(0.3)	1858.2(1.9)
	150	42.6(0.5)	786.2(109.2)	42.0(0.0)	131.9(5.2)	42.6(0.5)	670.1(1.0)	42.0(0.0)	3463.9(0.9)
	200	42.0(0.2)	768.9(71.7)	41.4(0.5)	175.0(6.9)	42.0(0.2)	698.8(1.2)	41.0(0.0)	4632.8(6.2)

solution quality is equally good or slightly worse and on protein sequences it is consistently better.

With regard to the runtime, the parameter sets obviously favor the architecture they were designed for. Using *setCPU* on the CPU and *setGPU* on the GPU results in much shorter runtimes than switching the parameter sets on the architectures.

When we compare the runtime of the CPU using the *setCPU* parameters with the runtime of the GPU using the *setGPU* parameters, the CPU is faster in all tests. In the DNA tests the CPU is faster than the GPU by a factor of 3.5 to 4.85 and in the protein tests by a factor of 4 to 6.8. This is because we compare the GPU to a multi-core CPU, not just to a single core.

Using the reverse parameter set the runtime drastically increases for the runs on the GPU with *setCPU* (3.3 to 6.6 times slower than *setGPU*). For the CPU runs with *setGPU* the runtime also increases. In this case the CPU becomes slower than the GPU using *setGPU*, up to a factor of 2.3, which resembles the results from the literature. We already argued that this comparison is not fair but in favor of the GPU. When each architecture uses its respective parameter set the multi-core CPU clearly outperforms the many-core GPU. Thus, we cannot confirm the trend documented in the literature for our use case.

6 Conclusions

In this work we analyzed the runtime behavior of a many-core GPU and a multi-core CPU. For our experiments we decided on an ACO for the longest common subsequence problem implemented on a many-core GPU in comparison to a multi-core CPU. We implemented the ACO in OpenCL, which allows parallel execution on the GPU as well as the CPU, which we considered as a requirement for a fair comparison. During the implementation we were able to improve the original ACO in terms of solution quality by adapting its heuristic function. We then determined fine-tuned settings for both architectures respectively—another requirement—and compared the runtime behavior according to these setting. As expected, our results showed that the parallel execution on the GPU outperforms a sequential execution on a single-core CPU in terms of wall-clock runtime. But the situation changes, when we execute the ACO on all CPU cores in parallel. In that case the many-core GPU could not catch up with the multi-core CPU runs.

References

1. Bai, H., OuYang, D., Li, X., He, L., Yu, H.: MAX-MIN ant system on GPU with CUDA. In: Proceedings of the 2009 Fourth International Conference on Innovative Computing, Information and Control, pp. 801–804. IEEE Press (2009)
2. Bergroth, L., Hakonen, H., Raita, T.: A survey of longest common subsequence algorithms. In: Proceedings Seventh International Symposium on String Processing and Information Retrieval, SPIRE 2000, pp. 39–48 (2000)
3. Blum, C.: Beam-ACO for the longest common subsequence problem. In: Proceedings of the 2010 IEEE Congress on Evolutionary Computation (CEC), pp. 1–8. IEEE Press (2010)
4. Klöckner, A., Pinto, N., Lee, Y., Catanzaro, B., Ivanov, P., Fasih, A.: PyCUDA and PyOpenCL: a scripting-based approach to GPU run-time code generation. Parallel Comput. **38**(3), 157–174 (2012)
5. Lee, V.W., Kim, C., Chhugani, J., Deisher, M., Kim, D., Nguyen, A.D., Satish, N., Smelyanskiy, M., Chennupaty, S., Hammarlund, P., Singhal, R., Dubey, P.: Debunking the 100X GPU vs. CPU Myth: an evaluation of throughput computing on CPU and GPU. ACM SIGARCH Comput. Architect. News **38**(3), 451–460 (2010)
6. Maier, D.: The complexity of some problems on subsequences and supersequences. J. ACM **25**, 322–336 (1978)
7. Pospichal, P., Jaros, J., Schwarz, J.: Parallel genetic algorithm on the CUDA architecture. In: Di Chio, C., Cagnoni, S., Cotta, C., Ebner, M., Ekárt, A., Esparcia-Alcazar, A.I., Goh, C.-K., Merelo, J.J., Neri, F., Preuß, M., Togelius, J., Yannakakis, G.N. (eds.) EvoApplicatons 2010, Part I. LNCS, vol. 6024, pp. 442–451. Springer, Heidelberg (2010)
8. Shyu, S.J., Tsai, C.Y.: Finding the longest common subsequence for multiple biological sequences by ant colony optimization. Comput. Oper. Res. **36**, 73–91 (2009)
9. Tabataba, F.S., Mousavi, S.R.: A hyper-heuristic for the longest common subsequence problem. Comput. Biol. Chem. **36**, 42–54 (2012)
10. Yang, J., Xu, Y., Shang, Y.: An efficient parallel algorithm for longest common subsequence problem on GPUs. Lect. Notes Eng. Comput. Sci. **2183**(1), 499–504 (2010)

Complexity Measures for Multi-objective Symbolic Regression

Michael Kommenda[1,2]($\boxtimes$), Andreas Beham[1,2], Michael Affenzeller[1,2],
and Gabriel Kronberger[1]

[1] Heuristic and Evolutionary Algorithms Laboratory, School of Informatics,
Communications and Media, University of Applied Sciences Upper Austria,
Softwarepark 11, 4232 Hagenberg, Austria
{michael.kommenda,andreas.beham,michael.affenzeller,
gabriel.kronberger}@fh-hagenberg.at
[2] Institute for Formal Models and Verification, Johannes Kepler University Linz,
Altenbergerstr. 69, 4040 Linz, Austria

Abstract. Multi-objective symbolic regression has the advantage that
while the accuracy of the learned models is maximized, the complexity
is automatically adapted and need not be specified a-priori. The result
of the optimization is not a single solution anymore, but a whole Pareto-
front describing the trade-off between accuracy and complexity.

In this contribution we study which complexity measures are most
appropriately used in symbolic regression when performing multi-
objective optimization with NSGA-II. Furthermore, we present a novel
complexity measure that includes semantic information based on the
function symbols occurring in the models and test its effects on several
benchmark datasets. Results comparing multiple complexity measures
are presented in terms of the achieved accuracy and model length to
illustrate how the search direction of the algorithm is affected.

Keywords: Symbolic regression · Complexity measures · Multi-
objective optimization · NSGA-II · Genetic programming

1 Introduction

Symbolic regression is a data-based machine learning method, where the relation
between several independent and one dependent variable is modeled. Contrary
to other modeling methods the structure of the learned model is not specified
a-priori, but determined during the algorithm execution. Symbolic regression
problems are commonly solved by genetic programming (GP) [6], because the
variable-length encoding used in GP is particularly suited for the evolution of the
model structure. An expression tree encoding is frequently used in GP for symbolic regression, where every leaf node represent either a variable or a numeric
constant and every internal node a mathematical function. Thus, every expression tree represents a mathematical formula that can be interpreted, validated
and easily incorporated in other programs [1].

© Springer International Publishing Switzerland 2015
R. Moreno-Díaz et al. (Eds.): EUROCAST 2015, LNCS 9520, pp. 409–416, 2015.
DOI: 10.1007/978-3-319-27340-2_51

The phenomenon of bloat in GP [7] (an increase in the average size of the individuals without an corresponding increase in fitness), overly complex and large individuals, or the excessive use of variables reduce the interpretability of symbolic regression methods. As bloat and introns are not specific to symbolic regression, but rather occur when using arbitrary-sized representations in evolutionary computation [8], several methods to limit the growth of GP individuals and to counteract bloat have been suggested previously. One approach is to specify static size and depth limits for the symbolic expression trees used in GP [10] that must not be exceeded. However, these two limits are highly problem-dependent, cannot be known a-priori and must be adapted for each problem so that the trees can grow large enough to model the data accurately while unnecessary complexity is avoided. Other methods of controlling the tree size range from dynamic size limits [11] or parsimony pressure methods [9] to controlling the distribution of tree sizes [3].

The previously mentioned methods have been developed to limit the growth of symbolic expression trees in GP and do not include any semantic information about the mathematical formulas represented by the expression trees when performing symbolic regression. Although complexity is to some extent correlated to size, it is not necessarily the case that the complexity of a formula is reflected in its size. For example the formula $f(x) = e^{\sin \sqrt{x}}$ consists of three operations, one variable, and one constant, while $f(x) = 7x^2 + 3x + 5$ consists of five operations, two variable, and three constants and is intuitively less complex.

A different approach for managing complexity and model size in symbolic regression is to use multi-objective optimization, where while maximizing the prediction accuracy the complexity is minimized [8,12]. Hence, no size limits or other complexity related parameters must be configured and the optimization algorithm is expected to automatically evolve solutions of appropriate length and complexity. In this contribution we compare the effects on algorithm performance of several complexity and size related quality criteria for multi-objective symbolic regression on benchmark problems.

2   Multi-objective Symbolic Regression

The nondominant sorting genetic algorithm II (NSGA-II) [2] is one of the most prominent algorithms for multi-objective optimization. It uses a novel selection mechanism based on the nondomination rank and crowding distance for selection to build a uniformly spread Pareto-optimal front. In the case of multi-objective symbolic regression the objectives to be optimized are the prediction accuracy and the complexity of the learned models. The prediction accuracy can be expressed by any error or correlation measure such as the coefficient of determination R^2, the mean squared error, or the mean absolute percentage error between the estimated and observed values.

The complexity of a symbolic regression model can be calculated as the *tree length* or the *expressional complexity* (visitation length) [5,12]. More sophisticated measures that also include semantics of the evolved models range from the number of included variables, or the *order of nonlinearity* [14] to the *functional complexity* [13]. While the *order of nonlinearity* and the *functional complexity* express the complexity of a symbolic regression model rather accurately, they are computationally expensive to calculate. On the other hand, measures such as the *tree length* or the *expressional complexity* are efficiently calculated, but do not include any information except the shape of the symbolic expression tree encoding the model.

We propose a new complexity measure that is easy to calculate and includes semantics about the regression model, so that the search direction of the multi-objective algorithm is altered towards simple and parsimonious models. The measure is calculated by recursive iteration over the symbolic expression tree and accumulates the individual complexity values for each subtree while taking into account different complexity values for the encountered function symbols. The mathematical definition for the calculation of this new complexity measure is given in Eq. 1, where n denotes a tree node and c a direct child node of n. The complexity of the whole symbolic expression tree encoding the regression model can then be calculated by recursive application of Eq. 1 starting at the root node.

$$\text{Complexity}(n) = \begin{cases} 1 & \text{if } n \equiv \text{constant} \\ 2 & \text{if } n \equiv \text{variable} \\ \sum \text{Complexity}(c) & \text{if } n \in (+, -) \\ \prod \text{Complexity}(c) + 1 & \text{if } n \in (*, /) \\ \text{Complexity}(c)^2 & \text{if } n \equiv \text{square} \\ \text{Complexity}(c)^3 & \text{if } n \equiv \text{squareroot} \\ 2^{\text{Complexity}(c)} & \text{if } n \in (\sin, \cos, \tan, \exp, \log) \end{cases} \quad (1)$$

In the following we explore the complexity differences of two exemplary models, $f_1(x) = e^{\sin \sqrt{x}}$ and $f_2(x) = 7x^2 + 3x + 5$. The corresponding symbolic expression trees representing these formulas are illustrated in Fig. 1. The tree length for $f_1(x)$ is 4 and 9 for $f_2(x)$, which indicates that representation of $f_1(x)$ is more compact. However, Fig. 1 also shows the calculation steps for the new complexity measure according to Eq. 1, which is iteratively applied starting at the leaf nodes. The complexity measure results in 65536 for $f_1(x)$ and 17 for $f_2(x)$, which reflects our intuition that $f_2(x)$ is less complex and easier to interpret than $f_1(x)$, whereas according to the tree length the contrary is true.

3   Experiments

We used an NSGA-II algorithm to test the effects of different complexity measures for multi-objective symbolic regression. The first objective for the algorithm is the Pearson's R^2 correlation describing the model accuracy. Varying complexity measures such as the number of used variables (*Variables*), the model length (*Tree Length*), the expressional complexity (*Visitation Length*) and the

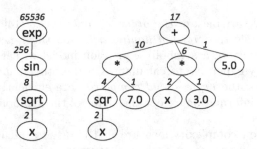

Fig. 1. Symbolic expression tree representation of $f_1(x) = e^{\sin \sqrt{x}}$ and $f_2(x) = 7x^2 + 3x + 5$, where the calculation steps for the complexity measure are indicated next to the arcs.

new complexity measure (*Complexity*) described in Eq. 1 have been used as second optimization objective. Despite maximizing the Pearson's R^2, the results regarding accuracy are presented in terms of the normalized mean squared error (NMSE), so that for both measures smaller values are better.

NSGA-II was configured to evolve models with a maximum tree length of 100 that are allowed to include arithmetic $(+, -, *, /)$, trigonometric $(\sin, \cos, \tan)$, power$(^2, \sqrt{})$ and exponential $(\exp, \log)$ symbols and stops when the termination criterion of $200,000$ model evaluations has been reached. The benchmark problems used for testing have been selected from [4,15] and the generating formulas are listed in Table 1.

When switching from single to multi-objective algorithms the result of an algorithm execution is not a single solution any more, but rather a Pareto-front showing the trade-off between accuracy and complexity of the models. An example of a Pareto-front generated by the NSGA-II is shown in Fig. 2, where besides the training qualities the models' accuracies on the test set are shown to evaluate their generalization capabilities. However, whole Pareto-fronts are hard

Table 1. Definition of benchmark problems.

Name	Function
Keijzer-5	$f(x_1, x_2, x_3) = 30x_1 x_3 / [(x_1 - 10)x_2^2]$
Vladislavleva-1	$f(x_1, x_2) = e^{-(x_1 - 1)^2} / [1.2 + (x_2 - 2.5)^2]$
Vladislavleva-2	$f(x_1) = e^{-x_1} x_1^3 \cos(x) \sin(x)(\cos(x) \sin^2(x) - 1)$
Vladislavleva-7	$f(x_1, x_2) = (x_1 - 3)(x_2 - 3) + 2\sin((x_1 - 4)(x_2 - 4))$
Pagie-1	$f(x_1, x_2) = 1/[1 + x_1^{-4}] + 1/[1 + x_2^{-4}]$
Poly-10	$f(x_1 - x_{10}) = x_1 x_2 + x_3 x_4 + x_5 x_6 + x_1 x_7 x_9 + x_3 x_6 x_{10}$
Friedman-1	$f(x_1 - x_{10}) = 0.1e^{4x_1} + 4/[1 + e^{-20x_2} + 10] + 3x_3 + 2x_2 + x_5 + N$
Friedman-2	$f(x_1 - x_{10}) = 10\sin(\pi x_1 x_2) + 20(x_3 - 0.5)^2 + 10x_4 + 5x_5 + N$
Tower	Real world data

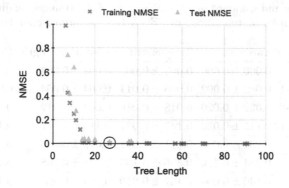

Fig. 2. Exemplary Pareto-front evolved by NSGA-II showing the trade-off between accuracy in terms of the NMSE and the model length. Every model contributes to two data points, one for training and one for test evaluation (if no test evaluation is shown, the NMSE exceeds 1.0). The *best* model, which is rather small but still accurate, is encircled.

to compare, especially in the case of symbolic regression where a high training quality doesn't necessary indicate a good model due to overfitting reasons (for example the largest models in Fig. 2 whose test NMSEs exceeds 1.0 and are not displayed at all). Hence, we used only single models of a Pareto-front for algorithm comparison and used the model with the highest training accuracy. A better way for model selection would be, if an additional validation partition is defined, to use the model with the highest accuracy on this partition.

4   Results

We have performed 50 repetitions of each NSGA-II configuration to account for the stochastic nature of the algorithm. We extracted the most accurate models, at the same time the most complex ones, from each generated Pareto-front and compared them against each other. In Table 2 the average and standard deviation of those models are displayed. Although for most of the problems the results are quite similar, there are some differences. The *Complexity* configuration obtains by far the best results with the smallest variation on the Poly-10 problem. The *Variables* configuration works best on the Friedman-2 problem and both configuration perfrom well on the Pagie-1 problem.

The generalization capabilities of the best models have been evaluated on a separate test partition and those results are shown in Table 3. Every configuration produces, at least on some problems, overfit models, which is indicate by an high average normalized squared error and high standard deviations. The *Tree Length* and *Visitation Length* perform equally well with the exception of the Vladislavleva-1 and Pagie-1 problem. It still holds that the *Complexity* and *Variables* algorithm runs produced the best models on the Poly-10 and Friedman-2 problem respectively. An interesting observation is that excluding

Table 2. Average and standard deviation ($\mu \pm \sigma$) of the training qualities (NMSE) of the best individual for 50 repetitions of NSGA-II with varying complexity measures.

Problem	Variables	Tree length	Visitation length	Complexity
Keijzer-5	0.000 ± 0.000	0.003 ± 0.003	0.002 ± 0.003	0.000 ± 0.000
Vladislavleva-1	0.002 ± 0.002	0.005 ± 0.011	0.004 ± 0.004	0.002 ± 0.002
Vladislavleva-2	0.022 ± 0.020	0.018 ± 0.016	0.014 ± 0.012	0.016 ± 0.013
Vladislavleva-7	0.111 ± 0.020	0.147 ± 0.077	0.116 ± 0.027	0.115 ± 0.027
Pagie-1	0.001 ± 0.003	0.011 ± 0.017	0.012 ± 0.018	0.007 ± 0.003
Poly-10	0.294 ± 0.126	0.356 ± 0.165	0.341 ± 0.168	0.202 ± 0.079
Friedman-1	0.140 ± 0.004	0.157 ± 0.019	0.163 ± 0.023	0.175 ± 0.021
Friedman-2	0.081 ± 0.031	0.134 ± 0.050	0.146 ± 0.038	0.143 ± 0.049
Tower	0.148 ± 0.025	0.148 ± 0.020	0.146 ± 0.016	0.140 ± 0.018

Vladislavleva-1 and Vladislavleva-2 the *Complexity* measure as second objective performs either better or equally well as the other configurations. A reason for this might be that those two problems consist of complicated formulas that have to be discovered and the algorithm is not able to build that complicated yet accurate formulas. The other complexity measure that do not include semantic information about the models, have no such limitations as long as the models are compact enough.

Table 3. Average and standard deviation ($\mu \pm \sigma$) of the quality of the best training individual evaluated on the test partition for 50 repetitions of the multi-objective symbolic regression algorithm with varying complexity measures.

Problem	Variables	Tree length	Visitation length	Complexity
Keijzer-5	0.000 ± 0.000	0.004 ± 0.003	0.002 ± 0.003	0.000 ± 0.000
Vladislavleva-1	1.568 ± 1.568	0.047 ± 0.062	1.460 ± 8.291	5.509 ± 12.00
Vladislavleva-2	0.112 ± 0.587	0.023 ± 0.022	0.019 ± 0.014	0.823 ± 3.193
Vladislavleva-7	0.529 ± 2.753	0.168 ± 0.099	0.138 ± 0.037	0.138 ± 0.125
Pagie-1	0.015 ± 2.174	0.445 ± 1.737	0.061 ± 0.087	0.028 ± 0.046
Poly-10	0.457 ± 0.211	0.558 ± 1.188	0.510 ± 0.626	0.301 ± 0.129
Friedman-1	0.150 ± 0.000	0.156 ± 0.019	0.169 ± 0.024	0.175 ± 0.021
Friedman-2	0.083 ± 0.032	0.143 ± 0.054	0.149 ± 0.039	0.140 ± 0.049
Tower	0.138 ± 0.026	0.144 ± 0.020	0.144 ± 0.019	0.138 ± 0.018

Next to the accuracy of the models their interpretability is of importance, because model interpretability is one of the major reasons to use symbolic regression. The lengths of the models generated by NSGA-II with varying complexity

Table 4. Average and standard deviation ($\mu \pm \sigma$) of the length of the best training individuals for 50 repetitions of NSGA-II with varying complexity measures.

Problem	Variables	Tree length	Visitation length	Complexity
Keijzer-5	86.3 ± 19.34	21.2 ± 13.30	22.7 ± 15.75	47.0 ± 18.59
Vladislavleva-1	91.8 ± 15.27	44.6 ± 22.72	41.7 ± 24.71	85.7 ± 22.22
Vladislavleva-2	88.7 ± 16.81	42.6 ± 23.47	37.7 ± 21.21	79.8 ± 21.77
Vladislavleva-7	94.4 ± 10.93	44.0 ± 29.41	48.4 ± 29.98	81.3 ± 24.08
Pagie-1	91.7 ± 16.50	51.7 ± 28.88	40.6 ± 23.34	72.4 ± 28.01
Poly-10	96.8 ± 7.320	53.0 ± 30.79	54.8 ± 30.06	72.7 ± 24.70
Friedman-1	90.5 ± 12.96	61.0 ± 26.81	55.1 ± 29.74	69.2 ± 26.53
Friedman-2	91.4 ± 12.00	47.1 ± 28.60	40.8 ± 25.30	68.3 ± 25.54
Tower	94.4 ± 8.860	59.8 ± 29.30	58.9 ± 27.02	78.2 ± 21.07

measures have been compared and the results are stated in Table 4. It is clear that the *Variables* configuration, which just counts the variable occurrences, generates by far the largest models as no selection pressure towards more parsimonious ones is applied. The *Tree Length* and *Visitation Length* produce the smallest models and no significant differences could be found between these two variations. Although no explicit parsimony pressure is applied to models created by NSGA-II with the new complexity measure, these are smaller than the ones produced by *Variables*, but still larger than those using explicitly the tree and visitation length for optimization.

5   Conclusion

In this publication we have investigated the effects of different complexity measures on multi-objective symbolic regression. Furthermore, we have presented a novel complexity measure based on the mathematical symbols occurring in the formulas. The differences with respect to the accuracies of the models on the tested benchmark problems were in most cases not significant. An exception is the new complexity measure that performs best on problems with simpler data generating formulas, but on the other hand fails to evolve well-fitting models on the most complex problems.

When comparing the length of the evolved models to give an indication of their interpretability, the algorithm configurations explicitly using the tree length as an optimization objective generated the most parsimonious models. As previously argued and used as motivation for the development of the new complexity measure, the length is only to some extend correlated to simplicity and interpretability and more research to illustrate the differences of the complexity measures has to be performed.

Acknowledgments. The work described in this paper was done within the COMET Project Heuristic Optimization in Production and Logistics (HOPL), #843532 funded by the Austrian Research Promotion Agency (FFG).

References

1. Affenzeller, M., Winkler, S., Kronberger, G., Kommenda, M., Burlacu, B., Wagner, S.: Gaining deeper insights in symbolic regression. In: Riolo, R., Moore, J.H., Kotanchek, M. (eds.) Genetic Programming Theory and Practice XI. Genetic and Evolutionary Computation, pp. 175–190. Springer, New York (2014)
2. Deb, K., Pratap, A., Agarwal, S., Meyarivan, T.: A fast and elitist multiobjective genetic algorithm: Nsga-ii. IEEE Trans. Evol. Comput. **6**(2), 182–197 (2002)
3. Dignum, S., Poli, R.: Operator equalisation and bloat free GP. In: O'Neill, M., Vanneschi, L., Gustafson, S., Esparcia Alcázar, A.I., De Falco, I., Della Cioppa, A., Tarantino, E. (eds.) EuroGP 2008. LNCS, vol. 4971, pp. 110–121. Springer, Heidelberg (2008)
4. Friedman, J.H.: Multivariate adaptive regression splines. Ann. Stat. **19**, 1–67 (1991)
5. Keijzer, M., Foster, J.: Crossover bias in genetic programming. In: Ebner, M., O'Neill, M., Ekárt, A., Vanneschi, L., Esparcia-Alcázar, A.I. (eds.) EuroGP 2007. LNCS, vol. 4445, pp. 33–44. Springer, Heidelberg (2007)
6. Koza, J.R.: Genetic Programming: On the Programming of Computers by Means of Natural Selection. MIT Press, Cambridge (1992)
7. Luke, S.: Issues in scaling genetic programming: breeding strategies, tree generation, and code bloat. Ph.D. thesis, Dept. of Computer Science. University of Maryland, College Park (2000)
8. Luke, S., Panait, L., et al.: Lexicographic parsimony pressure. In: GECCO 2002: Proceedings of the Genetic and Evolutionary Computation Conference, vol. 2, pp. 829–836 (2002)
9. Poli, R.: Covariant tarpeian method for bloat control in genetic programming. In: Riolo, R., McConaghy, T., Vladislavleva, E. (eds.) Genetic Programming Theory and Practice VIII 8, pp. 71–90. Springer, New York (2010)
10. Poli, R., Langdon, W.B., McPhee, N.F.: A field guide to genetic programming (2008). http://lulu.com
11. Silva, S., Costa, E.: Dynamic limits for bloat control in genetic programming and a review of past and current bloat theories. Genet. Program Evolvable Mach. **10**(2), 141–179 (2009)
12. Smits, G.F., Kotanchek, M.: Pareto-front exploitation in symbolic regression. In: O'Reilly, U.-M., et al. (eds.) Genetic Programming Theory and Practice II, pp. 283–299. Springer, New York (2005)
13. Vanneschi, L., Castelli, M., Silva, S.: Measuring bloat, overfitting and functional complexity in genetic programming. In: Proceedings of the 12th Annual Conference on Genetic and Evolutionary Computation, pp. 877–884. ACM (2010)
14. Vladislavleva, E.J., Smits, G.F., Den Hertog, D.: Order of nonlinearity as a complexity measure for models generated by symbolic regression via pareto genetic programming. IEEE Trans. Evol. Comput. **13**(2), 333–349 (2009)
15. White, D.R., McDermott, J., Castelli, M., Manzoni, L., Goldman, B.W., Kronberger, G., Jaskowski, W., O'Reilly, U.M., Luke, S.: Better GP benchmarks: community survey results and proposals. Genet. Program Evolvable Mach. **14**(1), 3–29 (2013)

Using Contextual Information in Sequential Search for Grammatical Optimization Problems

Gabriel Kronberger[1]($\boxtimes$), Michael Kommenda[1,2], Stephan Winkler[1,2], and Michael Affenzeller[1,2]

[1] Heuristic and Evolutionary Algorithms Laboratory, School of Informatics, Communications and Media, University of Applied Sciences Upper Austria, Hagenberg Campus, Softwarepark 11, 4232 Hagenberg, Austria
{gkronber,mkommend,swinkler,maffenze}@heuristiclab.com
[2] Institute for Formal Models and Verification, Johannes Kepler University Linz, Altenbergerstr. 69, 4040 Linz, Austria

Abstract. Automated synthesis of complex programs is still an unsolved problem even though some successes have been achieved recently for relatively contrived and specialized settings. One possible approach to automated programming is genetic programming, however, a diverse set of alternative techniques are possible which makes it rather difficult to make general assertions about characteristics or structure of automated programming tasks. We have therefore defined the concept of grammatical optimization problems for problems with an objective function and grammar constraint for valid solutions. The problem of synthesizing computer programs can be formulated as a grammatical optimization problem. In this contribution we describe our idea of using contextual information for guiding the search process. First, we describe how the search process can be described as a sequential decision process and show how Monte-Carlo tree search is one way to optimize this decision process. Based on the formulation as a sequential decision process we explain how lexical, syntactical, as well as program state can be used for guiding the search process. This makes it possible to learn problem structure in a way that goes beyond what is possible with simple Monte-Carlo tree search.

Keywords: Automated programming · Genetic programming · Monte-Carlo tree search · Sequential decision processes

1 Introduction

Automated synthesis of complex computer programs is not yet a reality even though a lot of research effort has been invested for solving this particularly hard problem. Recently, some successes have been achieved in rather contrived settings such as programming by example [1], automated correction of bugs [2–4], or super-optimization [5,6]. A generally applicable technology for the synthesis of complex programs in general is however not yet available [7].

© Springer International Publishing Switzerland 2015
R. Moreno-Díaz et al. (Eds.): EUROCAST 2015, LNCS 9520, pp. 417–424, 2015.
DOI: 10.1007/978-3-319-27340-2_52

One possible approach for automated programming propagated by John Koza is genetic programming (GP) which uses an evolutionary algorithm to generate computer programs that solve a given problem when executed [8]. GP relies on a simulated evolutionary process to generate computer programs.

We have previously introduced the notion of "grammatical optimization problems" [9] to refer to a class of problems, that are usually discussed in the context of grammar-guided GP. Examples for problem instances which can be formulated as grammatical optimization problem are symbolic regression, synthesis of controller programs, or synthesis of analog circuits. Instances of this type of optimization problems also occur in areas outside of genetic programming (e.g. in machine learning, cf. [10]). Automated synthesis of computer programs can also be described as a grammatical optimization problem using the syntax description of the target programming language. In a related contribution a declarative language for the specification of grammatical optimization problems has been defined to facilitate experimentation with different kinds of solvers [11].

In this contribution we focus on Monte-Carlo tree search (MCTS) [12,13] for solving grammatical optimization problems. The idea of using MCTS for expression or program synthesis is not new and has been applied effectively before e.g. for expression discovery [14] or for optimizing computation kernels [15]. In this contribution we take a more general approach and discuss the specific assumptions of MCTS – which is one particular form of a sequential search technique. The goal is to identify problem characteristics which make a problem easier or harder for GP or MCTS. Our central claim is that search efficiency can be improved by using contextual information in the search process.

We do not aim to answer the question whether the task of automated program synthesis actually exhibits these characteristics and whether using contextual information can increase the search efficiency and leave this question open for further research.

2   Motivation

It has been shown that the evolutionary approach to program synthesis of genetic programming works well for certain types of problems such as symbolic regression. For the more general goal of automated program synthesis genetic programming has also produced first successes at least for rather simple problems (see e.g. [16] and other recent publications of Helmuth and Spector). We hypothesize that automated programming problems that cannot be solved using GP might be solvable with alternative techniques, for instance Markov-chain Monte-Carlo or Monte-Carlo tree search techniques and that using contextual information is essential for solving harder problems.

3   Grammatical Optimization Problems

We formulate the task of automated program synthesis as a grammatical optimization problem [9]. The syntactical structure of the target programming language is specified using a context-free grammar and additionally an objective function is specified which expresses the quality of a generated program. We use an approach driven by examples or test cases where the inputs and the target outputs of the program must be specified. The goal is then to find a program that produces the correct output for all test cases. A simple objective function could just return the number of failed test cases which should be minimized. More elaborate test functions could incorporate more detailed information on the size of the error or how strongly the produced output deviates from the target output. As described in [9] the objective function encapsulates all language semantics and simply maps a valid sentence in the form of a sequence of symbols (the generated program) to an objective value. The objective value could be a scalar representing the correctness of the program measured through the test cases but could also be a vector that includes more information such as the length of the program or also the runtime of the program.

Solving a grammatical optimization problem means to find a valid sentence of the grammar (representing the synthesized program) that produces the correct output for all supplied test cases. Optimization in the context of grammatical optimization problems means to find an optimal sentence with regard to the potentially multiple objectives. Typically, that means to find a program that produces the correct output for all test cases and is the shortest of all such problems and eventually has the shortest runtime.

In the following, we use the terms as defined in the field of formal languages. The grammar has a specified sentence or root symbol from which all sentences are derived. The grammar also has a set of replacement rules for each non-terminal symbol. Derivation of a complete sentence from the sentence symbol means to repeatedly apply replacement rules on a chain of symbols (phrase) until reaching a terminal phrase containing only terminal symbols (terminal phrases are also called sentences). We are limiting our discussion to context-free grammars even though the presented techniques can also be applied to context-sensitive grammars.

4   Sequential Decision Processes

The derivation of a sentence is a sequential decision process. The process starts with a sequence containing only the sentence symbol and multiple decision steps are necessary where in each step one of the replacement rules is applied until a sequence containing only terminal symbols is found. Generally, multiple non-terminal symbols can be chosen for replacement but by only allowing left-canonical derivation only the left-most non-terminal can be replaced in any step. Generally, it is necessary to chose between multiple alternative replacement rules so a decision is necessary whenever multiple alternatives are available. Practically relevant grammars allow to generate an infinite set of valid sentences. For the purpose of program synthesis it is however useful to add a length constraint for sentences which has the effect that the number of derivation steps is limited for context-free grammars.

In reinforcement learning [17], which is concerned about learning to make optimal decisions in sequential decision processes, the process is augmented with a reward distribution function and when a sample of the decision process is realized a corresponding reward is sampled for each action taken. Rewards are dependent on the action and the current state in the process. One aim of reinforcement learning is to learn to make optimal decisions to collect the maximum total reward based on previous actions and observed rewards. If the decision process is finite and realizations can be repeatedly sampled by restarting the process the problem is called an episodic decision problem. The repeated derivation of sentences from a grammar is an example for an episodic decision problem.

For a given grammar all possible derivation paths form a graph where each node of the graph represents a phrase and the edges of the graph represent the application of replacement rules.

Figure 1 shows a visualization of a part of such a graph for the grammar $G(S) : S \rightarrow a|b|aS|bS$. For this particular grammar the phrase graph is a tree but generally phrases are connected in a graph when it is possible to reach a given phrase through multiple paths. As shown in Fig. 1 the root node of the tree represents the phrase S and four alternatives for the derivation of the phrase are possible. The indicated green path represents the full derivation $S \Rightarrow bS \Rightarrow baS \Rightarrow baaS \Rightarrow baab$.

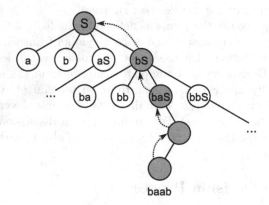

Fig. 1. Example for a MCTS search tree. Leaf-nodes in the tree represent complete sentences the internal nodes of the tree represent phrases visited in the derivation. It is important to note that the search tree is not directly related to the parse trees of sentences, as each leaf node of the search tree represents one sentence and its parse tree.

If full programs are synthesized using this mechanism then each produced program can be executed and tested on the test cases. The quality of the program (e.g. the number of correct test cases) is then used to calculate the reward received at the end of the decision process (when reaching a terminal node in the phrase graph). For simplicity we assume that the output of the programs is deterministic meaning that the reward for reaching a certain terminal phrase is also deterministic. We also assume that only full programs can be executed, this means that partial programs of internal nodes are not executed and that we cannot directly calculate a reward for reaching a non-terminal phrase (internal node). Obviously, we can derive an implicit value of internal nodes when back-propagating rewards from the leaf nodes as indicated in Fig. 1.

5   Monte-Carlo Tree Search

In Monte-Carlo tree search the idea is to visit and extend only those parts of the full search tree that lead to the best possible solutions. Starting from the root node the algorithm selects the actions with higher likelihood that seem best, based on previous rewards. When a leaf node of the search tree is reached the sentence is completed randomly if necessary and the finally achieved reward is propagated back to the root node. Leaf nodes that do not represent a terminal phrase are expanded only after they have been visited often enough to limit the memory requirements of the search tree.

In MCTS the search tree is extended in an unbalanced manner where branches leading to sentences of higher quality are visited more frequently and therefore the tree is expanded to a deeper level for those branches that appear to be most interesting.

For grammatical optimization problems the goal is to find a sentence reaching an optimal objective. If we assume that the synthesized programs are deterministic each node representing a terminal phrase must be visited only once as the reward is the same at later visits.

An important observation is that MCTS only considers information gained through sampling sentences with exactly the same beginning as the current sentence for the decision which action to use. Therefore, MCTS cannot reuse learned patterns from disconnected branches of the search tree. The algorithm rather learns which replacements are preferable starting from the beginning of the sentence instead of learning general replacement patterns which work well even for different sentence beginnings.

Generally, in a sequential decision process a number of states are visited where in each state a number of actions are possible and taking an action results in a new state. In the case of MCTS the state is equivalent to the full phrase and a value function for states is learned which expresses the value of visiting a given state. This is however problematic especially when the state space becomes very large which is the case for grammatical optimization problems. Therefore, algorithms that use value function approximations have been proposed which are frequently better suited for such problems [17,18]. A simple state value function is represented as a table storing the value for each state based on aggregated rewards received via this state. When using value function approximation, a set of basis functions is used instead to determine features for each state and the goal is to learn a model that estimates the value of states based solely on their features. The benefit of this approach is that information can be used more efficiently because it opens the possibility that of generalization to new, previously unseen states based on state similarity. As an example, a simple feature function for a phrase could return which replacement rule was applied to generate the current phrase. If the phrase $abaS$ was generated from abS using the replacement $S \rightarrow aS$ then the feature function would return $S \rightarrow aS$. At the end of the derivation a reward would be received and propagated back which would result in an update of the value function for the replacement rule $S \rightarrow aS$. This approach allows to calculate values for different alternative replacements for a non-terminal symbol[1]. In general, a large variety of features could be defined that describe a phrase. Ideally, the features are defined in such a way that they can be used to model the value of a state/phrase accurately.

6   Using Contextual Information

MCTS uses only the full phrase as pattern to select alternatives for replacements. This is sensible if a problem requires to get the full sequence of symbols exactly right i.e. if the complete solution cannot be decomposed into multiple smaller solutions which might be arranged in a different order, or if the solution cannot be composed of different complementary pieces in any ordering. Also MCTS is focused on finding the optimal beginning of a solution and does not work as efficiently if the beginning of the solution does not have a strong effect on the quality of the solution.

In contrast tree-based GP with sub-tree crossover works on the assumption that a solution can be created by combining parts of good solution candidates in random order. Therefore, tree-based GP should work better for problems that can be decomposed into several parts which can be combined in any ordering while MCTS should work better for problems where it is important to get the complete chain correct and the problem exhibits the characteristic that better solutions have the same beginning.

In grammatical optimization problems different kinds of contextual information are available. Beginning on the lowest level, the symbols occurring in an incomplete sentence are of course an important lead for the search process (lexical context). On the same level it might be useful to look at positional dependencies of symbols. On a higher level the current syntactical context (e.g. parts of sentences or partial syntactical constructs or the nesting depth of an expression) could be a useful lead for the search process.

However, the most important information is certainly hidden on the semantic level or in the execution state of the program. Obviously, it is possible that two different program fragments perform the same calculation. Then certainly both program fragments could be expanded with the same additional operations to complete the program. To detect such patterns it would be necessary to analyze program semantics. One naive idea is to interpret partial programs while expanding the programs left-canonically. Then the interpreter state encapsulates the complete semantic information of the program fragment. One problem with this approach is however that interpreter state depends on input values for the program and thus is not the equal for different test cases. So ideally, some kind of

---

[1] MCTS can be expressed as a special form of this approach where each state maps exactly to one feature representing this state.

semantic analysis or semantically-aware transformation to canonical form would be necessary. This could eventually be accomplished through data flow analysis and/or detection of independent program fragments. We are not aware of any previous work where value function approximation is used in combination with features encoding the semantics of the program or the execution state.

7   Summary

In this contribution we described how searching solutions for grammatical optimization problems can be formulated as an episodic sequential decision problem and discussed that Monte-Carlo tree search is one specific algorithmic approach for solving this type of problems. A crucial issue for the efficiency of approximate dynamic programming algorithms such as MCTS is that the value function for states can be learned quickly from reward realizations in order to guide the search process to find an optimal solution efficiently. We strongly believe that simple MCTS is limited because it uses a tabular state-value function which does not scale to very large state spaces. Instead, we argue that using value function approximations could be better suited for detecting important structural patterns in partial solutions. We also claim that it is necessary to include other contextual information e.g. information about the program execution state into the search process which can be easily accomplished when using value function approximation based on state features.

We have not discussed if automated program synthesis actually exhibits characteristics where such features are helpful for value approximation. Answering this question is left open for future work.

Acknowledgments. The authors would like to thank Tristan Cazenave for the helpful discussion which lead to improvements of this paper. The work described in this paper was done within the COMET Project Heuristic Optimization in Production and Logistics (HOPL), #843532 funded by the Austrian Research Promotion Agency (FFG).

References

1. Gulwani, S.: Synthesis from examples: interaction models and algorithms. In: 14th International Symposium on Symbolic and Numeric Algorithms for Scientific Computing (SYNASC), pp. 8–14 (2012)
2. Le Goues, C., Dewey-Vogt, M., Forrest, S., Weimer, W.: A systematic study of automated program repair: fixing 55 out of 105 bugs for $8 each. In: 2012 34th International Conference on Software Engineering (ICSE), pp. 3–13 (2012)
3. Weimer, W., Forrest, S., Le Goues, C., Nguyen, T.: Automatic program repair with evolutionary computation. Commun. ACM **53**, 109–116 (2010)
4. Weimer, W., Nguyen, T., Le Goues, C., Forrest, S.: Automatically finding patches using genetic programming. In: Proceedings of the 31st International Conference on Software Engineering, ICSE 2009, pp. 364–374. IEEE Computer Society, Washington, DC (2009)

5. Schkufza, E., Sharma, R., Aiken, A.: Stochastic optimization of floating-point programs with tunable precision. In: O'Boyle, M.F.P., Pingali, K. (eds.) PLDI, p. 9. ACM (2014)
6. Schkufza, E., Sharma, R., Aiken, A.: Stochastic superoptimization. In: Proceedings of the Eighteenth International Conference on Architectural Support for Programming Languages and Operating Systems, ASPLOS 2013, pp. 305–316. ACM, New York (2013)
7. Norvig, P.: Machine learning for programming. In: Proceedings of the Companion Publication of the 2014 ACM SIGPLAN Conference on Systems, Programming, and Applications: Software for Humanity, p. 3. ACM (2014)
8. Koza, J.R.: Genetic Programming: On the Programming of Computers by Means of Natural Selection, vol. 1. MIT Press, Cambridge (1992)
9. Kronberger, G., Kommenda, M.: Search strategies for grammatical optmization problems - alternatives to grammar-guided genetic programming. In: Borowik, G., Chaczko, Z., Jacak, W., Łuba, T. (eds.) Computational Intelligence and Efficiency in Engineering Systems. SCI, vol. 595, pp. 89–102. Springer, Heidelberg (2015)
10. Duvenaud, D., Lloyd, J.R., Grosse, R., Tenenbaum, J.B., Ghahramani, Z.: Structure discovery in nonparametric regression through compositional kernel search. arXiv preprint arXiv:1302.4922 (2013)
11. Kronberger, G., Kommenda, M., Wagner, S., Dobler, H.: GPDL: a framework-independent problem definition language for grammar-guided genetic programming. In: Proceeding of the Fifteenth Annual Conference Companion on Genetic and Evolutionary Computation Conference Companion, pp. 1333–1340. ACM (2013)
12. Kocsis, L., Szepesvári, C.: Bandit based Monte-Carlo planning. In: Fürnkranz, J., Scheffer, T., Spiliopoulou, M. (eds.) ECML 2006. LNCS (LNAI), vol. 4212, pp. 282–293. Springer, Heidelberg (2006)
13. Browne, C.B., Powley, E., Whitehouse, D., Lucas, S.M., Cowling, P.I., Rohlfshagen, P., Tavener, S., Perez, D., Samothrakis, S., Colton, S.: A survey of monte carlo tree search methods. IEEE Trans. Comput. Intell. AI Games 4, 1–43 (2012)
14. Cazenave, T.: Monte-carlo expression discovery. Int. J. Artif. Intell. Tools 22, 1–21 (2013)
15. de Mesmay, F., Rimmel, A., Voronenko, Y., Püschel, M.: Bandit-based optimization on graphs with application to library performance tuning. In: Proceedings of the 26th Annual International Conference on Machine Learning, ICML 2009, pp. 729–736. ACM, New York (2009)
16. Helmuth, T., Spector, L.: Word count as a traditional programming benchmark problem for genetic programming. In: Proceedings of the 2014 Conference on Genetic and Evolutionary Computation, GECCO 2014, pp. 919–926. ACM, New York (2014)
17. Szepesvári, C.: Algorithms for reinforcement learning. Synth. Lect. Artif. Intell. Mach. Learn. 4, 1–103 (2010)
18. Powell, W.B.: Approximate Dynamic Programming: Solving the Curses of Dimensionality. Wiley, Hoboken (2007)

A New Type of Metamodel for Longitudinal Dynamics Optimization of Hybrid Electric Vehicles

Christopher Bacher[1](✉), Günther R. Raidl[1], and Thorsten Krenek[2]

[1] Institute of Computer Graphics and Algorithms, TU Wien, Vienna, Austria
{bacher,raidl}@ac.tuwien.ac.at
[2] Institute for Powertrains and Automotive Technology, TU Wien, Vienna, Austria
thorsten.krenek@ifa.tuwien.ac.at

Abstract. Parameter optimization for Hybrid Electric Vehicles (HEVs) is very time consuming due to the necessity to evaluate a simulation model. This bottleneck is usually removed by using metamodels as surrogates for the simulation. We consider metamodels for longitudinal dynamics simulation, which simulate a vehicle following a given driving cycle. Typical "top-down" metamodels are parametrized by both the HEV model and the driving cycle. We propose a novel bottom up meta-modelling scheme only parametrized by the HEV model and discuss preliminary results.

Keywords: Hybrid electric vehicle · Optimization · Metamodel · Surrogate

1 Introduction

Hybrid Electric Vehicle (HEVs) and their related concepts—on the fringes just a few years ago—become increasingly common in automobiles today. Technically, HEVs combine aspects of conventional vehicles and electric vehicles. They possess an Internal Combustion Engine (ICE) using conventional fuel and one or more Electric Machines (EMs) with alternative energy storages. As energy storage systems batteries are most commonly used but also variants with fuel cells have been considered.

The reasons for the increasing popularity of HEVs are manifold. On one hand there are environmental considerations. HEVs are considered to be more environmentally friendly than conventional vehicles. Their ability to use EMs for propulsion leads to decreased pollutant emission. In the same breath increased fuel efficiency—and thereby cost reduction for the customer—is often named as a main benefit of HEVs, if not overshadowed by high initial costs.

On the other hand one finds that hybridization of vehicles is graded and can be found in many vehicles today. For example sports car manufacturers use EMs for boosting, i.e. faster acceleration in comparison to a common ICE.

© Springer International Publishing Switzerland 2015
R. Moreno-Díaz et al. (Eds.): EUROCAST 2015, LNCS 9520, pp. 425–432, 2015.
DOI: 10.1007/978-3-319-27340-2_53

In any use case the effective use of the hybrid components is critical for the performance and efficiency of a HEV. Proper sizes for the ICE, EMs, battery capacities and gear sets have to be chosen, as well as an effective operation strategy deciding which components are active under what circumstances.

One solution to this problem is to perform optimization using an accurate computer model for simulating the behaviour of the HEV under different circumstances. In the following we consider longitudinal dynamics simulations. This simulation type simulates the behaviour of the HEV on a driving cycle defining target velocities for each moment of the simulation.

The task of finding appropriate parameter settings for the according computer model poses a difficult continuous optimization problem. Manually establishing a good solution to this high-dimensional problem is neither effective nor efficient. Therefore metaheuristic algorithms are used for this purpose.

However the main drawback of their straight-forward use in this setting is the time-intensive evaluation of the objective function which involves the simulation of the chosen parameter configuration for the HEV. Simulation times for HEV models vary on their degree of detail and the length of the selected driving cycle, but can easily reach five to twenty minutes per test case in our experiments with high-detail models. A possible solution to this problem is the development of metamodels acting as surrogates for the simulation in the optimization process.

In the following sections we review related work, discuss the usage of metamodels in HEV optimization and outline their drawbacks. Afterwards we introduce a new metamodelling technique addressing these problems and provide results for preliminary experiments.

2   Related Work

Optimization of HEVs has been discussed by many authors. Johnson et al. [4] optimize the parameters of a real-time operational strategy. The optimization is carried out on a surrogate based on a surface fitting model obtained from a Design-Of-Experiments for the original simulation to deal with long simulation times. Multi-objective optimization is treated in [3] and more recently by Rodemann et al. in [6]. In both [3,4] the simulation software ADVISOR is used, whereas [6] uses Matlab/Simulink as simulation tool. Both [3,6] do not have to deal with long simulation times, as in both cases faster, less detailed models are used. This is explicitly stated in [6] and from the authors' experience this also holds true for ADVISOR models as used in [3].

Optimization of simulation models with high computation times is treated in [2,5]. There different regression models based on neural networks are used as surrogates in metaheuristics. Both works use GT Suite as simulation software which is also used for the experiments in Sect. 5.

3   Metamodels and HEV Optimization

To optimize HEVs we rely on metaheuristic approaches like Genetic Algorithms and Particle Swarm Optimization as described in [2]. The metaheuristics use the

HEV model by setting its parameters and simulating it according to a prespecified driving cycle. A driving cycle specifies a target velocity for any point in time which the vehicle has to match.

In the authors' previous work on parameter optimization for HEVs it became necessary to develop surrogates for the simulation. As the objective function relies on performing a simulation for any tested parameter configuration and to neglect the high time requirements to perform the simulation, it is inefficient to use the model directly. A better possibility is to develop a faster but coarse version of the HEV model for optimization. Manually developing such a model and calibrating it to match the original model or even the HEV itself would incur substantial time and financial costs. Moreover if the optimization is run as part of the development of an actual vehicle, keeping the different models synchronized with the changes would likely be prohibitive.

Therefore automatically deduced regression models are created as a replacement to the simulation. The regression models used in previous work are different variants of neural networks which are trained on results from a sampling phase during optimization. The inputs of the networks are all varied parameters of the HEV model and its output is a prediction of the according objective value. The results in [2] show that the use of these surrogates is effective and an altered optimization scheme in [5] seems to even improve the overall performance.

Nevertheless the use of neural networks as metamodels comes with a substantial drawback. The fitted metamodel is only valid for a single driving cycle. The time-expensive collection of training data hampers the usability of the metamodel as it has to be created anew for each driving cycle.

Though optimizing the HEV for a variety of driving cycles is deemed. Otherwise the final optimized parameter configuration might overfit the prespecified driving cycle resulting in poor performance in real usage scenarios. A better approach would be to optimize the vehicle over a weighted set of driving cycles which represent typical use cases of potential drivers. To this end we propose a new metamodelling scheme discussed in the next section.

4   Bottom-Up Metamodels for HEVs

To deal with the above-mentioned reusability issue we diverge from the "top-down" perspective of the regression models for HEVs simulation, where metamodels represent the simulation as an atomic unit. This viewpoint on regression lacks generalization across driving cycles.

In [1] several possibilities to enhance the prediction performance of the neural networks are explored. Notably two concepts—the Partial Simulation and the Time-Progressive Learning Ensemble (TPLE) approaches—try to split the prediction of the simulation into several parts. The Partial Simulation approach splits the driving cycle, uses the original model to simulate the first part of the cycle and passes the resulting fuel consumption along with the parameter configuration of the HEV to a neural network to predict the final objective value. TPLE on the other hand splits the driving cycle into several parts and trains separate regression models to predict the fuel consumptions for each part. Starting with the first part, the prediction result is iteratively passed to the next slice until a final objective value is obtained. Both variants show good prediction behaviour in experiments. Our bottom-up approach relies on similar decompositions and composes the final result from a chain of predictions for parts of a driving cycle.

4.1   Formal Description of Bottom-Up Metamodels

Formally let D be the driving cycle of length $|D|$ to be predicted and $\mathcal{S}$ be the set of all driving scenarios, and $\mathcal{S}_T \subset \mathcal{S}$ a set of driving scenarios chosen for training. Driving scenarios are short linear driving cycles acting as building blocks which we use to reconstruct the whole driving cycle D. A scenario s is defined by the triple (v_b, v_e, a) where v_b, v_e specify the start and end velocity of the scenario and a the respective acceleration. Observe that $\mathcal{S}_T$ can be chosen independently from D. Selection strategies for $\mathcal{S}_T$ will be discussed below.

Let $\mathcal{P}$ be the discretized search space of the optimization problem and $\mathbf{p} \in \mathcal{P}$ be a candidate solution. The continuous search space is discretized due to performance reasons and due to insignificant changes in the objective function. This matter is discussed in more detail in [2].

Let $\mathcal{P}_A$ be $\mathcal{P}$'s dimensions restricted to the set of operational parameters. Operational parameters are parameters which affect the HEVs operation strategy. The operation strategy $\mathcal{A} : \mathcal{P}_A \times \mathcal{M} \times \mathcal{I} \to \mathcal{M}$ determines the next operation mode $m \in \mathcal{M}$ of the HEV. A mode m defines the active components and their use during driving, e.g. pure electric, range extension, power split or recuperation. Modes for an exemplary vehicle are described in Sect. 5. Further $\mathcal{I}$ is the set of input signals to $\mathcal{A}$ on which a the mode switch depends, like State of Charge (SOC) of the battery, axle torque, or power demand. Observe that $\mathcal{A}$ forms a state machine with rule-based state changes. $\mathcal{I}$ itself is a subset of the metamodels outputs, i.e. $\mathcal{I} \subseteq \mathcal{O}$, as the state of $\mathcal{I}$ has to be predicted throughout the evaluation to determine the current operation mode.

Let $\mathcal{P}_s$ be the set of structural parameters. Structural parameters affect the simulation results of a driving scenario if the operation mode is fixed, e.g. gear ratios or engine sizing.

Finally let $\phi_{\mathcal{S}_T}^{\mathcal{A}} : \mathcal{P} \times \mathcal{D} \to \mathcal{O}$ be the bottom-up metamodel parametrized by the driving scenarios and the operation strategy to predict values of the output signals $\mathbf{o} \in \mathcal{O}$ for a given candidate solution $\mathbf{p}^* \in \mathcal{P}$ and a driving cycle $D \in \mathcal{D}$. The metamodel $\phi_{\mathcal{S}_T}^{\mathcal{A}}$ is trained by creating scenario models $\varphi_{\mathbf{p}_s, \mathbf{j}, s}^m :$ $\mathcal{P}_s \times \mathcal{J} \times \mathcal{S}_T \to \Delta\mathcal{O}$ by recording the results of simulating all combinations of $s \in \mathcal{S}_T$, $m \in \mathcal{M}$, a subset of $\mathbf{p}_s \in \mathcal{P}_s$, and a subset of $\mathbf{j} \in \mathcal{J}$. The inputs $\mathbf{j} \in \mathcal{J}$, $\mathcal{J} \subseteq \mathcal{O}$ are additional discretized signals affecting the simulation results, e.g. SOC or power demand. The subsets of $\mathcal{P}_s$ and $\mathcal{J}$ can be obtained by a properly chosen Design-of-Experiments (DoE), e.g. full factorial if the domains are small.

The scenario models $\varphi_{\mathbf{p}_s, \mathbf{j}, s}^m$ can then be used to predict the output vector $\mathbf{o}$ for given $\mathbf{p}_s^*$, $\mathbf{j}^*$ (not necessarily contained in the DoE), and a scenario $s^* \in \mathcal{S}$. The results of the single scenario models are then combined by a machine learning method $f_{\mathbf{p}_s^*, s^*} : \{\Delta\mathcal{O}\} \to \Delta\mathcal{O}$ such as k-Nearest-Neighbour or neural networks. The output of the bottom-up metamodel $\phi^{\mathcal{A}}_{\mathcal{S}_T}$ is obtained by the following recursion.

$$\phi^{\mathcal{A}}_{\mathcal{S}_T}(\mathbf{p}^*, D) = \mathbf{o}_{|D|-1} \tag{1}$$

$$\mathbf{o}_t = \mathbf{o}_{t-1} \oplus f_{\mathbf{p}^*, s_t}\left(\{\varphi^{m_t}_{\mathbf{p}_s, \mathbf{j}, s}(\mathbf{p}^*, \mathbf{o}_{t-1}, s_t) \mid \forall \mathbf{p}_s, \mathbf{j} \in \mathrm{DoE}(\mathcal{P}_s, \mathcal{J}), s \in \mathcal{S}_T\}\right) \tag{2}$$

$$m_t = \mathcal{A}(\mathbf{p}^*, m_{t-1}, \mathbf{o}_{t-1}) \tag{3}$$

$$s_t = (v_\mathrm{b}(D, t), v_\mathrm{e}(D, t+1), a(D, t)) \tag{4}$$

Basically the metamodel determines for each point in time t the active mode m_t, uses $f_{\mathbf{p}^*, s^*}$ and the scenario models to predict the change in the output signals and joins the results using $\oplus$ with the results from the previous time step. Depending on the predicted signal $\oplus$ might be a simple replacement or an addition. Of course sensible values for m_0 and $\mathbf{o}_0$ have to be chosen. Observe that depending on the implementation of $f_{\mathbf{p}^*, s^*}$ it is probably not necessary to evaluate all $\varphi^{m_t}_{\mathbf{p}_s, \mathrm{inf}, s}$ but only a small subset thereof.

4.2   Obtaining Training Scenarios

In the following we discuss the selection of training scenarios $\mathcal{S}_T$. From the explanations above it is clear that the choice of $\mathcal{S}_T$ is highly relevant to the performance of the metamodel. It is to be expected that a more fine grained set of scenarios produces more accurate results. Nevertheless if $\mathcal{S}_T$ is chosen too large then the simulation overhead can be significantly worse if compared to obtaining training data for top-down metamodels. Moreover the simulation time for the driving scenarios is without direct use to the optimization process as D is not evaluated. Therefore there are two major ways to choose $\mathcal{S}_T$.

1. Choose $\mathcal{S}_T$ s.t. a wide range of possible driving cycles can be approximated in future use, e.g. by equidistantly sampling the scenario space or some other DoE variant.
2. If the set of driving cycles $\mathcal{D}$ to be predicted is known beforehand, e.g. major standardized driving cycles used for official emission rating (US06, NEDC, WLTC3), then it is reasonable to trim $\mathcal{S}_T$ to yield higher accuracy on $\mathcal{D}$.

We propose a compression heuristic for the second case. Let $\varepsilon_a, \varepsilon_v$ be the minimal considered change in acceleration/velocity.

1. Split each cycle D into scenarios of duration Δt and categorize them in transient (acceleration, breaking) scenarios $\mathcal{S}_A$ and constant speed scenarios $\mathcal{S}_C$ (if $a \leq \varepsilon_a$).
2. Sort the constant velocity scenarios by velocity and collect all scenarios from s_0 to s_i greedily until

$$v(s_{i+1}) - (v(s_i) + \varepsilon_v) > \varepsilon_v \tag{5}$$

Then create a scenario with constant speed equal to the average speed of the collected scenarios, add it to the training set and proceed with $s_0 = s_i$.

3. The following is carried out for acceleration and breaking scenarios separately. Below the acceleration case is explained, the breaking case is analogous respective to some sign changes. Sort the transient scenarios by acceleration and split them into chunks whenever $|a(s_{i+1}) - a(s_i)| > \varepsilon_a$.

4. For each transient chunk scenarios are iteratively taken from both ends of the sorted list. Even numbered elements are taken from the left end and odd numbered elements from the right. A list of sets $\mathcal{X}_k$ is kept where each set is identified by the acceleration $a_k = a_i + \varepsilon_a$ of the scenario s_i first added to the set. For the current scenario s_i all sets are identified s.t. $|a_k - a_i| \le \varepsilon_a$. If no such set is found then a new set is created and s_i is added as its first element. Otherwise s_i is added to the set $\mathcal{X}_k$ whose duration

$$d_k = \frac{\max_{s \in \mathcal{X}_k}(v_e(s)) - \min_{s \in \mathcal{X}_k}(v_b(s))}{a_k} \tag{6}$$

changes least if s_i is added. After processing all scenarios, the scenario

$$\left(\min_{s \in \mathcal{X}_k}(v_b(s)), \max_{s \in \mathcal{X}_k}(v_e(s)), \operatorname{avg}_{s \in \mathcal{X}_k}(a(s)) \right) \tag{7}$$

is added to the training set for each $\mathcal{X}_k$.

5   Experiments

We implemented a prototype of the bottom-up metamodel for the HEV model used in [1,2] (Model A). For a more complete description the reader is advised to consult these sources. The vehicle possesses an ICE and two EMs coupled by a planetary gear set. There are four different propulsion modes and two recuperation modes available.

- **EV1/2** use only one or two EMs for propulsion and consume battery charge.
- **ER1** uses the larger EM for propulsion and the smaller one as a generator powered by the ICE. Consumes battery but also charges the battery. The amount of charging depends on the requested charge power which has been identified as an internal signal in $\mathcal{J}$ to be predicted by the metamodel.
- **ER2** is a power split mode using both the larger EM and the ICE for propulsion. Further the load point of the ICE is shifted to a higher, more efficient level. The resulting surplus energy is used to charge battery via the smaller EM. The load point shift is determined by the charge power signal.
- **Recup1/2** are recuperation modes, i.e. performing regenerative braking with a single or both EMs active respectively.

The twelve parameters forming $\mathcal{P}$ of the model are the same as in [1,2] with the same discretization levels. Of those parameters we identified the number of ring and sun teeth of the planetary gear set as the only structural parameters. The remaining parameters are considered operational parameters. The output

Table 1. MTOD results for US06 standard strategy experiments

(a) Results with $\varepsilon_a = 0.4, \varepsilon_v = 2.5$

k	obj.	fuel	SOC
1	0.2072	0.1743	0.2158
2	0.1898	0.1868	0.2189
3	0.2182	0.2380	0.2649
4	0.2251	0.2478	0.2629

(b) Results with $\varepsilon_a = 0.7, \varepsilon_v = 2.5$

k	obj.	fuel	SOC
1	0.2279	0.1615	0.2555
2	0.2182	0.1687	0.2522
3	0.2480	0.2302	0.2468
4	0.2483	0.2255	0.2478

Table 2. MTOD baseline errors for US06

(a) $\varepsilon_a = 0.4, \varepsilon_v = 2.5$

k	obj.	fuel	SOC
1	0.2920	0.1640	0.2834
2	0.2670	0.1207	0.2784
3	0.2791	0.2003	0.2981
4	0.2872	0.2750	0.3061

(b) $\varepsilon_a = 0.7, \varepsilon_v = 2.5$

k	obj.	fuel	SOC
1	0.2564	0.2622	0.2854
2	0.2383	0.1550	0.2696
3	0.2814	0.2830	0.3000
4	0.2845	0.3710	0.3114

(c) $\mathcal{S}_T = $ US06, $\Delta t = 4$sec

k	obj.	fuel	SOC
1	0.2111	0.1278	0.3253

set $\mathcal{O}$ has been identified to consist of the fuel consumption, SOC, charge power, power demand, and axle torque. The only signal in $\mathcal{J}$ is the requested charge power. For this signal five equidistantly spaced power levels have been chosen to be included in the coarse training set (explained below) and six for the more fine grained set. For the structural parameters $\mathcal{P}_s$ and the internal signals $\mathcal{J}$ a full factorial design has been chosen. All scenario models are evaluated prematurely and their results are cached for future use.

As combination method $f_{\mathbf{p}_s^*, s^*}$, a k-Nearest-Neighbour (kNN) model for every combination of mode, structural parameters and internal signal $\mathcal{J}$ is built, once for fuel consumption and once for SOC. The remaining output signals can be calculated directly by mathematical relationships with information from the previous time step.

To evaluate the quality of the fit, the Mean Total Order Deviation (MTOD) is considered. The optimization algorithms in [2] do not use the absolute objective values of candidate solutions to select among them but their ranks, e.g. by using tournament selection in genetic algorithms. MTOD takes this into account by ordering the sequence of expected output values and the sequence of the actual output values. Then for each candidate solution the percental shift between its positions in both lists is calculated. The mean of those percental shifts forms the MTOD which measures rank errors, but not the absolute deviation between the expected and actual output values.

The 903 evaluated candidate solutions are taken from Phase I in [2] s.t. the MTOD results for both model types are comparable. Simulations of random shuffling show an empirical MTOD of about 0.33. The experiments have been carried out with two different $\mathcal{S}_T$, one coarse and one more fine grained. Both sets are obtained by the procedure described in Sect. 4 by compressing the US06, NEDC, and WLTC3 with $\Delta t = 1$s all other units use km/h as base unit.

Table 1 depicts the MTOD for the objective function, the fuel consumption, and the SOC. It can be seen that low values for k yield better results and that the fine grained training set outperforms the coarse one. Nevertheless if compared to the results in [2] the MTOD of a simple neural network is only 0.0952. To discover the reason for this discrepancy, additional experiments have been run where the operation strategy is removed from the metamodel and the same mode switches as in the respective simulations are performed instead. An additional $\mathcal{S}_T$ is evaluated which consists of scenarios sampled at four second intervals from the US06 cycle without compression and predicted with $k = 1$. This results in a close reconstruction of the US06 driving cycle by the metamodel.

Table 2 shows these baseline errors, i.e. errors not resulting from a "wrong" mode switch. Surprisingly the results are worse than in the standard strategy variant. From the current state of experiments no conclusions about the reason for this behaviour can be made. The results are subject to further investigations.

6   Conclusion and Future Work

In this paper we introduce bottom-up metamodels for HEV optimization which are able to generalize over different driving cycles at no additional simulation costs. While those concepts appear to be highly promising, our preliminary experimental results for prediction performance are behind expectations for unclear reasons and under further investigation. In future work optimization techniques exploiting the metamodel structure shall be developed.

References

1. Bacher, C.: Metaheuristic optimization of electro-hybrid powertrains using machine learning techniques. Master's thesis, TU Wien, Vienna, Austria (2013)
2. Bacher, C., Krenek, T., Raidl, G.R.: Reducing the number of simulationsin operation strategy optimizationfor hybrid electric vehicles. In: Esparcia-Alcázar, A.I., Mora, A.M. (eds.) EvoApplications 2014. LNCS, vol. 8602, pp. 553–564. Springer, Heidelberg (2014)
3. Hu, X., Wang, Z., Liao, L.: Multi-objective optimization of HEV fuel economy and emissions using evolutionary computation. In: Society of Automotive Engineers World Congress and Exhibition, vol. SP-1856, pp. 117–128 (2004)
4. Johnson, V.H., Wipke, K.B., Rausen, D.J.: HEV control strategy for real-time optimization of fuel economy and emissions. Soc. Automot. Eng. Trans. 109(3), 1677–1690 (2000)
5. Krenek, T., Bacher, C., Lauer, T., Raidl, G.R.: Numerical optimisation of electro-hybrid powertrains. MTZ Worldwide 76(3), 46–52 (2015)
6. Rodemann, T., Narukawa, K., Fischer, M., Awada, M.: Many-objective optimization of a hybrid car controller. In: Mora, A.M., Squillero, G. (eds.) EvoApplications 2015. LNCS, vol. 9028, pp. 593–603. Springer, Heidelberg (2015)

Automatic Adaption of Operator Probabilities in Genetic Algorithms with Offspring Selection

Stefan Wagner[1]([⊠]), Michael Affenzeller[1,2], and Andreas Scheibenpflug[1,2]

[1] Heuristic and Evolutionary Algorithms Laboratory, School of Informatics,
Communications and Media – Campus Hagenberg, University of Applied Sciences
Upper Austria, Softwarepark 11, 4232 Hagenberg, Austria
{swagner,maffenze,ascheibe}@heuristiclab.com
[2] Institute for Formal Models and Verification, Johannes Kepler University Linz,
Altenbergerstr. 69, 4040 Linz, Austria

Abstract. When offspring selection is applied in genetic algorithms, multiple crossover and mutation operators can be easily used together as crossover and mutation results of insufficient quality are discarded in the additional selection step after creating new solutions. Therefore, the a priori choice of appropriate crossover and mutation operators becomes less critical and it even turned out that multiple operators reduce the bias, broaden the search, and thus lead to higher solution quality in the end. However, using crossover and mutation operators which often produce solutions not passing the offspring selection criterion also increases the selection pressure and consequently the number of evaluated solutions.

Therefore, we present a new generic scheme for tuning the selection probabilities of multiple crossover and mutation operators in genetic algorithms with offspring selection automatically at runtime. Thereby those operators are applied more frequently which were able to produce good results in the last generation, which leads to comparable solution quality and results in a significant decrease of evaluated solutions.

1 Introduction

In genetic algorithms (GAs) selection, crossover, and mutation are repeatedly executed to recombine the genetic information in solutions of above average quality in order to achieve even better solutions. Thereby solutions are encoded as for example vectors of bits, vectors of real numbers, or permutations. These data structures represent the genotypic information of solutions and the choice of an appropriate solution encoding depends on the tackled optimization problem. According to the chosen solution encoding, different crossover and mutation operators can be applied. Many different solution encodings and thus also crossover and mutation operators have been developed and applied for diverse optimization problems in the past. A comprehensive review of different encodings and operators for the Traveling Salesman Problem (TSP) has for example been published in [4]. It turned out that different encodings and operators

R. Moreno-Díaz et al. (Eds.): EUROCAST 2015, LNCS 9520, pp. 433–438, 2015.
DOI: 10.1007/978-3-319-27340-2_54

have different characteristics which significantly influence the performance of the search process. Therefore, the selection of an appropriate encoding and suitable crossover and mutation operators is an important and crucial step.

When using GAs together with offspring selection an appropriate choice of operators is less critical as due to the offspring selection step after crossover and mutation only those children are considered as successful which are able to outperform their parents. In terms of solution quality it is therefore not problematic if a crossover or mutation operator produces a worse child as this solution is simply discarded. It even turned out that applying multiple crossover and mutation operators together has a beneficial effect on performance as the bias of single operators is reduced and the search is broadened, leading to better solution quality in the end [3].

However, when studying the frequency of operator applications it can be seen that the success rate of operators changes over time during an algorithm run. An operator which is not very successful in an early phase of an algorithm run can become more successful later on and vice versa. This observation indicates that it is reasonable to adapt the selection probabilities of different crossover and mutation operators at runtime in such a way that more successful operators are chosen more frequently. By this means, the overhead of worse operators can be reduced which is important for applications where the evaluation of solutions is computationally complex and time-consuming.

In this paper we present a generic scheme for automatically adapting the application probabilities of multiple crossover and mutation operators in offspring selection GAs and present results that show its impact on the behavior of the algorithm in terms of solution quality and required effort. Furthermore, we show that this approach results in less selection pressure and therefore leads to a significant reduction of evaluated solutions.

2   Offspring Selection

Offspring selection introduced by Affenzeller and Wagner [1,2] is an enhanced selection scheme for GAs which aims at preventing premature convergence [5]. In a GA with offspring selection an additional selection step is included after creating a new solution by crossover and mutation which checks whether the quality of the child solution is better or worse than its parents. If it is better, the new solution is denoted as successful and is added to the next generation, otherwise it is discarded. Therefore, the search process is focused on those solutions which represent a beneficial combination of the parents' chromosomes. This counteracts the loss of relevant genetic information and prevents premature convergence.

One of the benefits of offspring selection is that it enables the application of multiple crossover and mutation operators. Even if operators of inferior quality are used, the search process is not handicapped as unsuccessful children are sorted out [2]. Actually not that well suited operators can even have a positive impact on the search, as long as they are able to produce successful offspring at least from time to time. The application of multiple crossover and mutation operators therefore leads to better maintenance of genetic diversity and consequently to better algorithm performance [3]. However, on the downside the required selection pressure and consequently the algorithm's runtime is also increased when more unsuccessful solutions are created. This aspect is especially critical for applications where the evaluation function is runtime-intensive and consequently the number of solution evaluations has to be kept as low as possible.

3   Automatic Adaption of Crossover and Mutation Operator Weights

In GAs with offspring selection it can be observed that different crossover and mutation operators do not perform constantly well. When tracing the operators that are able to produce successful offspring in each generation, it can be seen that the relative frequency of an operator can change significantly throughout an algorithm run. For example, Fig. 1 shows the relative frequency of six different crossover operators in a GA with offspring selection applied on the TSP instance "ch130" from TSPLIB [6].

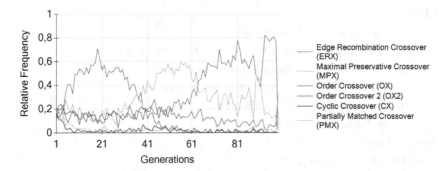

Fig. 1. Relative crossover operator frequency for successful offspring

In order to favor successful operators and to reduce the overhead of operators which are not performing well, we can use this information to adjust the selection probabilities of operators according to the rate of successes. We therefore check the offspring selection criterion after each application of an operator and count how many times an operator was able to produce a successful solution (i.e., a better solution) in the current generation. At the end of each generation we compute the success rate of each operator by dividing its number of improvements by the times how often the operator was applied in the current generation. Then we set this value for each operator as its new weight and select operators proportionally to their weights in the following generation.

Additionally, we have to take care that the weight of an operator is never set to 0, if an operator is not able to produce successful solutions in the current generation. Otherwise the operator will not be selected anymore and will never have a chance to become more successful again later on. We therefore define a lower limit of 0.02 for each operator weight to guarantee a non-zero selection probability.

4   Experimental Results and Analysis

For the evaluation and analysis of the automatic adaption of operator probabilities described in the previous section, we executed a series of tests[1] with HeuristicLab [7]. We used three different TSP instances from TSPLIB and compared the results of a genetic algorithm with offspring selection (OSGA) with and without automatic adjustment of operator weights. Table 1 shows the used parameter values which represent typical settings for solving TSP instances with OSGA.

Table 1. Algorithm parameter settings

Parameter	Value
Population Size	500
Elites	1
Selection Operator	Proportional
Crossover Operators	CX, ERX, MPX, OBX, OX, PMX
Mutation Operators	Insertion, Inversion, Swap2, Swap3, Translocation, Translocation & Inversion
Mutation Probability	5 % / 10 % / 20 %
Comparison Factor	1.0
Success Ratio	0.9 / 1.0
Max. Selection Pressure	500

In Table 2 the results in terms of solution quality and evaluated solutions are shown. We executed a series of 10 independent test runs for each parameter configuration and each problem instance. For each series the relative difference of the best found solution to the optimal solution in percent is given (column "Best"). Column "Med." shows the corresponding median value and the median number of evaluated solutions is stated in column "Eval. Sol.".

The results in Table 2 indicate that the automatic adaption of operator weights has neither a significant positive nor negative impact on the achieved solution quality. Both versions show similar values in the "Best" and "Med." columns. Significant differences can be seen for the number of evaluated solutions, though. Automatic adaption of operator weights obviously reduces the overhead of less successful operators which results in a reduction of evaluated

---

[1] All code and data required to reproduce these tests are published on http://dev.heuristiclab.com/AdditionalMaterial.

Table 2. Results of OSGA with and without automatic adaption of operator probabilities

Prob. Inst.	Succ. Ratio	Mut. Prob.	OSGA without op. adjust.			OSGA with op. adjust.			Change of Eval. Sol.
			Best	Med.	Eval. Sol.	Best	Med.	Eval. Sol.	
ch130	0.9	5 %	0.012	0.020	3,751,550	0.013	0.022	3,116,550	−**16.93** %
		10 %	0.019	0.023	3,828,600	0.016	0.027	3,231,550	−**15.59** %
		20 %	0.003	0.017	4,656,050	0.006	0.016	3,531,800	−**24.15** %
	1.0	5 %	0.007	0.038	2,782,600	0.013	0.031	2,141,700	−**23.03** %
		10 %	0.009	0.030	2,946,650	0.011	0.032	2,374,650	−**19.41** %
		20 %	0.012	0.025	3,385,450	0.005	0.031	2,471,100	−**27.01** %
kroA200	0.9	5 %	3.487	5.760	7,529,350	4.553	6.339	5,815,300	−**22.76** %
		10 %	2.530	5.159	7,448,550	3.119	6.999	5,362,550	−**28.01** %
		20 %	3.732	5.717	8,087,650	4.052	5.918	6,239,350	−**22.85** %
	1.0	5 %	3.500	7.355	4,850,550	7.484	10.479	3,555,250	−**26.70** %
		10 %	4.529	6.134	5,230,800	2.785	7.021	3,941,700	−**24.64** %
		20 %	2.847	5.724	5,862,000	4.668	7.878	4,181,800	−**28.66** %
gr666	0.9	5 %	1.906	2.002	7,229,400	1.855	2.034	5,451,350	−**24.59** %
		10 %	1.902	2.088	6,910,150	1.970	2.075	4,997,350	−**27.68** %
		20 %	2.086	2.194	6,761,850	2.040	2.172	4,875,250	−**27.90** %
	1.0	5 %	0.170	2.491	4,608,400	0.227	2.336	3,634,150	−**21.14** %
		10 %	2.340	2.501	4,750,500	2.222	2.422	3,308,250	−**30.36** %
		20 %	2.440	2.553	4,588,200	2.440	2.473	3,139,000	−**31.59** %

solutions by roughly 25 %. Adjusting the selection probabilities of operators using the generic scheme described in Sect. 3 is therefore very suitable for application scenarios in which the number of evaluated solutions has to be reduced to achieve a shorter algorithm runtime.

5   Summary and Conclusion

In this paper we described a new generic scheme to adjust the selection probabilities of operators automatically at runtime when using multiple crossover and mutation operators together in genetic algorithms with offspring selection. After each generation we thereby compute the success rate of each operator and adjust its weight accordingly. Each time when a crossover or mutation has to take place we then select an operator proportionally to its weight. By this means, operators which were able to produce good solutions in the last generation are chosen more frequently in the next generation.

In a series of tests with three TSP instances of different size we analyzed the effect of this adaption scheme in terms of solution quality and evaluated solutions. The presented results show that the automatic adjustment of operator probabilities leads to a significant reduction of evaluated solutions by roughly 25 % while achieving a comparable final solution quality. Therefore, the positive impact of applying multiple crossover and mutation operators in genetic algorithms with offspring selection is preserved but the required effort is reduced notably. These results highlight that the described scheme for tuning selection probabilities of operators is especially beneficial in application scenarios where solution evaluations are very time-consuming and consequently their number has to be kept as low as possible.

Acknowledgements. The work described in this paper was done within the COMET Project Heuristic Optimization in Production and Logistics (HOPL), #843532 funded by the Austrian Research Promotion Agency (FFG).

References

1. Affenzeller, M., Wagner, S.: SASEGASA: a new generic parallel evolutionary algorithm for achieving highest quality results. J. Heuristics - Spec. Issue New Adv. Parallel Meta-Heuristics Complex Probl. **10**, 239–263 (2004)
2. Affenzeller, M., Wagner, S.: Offspring selection: a new self-adaptive selection scheme for genetic algorithms. In: Ribeiro, B., Albrecht, R.F., Dobnikar, A., Pearson, D.W., Steele, N.C. (eds.) Adaptive and Natural Computing Algorithms. Springer Computer Series, pp. 218–221. Springer, Vienna (2005)
3. Affenzeller, M., Wagner, S., Winkler, S.: Effective allele preservation by offspring selection: an empirical study for the TSP. Int. J. Simul. Process Model. **6**(1), 29–39 (2010)
4. Larranaga, P., Kuijpers, C.M.H., Murga, R.H., Inza, I., Dizdarevic, D.: Genetic algorithms for the travelling salesman problem: a review of representations and operators. Artif. Intell. Rev. **13**, 129–170 (1999)
5. Pandey, H.M., Choudhary, A., Mehrotra, D.: A comparative review of approaches to prevent premature convergence in ga. Appl. Soft Comput. **24**, 1047–1077 (2014)
6. Reinelt, G.: TSPLIB - a traveling salesman problem library. ORSA J. Comput. **3**, 376–384 (1991)
7. Wagner, S., Kronberger, G., Beham, A., Kommenda, M., Scheibenpflug, A., Pitzer, E., Vonolfen, S., Kofler, M., Winkler, S.: Architecture and design of the heuristiclab optimization environment. In: Klempous, R., Nikodem, J., Jacak, W., Chaczko, Z. (eds.) Advanced Methods and Applications in Computational Intelligence. Topics in Intelligent Engineering and Informatics, vol. 6, pp. 197–261. Springer, New York (2014)

A Cluster-First Route-Second Approach for Balancing Bicycle Sharing Systems

Christian Kloimüllner[1]([✉]), Petrina Papazek[1], Bin Hu[2], and Günther R. Raidl[1]

[1] Institute of Computer Graphics and Algorithms, TU Wien, Favoritenstraße
9–11/1861, 1040 Vienna, Austria
{kloimuellner,papazek,raidl}@ac.tuwien.ac.at
[2] Mobility Department - Dynamic Transportation Systems,
AIT Austrian Institute of Technology, Giefinggasse 2, 1210 Vienna, Austria
bin.hu@ait.ac.at

Abstract. Public Bicycle Sharing Systems are booming all over the
world as they provide a green way of commuting in cities. However, it
is a challenging task to keep such systems in a balanced state, which
means that people can rent and return bikes where and when they want.
Usually, operators of these systems rebalance them actively by moving
bikes using vehicles with trailers. They plan routes around the city so
that technicians can move bikes from full stations to empty ones. In contrast to previous work we address this issue by a novel simplified problem
definition in conjunction with a Cluster-First Route-Second approach. It
is an exact algorithm utilizing *logic-based Benders decomposition* where
we solve an Assignment Problem as master problem and Traveling Salesman Problems as subproblems. Results show that we are able to solve
instances with up to 60 stations which was not possible with previous
problem definitions.

Keywords: Bike sharing · Vehicle routing · Cluster-first route-second ·
Logic-based Benders decomposition

1 Introduction

Many cities around the world augment their public transport by Bike-Sharing
Systems (BSS). They provide an ecofriendly way of traveling in the city and thus
reduce emissions by avoiding some of the city's motorized traffic. Last but not
least, BSS also motivate the population to do more sports and stay healthy [5].
An important factor to successfully run a BSS is the availability of bikes as
well as empty parking slots at each station at any time. Especially this aspect
is a major challenge and frequently a problem of existing BSS. Therefore, BSS
operators need to redistribute bikes among stations to increase user satisfaction.

This work is supported by the Austrian Research Promotion Agency (FFG), contract 831740. The authors thank Matthias Prandtstetter, Andrea Rendl and Markus
Straub from the Austrian Institute of Technology (AIT) for the collaboration in this
project.

R. Moreno-Díaz et al. (Eds.): EUROCAST 2015, LNCS 9520, pp. 439–446, 2015.
DOI: 10.1007/978-3-319-27340-2_55

Previous works aimed at providing a solution consisting of a route for every vehicle, and an accurate calculation of the loading operations at each stop of the vehicles. Although the computation of accurate loading instructions makes the problem more complex it seemed necessary to researchers and practitioners. We have also developed approaches for this problem definition in our previous work [8–10,12–14] but after applying our algorithms to the system of *Citybike Wien* in Vienna we got valuable feedback from their technicians. They told us that in practice the vehicle will almost never carry just a few bicycles. With small exceptions, only full vehicle loads will be picked up at a pickup station and completely delivered to a delivery station. In practice, achieving a "perfect" balance with respect to precise target numbers of bikes would be economically unreasonable; clearly too many vehicles and drivers would be needed without a substantial quality gain. Thus, in Citybike Wien's real setting, we can assume that there is always more than enough rebalancing work to do. In this work we exploit this information and neglect loading operations which substantially simplifies the problem. Instead, we classify each station as either a pickup or a delivery station and consider for each station how much vehicle loads we need to service it. Thus, we are using a Cluster-First Route-Second approach where we assign stations to vehicles, and then, solve the according routing problems.

2   Related Work

Over the last years several authors have addressed diverse problem definitions for Balancing Bicycle Sharing Systems (BBSS) with many different approaches. Most existing works rely on mixed integer programming (MIP) techniques. Benchimol et al. [1], Chemla et al. [2], Contardo et al. [3], Raviv et al. [15] all use various MIP approaches with decomposition techniques to solve the problem.

We have developed various metaheuristic approaches [9,10,12–14] working excellently on instances with up to 700 stations, which is substantially more than what can be handled with the MIP-based methods from the literature. Moreover, we also published an approach for the dynamic case [8].

Schuijbroek et al. [16] apply a Cluster-First Route-Second approach. In contrast to our work they define target intervals that must be met at the end of rebalancing and minimize the makespan. Instead of minimizing the makespan, we want to maximize the number of stations which we can serve as this is a more practical goal at least in the context of Vienna's bike sharing system *Citybike Wien*. Schuijbroek et al. implement their approach on a rolling horizon which means that they serve all stations of the system at a minimum service time. In contrast we consider a time limit corresponding to the shift time of the drivers. Schuijbroek et al.'s time-indexed MIP formulation for the routing part is expensive and does not seem practically important for solving the static case.

3   Problem Definition

Given is a set of nodes V representing the stations, and having associated a capacity C_v. Stations that need to be visited several times as multiple full loads need to be picked up or delivered are considered by including a respective number of copies of nodes in V. We define $V_{\text{pic}} \subseteq V$ as the set of all pickup stations and $V_{\text{del}} \subseteq V$ as the set of all delivery stations, i.e., $V = V_{\text{pic}} \cup V_{\text{del}}$. Furthermore, we add the node 0, representing the depot, and define $V_0 = V \cup \{0\}$. The arc set A represents the fastest connections between the nodes and every arc has associated a traveltime t_{uv}, and formally, $A = \{(u,v) \mid u \in V_{\text{pic}}, v \in V_{\text{del}}\} \cup \{(u,v) \mid u \in V_{\text{del}}, v \in V_{\text{pic}}\}$. Accordingly, we define the arc set $A_0 = A \cup \{(0,v) \mid v \in V_{pic}\} \cup \{(v,0) \mid v \in V_{del}\}$. The corresponding bipartite graph G is defined as $G = (V, A)$, and graph G_0, including the depot, accordingly as $G_0 = (V_0, A_0)$. By assumption, we are given a homogeneous vehicle fleet L with a common time budget $\hat{t}$ wherein technicians have to finish their routes. Additionally, all vehicles have a common capacity Z defining how many bikes they can transport at the same time. We assume, that all vehicles have to start empty at the depot and return empty to the depot. Every station is visited at most once.

Our aim is to service as many stations as possible within the time budgets of the drivers. Feasible solutions to the problem do not exceed the time budget for any driver, all routes start with a pickup station and end with a delivery station. Furthermore, the tour must alternate between pickup and delivery stations. Finally, the solution is represented by an alternating tour for every vehicle.

4   Logic-Based Benders Decomposition Scheme

The idea of classical *Benders decomposition* is to split the compact model into two parts, namely a *restricted master problem* and a *subproblem* by separating the variables and using LP duality. Logic-based Benders decomposition [6] aims at extending this approach to a "logical split" of the problem into a *master problem* and a *subproblem* where the subproblem yields Benders cuts through *logical deduction*. This means, Benders infeasibility cuts are added to the master problem whenever the solution of a subproblem is infeasible and the master problem is then resolved with these cuts.

The Assignment Problem (AP) deals with assigning stations to vehicles and serves as the master problem of this approach. Much work on the AP in conjunction with *Vehicle Routing Problems* is done with heuristic approaches (e.g., Genetic Algorithms) as it can be tough to find good routing costs approximation which can be formulated efficiently inside a MIP. In fact it turned out to be the biggest challenge to effectively encode the routing costs approximation into the MIP model. We need a lower bound on the TSP, because if we would overestimate the routing costs, obviously the subproblem would always be feasible as the optimal TSP tour would be lower than the estimation. Thus, our algorithm would terminate regardless whether the solution is optimal or not. Schuijbroek et al. [16] use a *Maximum Spanning Star* which they have proved to be an upper bound on the routing costs for their problem. However, in our case we need a lower bound, and thus, we ended up by using a single commodity flow formulation for computing a minimum spanning tree (MST) for approximating the routing costs in our MIP model. It has several advantages: It is a standard and well-known problem of graph theory, so it can be formulated very well inside the MIP and can be solved relatively efficiently. As preprocessing we calculate an upper bound ω on the assignment per cluster. Thus, we define a variable $t = 0$. Then, we seek for the pickup station with the least travel cost from the depot and the delivery station with the least travel cost to the depot and add these costs to t. Afterwards, we look for any lowest cost edges to add them also to t as long as $t < \hat{t}$. The number of nodes added during this procedure is an upper bound on the maximum assigned stations per cluster. This helps us to get some bound and our MIP model does not become quadratic (see Eq. 8 in the MIP).

Let $x_{vl} \, \forall v \in V_0, l \in L$ be 1 if v is assigned to vehicle l, 0 otherwise, $y_{uv}^l \, \forall (u, v) \in A_0, l \in L$ be 1 if there exists an edge from u to v in the MST for vehicle l, 0 otherwise, $f_{uv}^l \, \forall (u, v) \in A_0, l \in L$ the flow between nodes u and v for the MST in cluster l and h_l be the routing costs approximation for vehicle l. Moreover, we define the constant τ as the scaling factor for the MST in the objective function. This scaling factor is used to neglect any influence of the MST in the objective function because we only want to maximize the total assigned stations. The MST in the objective function is only used for routing costs approximation. Then our MIP model is formally defined as follows:

$$\max \quad \sum_{l \in L} \sum_{v \in V} x_{vl} - \sum_{l \in L} \tau \cdot h_l \tag{1}$$

subject to

$$\sum_{v \in V_0} x_{vl} \leq \omega \qquad\qquad \forall l \in L \tag{2}$$

$$x_{0l} = 1 \qquad\qquad \forall l \in L \tag{3}$$

$$\sum_{l \in L} x_{vl} \leq 1 \qquad\qquad \forall v \in V \tag{4}$$

$$\sum_{v \in V_{pic}} x_{vl} = \sum_{v \in V_{del}} x_{vl} \qquad\qquad \forall l \in L \tag{5}$$

$$\sum_{(0,v) \in A_0} f_{0v}^l = \sum_{v \in V} x_{vl} \qquad\qquad \forall l \in L \tag{6}$$

$$\sum_{(u,v) \in A_0} f_{uv}^l - \sum_{(v,u) \in A_0} f_{vu}^l = -1 \qquad\qquad \forall l \in L, u \in V \tag{7}$$

$$f_{uv}^l \leq y_{uv}^l \cdot \omega \qquad\qquad \forall l \in L, (u, v) \in A_0 \tag{8}$$

$$\sum_{(u,v) \in A_0} y_{uv}^l = \sum_{v \in V} x_{vl} \qquad\qquad \forall l \in L \tag{9}$$

$$y_{uv}^l \leq x_{vl} \qquad\qquad \forall l \in L, (u, v) \in A_0 \tag{10}$$

$$y_{uv}^l \leq x_{ul} \qquad\qquad \forall l \in L, (u, v) \in A_0 \tag{11}$$

$$h_l \geq \sum_{(u,v) \in A} y_{uv}^l \cdot t_{uv} \qquad\qquad \forall l \in L \tag{12}$$

$$h_l \leq \hat{t} \qquad\qquad \forall l \in L \qquad\qquad (13)$$

$$x_{vl}, y_{uv}^l \in \{0,1\} \qquad\qquad \forall v \in V_0, (u,v) \in A_0, l \in L \qquad (14)$$

$$h_l, f_{uv}^l \in \mathbb{R}^+ \qquad\qquad \forall (u,v) \in A_0, l \in L \qquad\qquad (15)$$

The objective function (1) maximizes the stations assigned to vehicles and minimizes the approximated costs by the spanning trees computed for each cluster. Note that not all stations may be assigned to a cluster as it is not possible to serve all stations within the given time limit. Inequalities (2)–(5) constitute the assignment of stations to the vehicles whereas inequalities (6)–(11) represent the spanning tree polytope. We restrict the maximum assigned stations per cluster for each vehicle $l \in L$ with the calculated upper bound by inequalities (2). Equalities (3) state that the depot 0 is included in every cluster. Inequalities (4) ensure that each station is assigned to at most one vehicle, and equalities (5) state that the number of assigned pickup stations must be equal to the number of assigned delivery stations for each cluster. The spanning tree is modeled by a single commodity flow formulation where the outgoing flow of the root node for each cluster must be the number of nodes assigned to that cluster which is ensured by equalities (6). For all other nodes except the root node, equalities (7) define that every node must consume 1 flow. Inequalities (8) restrict the maximum flow value of each cluster. Furthermore, these inequalities define the flow to be 0, if the edge is not chosen by the MST (i.e., $y_{uv}^l = 0$). Equalities (9) state that the total number of selected edges for the MST must be the number of stations assigned to that cluster. Equalities (10) and (11) state that the edge (u, v) can only be chosen by the MST, if both nodes u and v are contained in the cluster l. Equalities (12) are used to assign the approximated routing costs for each vehicle $l \in L$ to the variable h_l. Inequalities (13) ensure that the approximated routing costs lie within the time budget of each vehicle.

We can extract the assignment of stations from the x-variables. Note that the assignment may not necessarily be feasible as we only approximate the routing costs. The MST is a lower bound on the TSP, and therefore, the optimal routing costs may be higher than the time budget.

Traveling Salesman Problems have to be solved in our subproblems. After solving the AP we know which stations have to be serviced by which vehicle. Thus, we have to solve a TSP for each vehicle separately on the respective subgraph. As the TSP is already a well-studied problem, we use the State-Of-The-Art TSP solver *Concorde* [4]. However, Concorde is designed for solving only symmetric TSP instances on the complete graph. Thus, we transform our asymmetric instance into a symmetric one as shown in [7]. Infeasible edges (i.e., pickup to pickup and delivery to delivery stations) are modeled by very high routing costs so that these edges will not be used. Because of the maximum time limit of 480 min in our experiments, we get rather small TSP instances with about 25 stations for each subproblem. *Concorde* is able to solve those instances within milliseconds.

By using *Concorde* and translating the result back, we retrieve an alternating tour through all stations of the cluster starting and ending at the depot with minimal costs. We have to check if the costs of the optimal TSP tour are within the common time limit $\hat{t}$ of the vehicle. If this is the case, we have found a feasible solution. If this is not the case, we know that we have an infeasible assignment, because it is not possible to traverse all stations within the given time limit. Thus, we add a cut for this assignment and resolve the AP.

If all subproblems are feasible we have found a feasible and optimal solution to our problem and the algorithm terminates.

Benders infeasibility cuts are generated whenever we find a cluster which is not feasible due to the time limit of the vehicles. As we deal with a homogeneous vehicle fleet we can add this cut for each vehicle. Let C be the set of all cuts, then the *Benders cuts* are formally defined as: $\sum_{v \in c} x_{vl} \leq |c| - 1 \quad \forall c \in C, l \in L$. This means all sets $S \subseteq V_0$ where $\exists c \in C : S \supseteq c$ are discarded.

For improving the cuts we use the following additional heuristic: When we examine an infeasible assignment, we try to make the infeasible set smaller to cut off more infeasible assignments. Thus, we look for two stations, one pickup and one delivery station which have the least travel costs in the assignment. We remove these stations and try to resolve the TSP using *Concorde*. If the assignment stays infeasible we have found a better cut, and we can prune more infeasible assignments for the next run of the AP.

5   Computational Results

In this section we compare the logic-based Benders decomposition with the effective and powerful *Variable Neighborhood Search (VNS)* from [14]. For comparison, we also use the pre-processed instances for the VNS so that it produces alternating tours picking up and delivering as many bikes as possible.

As benchmark set we have chosen $|V| \in \{10, 20, 30, 60\}$, $|L| \in \{1, 2\}$ and $\hat{t} \in \{120, 240, 480\}$. The instances have been taken from [14] but now we only consider the type of the station rather than the exact fill levels.

The algorithm was implemented in C++ using GCC 4.8.2. For running our tests we used a single core of an Intel XEON E5540 with 2.53 GHz and 3 GB of memory. As MIP solver for the AP and Concorde we used CPLEX 12.6.

We set $\tau = 0.001$ for our experiments. The time limit for the logic-based Benders decomposition was 1 h and for the VNS we used half an hour. To compare to the VNS, we count the visited stations at the end of rebalancing. For every benchmark type we used 30 different instances and calculated the average.

Table 1 shows that small instances can easily be solved to optimality by the logic-based Benders decomposition. Furthermore, all instances up to 30 stations using 2 vehicles and 8 hours have been solved to optimality. In overall, we obtained optimal solutions for 66 % of the selected instance sets. In the third column of the logic-based Benders decomposition we show the *approximation quality* of the MST for the TSP. By *approximation quality* we measure how far off the estimated routing costs of the MST are compared to the optimal costs of the TSP. Generally, it looks that approximation quality becomes better with

Table 1. Results from our computational tests showing logic-based Benders decomposition

Inst. set			logic-based Benders decomposition						VNS	
$|V|$	$|L|$	$\hat{t}_{max}$	#Feasible [%]	obj	qual [%]	#iterations	#cuts	$\widetilde{t_{tot}}$ [s]	obj	diff
10	2	120	100.00	6.93	23.15	12.97	15.58	0.39	4.93	−2.00
10	2	240	100.00	8.20	24.56	1.20	0.76	0.06	8.07	−0.13
10	3	120	100.00	7.93	26.55	9.60	14.84	0.32	7.20	−0.73
20	2	120	86.67	7.92	22.97	71.88	149.04	48.98	5.37	−2.56
20	2	240	60.00	15.67	13.76	18.56	63.38	0.56	10.00	−5.67
20	3	120	56.67	11.76	20.82	65.59	163.84	197.22	8.13	−3.63
20	3	240	100.00	16.87	18.26	3.57	3.74	1.43	15.90	−0.97
30	2	120	40.00	8.00	22.98	14.58	14.27	829.56	5.10	−2.90
30	2	240	6.67	21.00	13.61	1.50	0.71	2851.00	9.53	−11.47
30	2	480	100.00	26.47	11.24	2.23	3.09	1.13	19.23	−7.23
30	3	120	10.00	12.00	24.14	1.00	0.00	3597.89	7.70	−4.30
30	3	240	30.00	23.78	14.39	8.00	5.96	7.79	17.53	−6.24
60	3	480	73.33	51.91	9.03	20.36	21.81	456.10	36.10	−15.81
			66.41	218.44	18.88				154.80	−63.64

bigger instances although we sometimes cannot solve all of the instances to optimality. In overall, we have achieved an approximation quality of 18 % with respect to the TSP. The number of iterations and cuts are moderate for the selected instances.

When comparing the exact logic-based Benders decomposition with the VNS, we noticed that differences between the exact algorithm and the metaheuristic become bigger when instance sets are larger although the VNS is most of the time not far off from the exact solution.

6   Conclusions and Future Work

We have proposed a novel problem definition for BBSS which is in some BSS practically highly relevant (e.g., Citybike Wien), but substantially simplifies the problem. For solving the problem we have come up with a logic-based Benders decomposition. The master problem is modeled as an AP and the subproblems as TSPs accordingly. It is possible to solve these subproblems with State-Of-The-Art methods, like *Concorde*, within milliseconds. Furthermore, we have shown that the Minimum spanning tree is a reasonable approximation for routing costs in the master problem. However, for bigger instances with more than 60 stations exact solutions are not always found within the time limit.

For future work it would be very interesting to investigate Branch-and-Check [17] as the subproblem can be solved very efficiently using *Concorde*. Furthermore, we would like to extend this approach to a heuristic Cluster-First Route-Second algorithm. If the AP would be solved heuristically, we could treat much bigger instances, probably even bigger instances than we have solved before (up to 700 stations in [14]). Moreover, as *Concorde* is very efficient for solving the TSP it would also be interesting to compare to a Route-First Cluster-Second algorithm as these approaches got very efficient during the last decade [11].

References

1. Benchimol, M., Benchimol, P., Chappert, B., De la Taille, A., Laroche, F., Meunier, F., Robinet, L.: Balancing the stations of a self service bike hire system. RAIRO - Oper. Res. **45**(1), 37–61 (2011)
2. Chemla, D., Meunier, F., Calvo, R.W.: Bike sharing systems: solving the static rebalancing problem. Discrete Optim. **10**(2), 120–146 (2013)
3. Contardo, C., Morency, C., Rousseau, L.M.: Balancing a dynamic public bike-sharing system. Technical report. CIRRELT-2012-09, Montreal, Canada (2012)
4. Cook, W.: Concorde TSP Solver (2011). http://www.math.uwaterloo.ca/tsp/concorde/. Accessed 06 May 2015
5. DeMaio, P.: Bike-sharing: history, impacts, models of provision, and future. Public Transp. **12**(4), 41–56 (2009)
6. Hooker, J.: Logic-based benders decomposition. Math. Program. **96**, 33–60 (1995)
7. Jonker, R., Volgenant, T.: Transforming asymmetric into symmetric traveling salesman problems. Oper. Res. Lett. **2**(4), 161–163 (1983)
8. Kloimüllner, C., Papazek, P., Hu, B., Raidl, G.R.: Balancing bicycle sharing systems: an approach for the dynamic case. In: Blum, C., Ochoa, G. (eds.) EvoCOP 2014. LNCS, vol. 8600, pp. 73–84. Springer, Heidelberg (2014)
9. Papazek, P., Kloimüllner, C., Hu, B., Raidl, G.R.: Balancing bicycle sharing systems: an analysis of path relinking and recombination within a GRASP hybrid. In: Bartz-Beielstein, T., Branke, J., Filipič, B., Smith, J. (eds.) PPSN 2014. LNCS, vol. 8672, pp. 792–801. Springer, Heidelberg (2014)
10. Papazek, P., Raidl, G.R., Rainer-Harbach, M., Hu, B.: A PILOT/VND/GRASP hybrid for the static balancing of public bicycle sharing systems. In: Moreno-Díaz, R., Pichler, F., Quesada-Arencibia, A. (eds.) EUROCAST. LNCS, vol. 8111, pp. 372–379. Springer, Heidelberg (2013)
11. Prins, C., Lacomme, P., Prodhon, C.: Order-first split-second methods for vehicle routing problems: a review. Transport. Res. C-Emer. **40**, 179–200 (2014)
12. Raidl, G.R., Hu, B., Rainer-Harbach, M., Papazek, P.: Balancing bicycle sharing systems: improving a VNS by efficiently determining optimal loading operations. In: Blesa, M.J., Blum, C., Festa, P., Roli, A., Sampels, M. (eds.) HM 2013. LNCS, vol. 7919, pp. 130–143. Springer, Heidelberg (2013)
13. Rainer-Harbach, M., Papazek, P., Hu, B., Raidl, G.R.: Balancing bicycle sharing systems: a variable neighborhood search approach. In: Middendorf, M., Blum, C. (eds.) EvoCOP 2013. LNCS, vol. 7832, pp. 121–132. Springer, Heidelberg (2013)
14. Rainer-Harbach, M., Papazek, P., Hu, B., Raidl, G.R., Kloimüllner, C.: PILOT, GRASP, and VNS approaches for the static balancing of bicycle sharing systems. J. Glob. Optim. **63**, 597–629 (2015)
15. Raviv, T., Tzur, M., Forma, I.A.: Static repositioning in a bike-sharing system: models and solution approaches. EURO J. Trans. Log. **2**(3), 187–229 (2013)
16. Schuijbroek, J., Hampshire, R., van Hoeve, W.J.: Inventory rebalancing and vehicle routing in bike sharing systems. Technical report. 2013–E1, Tepper School of Business, Carnegie Mellon University (2013)
17. Thorsteinsson, E.S.: Branch-and-check: a hybrid framework integrating mixed integer programming and constraint logic programming. In: Walsh, T. (ed.) CP 2001. LNCS, vol. 2239, pp. 16–30. Springer, Heidelberg (2001)

Computer Methods, Virtual Reality and Image Processing for Clinical and Academic Medicine

MATLAB/Simulink-Supported EMG Classification on the Raspberry Pi

Andreas Attenberger[✉] and Klaus Buchenrieder

Institut Für Technische Informatik, Universität der Bundeswehr München,
Neubiberg, Germany
{andreas.attenberger,klaus.buchenrieder}@unibw.de

Abstract. Patient satisfaction with body-powered myoelectric upper limb prostheses is limited, often resulting in device abandonment. Multifunctional hand prostheses are one potential solution to increase patient acceptance. These require sophisticated control schemes like pattern-recognition-based approaches involving classification of myoelectric signals (MES). To allow fast and flexible evaluation of prosthesis control approaches, a prototyping environment based on the Raspberry Pi and MATLAB/Simulink was created. It supports commonly applied features like RMS and zero crossings as well as classification methods like Naive Bayesian and Support Vector Machine classifiers. After classifier training with a custom MATLAB application, MES can be classified in real-time and the results employed for prosthesis actuation. The setup was tested with five participants for controlling a Michelangelo Hand. Over 90 % of movements were correctly identified for three classes from two channel EMG data.

Keywords: Electromyography · Pattern recognition · Prosthetic hands · Raspberry Pi

1 Introduction

Advanced hand prostheses with multiple degrees of freedom like the Michelangelo hand available from Otto Bock or the bebionic3 hand developed by RSLSteeper offer sophisticated control over a wide array of hand positions [14]. However, the underlying control strategies have not experienced a continuing revolution [9] and modern myoelectric prostheses are still not widely accepted by patients [3,13]. Several issues, such as system complexity, reduced robustness or the absence of feedback and proportionality have previously been identified as a reason [9,12]. Clearly, a higher number of test cycles in the development process could resolve the issues of system reliability and patient acceptance for myoelectric prostheses. In the scope of this work, we present a classification system that combines the flexibility of MATLAB/Simulink-based control models with a low-cost hardware platform, the Raspberry Pi. This allows for faster testing of prosthesis control approaches with a significant amount of users. It offers higher system performance than previous approaches employing Arduino devices [2], which permits

© Springer International Publishing Switzerland 2015
R. Moreno-Díaz et al. (Eds.): EUROCAST 2015, LNCS 9520, pp. 449–456, 2015.
DOI: 10.1007/978-3-319-27340-2_56

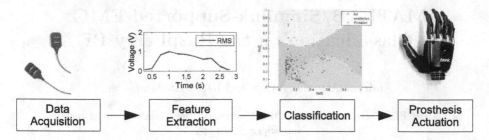

Fig. 1. The classification process as implemented in the Raspberry Pi-based proto-type including sensor signal acquisition, feature extraction and classification as well as prostheses actuation.

the implementation and the comparison of various pattern recognition methods. Tight-loop development cycles, incorporating these methods for embedded targets are especially suitable for the modern multifunctional hand prostheses at present available commercially [15].

2 Myoelectric Signal Classification

The prototype integrates the basic steps of the classification process as devised by Englehart et al. [7] and illustrated in Fig. 1. The first step is signal acquisition employing electromyography (EMG), which is the predominant sensing technology currently applied in upper limb prosthetics [9,14]. EMG sensors placed on the skin surface detect changes in electrical potential caused by activity in the observed muscles. These signals range from $10\,\mu V$ to $10\,mV$ and are subsequently amplified and filtered [11]. Characteristic features are extracted from the conditioned signal, which are then applied to train a classifier model. The following feature algorithms are currently implemented in our prototype:

Root Mean Square (RMS): The average strength of a muscle contraction can be calculated with the root mean square value for N samples $x_1, ..., x_n$ with [5]:

$$RMS(x) = \sqrt{\frac{1}{N} \sum_{i=1}^{N} x_i^2}$$

Zero Crossings (ZC): The zero crossing feature extracts the amount of times the signal value changes sign. It gives a basic indication of the frequency of the signal [8]. For N samples and a threshold T, it is denoted by:

$$ZC(x) = \sum_{k=1}^{N-1} g_{ZC}(x_k)$$

with

$$g_{ZC}(x) = \begin{cases} 1 \text{ if } sgn(-x_k \cdot x_{k+1}) \wedge (|x_k - x_{k+1}|) \geq T \\ 0 \text{ otherwise} \end{cases}$$

and

$$sgn(x) = \begin{cases} true & \text{if } x \geq 0 \\ false & \text{else} \end{cases}$$

Mean Absolute Value (MAV): Besides the RMS feature values, the mean absolute value (MAV) feature can also be used to gauge muscle contraction strength [6]. For N samples it is determined by the following formula:

$$MAV(x) = \overline{X} = \frac{1}{N} \sum_{i=1}^{N} |x_i|$$

During training, the calculated feature values denoting muscle activity of different hand movements are fed to the classifier with respective class labels. In the operational phase of the classifier, features are extracted from acquired signals and classified into the previously trained movement classes. At the moment, Support Vector Machine (SVM), Naive Bayesian (NBC) and Linear Discriminant Analysis (LDA) classifiers are supported by the prototype.

Linear Discriminant Analysis (LDA): During LDA, feature vectors are assigned a class through a discriminant function with weight vector w and a bias w_0. For two classes, this is expressed by [4]:

$$y(x) = \omega^T \cdot x + \omega_0 = 0$$

Multiple classes can be classified by partitioning the feature space into binary classification problems.

Naive Bayes Classifier (NBC): The NBC assumes statistical independence of features, which is especially important for bigger sets of samples [16]. In the case of feature vectors x_j, $j = 1, 2, ..., l$, this results in:

$$p(x \mid \omega_i) = \prod_{j=1}^{l} p(x_j \mid \omega_i), i = 1, 2, ..., M$$

Unlabeled feature values $x = [x_1, x_2, ..., x_l]^T$ are then classified employing the following equation:

$$\omega_m = \arg\max_{\omega_i} \prod_{j=1}^{l} p(x_j \mid \omega_i), i = 1, 2, ..., M$$

Support Vector Machine (SVM): SVM classifiers separate classes with hyperplanes [16]. In the case of two classes and feature sample vectors x_i with $i = 1, 2, ..., n$, a hyperplane is denoted by:

$$g(x) = \omega^T \cdot x + \omega_0 = 0$$

Analogous to LDA, a combination of binary classification problems results in multiple-class classification.

While it is possible to integrate feature selection into the prototype, it is not supported in the presented version. This is due to the low dimensionality of the time-domain features currently implemented, which do not necessarily mandate feature selection in contrast to higher-dimensional features like wavelet transform coefficients [15].

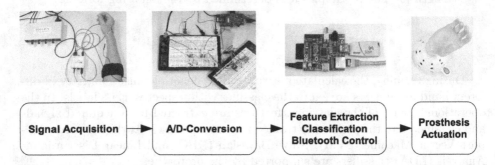

Fig. 2. After signal acquisition and A/D conversion, EMG features are extracted and classified with a MATLAB/Simulink model executed on the Raspberry Pi. At the end of the process chain, control information is generated for prosthesis actuation.

3   Raspberry Pi Prototype

As shown in Fig. 2, the system includes the necessary hard- and software components for pattern-recognition-based prosthesis control schemes [7]. The output from the sensing and digitization components is subsequently processed on the Raspberry Pi for hand movement classification.

3.1   Hardware Setup

The myoelectric signals are acquired with a Delsys Bagnoli EMG system including single differential EMG electrodes[1]. After range adjustment the signals are input to an MCP3208 analog-digital converter (ADC). The MCP3208 offers 12-bit resolution with a maximum speed of 100 ksps [10]. It is controlled through a Serial Parallel Interface (SPI) with a C++ application on the Raspberry Pi[2]. Converted data is transferred via UDP to either the localhost interface for stand-alone classification or over the Ethernet port to a host equipped with MATLAB for signal verification and classification model creation. After GUI-supported classifier training, the resulting classifier model is transferred to the Raspberry Pi. Results for the hand movement can either be displayed on an LED bar graph or converted to Bluetooth control commands for the physical Michelangelo hand. Bluetooth connectivity is made available through a USB Bluetooth adapter.

---

[1] http://www.delsys.com/products/desktop-emg/bagnoli-desktop/.
[2] http://hertaville.com/2013/07/24/interfacing-an-spi-adc-mcp3008-chip-to-the-raspberry-pi-using-c/.

3.2 Feature Extraction and Classifier Training

The supported classification methods can be trained employing the MATLAB GUI shown in Fig. 3. Currently, RMS, MAV, ZC features and LDA, NBC, SVM classifiers are available through pull-down menu selection. The classifier implementation is taken from the NaN-toolbox[3] and customized to allow code generation for stand-alone model deployment[4]. To train the system, first, the analog-digital conversion process has to be started on the Raspberry Pi, which must be connected to the same network as the computer running MATLAB. Once A/D-converted data is available, a threshold can be determined automatically and manually adjusted for the selected feature. Maximum amplitude values can also be detected for subsequent normalization of the feature data. Currently, the prototype can be trained with two sensors and three different hand movements: wrist extension, wrist flexion and fist motions. Feature data are displayed at the

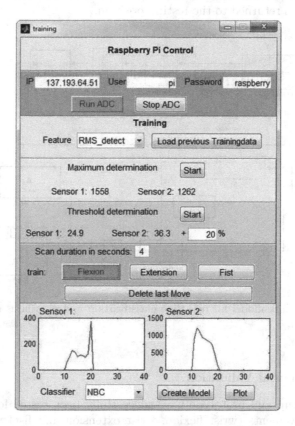

Fig. 3. The MATLAB GUI for training the classifier, supporting selection of feature extraction and classification methods as well as automatic threshold and maximum value detection.

[3] http://pub.ist.ac.at/~schloegl/matlab/NaN/.
[4] http://mathworks.com/hardware-support/raspberry-pi-simulink.html.

bottom of the GUI allowing for deletion of a recorded movement in case of error. Finally, a classifier model can be generated for one of the available classifiers. A class boundary plot is available for inspection by the user.

3.3 Classifier Operation and Prosthesis Actuation

Once the classifier model has been generated, it is transferred to the Raspberry Pi for standalone, real-time classification. The corresponding Simulink model is shown in Fig. 4. Here, the selected feature is extracted from the converted sensor signal values, subjected to the determined threshold and then input to the classifier. The output is then transferred to the Michelangelo Hand control model from which the command sequences for the Bluetooth transmission are generated. The hand is controlled with a simple state machine that activates a recognized hand position on successful recognition. If it is already actuated to the position, it is returned to the resting position.

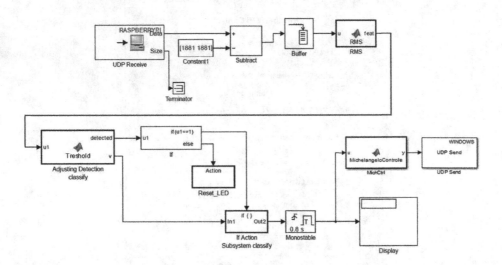

Fig. 4. The Simulink model for real-time classification and prosthesis actuation with the Raspberry Pi.

3.4 Experimental Validation

The current setup and prototype have successfully been tested for recognizing three hand movements (wrist flexion, wrist extension and fist) with an NBC classifier and two EMG sensors. The two sensors were positioned over the flexor and extensor muscle group of the right forearm of five participants. After sampling the sensor signals with a sampling frequency of 1 kHz, the RMS feature was calculated with a window size of 256 and an increment of 128 samples. After five repetitions for each movement, the NBC model was generated and transferred to the Raspberry Pi for standalone real-time classification. For classifier validation, participants performed three sessions each with a sequence of a wrist flexion, a wrist extension and a fist in three sets with adequate rest in between. This resulted in a total of 27 movements. Overall, 90.4 % of all movements were classified correctly, with marked differences between individuals ranging from only 27 % up to 100 % correctly identified motion patterns. While incorrect threshold settings are suspected as the reason for pronounced misclassification in some users, further tests have to be conducted for confirmation.

4   Conclusion and Future Work

This paper presented a prototype setup for testing pattern-recognition-based prostheses control approaches created with MATLAB/Simulink on a Raspberry Pi. Basic time-domain features like RMS or ZC are supported at the time of this publication. Furthermore, popular classification methods like NBC and SVM are available for standalone classification in real-time. The integration of Simulink models and the open-source NaN-toolbox for code generation allows for fast prototyping and real-time testing of the designed control approaches. The current setup has successfully been tested for recognizing three different hand movements (wrist flexion, wrist extension and fist) utilizing a NBC classifier. In the conducted study with five probands, correct recognition of over 90 % of all movements was achieved for two channel EMG data as expected. Due to the modular construction of the individual components, it is possible to replace different parts of the system. For example, small portable EMG sensors can serve as input for analog-digital conversion and other prostheses like the bebionic3 hand. Generally, wired and wireless prostheses alike can be controlled with the Raspberry Pi. If the chosen classification algorithms do not mandate high system performance, the Raspberry Pi can also be replaced with an Arduino while employing the same Simulink model and MATLAB training application.

Acknowledgement. We are grateful to M.Sc. Lars Achterberg for his work in implementing the Raspberry Pi ADC software and MATLAB/Simulink model [1]. Furthermore, we like to thank M.Sc. Sebastian Preibisch, M.Sc. Steve Wilhelm and mgr inż Sławomir Wojciechowski for taking part in the study.

References

1. Achterberg, L.: Mikrocontroller-Implementierung eines MATLAB-Klassifizierers für EMG-Signale. Master's thesis, Universität der Bundeswehr München (2014)
2. Attenberger, A., Buchenrieder, K.: An arduino-simulink-control system for modern hand protheses. In: Rutkowski, L., Korytkowski, M., Scherer, R., Tadeusiewicz, R., Zadeh, L.A., Zurada, J.M. (eds.) ICAISC 2014, Part II. LNCS, vol. 8468, pp. 433–444. Springer, Heidelberg (2014)
3. Biddiss, E.A., Chau, T.T.: Upper limb prosthesis use and abandonment: a survey of the last 25 years. Prosthet. Orthot. Int. **31**(3), 236–257 (2007). http://poi.sagepub.com/content/31/3/236.abstract

4. Bishop, C.: Pattern Recognition and Machine Learning. Information Science and Statistics. Springer, New York (2006). http://books.google.de/books?id= kTNoQgAACAAJ

5. Buchenrieder, K.: Dimensionality reduction for the control of powered upper limb prostheses. In: Proceedings of 14th Annual IEEE International Conference and Workshops on the Engineering of Computer-Based Systems (ECBS 2007), pp. 327–333, March 2007

6. Clancy, E.A., Hogan, N.: Theoretic and Experimental Comparison of Root-Mean-Square and Mean-Absolute-Value Electromyogram Amplitude Detectors (1997). http://www.scopus.com/inward/record.url?eid=2-s2.0-0031293539& partnerID=40&md5=8010dd988aa99b6acccb57ec5bece461

7. Englehart, K., Hudgins, B., Parker, P., Stevenson, M.: Classification of the myoelectric signal using time-frequency based representations. Med. Eng. Phys. **21**(6–7), 431–438 (1999)

8. Herrmann, S., Buchenrieder, K.: Advanced control schemes for upper limb prosthesis. Adv. Med. Biol. **15**, 377–408 (2011)

9. Jiang, N., Dosen, S., Müller, K., Farina, D.: Myoelectric control of artificial limbs: is there the need for a change of focus? IEEE Signal Process. Mag. **152**, 1–4 (2012). doi:10.1109/MSP.2012.2203480. http://www.bfnt-goettingen.de/ Publications/articlereference.2013-09-25.4943665964

10. Microchip Technology Inc.: MCP3204/8 Datasheet. Microchip Technology Inc. (2008)

11. Muzumdar, A.: Powered Upper Limb Prostheses: Control, Implementation and Clinical Application. Springer, New York (2004)

12. Paredes, L., Graimann, B.: Advanced myoelectric control of prostheses: requirements and challenges. In: Pons, J.L., Torricelli, D., Pajaro, M. (eds.) Converging Clinical and Engineering Research on Neurorehabilitation, Biosystems & Biorobotics, vol. 1, pp. 1221–1224. Springer, Heidelberg (2013). http://dx.doi.org/10.1007/978-3-642-34546-3_202

13. Peerdeman, B., Boere, D., Witteveen, H.J.B., Huis in 't Veld, M.H.A., Hermens, H.J., Stramigioli, S., Rietman, J.S., Veltink, P.H., Misra, S.: Myoelectric forearm prostheses: state of the art from a user-centered perspective. J. Rehabil. Res. Dev. **48**(6), 719–738 (2011)

14. van der Riet, D., Stopforth, R., Bright, G., Diegel, O.: An overview and comparison of upper limb prosthetics. In: AFRICON 2013, pp. 1–8, September 2013

15. Scheme, E., Englehart, K.: Electromyogram pattern recognition for control of powered upper-limb prostheses: state of the art and challenges for clinical use. J. Rehabil. Res. Dev. (JRRD) **48**(6), 643–660 (2011). http://www.rehab.research.va.gov/jour/11/486/scheme486.html

16. Theodoridis, S., Koutroumbas, K.: Pattern Recognition, 4th edn. Academic Press (2008)

Applicability of Patient-Specific Simulation

Andrzej Wytyczak-Partyka[1]([✉]), Jan Nikodem[2], and Ryszard Klempous[1]

[1] Department of Control Systems and Mechatronics,
Wroclaw University of Technology, Wroclaw, Poland
{andrzej.wytyczak-partyka,ryszard.klempous}@pwr.edu.pl
[2] Department of Computer Engineering,
Wroclaw University of Technology, Wroclaw, Poland
jan.nikodem@pwr.edu.pl

Abstract. Patient-specific surgical simulation is a new and important trend in surgical simulation that creates new possibilities for increasing patient safety by giving the surgeons an opportunity to practice before real procedures using the patient's simulated anatomy. The following paper discusses the current state of patient-specific simulation, its drawbacks and possible applications as well as describes a prototype system.

Keywords: Laparoscopic surgery · Surgical simulation · Patient-specific simulation

1 Background

Simulation has been already widely adopted in the area of laparoscopic surgery and has shown positive impact on performance in the operating room [1–4]. Simulation is especially appreciated in the early part of training, during the development of basic skills, as outlined in [5]. It becomes more requiring in case of experienced surgeons, who already mastered the basic skills and have higher expectations of a simulator, which should either help them improve their skills further or in other ways increase the patient's safety. An important area of applications of simulation is the preoperative planning, which in case of more complicated procedures and in the face of anatomical variations can significantly improve patient's safety during surgical procedures. Sometimes dubbed Patient-Specific Virtual Reality [6], the area of preoperative planning and simulation tailored to the specific patient's case and anatomy is becoming more and more important [7]. It is also becoming more and more feasible thanks to the ubiquitous CT and MRI scanners, which are currently available in almost every larger hospital. These devices can serve as a non-invasive source for data required for visualisation of the specific patient's anatomy used in the VR simulator. However it still remains unclear as to how to embed patient-specific VR in current medical procedures (both - formally and practically) - it can undoubtly bring a new level of patient safety and therefore should be investigated in depth.

© Springer International Publishing Switzerland 2015
R. Moreno-Díaz et al. (Eds.): EUROCAST 2015, LNCS 9520, pp. 457–462, 2015.
DOI: 10.1007/978-3-319-27340-2_57

2 Simulator

The most important parts of a laparoscopic simulator are the 3D graphics engine, human-computer interface used to control the engine, the knowledge-base that contains the training scenarios and 3D models and the assesment engine that evaluates the performance in real time [8]. In case of patient-specific simulation the knowledge-base has to be fed with real data obtained from patient's CT or MRI scan taken immediately before the procedure, Fig. 1.

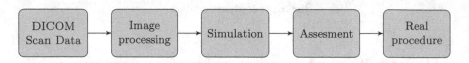

Fig. 1. The image processing and surface reconstruction steps

3 Data Sources

The most prominent data sources for Virtual Reality simulation are the MRI and CT imaging techniques. The datasets produced using these modalities (at least with recent generations scanners) provide enough data for high-fidelity visualisations of the anatomy. The main concern for applications of this data is the image segmentation step, which should extract particular anatomical structures from the cross-section images. It is a difficult task, which rises doubts even among experienced radiologists. Several classes of methods exist with varying complexity and different level of required human attention [9]. Fully automatic segmentation and classification of anatomical structures is still rarely possible, which we consider as one of the main obstacles for wider adoption of patient-specific surgical simulation. The amount of data registered in a CT or MRI scan is too large for manual segmentation, even semi-automatic methods, which require a very limited attention of a medical proffesional, will still make the simulation useless for urgent procedures. Therefore it seems reasonable to enable different segmentation modes:

– high-fidelity segmentation,
– high-speed segmentation.

3.1 High-Fidelity Segmentation

The high-fidelity segmentation mode should be used in non-urgent cases, where time can be taken to conduct proper segmentation and where the high level of detail plays an important role, e.g. in tumor resection procedures or when operating in vicinity of very sensitive structures.

3.2   High-Speed Segmentation

This segmentation mode should be used for pre-operative simulation in urgent cases, when only a general understanding of the operating area is required, e.g. in appendectomy or cholecystectomy. However, special caution should be taken in these cases and conversion to the high-fidelity mode should be considered if there are any signs indicating a difficult or uncommon case.

3.3   Image Processing Pipeline

Currently a modified version of the image processing pipeline described in [10] is used to provide the high-speed mode of automatic segmentation and reconstruction of 3D constraints of anatomical structures - Fig. 2. Further development is underway in the area of high-fidelity segmentation, based on region-growing methods. The surface reconstruction part of the process has been optimized to work in parallel on a GPU and therefore is very fast. The final product of the pipeline is a 3D surface model of a structure, that further needs to be converted to a common interchange format, e.g. STL, Wavefront OBJ or Autodesk FBX that will be ingested by the simulation engine.

4   Simulation Engine

The selection of a 3D simulation engine is very important in order to provide high level of detail and realism. We selected freely available engines supporting soft-body dynamics required for realistic simulation of interaction between the laparoscopic instruments and anatomical structures. The engines explored include:

- Nvidia PhysX
- Unreal Engine (PhysX based)
- Sofa framework
- Ogre3D + Bullet
- LibGDX + Bullet.

The Nvidia PhysX and the Unreal Engine, which seemed very promising have eventually turned out to be useless because of the state of soft-body implementation in the current version of PhysX (3.3) - as a regression from the previous version, soft-body simulation has almost completely disappeared from the 3.3 version and is described as "under development" by Nvidia.

The Sofa framework [11]- another promising project, with the advantage of easily defined simulation scenarios and proper implementation of deformable soft-bodies has rendered problems with importing 3D models with skeletal animation (e.g. the models of laparoscopic instruments) and shown unstable performance of the ODE solver which is the workhorse of the soft-body implementation.

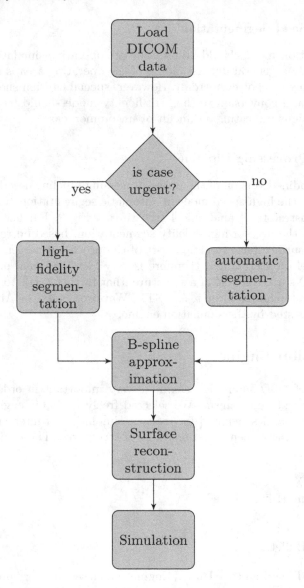

Fig. 2. The image processing and surface reconstruction steps

Ogre3D and Bullet combination was a very close match, however the level of integration between Ogre3D and Bullet was insufficient for further rapid prototyping of the system as well as the availability of APIs for painless importing of 3D models from tools like Blender and lack of good documentation. Finally the pair of LibGDX (Fig. 3) together with Bullet Physics engine has been chosen for further work due to their close integration, availability of examples and documentation.

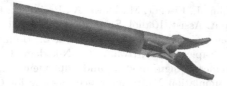

Fig. 3. A laparoscopic instrument rendered in LibGDX

5   Conclusions

Patient-specific simulation by means of Virtual Reality is becoming an important trend in surgical simulation. There are several obstacles that were identified in this article that need to be addressed for wider adoption of such simulations - the time required for attending semi-automatic segmenation methods vs. the infidelity of models produced through automated segmenation, the disputable application of pre-operative planning in urgent surgical cases, where time is a major factor, finally the level of realism in reflecting the haptic features of internal structures. Some of these arise due to technical issues that can be overcome, some need to be evaluated in terms of cost-benefit ratio in every case and we have proposed several methods of dealing with these obstacles.

Acknowledgements. This work has been supported by the National Science Center under grant: 2012/07/B/ST7/01216.

References

1. Aggarwal, R., Grantcharov, T.P., Eriksen, J.R., Blirup, D., Kristiansen, V.B., Funch-Jensen, P., Darzi, A.: An evidence-based virtual reality training program for novice laparoscopic surgeons. Ann. Surg. **244**(2), 310–314 (2006)
2. Seymour, N.E., Gallagher, A.G., Roman, S.A., OBrien, M.K., Bansal, V.K., Andersen, D.K., Satava, R.M.: Virtual reality training improves operating room performance: results of a randomized, double-blinded study. Ann. Surg. **236**(4), 458–464 (2002)
3. Zendejas, B., Brydges, R., Hamstra, S.J., Cook, D.A.: State of the evidence on simulation-based training for laparoscopic surgery: a systematic review. Ann. Surg. **257**(4), 586–593 (2013)
4. Grantcharov, T.P., Kristiansen, V.B., Bendix, J., Bardram, L., Rosenberg, J., Funch-Jensen, P.: Randomized clinical trial of virtual reality simulation for laparoscopic skills training. Br. J. Surg. **91**(2), 146–150 (2004)
5. Vassiliou, M.C., Ghitulescu, G.A., Feldman, L.S., Stanbridge, D., Leffondre, K., Sigman, H.H., Fried, G.M.: The MISTELS program to measure technical skill in laparoscopic surgery. Surg. Endosc. Other Intervent. Tech. **20**(5), 744–747 (2006)
6. Willaert, W.I.M., Aggarwal, R., Van Herzeele, I., Cheshire, N.J., Vermassen, F.E.: Recent advancements in medical simulation: patient-specific virtual reality simulation. World J. Surg. **36**(7), 1703–1712 (2012)

7. Boehm, A., Dornheim, J., Fischer, M., Dietz, A., Preim, B.: Patient Specific Modelling. Int. J. Comput. Assist. Radiol. Surg. 4(S1), 222–224 (2009)
8. Rozenblit, J.W., Feng, C., Riojas, M., Napalkova, L., Hamilton, A.J., Hong, M., Berthet-Rayne, P., Czapiewski, P., Hwang, G., Nikodem, J., et al.: The computer assisted surgical trainer: design, models, and implementation. In: Proceedings of the 2014 Summer Simulation Multiconference, Society for Computer Simulation International, pp. 211–220 (2014)
9. Pham, D.L., Xu, C.Y., Prince, J.L.: Current methods in medical image segmentation. Ann. Rev. Biomed. Eng. 2, 315–337 (2000)
10. Wytyczak-Partyka, A.: Organ Surface Reconstruction using B-Splines and Hu Moments. Acta Polytech. Hung. 11(10), 151–161 (2014)
11. Allard, J., Cotin, S., Faure, F., Bensoussan, P.J., Poyer, F., Duriez, C., Delingette, H., Grisoni, L., et al.: Sofa-an open source framework for medical simulation. Medicine Meets Virtual Reality, MMVR 15. IOP Press, Amsterdam (2007)

Application of Image Processing and Virtual Reality Technologies in Simulation of Laparoscopic Procedures

Jan Nikodem[1]([✉]), Andrzej Wytyczak-Partyka[2], and Ryszard Klempous[2]

[1] Department of Computer Engineering, Wroclaw University of Technology,
Wroclaw, Poland
jan.nikodem@pwr.edu.pl
[2] Department of Control Systems and Mechatronics,
Wroclaw University of Technology, Wroclaw, Poland
{andrzej.wytyczak-partyka,ryszard.klempous}@pwr.edu.pl

Abstract. In this paper we focus on developing the simulators of laparoscopic surgery procedures. We propose expanding the role of video channel, which allows to reduce the mechatronic systems providing information about the spatial position of instruments. The mechatronic structure is indispensable in order to achieve the effect of haptic feedback, however in the proposed solution it is much simpler, than as in the case of currently occurring solutions. In proposed issue, mechatronic consists of actuators with a simple control software only. Entire perception (data acquisition) for the realization of haptic feedback is implemented using the video channel. Moreover, haptic feedback effect is supported by the dynamics calculations made in the graphics software. While calculating of the movement of the objects, their collisions and associated with that deformations, the physics engine purveyed current value of forces, torques, speed or acceleration to haptic feedback fittings.

Keywords: Laparoscopic skill trainer · Virtual reality · 3D graphics · Image processing

1 Introduction

There are plenty of articles in the literature [3,8,10] on a laparoscopic surgery training simulators. Although an objective evidence is relatively sparse, there is no doubt that such simulation must be an important part of surgeons education for the future [5,9,11]. Accordingly, a new laparoscopic surgery training simulators appear at any time on the market. Currently, there are three different general categories of simulators for surgeons and residents to train their technical skills:

– *simple boxtrainers*, equipped with camera and laparoscopic instruments. The camera shows the movement of the instruments within the box, and surgeons train their skills working on human organ models.

© Springer International Publishing Switzerland 2015
R. Moreno-Díaz et al. (Eds.): EUROCAST 2015, LNCS 9520, pp. 463–470, 2015.
DOI: 10.1007/978-3-319-27340-2_58

- *virtual reality trainers.* Use computer to generate images of organs and instruments allowing the trainee to navigate these images by using laparoscopic joysticks as controllers. Equipped with sophisticated mechatronic systems, providing smooth haptic interactions, the collision detection, or measuring the torque and force applied by a surgeon during laparoscopic tasks.
- *augmented reality trainers.* Virtual reality trainers enhanced by 3D image processing to obtain the 3D models of anatomical structures from real patient ultrasonography data, Magnetic Resonance Imaging, and Computed Tomography scans.

Due to the diverse range of prices and capabilities, presence in the market of all three types of simulators is substantiated. Relatively cheap *simple boxtrainers* generally are sufficient to train such skills as the eye-hand coordination, depth perception, and efficiency of instrument movement due to the fulcrum effect. Therefore, probably still for a long time it will be available on the market.

At the same time, emerged two development trends towards the implementation of IT technology to laparoscopic surgery simulators. The first, *striving for active control* of instrument's trajectory during surgery training (forcing the desired trajectory of instrument, as it is realized for surgery robots).

The second, *focusing on the anatomy* of human organs used in simulations. Acceptance of standard anatomical model is useful for simulation of laparoscopic surgery. Nonetheless, if the simulation exercises should prepare the surgeon to the actual operation on the patient, an even better solution is a modeling of diseased organ of the patient who will be treated. The shape, the bodily structures, and location of diseased organs often deviate from the standard model. Hence in the simulator it is preferable to use a personalized model of the concrete patient's anatomy, which will be a close representation of what the surgeon will encounter in the operating room.

In the simulation of laparoscopic surgery we need to control the movement of instruments not in the active manner (forcing the correct position of the instrument), but in the passive manner when simulator signals undesirable position of the instrument. Therefore below, we leave the idea of active control and we will focus on features common for both trends, i.e. increased participation of 3D graphic engine technologies and software image processing in the final product, which is a simulator of laparoscopic surgery procedures.

2 Developing a Laparoscopic Simulators for the Future

2.1 Software Should Dominate Hardware

All commercially available simulators, as well as those described in literature, show a common trend of emphasizing the role of software. Thanks to that the mechatronic systems can be simpler, and the overall product easier to maintain, more reliable and significantly cheaper. Instead the development effort is put into enhancing the user (human) interface in order to increase the simulator's efficiency and user experience.

2.2   Minimally Invasive Surgery Simulators Cultivate Human Brain

We build simulators as a technical devices supported by computers and their software. But let's try to answer the question: what these simulators are for? We are arguing that simulators are designed to adapt psycho-motor skills of trainees, to situations occurring during the implementation of laparoscopy surgery in real world. Simulator improves the psycho-motor dexterity of surgeons, their work efficiency, maintaining the regularity of stimuli perception, decision making and muscle actuation response. Training on simulators allow the trainees to cultivate their brain connectome (Seung) characteristic for laparoscopic surgeon. Therefore, next several sentences we will devote to the brain and its communication channels, which are used by the surgeon during surgery on a patient.

2.3   Visual Channel Is the Most Important

People trained on the simulator uses information transmitted to the brain by three channels: visual, sensory and auditory. The first two of them are especially used in laparoscopic simulation, but the visual channel is used the most intensively. The surgeon receives haptic and auditory stimuli, but his brain analyzes them in the visual context, which the eyes provide to it. A simple experiment, which switch off the individual channels of information, leads to the conclusion that exercising deprived of auditory information or haptic stimuli, can perform the exercises correctly based only on the image of what he sees. However, turning off the video channel evidently stops execution of the exercise. Visual channel is really crucial. During the exercises on the simulator, the brain of exerciser is the main processor of information received from visual channel (even these, relating to the feedback level) and the results of this processing are passing on, to the human motoric system's actuators [1,2].

To focus on enhancement of the role of visual channel, that is our idea for the development of laparoscopic simulators. The image provides an extremely high degree of aggregation of information. In case of simulation, the visual channel with this kind of aggregation is a very desirable feature. Firstly, we have a wide range of software for image processing and 3D graphics, furthermore we have at our disposal a specialized hardware (graphic cards) supporting 3D visualization. Secondly, the brain can process visual information even more efficiently than are able to perform it modern computers.

2.4   Scope of Data Extraction

The simulator will be perfect, if the scope of information provided by it will be identical to what the surgeon receives during actual operations. However, it is possible to achieve the same effect simpler. Information, provided to the brain by the eye, are selectively analyzed in accordance with the arrangement of worked out connectome. Due to this brain selectivity, we should concentrate on processing only these elements, that are human perceivable and have a significant impact on the realism of the simulation. Therefore, the scope of the information provided by a visual channel can be restricted to the extent necessary for proper decision-making by a people training on the simulator.

2.5   Tracking the Instrument Movement

Visual channel carries (among other things) information about the instruments position in the operating field. The scope of this information is sufficient for the surgeon to take the right decisions regarding the 3D movement of instruments. In operating room, the specification of the exact surgical instrument position in Cartesian or polar coordinates is necessary only for mechatronics, but in our implementation all necessary complex algorithmic calculations are replaced with the trainee's brain activity.

In respect to 2D space, navigation by practicing laparoscopic instrument movements will be identical as using the mouse in computer system. Information about the third dimension (so-called depth perception) is achieved through observation of relative to neighbour objects position, the perspective and shadow observations.

The presented in literature [1, 4, 7], existing systems, use the metric method for handling location and tracking the movement of laparoscopic instrument. Position of the instrument's tip is determined by the triple of coordinates $< x, y, z >$. You'll notice, however, that people are moving quite smoothly in an environment without using any numbers (see the cursor movement using computer mouse). Humans instead of metric reference system use a topological arrangement.

To determine the position of the instrument, the human brain prefers relations to other objects (before, behind, beside, on the right, between, on the left) than calculations of coordinate values. We specify visually a distance or speed of the movement, thinking about it in terms of such concepts as: close, far, fast, slow. In order to efficiently navigate the laparoscopic instrument and avoid collisions, it is not important for surgeon to knew the exact value, expressed in numbers. His way of instrument navigation, bases on knowledge of the operating field topology.

In contrast to the human brain, the computer processing is optimized for numbers instead of symbols. Hence, simulators of minimally invasive surgery handle location by the help of computer calculation supported by sensors, resolvers, opto-mechanical and electronic systems. But it is evident that we are building simulators for the people not for computers. For surgeons, digital determination of the instrument position is not necessary for its correct navigation in the operating field. On the contrary, the presentation on the monitor the numbers determining these positions, met with strong opposition of trainees. They see the effects of their activity just watching the screen, and they amend the action, but they do not calculate any formulas.

3   Virtual Reality in Laparoscopic Surgery Simulations

In the context of the use of virtual reality software, for the simulation of laparoscopic procedures, two major sub-topics are crucial; image processing, and 3D graphics rendering engine coupled with real time physics simulation.

3.1   Image Processing for Instrument Position Identification

Image processing is a legacy of computer graphics [6,11] which allows as to forgo most of the complex mechatronic systems, sensor units and encoders. We eliminate these elements, that served for tracking the laparoscopic instruments movement realized by the trainee. To preserve the original functionality, we replace that hardware by a camera, and use the Open Source Computer Vision (*openCV*) library, in scope of real time object tracking. In this regard, we make the transformation similar to that which took place in the past, when the mechanical mice have been swapped with optical, and have been supported by image processing software.

Listing 1.1. Instrument position identification algorithm (using *openCV* library)

```
1. Convert a frame from RGB to HSV colorspace.
2. Filter HSV image between min/max threshold values and store
     filtered image to threshold matrix.
3. Perform morphological operations on thresholded image to
     eliminate noise and emphasize the filtered object(s)
   a) create structuring element that will be used to dilate
       and erode image,
   b) Erode twice with element chosen as a [3,3] pixels rectangle,
   c) Dilate is performed twice, with larger [8,8] element,
       so make sure object is nicely visible.
4. On the obtained in previous step (3) frame, perform object
     tracking function, which will return the x and y coordinates
     of the filtered object.
   a) find contours of filtered image using openCV findContours
       function.
   b) use moments method to calculate the x and y coordinates
       of the filtered object.
```

For the purposes of transfer the movement of laparoscopic instruments into the virtual reality world we will use the image obtained from the camera. Each frame taken from a camera we use to determine the current position of the instruments in simulator. Then, in virtual reality, we put the model of the instrument according to a determined position. Carrying out these operations with the frequency of the occurrence of image frames (30–50 fps), on the monitor screen we get a real-time projection of the instrument movement.

As a starting point, for the camera used in simulator, we make a software based correction of radial distortion, using the Brown-Conrady model. For this purpose we use a 2D monitor check chart, because the frame with perspective distortion, which creates a sense of a scene being deep or shallow, can not be use as it carries the 3D information, about the depth of objects in the scene. For this 2D monitor check chart we calculate radial distortion coefficients, taking into account a low order radial components (3–5). If their values are significant, we make image corrections. After such calibration we obtain a table of camera/frame transfer functions, which we apply to every frame.

For each corrected frame, using the ready-made procedures offered by the *openCV* library, we determine the positions of the tip of the laparoscopic instrument (Listing 1.1.). The second point, that allows us to calculate instrument position in the operating field, is the point where trocar is placed through the abdomen during laparoscopic surgery.

3.2   3D Graphics Rendering Engine and Real-Time Physics

As a result of using the graphics routines from *openCV* library we obtain data about the current position of laparoscopic instruments in the simulator. Next, we have apply it in virtual reality environment. *Ogre3D* graphic rendering engine helps us in this. Its main purpose is to provide a general solution for a scene-oriented, real-time *3D* graphics rendering.

There are two different categories of instruments. If it is a camera, showing the human abdomen cavity and organs which can be found beneath the surface of the patient skins, then we assign its position to a virtual camera, which observe the scene. In the case of the other laparoscopic instruments, information about their position, decide about placing the models of these instruments in the virtual operating field.

All models exported to *Ogre3D*, are performed by *Blender* graphics and animation software. *Ogre3D* integrates virtual instruments with data about the position of real instruments. It causes that instrument models move in virtual reality exactly as their counterparts in nature. Furthermore, *Ogre3D* arranges the scene, in the likeness of the human abdomen cavity. Provides a virtual trocar's entry points through abdominal tissues of the patient and performs lighting of the virtual operating field, coupled with the camera movement.

One of the main advantages of virtual reality is the possibility to use the virtual models of a human internal organs in the simulation of laparoscopic surgery. Such models, as well as models of instruments, are created in the *Blender* graphics and next we export such features as:

- *mesh*; shape object stored using tessellation grid (verts, normals, uv) as xml files,
- *material*; textures data enhanced with diffuse color, ambient intensity, emission parameters, multiple materials etc.,
- *skeleton*; it consist data of bones forming skeleton and their animation.

We model human organs as *soft body*, while *rigid body* is employed for modeling the laparoscopic instruments.

Models of instruments and organs are placed on the virtual scene, on which we lack only the physical interactions between them. For this reason, we use professional-grade library, *Bulllet Physic* engine, integrated with *Blender* and *Ogre3D*, which provides us:

- *rigid body* dynamics constraint solvers,
- continuous and discrete collision detection,
- *soft body* dynamics for deformable volumes,
- objects' updated world transform.

For each object we provide such parameters as; collision shape, mass (0 if static), physical material properties (frictional coefficient and coefficient of restitution) thereby creating *collision object*. At the end of the process of defining a physical dependencies, the *MotionState* properties of all objects are determine.

Listing 1.2. Dependiencies of cooperation betweem *Ogre3D* and *Bullet*

```
1.   Ogre3D, for ongoing frame, uses 30 Hz rendering frequency
          calls stepSimulation on dynamic Bullet's world.

2.   Bullet manages its physics objects and constraints,
          uses internal Bullet Physics, fixed time-step
          of 60 Hz

3.   Bullet, for ongoing frame, uses 30 Hz rendering frequency
          performs the update of all objects.

4.   Ogre3D uses dynamic Bullet's world to render
          with 30 Hz frequency.
```

4   Conclusion

In proposed solution, the mechatronic systems providing information about the instrument position in simulations of laparoscopic surgery, have been replaced with video channel. The obtained effects are, in addition to significant simplification of the system design, also lower implementation costs and greater operational reliability. In practice, compared with the other simulators that use virtual reality, the changes made are not noticeable from the user perspective. While working on the simulator, user does not feel any signals that might distinguish the work of mechatronic or video interface.

But we must remember that mechatronic structure is indispensable in order to achieve the effect of haptic feedback. However, in the proposed solution it can be much simpler, than it is in the case of currently occurring solutions. In proposed issue, mechatronic consists of actuators with a simple control software. Entire perception (data acquisition) for the realization of haptic feedback can be implemented using video channel. Moreover, haptic feedback effect can be supported by the dynamics calculations made in the graphics software. Calculating a movement of the objects, their collisions and associated with this deformation, *Bullet Physics* purvey the current value of forces, torques, speed or acceleration.

We realize that our proposals encumber the software for processing the data in video channel, increasing requirements for simulator computing efficiency. But there are two reasons convincing us that we can do that:

- big computational opportunities of contemporary graphic cards (multi-core, parallel computing, effective processing techniques of matrix or broad set of professional-grade libraries for image and 3D graphic processing).

- very high and tangible benefits of using an augmented reality. Use of a models for skill acquisition and refinement allows the trainee to work with tissue prior to doing so surgically in a human. However, the performance of surgical procedures on live animals has been prohibited in many countries. Furthermore, due to high financial costs, only a few have either ready lab or money necessary to use artificial models in regular training courses. Realization of a 3D model of the human organ requires a lot of work and it is not cheap. However, once made 3D graphic model can be shared by many centers all over the world. It has not been destroy during the exercises, and so it can be used repeatedly.

References

1. Basdogan, C., De, S., Kim, J., Muniyandi, M., Kim, H., Srinivasan, M.A.: Haptics in minimally invasive surgical simulation and training. IEEE Comput. Graph. Appl. **24**(2), 56–64 (2004)
2. Bell, A.K., Cao, C.G.: Effects of artificial force feedback in laparoscopic surgery training simulators. In: Proceedings of SMC, pp. 2239–2243 (2007)
3. Botden, S.M.B.I., Buzink, S.N., Schijven, M.P., Jakimowicz, J.J.: Augmented versus virtual reality laparoscopic simulation: what Is the difference? World J. Surg. **31**(4), 764–772 (2007). doi:10.1007/s00268-006-0724-y
4. Feng, C., Rozenblit, J.W., Hamilton A.J.: A hybrid view in a laparoscopic surgery training system. In: Proceedings of the 14th IEEE International Conference and Workshops on the Engineering of Computer Based Systems (ECBS 07), pp. 339–348 (2007)
5. Grantcharov, T.P., Kristiansen, V.B., Bendix, J., Bardram, L., Rosenberg, J., Funch-Jensen, P.: Randomized clinical trial of virtual reality simulation for laparoscopic skills training. Br. J. Surg. **91**(2), 146–150 (2004)
6. Klempous, R., Nikodem, J., Wytyczak-Partyka, A.: Application of simulation techniques in a virtual laparoscopic laboratory. In: Moreno-Díaz, R., Pichler, F., Quesada-Arencibia, A. (eds.) EUROCAST 2011, Part II. LNCS, vol. 6928, pp. 242–247. Springer, Heidelberg (2012)
7. Rozenblit, J.W.: Models and techniques for computer aided surgical training. In: Moreno-Díaz, R., Pichler, F., Quesada-Arencibia, A. (eds.) EUROCAST 2011, Part II. LNCS, vol. 6928, pp. 233–241. Springer, Heidelberg (2012)
8. Schreuder, H.W.R., van Dongen, K.W., Roeleveld, S.J., Schijven, M.P., Broeders, I.A.M.J.: Face and construct validity of virtual reality simulation of laparoscopic gynecologic surgery. Am. J. Obstet. Gynecol. **200**(5) (2009). doi:10.1016/j.ajog.2008.12.030
9. Seymour, N.E., Gallagher, A.G., Roman, S.A., OBrien, M.K., Bansal, V.K., Andersen, D.K., Satava, R.M.: Virtual reality training improves operating room performance: results of a randomized, double-blinded study. Ann. Surg. **236**(4), 458–464 (2002)
10. Thijssen, A.S., Schijven, M.P.: Contemporary virtual reality laparoscopy simulators: quicksand or solid grounds for assessing surgical trainees? Am. J. Surg. **199**(4), 529–541 (2010). doi:10.1016/j.amjsurg.2009.04.015
11. Zendejas, B., Brydges, R., Hamstra, S.J., Cook, D.A.: State of the evidence on simulation-based training for laparoscopic surgery: a systematic review. Ann. Surg. **257**(4), 586–593 (2013)

Differential Evolution Multi-objective Optimisation for Chemotherapy Treatment Planning

Ewa Szlachcic$^{(\boxtimes)}$ and Ryszard Klempous

Department of Control Systems and Mechatronics, Wroclaw University
of Technology, ul. Janiszewskiego 11/17, 51-570 Wroclaw, Poland
{ewa.szlachcic,ryszard.klempous}@pwr.edu.pl
http://www.weka.pwr.edu.pl

Abstract. Differential evolution is currently one of the most popular
population based stochastic meta-heuristics. In the paper, we propose
an extension of the Differential Evolution algorithm for multi-objective
optimization problem with constraints of chemotherapy scheduling for
a medical treatment. The differential evolution idea is used with some
significant improvements concerning the DE strategies and parameters
adaptation. The numerical results show that the proposed algorithm
is stable and robust in handling medical applications especially for a
chemotherapy planning process.

Keywords: Differential evolution meta-heuristics · Multi-objective
approach · Optimisation algorithm · Chemotherapy dose schedules

1 Introduction

The Differential Evolution approach is nowadays in great interests. The simplicity and the effectiveness in solving many multi-dimensional and multi-objective constrained optimization problems gives the great popularity to this approach [1,2,11,16,17]. The main idea is to construct, at each generation of the algorithm, a mutant vector for each element of the population. The gradient information could be available in this moment. The new mutant vector is constructed adding differences between randomly selected individuals to another individual. The proposed mutation operator allows a gradual exploration on the search space.

The quick convergence and robustness of differential evolution (DE) approach has turned to be one of the best evolutionary algorithms in many areas [4,6,15, 20,21]. In many papers [5,11,12,20] it has been stated that fixed values of DE control parameters is a poor idea. The limitations on DE structure had inspired many researchers to propose modifications to the original DE approach. With Differential Evolution being so popular and efficient algorithm, self-adaptation of key parameters in crossover and mutation operations has been investigated to make it even better and easier to use on various single- and multi-objective optimization problems [2,11,18,20].

© Springer International Publishing Switzerland 2015
R. Moreno-Díaz et al. (Eds.): EUROCAST 2015, LNCS 9520, pp. 471–478, 2015.
DOI: 10.1007/978-3-319-27340-2_59

Wide surveys of the research in the field of differential evolution were recently published [1,2,11,12,22]. Often current knowledge on differential evolution and its parameters values is based on empirical observations, not on a theoretical analysis. So in the DE field for chemotherapy treatment planning it is necessary to extract from numerical experiments some empirical rules on the algorithm behavior. In the paper we propose an extension of the Differential Evolution algorithm for multi-objective optimization problem with constraints of chemotherapy scheduling for a medical treatment planning.

2 Multi-objective Nature of Chemotherapy Process

A chemotherapy is a treatment of cancer using set of cytotoxic drugs to control and eradicate a cancer. The application of very toxic drugs reduces a tumor meanwhile leading to damage to the immune system and giving unacceptable effects to the patient. The drugs are administered to the body using schedules of multi-drugs and drug doses in time intervals. The drugs create a certain concentration in the bloodstream, which will systematically kill both cancerous and normal healthy cells [3,8,13]. The toxic drugs have great influence on a Patient Survival Time (PST) and it is very important to define very precisely the feasible set of constraints.

The aim of a chemotherapy treatment depends on maintaining the effective damage to the tumor burden while managing the toxic effects on the human body. Looking for the best schedule for drugs and drug doses in time intervals to be given with minimization of tumor burden and minimization of toxic side-effects determines the balance between killing cancer cells and limiting the damage of human body.

Mathematical model of tumour growth and reduction is based on most popular approach, taking under consideration the Gompertz growth model with a linear cell-loss effect [10,13]. The model takes the following form:

$$\frac{dn(x,t)}{dt} = \Lambda n(x,t)\, ln(\frac{\theta}{n(x,t)} - n_c(x,t), \tag{1}$$

where $n(x,t)$ represents the number of tumor cells in time t for a variables vector x. The vector $x = [x_{11}, x_{12}, ..., x_{ij}, ..., x_{ND}]$ is a template of drug doses for i defined as index of time interval, $i \in 1, ..., N$ and j is an index of j drug, for indexes $j \in 1, ..., D$. Each dose is a cocktail of D drugs characterized by a concentration level $c_1(x,t)$ of drug j at N switching periods of time in the bloodplasma. The variable x_{ij} determines a schedule of drug j at time interval t_i, the two coefficients define the tumor parameters, $n_c(x,t)$ describes a cell-kill effect of the multiple drugs on a cancer.

2.1 Constraints of an Chemotherapy Optimization Problem

The cancer chemotherapy treatment influences at a tumor site but also for the normal organs. We have to ensure that the human body tolerates anticancer drugs toxic side-effects. The drugs cause damage to sensitive tissues elsewhere in the body. So the toxicity constraints play the very important role in the cancer chemotherapy treatment and the constraint concerning the tumor size must be maintained below a lethal level.

The constraints of chemotherapy treatment process will be as follows:

1. The rate of drug j accumulation in urine is directly proportional to $c_{1j}(x,t)$ and must not exceed the fixed value C_{maxj} for each drug:

$$c_{1j}(x,t) \le C_{maxj} \ for \ i \in 1, ..., N \tag{2}$$

2. The White Blood Cells (WBC) count must be not less then a fixed down level W_D:

$$w_j(x,t_i) \ge W_D \ for \ i \in 1, ..., N \tag{3}$$

3. An additional constraint concerns the time $t_u(x, T_{max})$ over which the White Blood Cells count $w(x,t)$ remains below a fixed upper level W_u, to be less than time T_u:

$$t_u(x, T_{max}) \le T_u \ for \ i \in 1, ..., N \tag{4}$$

4. Maximum feasible size $n(x,t)$ of the tumor has not be greater then N_{max}:

$$n(x,t) \le N_{max}. \tag{5}$$

The set X of constraints of chemotherapeutic treatment process is represented by the relations (2)–(5). The chemotherapy schedule determines the dosages and drug combinations at each time interval throughout the whole treatment period.

2.2 Treatment Objectives in a Chemotherapy Optimization Problem

The first objective function, concerning the curative treatments attempt to eradicate the cancer tumor burden. The eradication means a reduction of the tumor from an initial size of around 10^9 cells to below 10^3 cells. The tumor burden, equal 10^9 is the minimum detectable tumour size [13]. The first objective function is to minimize the number of tumor cells $n(x,t)$ at a fixed period of time:

$$min_{x \in X} \ n(x,t) \tag{6}$$

The cells loss is proportional to the number of tumor cells and to the concentration $c_1(x,t)$ of toxic drugs. One commonly used performance measure of controlling treatment is toxic side-effect of anti-cancer drugs on human body, which is equivalent to maximizing a Patient Survival Time, defined by minimization of a concentration of toxic drugs in plasma in the form:

$$min \sum_{i \in 1,..,N} \sum_{j \in 1,..,D} c_{1j}(x_{ij}, t_i). \tag{7}$$

The two presented objectives on the set of constraints (2)–(5) character-ize the cancer chemotherapy treatment as a complex treatment process. These two objectives functions conflict with each other, due to the toxicity of used anti-cancer drugs. The specific chemotherapy treatment with different objectives defined on a complex set of constraints is an interesting and difficult domain for a multi-objective optimization approach.

3   Multi-objective Optimization with Differential Evolution Approach

Multi-objective optimization problem is to find a set of optimal vectors $x*$ opti-mizing a set of objective functions on the set X of all feasible solutions using Differential Evolution approach [5,7,9,12]. The minimum is taken in the sense of the standard Pareto order on an objective functions space. Thus, the idea of Pareto-dominance is used. A solution is said to be dominated, if another solu-tion exists in the search space with better performance on at least one objec-tive. At each step of the optimization process in a multi-objective differential evolution approach a set of solutions is constructed and we try to designate non-dominated points among evaluated dominated solutions. Differential Evo-lution (DE) for multi-objective (MO) optimization combines the MO algorithm NSGA-II [5,17,18] with the strength and simplicity of the differential evolution algorithm. DE is a new floating point encoded evolutionary algorithm for global optimization, owing to the special kind of differential operator which create new offspring from parents chromosomes instead of classical crossover and mutation. The unique in the DE approach is a reproduction procedure. The Differential Evolution algorithm aims evolving a population of NP $(N * D)$-dimensional individual vectors in the population t as below:

$$x^i(t) = [x^k_{11}, \ x^k_{12}, ..., x^k_{ND}] \ \ for \ k \in 1, ..., NP \tag{8}$$

In the initial population the ijth variable of the kth individual takes the following form:

$$x^k_{ij}(0) \ = \ L_{ij} \ + \ rand_{ij}(0, 1) \ (U_{ij} - L_{ij}) \tag{9}$$

where L_{ij} and U_{ij} determine the lower and upper bounds of variable ij and $rand_{ij}(0, 1)$ is a uniformly distributed random variable from the range [0,1].

3.1   Differential Mutation and Crossover Operators

New candidate solutions are created by combining the parent individuals and several other individuals of the same population. At each generation and for each individual DE employs mutation and crossover operations to produce a donor vector in the current population. There are many variants of offspring creation procedures. These strategies diversify by the way how to choose three vectors from the current population. The often applied mutation scheme uses a randomly selected vector $x^p(t)$. Only one weighted difference vector with the coefficient F is used to perturb the received mutant vector $v^i(t)$ in the form:

$$v^i(t) = x^p + F\left(x^r(t) - x^s(t)\right) \tag{10}$$

where p, r, $s \in [1, ..., NP]$. The difference between two randomly chosen vector makes the mutation operation self-adaptive according to the decreasing mutation step. The parameter F also influence on the mutation step and typically takes the value from the range [0,1]. The mutation scheme is referred as $DE/base/num/cross$, where DE stands for Differential Evolution idea, $base$ represents a string denoting the vector to be perturbed (usually a random or the best individual), num is the number of difference vectors considered for perturbation of base and cross stands for the type of crossover being used. The parameter base can be randomly selected or it is the best vector in the population with respect to fitness value. DE can use two kinds of crossover scheme: exponential or binomial to increase the potential diversity of the population. After the mutation phase the crossover operation, namely binomial or exponential, is used. The mutant vector with an individual x^i_j create the new vector $u^i_j(t)$ in the following form:

$$u^i_j(t) = v^i_j(t) \tag{11}$$

in the case, when

$$rand_j(0,1) \leq C_r \ or \ j = j_{rand} \tag{12}$$

where C_r defines the crossover probability. Otherwise the new vector: $u^i_j(t) = x^i_j(t)$. The crossover operator determines, which variable $x^i_j(t)$ or $v^i_j(t)$ will correspond to the trial vector $u^i_j(t)$.

We try to improve the strength Pareto differential evolution approach for multi-objective optimization algorithm for design and optimization of a chemotherapy treatment planning. The non-dominated optimal solutions are found using modified differential evolution algorithm for bi-criteria optimization problem with the help of standardization of constraints and constrained dominance operator. In discussed problem the range of values for modified parameters is very narrow for binomial crossover, but in the case of exponential crossover it is impossible to identify it.

In a cancer chemotherapy optimization problem given schedules of drugs doses can minimize a tumor size determining minimal toxic effects on human body. A schedule of medical treatment plan can be calculated based on a mathematical growth model described by a set of differential equations, when used in conjunction with an differential evolution approach. The drugs should be scheduled to ensure that the patients will tolerate its toxic side effects.

3.2   Chemotherapy Treatment Planning

The non-dominated optimal solutions are found with the help of proposed multi-objective differential evolution algorithm using differential mutation algorithm and differential crossover operator DE/rand/1/bin. The computer-based system,

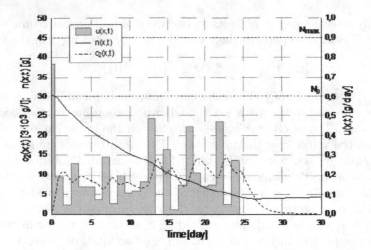

Fig. 1. The number of tumor cells n(x,t) and toxicity effects $c_2(x, t)$, based on optimal drug doses schedule u(x,t) on 25 days treatment period.

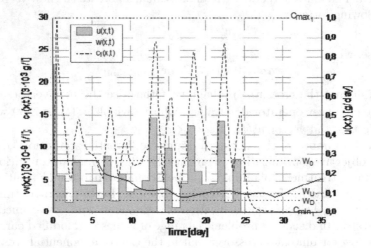

Fig. 2. The effective drug concentration $c_1(x, t)$ and the constraint White Blood Cells count $w(x, t)$ on optimal drug dose schedule during 25 days treatment interval.

which supports the physicians, allow an user to input treatment and patient parameters [19]. The system has to analyze very carefully a feasibility of constraints, because of the threat to life. For the problem of multi-objective chemotherapy optimization it is very difficult to determine the true Pareto front of nondominated solutions. The system contains a database of chemotherapy treatment for simulation and optimization of drug doses and schedules. The difficulties in fulfilling the constraints are observed during numerical tests. Sometimes it is more important to receive the feasible point, not Pareto-optimal to give the patient the quarantee of life. The parameters of the experimental treatment process concern the curative regime for 25 days of treatment with calculated drug doses. The Fig. 1 shows the first objective function $n(x, t)$ the reduction of the number of tumor cells during the time t_N described by optimal drug doses shown as $u(x, t)$. The second objective function $c_1(x, t)$, the constraint White Blood Cells count $w(x, t)$ and optimal dose schedule are shown on the Fig. 2 [14]. The drug concentration $c_1(x, t)$ is going to the minimal value on the end of treatment process, but in the time intervals with great drug doses the toxic drug concentration increases, but below the maximum allowed concentration value equal C_{min}. The WBC count remains controlled at level higher than a fixed down level W_D.

The most difficult constraint to be fulfilled concerns the time t_u, shown in the relation (4), which ensures the necessary protection from leukopenia. The time $t_u(x, T_{max})$ over which WBC count $w(x, t)$ remains below a fixed upper level W_u, has to be less than the time T_u. It is necessary to underline that the different simulation results we can obtain for different patients, according to their own properties. For some people the time T_u ought to be changed according the individual features of a patient and according to the upper level for time t_u.

4   Conclusion

The multi-objective optimization of chemotherapy treatment planning based on differential evolution approach demonstrates the high capabilities that can be effectively used especially for the complex set of constraints and objective functions, describing the cancer treatment procedure. In the process the user has the possibility to change input parameters in the search for a better optimization result. This search may be very time-consuming, depending on patient medical parameters, the experience of physicians and the complexity of the case. All numerical results show that the proposed algorithm is stable and robust in handling medical applications especially for a chemotherapy planning process.

References

1. Ali, M., Siarry, P., Pant, M.: An efficient differential evolution based algorithm for solving multi-objective optimization problems. Eur. J. Oper. Res. **217**(2), 404–416 (2012)
2. Amirian, H., Sahraeian, R.: Multi-objective evolution algorithm for the flow shop scheduling problem with a modified learning effect. IJE. Trans. C: Aspects **27**(9), 1395–1404 (2014)
3. Barbour, R., Corne, D., McCall, J.: Accelerated optimization of chemotherapy dose schedules using fitness inheritance. In: IEEE Congress on Evolutionary Computation (2010)
4. Beji, N., Jarboui, B., Siarry, P., Chabchoub, H.: A differential evolution algorithm to solve redundancy allocation problems. Int. Trans. Oper. Res. **19**, 809–824 (2012)

5. Cichon, A., Szlachcic, E.: Multi-objective differential evolution algorithm with self-adaptive learning process. In: Fodor, J., Klempous, R., Suárez Araujo, C.P. (eds.) Recent Advances in Intelligent Engineering Systems. SCI, pp. 131–150. Springer, Heidelberg (2010)
6. Das, S., Suganthan, P.N.: Differential evolution: a survey of the state-of-the-art. IEEE Trans. Evol. Comput. **15**(1), 4–31 (2009)
7. Ehrgott, M.: Multi-Criteria Optimization, 2nd edn. Springer Verlag, Berlin (2005)
8. Fdes-Olivares, J., Castillo, L., Czar, J.A., Prez, O.G.: Supporting clinical processes and decisions by hierarchical planning and scheduling. Comput. Intell. **27**(1) (2011)
9. Gong, W., Cai, Z.: A multi-objective differential evolution algorithm for constrained optimization. In: IEEE Congress on Evolutionary Computation, pp. 181–188. IEEE (2008)
10. Iliades, A., Barbalosi, D.: Optimizing drug regimes in cancer chemotherapy by an efficacy-toxicity mathematical model. Comput. Biomed. Res. **33**, 211–226 (2000). Academic Press, France
11. Wang, L., Qu, H., Chen, T.: An effective hybrid self-adapting differential evolution algorithm for the joint replenishment and location-inventory problem in a tree-level supply chain. Sci. World J. **2013**, 11 (2013). Article ID 270249
12. Neri, H., Tirronen, V.: Recent advances in differential evolution: a survey and experimental analysis. Artif. Intell. Rev. **33**(1–2), 61–106 (2010)
13. Petrovski, A., McCall, J., Sudha, B.: Multi-objective optmimization of cancer chemotherapy using swarm intelligence. School of Computing, The Robert Gordon University, AB25 3UE, UK
14. Porombka, P.: A meta-heuristic approach for the medical treatment planning, M.Sc. thesis, Wroclaw University of Technology, Wroclaw (2010)
15. Price, K.V., Storn, R.M., Lampinen, J.A.: Differential Evolution: A Practical Approach to Global Optimization. Springer, Heidelberg (2005)
16. Qian, W., Li, A.: Adaptive differential evolution algorithm for multi-objective optimization problems. Appl. Math. Comput. **201**(1–2), 431–440 (2008)
17. Robič, T., Filipič, B.: DEMO: differential evolution for multiobjective optimization. In: Coello Coello, C.A., Hernández Aguirre, A., Zitzler, E. (eds.) EMO 2005. LNCS, vol. 3410, pp. 520–533. Springer, Heidelberg (2005)
18. Santana-Quintero, L.V., Hernandez-Diaz, A.G., Molina, J., Coello-Coello, C.A., Caballero, R.: DEMORS: a hybrid multi-objective optimization algorithm using differential evolution and rough set theory for constrained problems. Comput. Oper. Res. **37**, 470–480 (2009). Elsevier
19. Szlachcic, E., Porombka, P.: Decision support system for cancer chemotherapy schedules. In: Moreno-Díaz, R., Pichler, F., Quesada-Arencibia, A. (eds.) EUROCAST. LNCS, vol. 8112, pp. 226–233. Springer, Heidelberg (2013)
20. Tang, L., Zhao, Y., Liu, J.: An improved differential evolution algorithm for practical dynamic scheduling in steelmaking-continuous casting production. IEEE Trans. Evol. Comput. **18**(2), 209–225 (2014)
21. Zaharie, D.: Influence of crossover on the behavior of differential evolution algorithms. Appl. Soft Comput. **9**(3), 1126–1138 (2009)
22. Zaharie, D.: Differential evolution: from theoretical analysis to practical insights (2012)

Automatic Selection of Video Frames
for Hyperemia Grading

L. Sánchez-Brea[1]([⊠]), N. Barreira-Rodríguez[1],
A. Mosquera-González[2], C. García-Resúa[3], and E. Yebra-Pimentel[3]

[1] VARPA Group, Department of Computer Science,
University of A Coruña, A Coruña, Spain
luisa.brea@udc.es
[2] Articial Vision Group, Department of Electronics and Computer Science,
University of Santiago de Compostela, Santiago de Compostela, Spain
[3] Optometry Group, Department of Applied Physics,
University of Santiago de Compostela, Santiago de Compostela, Spain

Abstract. Hyperemia, also called erythema or conjunctival injection,
is the occurrence of redness in the conjunctiva. It is produced by the
engorgement of conjunctival blood vessels, as blood accumulates and
gives the tissues a red coloration. Depending on factors such as how
strong the coloration is and where it is located, hyperemia serves as
an indicator of the presence of several pathologies; some examples are
allergical conjunctivitis, dry eye syndrome, or contact lenses complications. Hyperemia level is, therefore, a relevant parameter for diagnosis
in Optometry.

Keywords: Hyperemia grading · Image processing

1 Introduction

Hyperemia is the occurrence of redness in a certain tissue. When vessels engorge,
the accumulated blood causes this red coloration. Hyperemia can affect the conjunctiva, a thin transparent membrane which covers both the inner surface of the
eyelids (tarsal conjunctiva) and the sclera (bulbar conjunctiva) (Fig. 1). There
is also a joint between the two areas which is known as fornix conjunctiva. The
function of this membrane is helping the lubrication and the prevention of the
entrance of microbes into the eye.

There are various causes for the presence of conjunctival injection, some of
them related to pathologies such as different types of conjunctivitis, dry eye
syndrome, allergies, contact lenses complications, or glaucoma [5,7]. Therefore,
the level of hyperemia is a relevant parameter to diagnose these pathologies, and
also to measure their progression or their reaction to a certain treatment.

In order to grade the hyperemia level of a patient, optometrists first capture a video of the patient eye with a biomicroscope. It is common to capture
several videos from different angles of each eye, allowing the expert to examine

© Springer International Publishing Switzerland 2015
R. Moreno-Díaz et al. (Eds.): EUROCAST 2015, LNCS 9520, pp. 479–486, 2015.
DOI: 10.1007/978-3-319-27340-2_60

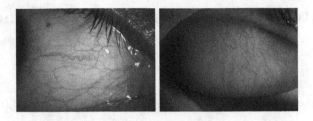

Fig. 1. Bulbar and tarsal conjunctiva.

the conjunctiva surface in detail. Once the videos have been recorded, specialists inspect each one of them, searching for the most suitable frame for grading. In order to do that, they take into account several features of the video. A good illumination is required, as well as a frame that comprises most of the conjunctival area and that shows clearly the conjunctival background. After the frame is selected, specialists measure the hyperemia level. For that purpose, there are several parameters that they take into account. Besides the sclera coloration, the number of vessels, their distribution, and their width [6].

Optometrists do not state the hyperemia level of a patient as a number, but as a value in a certain scale. There are several grading scales that had been developed with this purpose. Among them, CCLRU and Efron are two of the most well-known and widely used [1]. Scales are collections of images, photographies or pictures, that establish levels of severity. Specialists compare a patient image with the scale prototypes and assign a level depending on which image of the scale is the most similar. As it is shown in Fig. 2, different scales depict different areas of the conjunctiva, and take into account different features of the eye. This implies that, depending on the scale, the features the specialists analyze may vary.

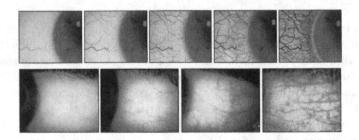

Fig. 2. From top to bottom: Efron grading scale and CCLRU grading scale for bulbar conjunctiva hyperemia.

The first step for hyperemia grading, this is, obtaining the best frame of the video sequence, is a time consuming and tedious process that has to be done manually. There are several works in the field of hyperemia grading, constructing new grading scales [8] or automatizing some steps of the process [4,11]. However, these works do not tackle the issue of automatically extracting a frame from a video sequence. In regard to this problem, we can find works in other fields that propose automatic methodologies for frame selection. Wolf [10] proposes an algorithm for identifying key frames in video sequences using the local minima of the motion. Erol and Kossentini [2] propose also a key frame detection algorithm, but using shape information instead of motion. Even though these approaches provide interesting solutions for the frame selection problem, they show a strongly domain dependence.

The present work proposes a method to perform the frame selection automatically, which will serve as a first step for the development of an automatic methodology for the hyperemia level calculation. This way, our system receives a video and automatically obtains the most suitable frame for hyperemia grading.

This work is focused on bulbar hyperemia grading. Our video database has a similar structure, starting with several black frames. The illumination progressively increases up to a peak, and then decreases again. In some videos, the last frames of the sequence are also black, due to the absence of illumination. Figure 3 depicts an example of the video illumination through time. This way, our approach is mainly based on lightness.

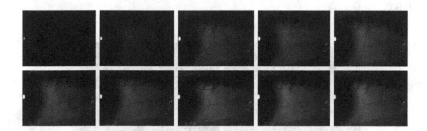

Fig. 3. Ten frames from a hyperemia video at different points of the video sequence. The illumination variability hinders the selection of a frame.

This work is structured as follows. Section 2 details the developed methodology. Section 3 explains the conducted experiments and results. Finally, Sect. 4 depicts our conclusions and future work.

2   Methodology

Our methodology receives a video of the patient's eye as input. Then, certain metrics are computed in each input frame in order to select the most suitable frame for further processing. Lightness, non-blurriness, or high contrast are some desirable features for the selected frame.

Taking into account the properties of the test set (Fig. 3), the first metric is focused on measuring the lightness of the image. To this end, we analyze lightness in several color spaces: luminance from RGB, V-channel from HSV, L-channel from HSL and L-channel from L*a*b*. In RGB, the luminance can be computed from the R, G, B channels using the following equations:

$$L_1 = 0.2126 * R + 0.7152 * G + 0.0722 * B \tag{1}$$

$$L_2 = 0.299 * R + 0.587 * G + 0.114 * B \tag{2}$$

$$L_3 = \sqrt{0.299 * R^2 + 0.587 * G^2 + 0.114 * B^2} \tag{3}$$

The lightness was calculated for each pixel in order to obtain the mean value for the complete image:

$$\bar{L}(i) = \frac{\sum L(x, y)}{NM} \tag{4}$$

where x, y, are the coordinates of the pixel in the frame i, L is the lightness measure, N is the width of the image, and M, its height. Since we look for the brightest frame, we select the frame with the highest lightness value:

$$F = \arg \max_i \bar{L}(i) \tag{5}$$

where i is a frame of the video. Figure 4 shows the best frames obtained for each color space.

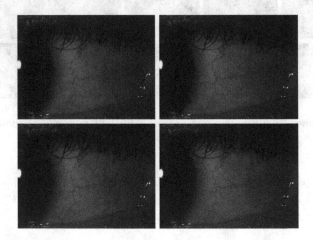

Fig. 4. Selected frames using different color spaces. From left to right and top to bottom: RGB, HSV, HSL and L*a*b* (Color figure online).

The results were accurate in most cases taking only into account lightness. However, some of the selected frames presented a recurring issue: the features of the image appeared blurry, making it hard to distinguish between a red hue on the conjunctiva and a healthy vessel. To solve this problem, we considered several blurriness metrics such as modified Laplace, normalized variance, and Tenenbaum gradient [9].

The modified Laplace computes the sum of the absolute values of the convolution of an image with Laplacian operators:

$$F_{SML} = \sum_M \sum_N |L_x(x,y)| + |L_y(x,y)| \tag{6}$$

where L_x and L_y are the Laplacian operators in each direction.

The normalized variance calculates variations in grey level among the image pixels. In order to do that, it uses the power function, so it will emphasize larger differences from the mean intensity μ. Differences in average intensities among several images are compensated by dividing the variance by μ:

$$F_{normVar} = \frac{1}{MN\mu} \sum_M \sum_N (I(x,y) - \mu)^2 \tag{7}$$

where I represents the intensity in each pixel and μ, the mean intensity.

Finally, Tenenbaum gradient uses the Sobel operator to compute the image sharpness function:

$$F_{Tenengrad} = \sum_M \sum_N S_x(x,y)^2 + S_y(x,y)^2 \tag{8}$$

where S_x and S_y are the Sobel derivatives in each direction.

We can observe in Fig. 5 how the use of this new information improves the result. In order to enhance the efficiency of the method, the blurriness is not computed for all the frames of the image, but for a set of frames with the highest lightness values. Also, there are some areas in the image that are not relevant, such as eyelashes and eyelids. In order to get rid of some of this elements, we applied a binary threshold. This computationally efficient operation restricts the blurriness measure to the conjunctiva and its surroundings.

3   Results

This methodology was tested with 50 videos captured in the Optometry Group from the University of Santiago de Compostela. The videos are about 20 s long,

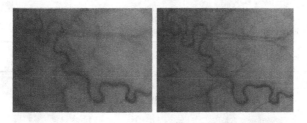

Fig. 5. Measuring the blurriness of the image. Left: best frame without applying blur measures. Right: best frame taking into account image blur.

and their frame rate is 7 fps. They were taken from both side views of the eye and both eyes.

Regarding the lightness measure, even though the results are quite similar, The L*a*b* colorspace was selected since it offers the closest representation to human vision [3].

About the blurriness calculation measure, the normalized variance method is faster (it takes barely 0.01 s to process a frame, more than 10 times faster than the other methods), but it presents problems in some images, such as the one depicted in Fig. 6. In view of the algorithms, this was expected, as statistic methods such as normalized variance measure the differences in intensity in the image. In our test set, those differences are too similar for blurry and sharp images, which worsens the results. On the contrary, Sobel and Laplace operators are focused on edge transitions, assuming that neighboring pixels in a blurry image will have less drastic changes in those edges. This causes that these methods provide good results in most of the images with a similar efficiency. The tests in this work were conducted using the Tenenbaum gradient algorithm.

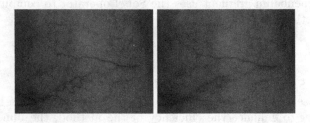

Fig. 6. Applying different blur measures. Left: best frame using Tenengrad algorithm. Right: best frame using normalized variance algorithm.

The results of the frame extraction procedure were validated by two specialists. The specialists watched the video and the best frame selected by the system. They had to decide if the selected frame was the best video frame and, otherwise, if it was still suitable for hyperemia grading. The results are depicted in Fig. 7. The column *Video issues* reflects those cases where the specialists reported problems with the video due to bad illumination or other circumstances. In these cases, the video was inadequate for grading.

Specialist	Best frames	Suitable frames	Non suitable frames	Video issues
E1	48	0	2	0
E2	43	4	0	3

Fig. 7. Results for the expert validation.

In view of the data, the system obtains the best frame in more than 90 % of the videos. Most of the discarded frames were also suitable for grading, though not the best ones of their video sequences. One of the specialists also discarded three of the videos because of poor illumination, as he could not find a good enough frame for grading. We can therefore conclude that the methodology provides good results and can be applied in diagnosis aid systems.

Regarding computational efficiency, videos were processed in 44.7 s on average in an Intel Core 2 Quad CPU (2.83 GHz) and 4 GB of RAM. The methodology was implemented in C++ and OpenCV library was used for the image processing operations.

4   Conclusions and Future Work

Hyperemia grading is a tedious and time-consuming work. Specialists need to invest a lot of time inspecting the videos in search of the frame most suitable for grading, which makes the grading process even longer. In this work, we propose a methodology to automatize the frame selection, which will serve as a first step to automatize the whole process of hyperemia grading. The methodology receives a video as input and selects the frame with the best illumination and the lowest blurriness. It can also return more candidates if the first one does not satisfy the specialist criteria. Results show that the method provides the best frame in most cases or, otherwise, it returns a frame suitable for grading. Besides, the results are objective and repeatable, and the computation time is low. Using this approach, we significantly reduce the time and effort invested for the specialists in the diagnosis. Furthermore, we achieve a repeatable and objective setup for the automatic hyperemia grading.

Nevertheless, there is other video features that could be analyzed in future refinements of the methodology. In some videos, we perceive a significant oscillation and the conjunctiva is not always in the center of the image. Although there is some margin and the eye does not get cut, it is a situation that may be useful to track. Moreover, the proposed methodology should be tested on videos acquired with different devices or different illumination conditions in order to prove its robustness.

References

1. Efron, N., Morgan, P.B., Katsara, S.S.: Validation of grading scales for contact lens complications. Ophthalmic Physiol. Opt. **21**(1), 17–29 (2001)
2. Erol, B., Kossentini, F.: Automatic key video object plane selection using the shape information in the mpeg-4 compressed domain. IEEE Trans. Multimedia **2**(2), 129–138 (2000)
3. Fairchild, M.D.: Color Appearance Models. Wiley, New York (2013)
4. Fieguth, P., Simpson, T.: Automated measurement of bulbar redness. Invest. Ophthalmol. Vis. Sci. **43**(2), 340–347 (2002)
5. Murphy, P.J., Lau, J.S.C., Sim, M.M.L., Woods, R.L.: How red is a white eye? Clinical grading of normal conjunctival hyperaemia. Eye **21**(5), 633–638 (2006)
6. Peterson, R.C., Wolffsohn, J.S.: Objective grading of the anterior eye. Optom. Vis. Sci. **86**(3), 273–278 (2009)

7. Rolando, M., Zierhut, M.: The ocular surface and tear film and their dysfunction in dry eye disease. Surv. Ophthalmol. **45**(Supplement 2(0)), S203–S210 (2001)

8. Schulze, M.M., Jones, D.A., Simpson, T.L.: The development of validated bulbar redness grading scales. Optom. Vis. Sci. **84**(10), 976–983 (2007)

9. Sun, Y., Duthaler, S., Nelson, B.J.: Autofocusing algorithm selection in computer microscopy. In: 2005 IEEE/RSJ International Conference on Intelligent Robots and Systems, (IROS 2005), pp. 70–76. IEEE (2005)

10. Wolf, W.: Key frame selection by motion analysis. In: 1996 IEEE International Conference on Acoustics, Speech, and Signal Processing, ICASSP 1996. Conference Proceedings, vol. 2, pp. 1228–1231, May 1996

11. Wolffsohn, J.S., Purslow, C.: Clinical monitoring of ocular physiology using digital image analysis. Contact Lens Anterior Eye **26**(1), 27–35 (2003)

A Texture-Based Method for Choroid Segmentation in Retinal EDI-OCT Images

Ana González-López[1], Beatriz Remeseiro[1]([⊠]), Marcos Ortega[1],
Manuel G. Penedo[1], and Pablo Charlón[2]

[1] Departamento de Computación, Universidade da Coruña, A Coruña, Spain
{ana.gonzalez,bremeseiro,mortega,mgpenedo}@udc.es
[2] Instituto Oftalmológico Victoria de Rojas, A Coruña, Spain
pcharlon@sgoc.es

Abstract. Retinal layers can be identified by ophthalmologists using OCT images, which is useful for the diagnosis of different diseases. Recent EDI-OCT technique allows to explore the choroid layer, whose segmentation has become one of the hottest topics in the field of retinal imaging. In this sense, and taking into account that the choroid layer has different visual properties than the other retinal layers, a methodology based on textural information is presented in this paper to segment the choroid. From a retinal EDI-OCT image, a region of interest is detected and its low-level features are extracted, generating a feature vector that describes it, to finally segment the choroid. This paper includes several texture analysis methods to calculate the feature vectors. Results provided by the proposed methodology showed that the approach is adequate for the problem at hand, since it allows to segment the choroid layer with promising results.

Keywords: EDI-OCT · Retinal images · Choroid layer · Texture analysis · Image segmentation

1 Introduction

Enhanced Depth Imaging Optical Coherence Tomography (EDI-OCT) images acquired from the retina are used by ophthalmologists to diagnose several diseases, since they provide useful information of the eye processes and allow to explore the choroid layer. The choroid is the vascular tissue located between the retina and the sclera, and provides oxygen and nourishment to the outer layers of the retina [1]. Changes in this layer are of critical importance in several retinal diseases, including glaucoma [2] and retinitis pigmentosa [3]. Thus, the automatic segmentation of this layer in retinal EDI-OCT images is important in order to understand the natural processes of the eye, and to facilitate an early diagnosis of eye diseases.

Different approaches have been studied to segment retinal layers, such as graph-based [4] and shortest path-based [5] techniques which provided promising

© Springer International Publishing Switzerland 2015
R. Moreno-Díaz et al. (Eds.): EUROCAST 2015, LNCS 9520, pp. 487–493, 2015.
DOI: 10.1007/978-3-319-27340-2_61

results. The use of active contours was proposed in [6,7], which also provide appropriate segmentation; and in [8], which additionally included a correction phase to eliminate possible mistakes that typically appear in presence of vessel shades or in case of altered layers. In this paper, a novel approach is proposed for choroid segmentation based on texture analysis, since previous research [9] demonstrated the adequacy of using textural properties to discriminate regions which belong to the choroid layer and regions do not.

This paper is organized as follows: Sect. 2 explains the methodology designed for the segmentation of the choroid, Sect. 3 presents the experimental results, and Sect. 4 includes the conclusions and future lines of research.

2   Research Methodology

A 3-step methodology has been designed to segment the choroid layer: (1) the input image is preprocessed and the region of interest is determined, (2) textural information is used to characterize the choroid, and (3) the choroid is segmented. Each stage is subsequently explained in depth.

2.1   ROI Extraction

In order to establish the region of interest (ROI), in which the further analysis will take place, upper boundary of choroid is segmented using the active contour-based process described in [8]. Once the ROI is located, borderline between choroid and sclera (see Fig. 1(a)) must be determined. To do that, sampled windows of $w \times h$ are obtained from the ROI and their texture descriptors are computed as following explained.

2.2   Texture-Based Characterization

Texture is used for choroid characterization by discriminating between regions which belong to the choroid from those which do not. Thus, texture descriptors are extracted from the ROI and then a process of classification is performed using marks provided by specialists. Several techniques for texture analysis could be applied and, in this study, five popular methods were tested in order to extend previous research [9]: Butterworth filters, Gabor filters and the discrete wavelet transform as signal processing methods; Markov random fields as a model based method; and co-occurrence features as an statistical method.

Butterworth Band-Pass Filters. [10] are frequency domain filters that have a flat response in the band-pass frequency, which gradually decays in the stopband.

A bank of 9 s order filters, designed to cover the whole frequency spectrum, is used in this research. By that means, the filter bank maps each input image into 9 filtered images, one per frequency band.

The results of each frequency are normalized, and then the uniform histograms of their output images are computed. The uniform histograms are obtained as follows: given all the filtered images of an specific frequency band, the limits of the histogram are defined so that each bin contains a maximum of $\frac{N}{N_{bins}}$ pixels, where N is the number of pixels in the corresponding frequency and N_{bins} the number of histogram bins.

Gabor Filters. [11] are complex exponential signal modulated by Gaussian functions widely used in texture analysis.

A bank of filters is created with 16 Gabor filters centered at 4 frequencies and 4 orientations. Thus, the filter bank maps each input image to 16 filtered images, one per frequency-orientation pair. Using the same idea as in Butterworth filters, the feature vector is created by generating the uniform histogram with non-equidistant bins.

Discrete Wavelet Transform. [12] generates a set of wavelets by scaling and translating a *mother wavelet* to create high-pass (H) or low-pass (L) filters.

The wavelet decomposition of an image consists in applying wavelets horizontally and vertically in order to generate 4 subimages at each scale (LL, LH, HL and HH), which are then subsampled by a factor of 2. After the decomposition of the input image, the process is repeated $n - 1$ times over the LL subimage, where n is the number of scales considered.

Some statistical measures are used to create the feature descriptor, which is composed of the mean and the absolute average deviation of the input and LL images, and the energy of the LH, HL and HH images. Note that in this study, the simplest nontrivial walevet Haar was used as mother wavelet.

Markov Random Fields. (MRF) [13] construct an image model whose parameters capture the essential perceived qualities of the texture. They generate a texture model by expressing the gray values of each pixel in an image as a function of the gray values in its neighborhood.

The concept of neighborhood is defined as the set of pixels within a distance d and, in this paper, the Chebyshev distance is considered. Additionally, the Markov process for textures is modeled using a Gaussian MRF, and the descriptor of an input image is composed of the directional variances [14].

Co-occurrence Features. [15] is a popular and effective texture descriptor based on the computation of the conditional joint probabilities of all pairwise combinations of gray levels, given an interpixel distance and an orientation.

Using the *Chebyshev* distance, the method generates a set of gray level co-occurrence matrices, and computes 14 statistical measures from their elements [15]. Finally, the mean and the range of these 14 statistics are calculated across matrices and a set of 28 features composes the texture descriptor.

2.3 Choroid Segmentation

In this stage, and taking into account the marks made by the experts, a classifier is used to discriminate between regions belonging to choroid from those corresponding to sclera. More specifically, a support vector machine (SVM) [16] is used to determine if they belong to choroid or not by using the textural information previously computed. Note that, in this step and for efficiency reasons, the image is sub-sampled and not all its windows are analyzed.

Next, the contour of the biggest area in the image corresponding to pixels classified as choroid is searched. In order to eliminate spurious pixels from further analysis, the morphological operator *closing* [10] is applied. Therefore, choroid is determined by upper boundary detected in Sect. 2.1 and the lower boundary of the detected contour, which is fitted to a curve in order to smooth the data.

3 Results

This method has been tested over a dataset of 63 two-dimensional EDI-OCT images of the retina extracted with a Spectralis OCT scanner, with an axial resolution of 5 μm. Windows extracted from the ROI have a size of 31 × 31 pixels according to previous experimentation [9]. Regarding the classification procedure, a SVM with radial basis kernel and automatic parameter estimation was trained [17], and a 10-fold cross validation [18] was performed. Different parameter configurations were considered to analyze the performance of the five textural descriptors considered, and so five experiments were carried out.

The first experiment was performed using a bank of 9 Butterworth filters, and 16-bin histograms. Table 1 shows the results obtained for each frequency band separately and, as can be seen, the results are quite stable since all the frequencies provide accuracies over 80 %. However, the lowest frequencies are the most discriminative ones with maximum accuracy over 87 %.

The second experiment was performed using Gabor filters, and different number of bins to create the uniform histograms. Table 2 depicts the results for the different histogram sizes considered. In this case, it should be highlighted the effectiveness of this method for the problem at hand, since it provides accuracies over 95 % regardless of the number of bins.

Table 1. Butterworth filters: SVM accuracy (%) for different frequency bands.

1	2	3	4	5	6	7	8	9
86.98	**87.59**	86.07	84.55	84.47	84.14	83.92	81.53	81.25

Table 2. Gabor filters: SVM accuracy (%) for different numbers of bins.

3	5	7	9	11
95.28	**95.81**	95.73	95.59	95.67

Table 3. Discrete wavelet transform: SVM accuracy (%) for different scales.

1	2	3	4
91.17	**94.50**	89.33	86.31

Table 4. Markov random fields: SVM accuracy (%) for different distances.

1	2	3	4	5	6	7
75.86	84.75	**86.76**	83.37	81.07	79.85	79.02

Table 5. Co-occurrence features: SVM accuracy (%) for different distances.

1	2	3	4	5	6	7
96.54	**96.88**	96.60	96.46	96.29	95.91	96.07

The third experiment was performed with the discrete wavelet transform and aimed at analyzing different number of scales. Table 3 illustrates the results and demonstrates the adequacy of using a lower number of scales. Concretely, the best result is obtained when using 2 scales, with an accuracy over 94 %.

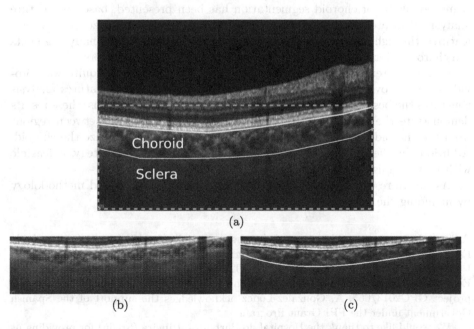

Fig. 1. Delimitation of the choroid: (a) a representative EDI-OCT image with the layers marked in yellow, and the extracted ROI squared with a red-dot line, (b) the pixels of the zoomed ROI classified as choroid (red) or not (green), and (c) the final choroid delimitation (Color figure online).

The fourth experiment was carried out using Markov random fields and aimed at comparing different neighborhoods. Table 4 presents the results for each distance individually and, as can be seen, the intermediate distances are more discriminative than the lowest and highest ones. Note that the best result surpasses the 86 % of percentage accuracy.

The fifth experiment was related to co-occurrence features, and its target is to analyze the impact of using different distances. Table 5 shows the results and, as well as Gabor filters, co-occurrence features technique is very appropriate for this problem since it provides accuracies over 95 % regardless of the distance considered. However, the best accuracy obtained in this case is over 96 % and so this method outperforms all previous results.

Regarding the choroid characterization, Fig. 1(a) depicts a representative sample EDI-OCT image, in which the choroid has been identified and its ROI extracted (see the red-dot line). Then, Fig. 1(b) shows the results of the classification performed over sample pixels in the zoomed ROI. Finally, Fig. 1(c) presents the layer segmentation obtained after applying the steps described in Sect. 2.3. As can be seen in these figures, this approach provides reliable results and so it is suitable for the choroid segmentation task.

4   Conclusions

A methodology for choroid segmentation has been presented, based on texture analysis. It locates the region of interest of an input image, analyzes its low-level features through different texture extraction techniques, and finally segments the choroid layer by means of a SVM and morphological operators.

In general terms, all the texture analysis methods perform quite well providing results over the 85 % in some cases, but co-occurrence features analysis generates the best results with maximum accuracy over 96 %. Thus, these results demonstrate the adequacy of texture analysis to discriminate between regions from the choroid and regions from other layers, i.e. to characterize the choroid. Additionally, the choroid segmentation, with the developed strategy, is feasible with very promising results.

As future research, the authors plan to improve the proposed methodology by including the information between frames in the sequence.

Acknowledgements. This research has been partially funded by the Secretaría de Estado de Investigación of the Spanish Government and FEDER funds of the European Union through the research project PI14/02161, and by the Consellería de Cultura, Educación e Ordenación Universitaria of the Xunta de Galicia through the research project GPC2013/065. A. González-López acknowledges the support of the Spanish Government under the FPI Grant Program.

We would like to thank the Hospital do Barbanza, Ribeira (Spain) for providing us with the image dataset.

References

1. Bill, A., Sperber, G., Ujiie, K.: Physiology of the choroidal vascular bed. Int. Ophthalmol. **6**(2), 101–107 (1983)
2. Yin, Z.Q., Vaegan, T.J., Millar, T.J., Beaumont, P., Sarks, S.: Widespread choroidal insufficiency in primary open-angle glaucoma. J. Glaucoma **6**(1), 23–32 (1997)
3. Dhoot, D.S., Huo, S., Yuan, A., Xu, D., Srivistava, S., Ehlers, J., Traboulsi, E., Kaiser, P.K.: Evaluation of choroidal thickness in retinitis pigmentosa using enhanced depth imaging optical coherence tomography. Br. J. Ophthalmol. **97**(1), 66–69 (2013)
4. Garvin, M.K., Abràmoff, M.D., Wu, X., Russell, S.R., Burns, T.L., Sonka, M.: Automated 3-D intraretinal layer segmentation of macular spectral-domain optical coherence tomography images. IEEE Trans. Med. Imaging **28**(9), 1436–1447 (2009)
5. Yang, Q., Reisman, C.A., Chan, K., Ramachandran, R., Raza, A., Hood, D.C.: Automated segmentation of outer retinal layers in macular oct images of patients with retinitis pigmentosa. Biomed. Opt. Express **2**(9), 2493–2503 (2011)
6. Yazdanpanah, A., Hamarneh, G., Smith, B., Sarunic, M.: Intra-retinal layer segmentation in optical coherence tomography using an active contour approach. In: Yang, G.-Z., Hawkes, D., Rueckert, D., Noble, A., Taylor, C. (eds.) MICCAI 2009, Part II. LNCS, vol. 5762, pp. 649–656. Springer, Heidelberg (2009)
7. Mishra, A., Wong, A., Bizheva, K., Clausi, D.A.: Intra-retinal layer segmentation in optical coherence tomography images. Opt. Express **17**(26), 23719–23728 (2009)
8. González-López, A., Ortega, M., Penedo, M.G., Charlón, P.: Automatic robust segmentation of retinal layers in oct images with refinement stages. In: Campilho, A., Kamel, M. (eds.) ICIAR 2014, Part II. LNCS, vol. 8815, pp. 337–346. Springer, Heidelberg (2014)
9. González, A., Remeseiro, B., Ortega, M., Penedo, M.G.: Choroid characterization in EDI OCT retinal images based on texture analysis. In: 7th International Conference on Agents and Artificial Intelligence (ICAART 2015), vol. 2, pp. 269–276 (2015)
10. Gonzalez, R., Woods, R.: Digital Image Processing. Pearson/Prentice Hall, Upper Saddle River (2008)
11. Gabor, D.: Theory of Communication. J. Inst. Electr. Eng. **93**, 429–457 (1946)
12. Mallat, S.G.: A theory for multiresolution signal decomposition: the wavelet representation. IEEE Trans. Pattern Anal. Mach. Intell. **11**, 674–693 (1989)
13. Besag, J.: Spatial interaction and the statistical analysis of lattice systems. J. Roy. Stat. Soc. Ser. B **36**, 192–236 (1974)
14. Çesmeli, E., Wang, D.: Texture segmentation using gaussian-markov random fields and neural oscillator networks. IEEE Trans. Neural Networks **12**(2), 394–404 (2001)
15. Haralick, R.M., Shanmugam, K., Dinstein, I.: Texture features for image classification. IEEE Trans. Syst. Man Cybern. **3**, 610–621 (1973)
16. Burges, C.: A tutorial on support vector machines for pattern recognition. Data Min. Knowl. Disc. **2**(2), 1–47 (1998)
17. Chang, C., Lin, C.: LIBSVM: a library for support vector machines. ACM Trans. Intell. Syst. Technol. **2**, 1–27 (2011)
18. Rodriguez, J., Perez, A., Lozano, J.: Sensitivity analysis of k-fold cross-validation in prediction error estimation. IEEE Trans. Pattern Anal. Mach. Intell. **32**, 569–575 (2010)

Analysis of Global and Local Intensity Distributions for the Segmentation of Computed Tomography Images

Miguel Alemán-Flores[1]([✉]), Patricia Alemán-Flores[2],
and Rafael Fuentes-Pavón[2]

[1] Departamento de Informática y Sistemas,
Universidad de Las Palmas de Gran Canaria, 35017 Las Palmas, Spain
maleman@dis.ulpgc.es
[2] Servicio de Radiodiagnóstico,
Hospital Universitario Insular de Gran Canaria, 35016 Las Palmas, Spain

Abstract. The segmentation of Computed Tomography images is an extremely challenging task due to the heterogeneities of the regions, their textured intensities, the presence of noise and the blurred edges which define the limits of the different areas. In this work, we propose a method for obtaining a segmentation of the abdominal region in Computed Tomography images based on the analysis of the global distribution of the intensity values in the whole data set and the local distribution within the neighborhood of each pixel. The global information is used to obtain an initial approximation, whereas the local data are analyzed to extract a much more accurate and complete segmentation. The combination of both scales allows obtaining a quite satisfactory segmentation in an automatic way.

1   Introduction

Computed Tomography (CT) is an imaging technique which processes X-rays in order to generate cross-sectional images (slices) of a part of the body or an object. These images are widely used for diagnostic purposes in numerous medical disciplines. The pixels corresponding to the different tissues and structures are shown according to their radiodensity on the Hounsfield scale (from -1024 to $+3071$ Hounsfield units).

Different approaches have been proposed to perform the segmentation of several types of images, from graph-based algorithms [1] to atlas-based systems [2] and region-growing schemes [3]. Active contours are one of the most commonly used approaches for the segmentation of textured regions and areas without clearly defined edges, using region descriptors or statistical information [4–6]. If we focus on medical images, texture descriptors and statistical information have been applied in [7].

In this work, we propose a method for obtaining a segmentation of the different tissues and organs of the abdominal region in Computed Tomography

© Springer International Publishing Switzerland 2015
R. Moreno-Díaz et al. (Eds.): EUROCAST 2015, LNCS 9520, pp. 494–501, 2015.
DOI: 10.1007/978-3-319-27340-2_62

images combining two types of information. On the one hand, the analysis of the global distribution of the intensity values in the whole data set provides an initial approximation of the regions in the image collection. On the other hand, the local distribution within the neighborhood of each pixel (or voxel) allows refining the segmentation and gradually discriminating the uncertain cases.

First, the images are filtered to reduce noise and homogenize the regions. The noise reduction stage is based on Perona-Malik filtering [8], a partial differential equation in which diffusion is not performed isotropically, but depending on the gradient, so that the boundaries of the regions are preserved while noise is diffused and reduced. Afterward, an initial classification of the most clearly defined regions is performed using the global analysis. It basically consists in extracting the most relevant values from the intensity histogram of the whole data set, but considering the filtered data and smoothing the results to eliminate the false maxima. Then, the uncertain pixels are associated to one of the labels (regions) according to their similarity and proximity to the already classified neighbors. This process is a modified statistical mode in which the scores in the voting scheme take into account how close two points are located and how similar their intensities are. Finally, a regularizing morphological filter is applied to obtain a smoother segmentation. Even if the regions are heterogeneous or the contours are not well defined, we are able to extract a segmentation of the different elements.

The rest of the paper is structured as follows: In Sect. 2, the anisotropic filter is explained. Section 3 describes the global analysis, whereas Sect. 4 explains the local one. Section 5 presents the morphological filter used to regularize the results. Finally, Sect. 6 includes some results and our main conclusions.

2   Anisotropic Filtering

This first stage aims to reduce irrelevant or spurious edges by decreasing the amount of noise, but preserving the important edges. Furthermore, we try to homogenize the textured regions to make them more suitable for an automatic segmentation. With this purpose, we apply a 3D adaptation of Perona-Malik filtering [8]:

$$u_t = div \left(k \left(\|\nabla u\| \right) \nabla u \right), \tag{1}$$

where we use:

$$k \left(x \right) = e^{-\beta x}. \tag{2}$$

Since we work with a series of uniformly spaced slices in the tomography, we can apply this filter in three dimensions, so that it also takes into account the neighbors in the previous and next images in the CT, i.e., the values at the same position in the neighboring images. However, the distance between two consecutive images is usually different to the distance between the pixels within a single image, and different weights must be assigned to the neighbors in the different coordinates. This way, we filter the 3D image as a whole, and not each slice separately.

Depending on the similarity of the various elements in the 3D image, their contrast and texture, the value of β in (2) can be adapted, as well as the number of iterations in the following discrete approach:

$$u_{i,j,k}^{n+1} = u_{i,j,k}^n + \frac{dt}{2\,(dh)^2} M\left(u_{i,j,k}^n\right), \tag{3}$$

where $M\left(u_{i,j,k}^n\right)$ is the result of convolving at each point (i, j, k) in the iteration n with the $3 \times 3 \times 3$ mask, whose coefficients are:

$$
\begin{aligned}
C_{i+a,j,k} &= k_{i+a,j,k} + k_{i,j,k} \\
C_{i,j+a,k} &= k_{i,j+a,k} + k_{i,j,k} \\
C_{i,j,k+a} &= k_{i,j,k+a} + k_{i,j,k} \\
C_{i,j,k} &= -k_{i+1,j,k} - k_{i-1,j,k} - k_{i,j+1,k} \\
&\quad -k_{i,j-1,k} - k_{i,j,k+1} - k_{i,j,k-1} - 6k_{i,j,k}
\end{aligned}
\tag{4}
$$

and $a \in \{-1, 1\}$. The values of $k_{i,j,k}$ are obtained from (2) as follows:

$$k_{i,j,k} = e^{-\beta \|\nabla u\|_{i,j,k}}. \tag{5}$$

An increase of β preserves more edges, but also noise. Therefore, its value must be adapted to the amount of noise present in the image and the relevance of the edges to be considered. Figure 1 shows the effects of this type of filtering in a slice of a tomography.

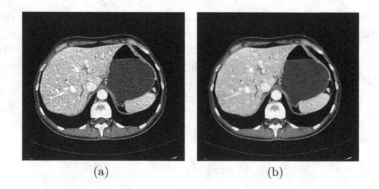

(a)   (b)

Fig. 1. Anisotropic filtering: (a) original image, (b) filtered image.

3   Global Segmentation

The Hounsfield scale is a quantitative scale for describing radiodensity. This scale defines a range of values to measure the density of the tissues and substances from -1024 to $+3071$ (we rescale these values into a range from 0 to 255). However, the regions are not completely uniform and homogeneous and each tissue has a range of values for its density in this scale, which means that the intensity of the pixels varies from one region to another within the same organ or tissue. Nevertheless, a reference value can be extracted from the images in the series in order to consider it as a class representative of the density values of the organ.

The second stage of our method focuses on determining the most significant intensities in the data set and grouping together those points where the radiodensity (intensity) is close to a certain class representative. By analyzing the intensity histogram, a series of concentration values which act as representatives of the regions, as well as their corresponding attraction ranges (intervals which converge toward those values) are extracted. In order to obtain the most suitable values, instead considering a single image, we calculate the combined histogram of the whole series, in such a way that the same representatives are used for all the images. Furthermore, the histogram is smoothed by averaging the values in the histogram with the neighbor bins so that small oscillations do not generate false maxima. From this smoothed histogram, we extract the maxima and a range around each one of them. Usually, four or five different intensity ranges are extracted.

As observed in Fig. 2, after having applied the anisotropic filter described in the previous section, the shape of the histogram is much more suitable for our purpose and, after smoothing it, the maxima are more clearly defined.

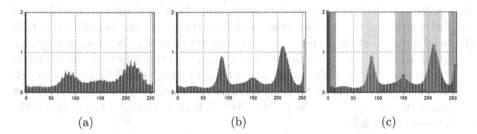

      (a)   (b)   (c)

Fig. 2. Extraction of the region representatives: (a) histogram of the initial series, (b) histogram after applying the anisotropic filter, and (c) smoothed histogram with the representatives and the ranges. The horizontal axis corresponds to the intensity while the vertical axis represents the percentage of pixels with each intensity value.

Since the ranges of intensities corresponding to different tissues may overlap, we use narrow ranges to label only the most reliable points. As illustrated in

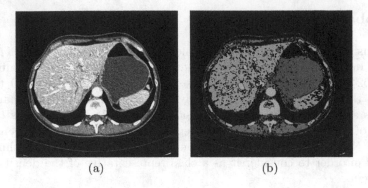

(a) (b)

Fig. 3. Initial segmentation: (a) original image, (b) labeling of the pixels within the different ranges.

Fig. 3, using these ranges, we classify the pixels and obtain an initial approximation. However, this initial classification of the points leads to some misclassified sections, and regions which are quite uncertain to be labeled. Therefore, a further process must be applied, as described in the next section.

4   Local Analysis

Using the intensity of a single pixel to determine to which region it belongs is frequently misleading. The textures, irregularities and noise present in this type of images cause the misclassification of several pixels. Therefore, it is imperative that the information of the neighborhood be used to improve this labeling process.

This third stage improves the initial approximation by using local statistics. A weighted mode is calculated for every pixel. This consists in an analysis of the distribution of the labels (classes to which the pixels are associated) within the neighborhood of each pixel, but weighting the contribution of each neighbor according to the distance to the reference pixel and the difference in intensity. The closer the pixels and the more similar their intensities, the higher the contribution of the corresponding label to calculate the local distribution. Thus, when analyzing the mode around the pixel p, its neighbor n adds the following weight to the score of its label:

$$w_n^p = e^{-k_1 s(p,n)} e^{-k_2 d(p,n)}, \tag{6}$$

where $s(p, n)$ is the distance between both pixels, $d(p, n)$ is the difference between their intensities, and k_1 and k_2 are balancing factors.

If the score of the weighted mode (label with the highest score) exceeds a given threshold, this is considered the most reliable value for the label of this point. If no label reaches the required score, the point is not labeled in this iteration, and left for a subsequent one. This results in a propagation scheme from the most reliable areas to the most uncertain ones. This method allows

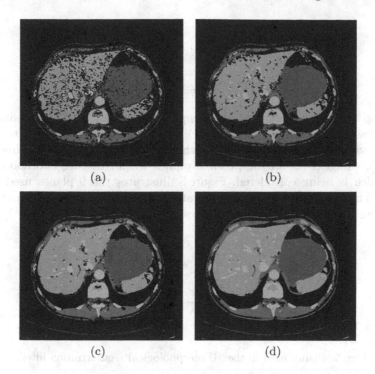

(a) (b)

(c) (d)

Fig. 4. Evolution of the segmentation when the weighted mode is applied: from (a) to (d), examples of several iterations in the labeling process using local information.

extracting an initial approximation for different structures, such as the bones, the liver, the spleen, the stomach or the vessels, as observed in Fig. 4, where the evolution of the regions is shown. As observed, the weighted local mode allows aggregating the uncertain pixels to the right regions and even correcting the misclassified ones.

5   Regularization

With the goal of smoothing the edges and filling the small holes remaining in the segmentation, thus avoiding an extremely irregular contour, we apply a regularizing morphological filter. This filter, based on the equivalent one described for two dimensions in [9,10], controls the curvature of the contour as follows:

$$\frac{\partial u}{\partial t} = g(I) \, \|\nabla u\| \left(div \left(\frac{\nabla u}{\|\nabla u\|} \right) \right). \tag{7}$$

In order to implement this kind of regularization, we consider the SI_d and IS_d operators:

$$(SI_du)(x) = \sup_{S \in B} \left(\inf_{y \in x+hS} u(y) \right)$$

$$(IS_du)(x) = \inf_{S \in B} \left(\sup_{y \in x+hS} u(y) \right)$$

(8)

where sup is the supremum or least upper bound and inf is the infimum or greatest lower bound (h is a scale factor). The base B is a set of 9 planes (since we work with a 3D image, we deal with 9 planes instead of the 4 lines used in [9,10]), which cover all the possible planes within the neighborhood of the point which is being considered. Figure 5 illustrates the 9 planes used in this process. The combination of both operators generates a smoother contour by performing erosion and dilation processes.

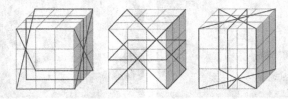

Fig. 5. Planes used in the 3D morphological regularization filter.

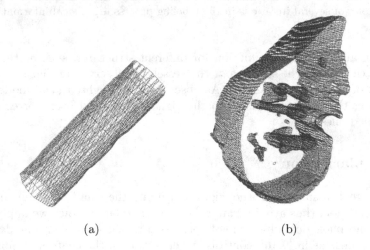

(a)   (b)

Fig. 6. Three-dimensional reconstruction of (a) a part of the aorta and (b) a section of the liver.

6   Results and Conclusion

After the regularization process described in the previous section, we can combine the set of voxels associated to a particular label (range of intensities) and extract a three-dimensional reconstruction of a section of an organ or a tissue. Figure 6 illustrates the reconstruction of a section of the aorta and a section of the liver, with the vessels which cross through it. As observed in this wire-frame model, the segmentation is satisfactory and useful to analyze the shape of the corresponding organ and detect possible abnormalities or pathologies that may appear.

The method which has been proposed is able to cope with the segmentation of this challenging type of images. The combination of two scales, the global ranges provided by the whole series of images and the detailed information obtained from the local neighborhood, allows segmenting the regions with no prior initialization of manual delimitation. In addition, the previous filtering process and the subsequent regularization improve the segmentation and generate more robust results.

References

1. Grady, L.: Random walks for image segmentation. IEEE Trans. Pattern Anal. Mach. Intell. **28**(11), 1768–1783 (2006)
2. Okada, T., Yokota, K., Hori, M., Nakamoto, M., Nakamura, H., Sato, Y.: Construction of hierarchical multi-organ statistical atlases and their application to multi-organ segmentation from CT images. In: Metaxas, D., Axel, L., Fichtinger, G., Székely, G. (eds.) MICCAI 2008, Part I. LNCS, vol. 5241, pp. 502–509. Springer, Heidelberg (2008)
3. Couprie, C., Grady, L.J., Najman, L., Talbot, H.: Anisotropic diffusion using power watersheds. In: Proceedings of the International Conference on Image Processing, ICIP 2010, 26–29 September, Hong Kong, China, pp. 4153–4156 (2010)
4. Chan, T.F., Sandberg, B.Y., Vese, L.A.: Active contours without edges for vector-valued images. J. Vis. Commun. Image Represent. **11**(2), 130–141 (2000)
5. Cremers, D., Tischhäuser, F., Weickert, J., Schnörr, C.: Diffusion snakes: introducing statistical shape knowledge into the mumford-shah functional. Int. J. Comput. Vis. **50**(3), 295–313 (2002)
6. Sagiv, C., Sochen, N.A., Zeevi, Y.Y.: Integrated active contours for texture segmentation. IEEE Trans. Image Process. **15**(6), 1633–1646 (2006)
7. Alemán-Flores, M., Álvarez-León, L., Caselles, V.: Texture-oriented anisotropic filtering and geodesic active contours in breast tumor ultrasound segmentation. J. Math. Imaging Div. **28**(1), 81–97 (2007)
8. Perona, P., Malik, J.: Scale-space and edge detection using anisotropic diffusion. IEEE Trans. Pattern Anal. Mach. Intell. **12**(7), 629–639 (1990)
9. Álvarez, L., Baumela, L., Márquez-Neila, P., Henríquez, P.: A real time morphological snakes algorithm. IPOL J. **2**, 1–7 (2012)
10. Álvarez, L., Baumela, L., Henríquez, P., Márquez-Neila, P.: Morphological snakes. In: The Twenty-Third IEEE Conference on Computer Vision and Pattern Recognition, CVPR 2010, San Francisco, CA, USA, 13–18 June 2010, pp. 2197–2202 (2010)

Complexity Analysis of HEVC Decoding for Multi-core Platforms

Paulo J. Cordeiro[1,2,3]([✉]), Pedro Assuncao[1,2], and Juan A. Gómez-Pulido[3]

[1] Instituto Politécnico de Leiria/ESTG, Leiria, Portugal
[2] Instituto de Telecomunicações, Leiria, Portugal
[3] Universidad de Extremadura, Cáceres, Spain
paulojorgecordeiro@gmail.com

Abstract. The High Efficiency Video Coding (HEVC) is the latest standard, providing the same quality as its predecessor H.264/AVC at about half of the bit-rate. An increasing demand for higher quality and better resolutions in mobile applications require the use of more efficient video codecs, but the high computational complexity of HEVC poses problems to resource-constrained devices and portable equipment with limited batery-life. Despite the fact that video coding complexity is much higher than decoding, in most user devices, video decoding is used more often than encoding, thus particular attention must also be given to HEVC decoders. This paper presents an experimental study and complexity analysis of the HEVC decoder's behaviour when decoding 4k ultra high definition (UHD) and HD video sequences on multi-core platforms, such as those of the most recent mobile devices. It is shown that when tile partitioning is used, different tiles have different decoding complexities. These findings are relevant for devising dynamic tile partitioning schemes capable of achieving load balancing in video decoders running on multi-core platforms.

Keywords: Video decoding · HEVC complexity · Video complexity-map

1 Introduction

Recent studies concluded that video data is becoming the major part in consumer internet traffic with a predicted share between 80 %–90 % by 2018 [1]. This is supported by mobile devices where increasing screen resolutions enable them to playback high definition (HD) video, which is usually streamed or downloaded over mobile networks. Besides, there are already broadcast services using 4 K ultra-high definition (UHD) video delivered over TV networks, reaching different types of usage environment, such as multiscreen, interactive, etc.

This fast evolution requires the use of more efficient video codecs that are able to deal with increased video resolutions, without too much computational complexity. The High Efficiency Video Coding Standard (HEVC) [2] is the most recent standard. It is able to reduce the bitrate by 50 % in comparison with

© Springer International Publishing Switzerland 2015
R. Moreno-Díaz et al. (Eds.): EUROCAST 2015, LNCS 9520, pp. 502–509, 2015.
DOI: 10.1007/978-3-319-27340-2_63

H.264/MPEG4-AVC (for the same quality), but its computational complexity can be more than 10 times greater [3].

In the development phase of HEVC it was taken into account that contemporary and future mobile architectures are parallel (multi- and many-core). As a consequence, built-in parallelism is now offered by the standard. By distributing the workload of HEVC decoder on multiple cores, the total decoding computational complexity can be reduced in order to potentially improve the overall energy efficiency, leading to increased battery-life in the mobile user devices. For high-level parallelism, HEVC currently supports different picture partition strategies such as entropy slices, wavefront parallel processing (WPP) and tiles to fulfil these requirements [4–6].

In this paper, the tile partitioning mechanism supported by HEVC is analyzed in regard to its decoding complexity for the purpose of load-balancing in multi-core platforms. A complexity model is devised and computed for each frame generating a decoding-complexity map, which demonstrates that load-balancing may benefit from dynamic tile partitioning. The paper is organized as follows. Section 2 presents a complexity model for HEVC decoding, based on computational complexity. Section 3 presents HEVC parallel tools with special emphasis on tile partitioning. Section 4 analyzes load-balancing of HEVC decoders based on a tile partitioning scheme using a dynamic frame-based complexity map to define the best tiles for encoding. Finally, Sect. 5 concludes the paper.

2   Complexity Model for HEVC Decoder

In order to identify the most time-consuming modules in the HEVC decoder, two different methods were used: the decoding time, measuring the execution time of each functional module with the help of the code profiler Intel Vtune Amplifier XE 2015; and Pixel Level Complexity (PLC), which is a complexity measurement method agreed by the experts in the AHG [9]. It consists in counting the number of pixels affected by each of the main functional modules during the decoding process. The main modules are Inter (Motion Compensation), Intra, Inverse Transform, Deblock Filter and SAO filter.

The profiling setup was composed by reference decoder HM 15.0 running on Intel i7-2400 2.4 GHz CPU with 24 GByte memory under the operating system of Microsoft Windows 7. All tests were conducted following common HEVC tests conditions and software reference configurations defined in [10]. The tests were performed for three types of coding configurations:

- All Intra: The main goal of intra coding in HEVC is to compress each frame on its own by finding the best predictions on a block-by-block basis using only information contained within the same frame;
- Random access: A configuration set for applications or services requiring relatively frequent (approximately 1 s) random access refreshes (representing such applications as broadcast video), This configuration emulates what may be used in a broadcasting environment;

– Low delay: This is intended for applications or services requiring low algorithmic delay (representing video usage for real-time communication with no
picture reordering between decoder processing and output). In this work only
low delay using B slices were used. This configuration is particularly suitable
for videoconferencing.

Test sequences with two different resolutions have been used: HD
(1920 × 1080 or 1080p) which is representative for current high definition systems, and 4k (UHD-1 or 3840 × 2160 or 2160p) which is representative for the
next generation of high quality video. For 1080p, the five class B sequences from
the JCT-VC test set have been used with frame rates of 24, 50 and 60 frames
per second (fps).

For 2160p120, two sequences from the Tampere University UHD-1 test set
have been selected, namely HoneyBee and Bosphorus. To get some insight about
the decoding complexity of different configurations, Table 1 presents the total
decoding time (sec.) measured for various sequences.

Table 1. Total decoding for ALL Intra (AI), Random Access (RA) and Low Delay B
(LB) using different QP, e.g., AI27 stands for All Intra with QP = 27.

Sequence	Time (s)					
	AI27	AI32	RA27	RA32	LB27	LB32
Kimono	35.1	32.3	22.3	21.1	23.1	19.4
ParkScene	51.1	43.2	22.7	21.1	24.1	19.7
Cactus	103.2	89.0	43.0	35.2	43.1	33.5
Basketball Drive	92.3	76.2	47.3	42.2	52.1	46.0
BQTerrace	145.2	119.1	55.3	38.7	57.6	48.2
Bosphorus	382.5	353.2	265.49	186.6	203.0	175.2
HoneyBee	345.0	310.1	248.7	268.2	198.2	155.2

Table 2 shows the decoding complexity obtained by using the two complexity
measurement methods described earlier. The first column presents the main
functional modules of HEVC decoder. Column PLC represents the number of
pixels processed by each of the corresponding modules. Since this method only
counts pixels for the five main functions shown in the Table, the class *Others* is
not used in this column. The next column to the right shows the percentage of
time spent in each functional module, followed by the respective time in seconds.
The fifth column shows the ratio time/pixel, i.e., the estimated time that takes
to process each pixel in each particular function. Finally *Normalized K* shows
five constants normalized to Intra Prediction Time/Pixel time. These constants
are utilized to calculate the complexity of each CU within a frame, that will be
used to generate a frame's complexity map.

Then, the average K for all sequences per functional module is calculated.
Table 3 shows the result of this average for each decoder's module.

Table 2. Results for sequence Kimono (1920 × 1080@24 Hz, QP27.

Modules	PLC	T(%)	T(s)	T/Pel(s)	Normalized K
Motion Compensation	458551808	51 %	11.37	2.48E−08	Kinter=1.45
Intra Prediction	39112192	3 %	0.67	1.71E−08	Kintra=1.00
Inverse Transform	120137328	5 %	1.12	9.28E−09	Ktransf=0.54
Deblocking Filter	75534608	14 %	3.12	4,13E−08	Kdeblock=2.42
SAO Filter	67434068	4 %	0.89	1,32E−08	Ksao=0.77
Others	−−	23 %	−−	−−	−−

The K values are then used to compute the total complexity of each CU on a frame-by-frame basis, according to Eqs. 1 and 2, where CU_c is the estimated complexity of a CU, $Pels(m)$ is the number of pixels processed by the functions of module m and $K(m)$ is the corresponding K value indicated in Table 3 for the module m.

Table 3. Average k value for each decoding functional module.

	INTER	INTRA	TRANSFORM	DEBLOCK	SAO
K	0.81	1	0.47	1.79	0.36

$$CU_c = \sum_{m \in M} Pels(m).K(m) \tag{1}$$

$$M = \{INTER, INTRA, TRANSFORM, DEBLOCK, SAO\} \tag{2}$$

Estimation of a complexity map is obtained for each frame by summing all CU_c of that frame as given by Eq. 3, where $Frame_c$ represents the sum of all CU_c starting from the beginning of the frame until reaching the maximum number (MAX) of CUs.

$$Frame_c = \sum_{i=1}^{i=MAX} (CU_c)_i \tag{3}$$

Using this model we can obtain the complexity map of each frame in a sequence, as is shown in Fig. 1 for a BasketballDrive sequence's frame. Section 4 presents an application scenario using this complexity map.

3   HEVC Tools for Parallel Processing

Parallelism support by video codecs is essential nowadays, since they require high computational effort as both the video resolution and complexity of coding/decoding algorithms are always increasing. Additionally, the dissemination

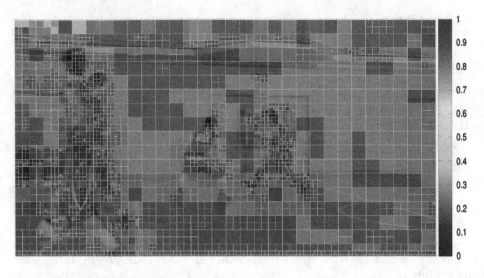

Fig. 1. Complexity map, where different CUs have different decoding complexity.

of parallel architectures on consumer multimedia device market encourages the development of solutions that exploit parallel processing. To correctly perform parallel processing HEVC has laid down three mechanisms pertaining to data partitioning and processing: Slices, Wavefront Parallel Processing (WPP) and Tiles. Encoder application context is the deciding factor that influences the choice of the best mechanism to use in each case. Slices are data structures that were already adopted by the previous H.264/AVC standard, and are also present in the HEVC standard. Its main objectives are resynchronization in the case of data loss and packetized transmission [11].

WPP of the Coding Tree Unit (CTU) is a straightforward approach to achieve parallelism for encoding and decoding, where slices are segmented into many rows of CTUs which then undergo processing in accordance with the algorithm shown in Fig. 2. The encoding of second CTU row begins only after completion of encoding of first 2 CTU in the first row. The encoding of third CTU row begins after completion of 2 first CTUs of second row and the process continues in this manner.

Tiles consist of rectangular partitions in a frame that are created by defining horizontal and vertical boundaries across a picture [5]. These boundaries must coincide with the Coding Tree Blocks (CTB) boundaries, as can be seen in Fig. 3. Tiles can be either uniform or non-uniform spaced. In uniform tiles, the number of CTBs are evenly distributed by the encoder inside the partitions, while in non-uniform tiles the number of CTBs per tile can be user-defined, despite the definition of multiple tile partitions per frame has a size restriction, where the minimum size defined is 256×64 samples per tile [12]. For instance, the maximum size of a CTB is considered (i.e., 64×64 samples), the minimum tile size is four CTBs wide per one CTB high [12].

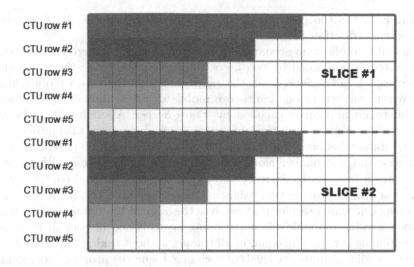

Fig. 2. Wavefront Parallel Processing encoding order.

This work is focused on the tiles mechanism. Next section presents a a scenario application where the frame complexity map is used in order to balance non-uniform tile partitioning according to decoding complexity.

4   Tile Partitioning for Load Balancing

As stated before, it is beneficial to employ the built-in parallelism offered by the HEVC standard, taking into account that current and future mobile architectures are parallel (multi- and many-core). Distributing the workload of HEVC decoder on multiple cores, can be done based on the proposed complexity map,

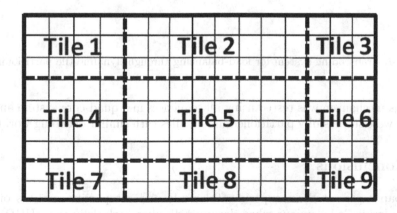

Fig. 3. A frame divided into 9 Tiles.

applying it to the tile partitioning of each frame, considering its unbalanced complexity distribution nature.

A possible application scenario is presented in Fig. 4, where the endpoints of the system is composed by two users, on the left hand side there is a video encoder, called *Video Server*. On the right hand side there is a mobile multi-core environment where one multi-core mobile device is intended to decode a video bitstream previously encoded by *Video Server*. Assuming that the first HEVC encoder used an agnostic configuration, which does not take into account the computational effort required to the decoder, there might be useful to insert some transcoding mechanism along the communication path, to modify the original bitstream in order to decrease the required computational complexity for decoding and/or to provide load balancing among several cores. Such transcoder could be a cloud-based service that receives the original bitstream, decode it and re-encode it using dynamic tile partitioning as explained in Sect. 3. In general tile partitioning is fixed and equal in all frames, without taking into account the different decoding complexity levels of each one. Using the proposed mechanism, a complexity map is generated when decoding the original bitstream and this information is passed to the HEVC encoder of the transcoder that will re-encode it by adapting the tile size according to its decoding complexity. In this manner the workload of each decoder core can be very similar, making it more suitable and power efficient when running in multi-core devices.

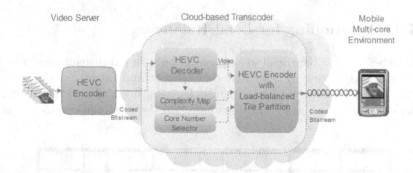

Fig. 4. Transcoding system for load-balancing through dynamic tile partitioning

This mechanism was tested using all sequences in a quad-core system and all frames were successfully partitioned in four tiles with similar decoding workload.

5   Conclusions

This paper presented an experimental study and complexity analysis of the HEVC decoder's behaviour when decoding 4k ultra high definition (UHD) and HD video sequences. It is proposed a mechanism to balance the workload of a multi-core system according to the decoding complexity of each frame. This mechanism makes use of the novel tile partitioning mechanism offered by HEVC and the complexity map calculated by our method. The results show that it is possible split a frame in tiles of different size but with similar decoding complexity. This is particularly useful to improve the decoder performance in multi-core platforms.

References

1. Cisco: Visual Networking Index (VNI) Forecast and Methodology, 2014–2019 (2014)
2. Bross, B., Han, W.J., Ohm, J.R., Sullivan, G.J., Wang, Y.K., Wiegand, T.: High Efficiency Video Coding (HEVC) text specification draft 10 (for FDIS & Last Call). In: document JCTVC-L1003 of JCT-VC, Geneve (2013)
3. Viitanen, M., Vanne, J., Hamalainen, T.D., Gabbouj, M., Lainema, J.: Complexity analysis of next-generation HEVC decoder. In: 2012 IEEE International Symposium on Circuits and Systems (ISCAS), pp. 882–885 (20–23 May 2012)
4. Henry, F., Pateux, S.: Wavefront parallel processing. Tech. rep. JCTVC-E196 (March 2011)
5. Fuldseth, A., Horowitz, M., Xu, S., Segall, A., Zhou, M.: Tiles in Proceedings of JCT-VC F335, 6th Meeting of Joint Collaborative Team on Video Coding (JCT-VC) of ITU-T SG16WP3 and ISO/IEC JTC1/SC29/WG11, Torino, Italy (2011)
6. Misra, K., Zhao, J., Segall, A.: Lightweight slicing for entropy coding. Tech. rep. JCTVC-D070 (January 2011)
7. JCT-VC: Subversion repository for the HEVC Test Model (HM) (2014). https:// hevc.hhi.fraunhofer.de/svn/svn_HEVCSoftware/tags/
8. Bossen, F.: Document of joint collaborative team on video coding. In: document JCTVC-G757 of JCT-VC, Geneve (2011)
9. Wien, M., Budagavi, M., Mishra, K., Ugur, K., Xiu, X.: JCT-VC AHG report: single-loop scalability (AHG16). Tech. rep. JCTVC-O0016, Geneva, CH, 15th meeting (2013)
10. Bossen F.: Common HM test conditions and software reference configurations (JCTVC-H1100), JCT-VC. 8th Meeting: San Jose, USA (2012)
11. Fuldseth, A., Horowitz, M., Shilin X., Misra, K., Segall, A., Minhua, Z.: Tiles for managing computational complexity of video encoding and decoding. Picture Coding Symposium (PCS) (2012)
12. Bross, B., Han, W.-J., Ohm, J.-R., Sullivan, G.J., Wang, Y.-K., Wiegand, T.: "High efficiency video coding (HEVC) text specification draft 10 (for FDIS & Last Call)", document JCTVC-L1003 of JCT-VC (2013)

Signals and Systems in Electronics

On the Sensitivity Degradation Caused by Short-Range Leakage in FMCW Radar Systems

Alexander Melzer[1](✉), Alexander Onic[2], and Mario Huemer[1]

[1] Institute of Signal Processing, Johannes Kepler University, Linz, Austria
Alexander.Melzer@jku.at
[2] DICE Danube Integrated Circuit Engineering GmbH & Co. KG, Linz, Austria

Abstract. Frequency modulated continuous wave (FMCW) radar systems suffer from permanent leakage due to their continuous operation. Especially in integrated circuits this leads to the well known issue of on-chip leakage due to limited isolation between transmit and receive circuitry. In addition, we investigate *short-range* (SR) leakage resulting from signal reflections of an unwanted close object located a few centimeters distant from the antennas. We carry out an in-depth analysis of the SR leakage and show that its residual phase noise in the intermediate frequency signal exceeds the total noise floor of the system, hence degrading the target detection sensitivity. We prove our analytical derivations with a complete FMCW radar system simulation.

1 Introduction

Automotive distance measurement and safety systems are typically realized with frequency modulated continuous wave (FMCW) radars. In contrast to pulse based systems, the FMCW principle uses a linear chirp sequence as transmit signal. The distance information is extracted by downconverting the reflected waves with the instantaneous transmit signal. For a single static object in the channel, this results in a sinusoid with constant frequency, which is termed *beat frequency*. It is proportional to the round-trip delay time (RTDT) of the radio waves and therewith also to the target distance.

The main advantage of the FMCW radar principle is that the instantaneous transmit power can be significantly reduced compared to pulse based systems. However, it suffers from permanent leakage of the transmit into the receive path. Especially in semiconductors this is an issue since isolation between transmitter and receiver circuitry is limited. The resulting *on-chip leakage* generates a beat frequency close to zero, which is why it is often also termed *DC-offset issue*. There is a vast literature on the leakage cancelation of such [1–4]. Several contributions analyze the impact of other non-idealities in FMCW radar systems, such as phase noise (PN) or the non-linearity of the chirp [6–8]. It is shown that these artifacts have a severe impact on the overall system performance.

Differently, in this work we consider a setup with a fixed target in front of the radar antennas, e.g. a fixture or cover, whose intermediate frequency (IF)

R. Moreno-Díaz et al. (Eds.): EUROCAST 2015, LNCS 9520, pp. 513–520, 2015.
DOI: 10.1007/978-3-319-27340-2_64

impact is unwanted and possibly interferes with the IF of other targets. We analyze the effects of the *short-range* (SR) leakage on the IF signal spectrum and show that the *decorrelated phase noise* (DPN) of the SR leakage exceeds the additive white Gaussian noise (AWGN) from the channel, hence the detection sensitivity is degraded significantly. Additionally, we point out the difficulties arising when seeking for an SR leakage cancelation concept. Finally, we carry out a full FMCW radar system simulation to evidence our analytical derivations.

The paper is structured as follows. In Sect. 2 the system model including the on-chip and SR leakage is introduced. Then an analytical analysis on the impact of the SR leakage is given in Sect. 3. Finally, in Sect. 4 the simulation results are presented.

2 System Model

The FMCW radar system model including the on-chip and SR leakage is depicted in Fig. 1. The PLL generates the chirp over a bandwidth B and duration T that is used as transmit signal defined as

$$s(t) = A \cos \left(2\pi f_0 t + \pi k t^2 + \varphi(t) + \Phi \right), \tag{1}$$

for $t \in [0, T]$. The peak amplitude is A and the chirp start frequency is f_0, $k = \frac{B}{T}$ is the sweep slope, $\varphi(t)$ is the instantaneous PN and Φ is a constant initial phase.

The channel comprises of the unwanted SR leakage as well as the targets that are to be detected. The SR leakage is modeled with an RTDT τ_S and a reflection factor A_S. Equivalently, targets are modeled with τ_{Tm} and A_{Tm} for $m = 1, \ldots, M$, where M is the number of targets in the channel. The channel noise $w(t)$ is modeled as white Gaussian noise and added to the receive signal prior to amplification by the low noise amplifier gain G_L. Lastly, the on-chip leakage is modeled with an isolation factor A_L and a delay τ_L. Note that due to the physical setup we have $\tau_L < \tau_S < \tau_{Tm}$.

The receive signal is a superposition of the on-chip leakage, the SR leakage, the target reflections and the channel noise, that is

$$r(t) = \underbrace{G_T A_L G_L \, s(t - \tau_L)}_{\text{On-chip leakage}} + \underbrace{G_T A_S G_L \, s(t - \tau_S)}_{\text{SR leakage}}$$

$$+ \underbrace{\sum_{m=1}^{M} G_T A_{Tm} G_L \, s(t - \tau_{Tm})}_{\text{Target reflections}} + G_L \, w(t), \tag{2}$$

where G_T is the transmission power amplifier gain. Since the reflected signal power decays steeply with the distance and the SR target is assumed to be only a few centimeters away from the radar antennas, A_S is in general significantly larger than A_L and A_{Tm}.

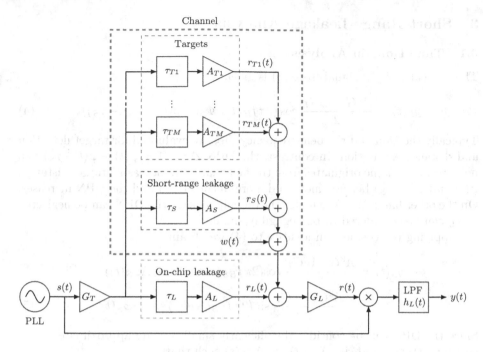

Fig. 1. System model with targets, on-chip leakage and SR leakage.

The receive signal is downconverted with the instantaneous transmit signal and lowpass filtered subsequently. Setting the initial phase $\Phi = 0$ for simplicity it is easy to show that the resulting IF signal is given as

$$
\begin{aligned}
y(t) &= [s(t)\, r(t)] * h_L(t) \\
&= \frac{A^2 G_T A_L G_L}{2} \cos\left(2\pi f_{BL} t + \Phi_L + \varphi(t) - \varphi(t - \tau_L)\right) \\
&\quad + \frac{A^2 G_T A_S G_L}{2} \cos\left(2\pi f_{BS} t + \Phi_S + \varphi(t) - \varphi(t - \tau_S)\right) \\
&\quad + \sum_{m=1}^{M} \frac{A^2 G_T A_{Tm} G_L}{2} \cos\left(2\pi f_{BTm} t + \Phi_{Tm} + \varphi(t) - \varphi(t - \tau_{Tm})\right) \\
&\quad + w_L(t),
\end{aligned}
\tag{3}
$$

where $h_L(t)$ is the impulse response of a lowpass filter that eliminates the image originating from the mixing process, $f_{BL} = k\tau_L$, $f_{BS} = k\tau_S$, $f_{BTm} = k\tau_{Tm}$ are the beat frequencies and $\Phi_L = 2\pi f_0 \tau_L - k\pi \tau_L^2$, $\Phi_S = 2\pi f_0 \tau_S - k\pi \tau_S^2$, $\Phi_{Tm} = 2\pi f_0 \tau_{Tm} - k\pi \tau_{Tm}^2$ are constant phase terms. The respective channel noise in the IF domain is described as $w_L(t) = [s(t)\, G_L\, w(t)] * h_L(t)$.

Building on the introduced system model, an analysis of the SR leakage in time and frequency domain is given in the next section.

3 Short-Range Leakage Analysis

3.1 Time-Domain Analysis

The SR leakage's IF signal from (3) is given as

$$y_S(t) = \frac{A^2 G_T A_S G_L}{2} \cos\left(2\pi f_{BS} t + \Phi_S + \varphi(t) - \varphi(t - \tau_S)\right). \tag{4}$$

Typically the gain and the beat frequency f_{BS} are evaluated for target detection and distance estimation. In contrast, the DPN $\Delta\varphi_S(t) = \varphi(t) - \varphi(t - \tau_S)$ is a noise term. Its name originates from the fact that with increasing target distance, $\varphi(t)$ and $\varphi(t - \tau_S)$ become more and more uncorrelated and the DPN increases. On the other hand, that is why for the on-chip leakage the DPN can be neglected as τ_L can be considered to be negligibly small.

Applying the cosine sum identity to (4) we obtain

$$y_S(t) = \frac{A^2 G_T A_S G_L}{2} \cos(2\pi f_{BS} t + \Phi_S) \cos(\Delta\varphi_S(t))$$
$$- \frac{A^2 G_T A_S G_L}{2} \sin(2\pi f_{BS} t + \Phi_S) \sin(\Delta\varphi_S(t)). \tag{5}$$

Since the DPN can be considered sufficiently small, we can approximate $\cos(\Delta\varphi_S(t)) \approx 1$ and $\sin(\Delta\varphi_S(t)) \approx \Delta\varphi_S(t)$ such that

$$y_S(t) \approx \underbrace{\frac{A^2 G_T A_S G_L}{2} \cos(2\pi f_{BS} t + \Phi_S)}_{y_{S1}(t)}$$
$$\underbrace{- \frac{A^2 G_T A_S G_L}{2} \sin(2\pi f_{BS} t + \Phi_S)\, \Delta\varphi_S(t)}_{y_{S2}(t)}. \tag{6}$$

The first summand $y_{S1}(t)$ in (6) is the actual beat frequency signal while the second summand $y_{S2}(t)$ is a noise term caused by the DPN $\Delta\varphi_S(t)$. These two summands are individually depicted in Fig. 2. Therein, the system parameters were chosen according to a typical automotive application scenario, that is a transmit power of 0 dBm, $G_T = 10$ dB, $A_S = -8$ dB, $\tau_S = 1$ ns and $G_L = 20$ dB. The PN is generated based on a typical PN power spectrum of a 77 GHz PLL. Note that in Fig. 2 the second summand is scaled for a better visibility of the DPN's effect. It can be observed that since the $\sin(\cdot)$ term is 90° phase shifted to the actual beat frequency signal, the second summand is largest at the zero-crossings and smallest for the peak amplitude of $y_{S1}(t)$.

3.2 Frequency-Domain Analysis

With the approximation from (6) the DPN term $\Delta\varphi_S(t)$ was extracted from the $\cos(\cdot)$ term. From the auto-correlation of the DPN, that is

$$c_{\Delta\varphi_S \Delta\varphi_S}(u) = \mathrm{E}\{\Delta\varphi_S(t)\Delta\varphi_S(t + u)\}, \tag{7}$$

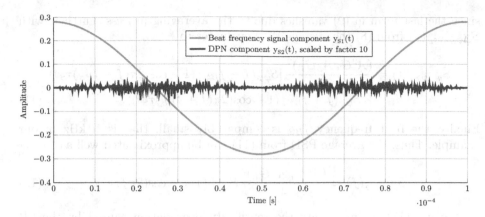

Fig. 2. Short-range leakage signal components in digital IF domain (approximation) over a single chirp for $\tau_S = 1\,\mathrm{ns}$ ($d_S \approx 15\,\mathrm{cm}$).

its power spectral density (PSD) can be computed with the *Wiener-Khintchine-Theorem* and is well known to be [5]

$$S_{\Delta\varphi_S\Delta\varphi_S}(f) = 2\,S_{\varphi\varphi}(f)\,(1 - \cos(2\pi f\tau_S)). \tag{8}$$

To determine the PSD of the overall error signal $y_{S2}(t)$ containing the DPN we compute its auto-correlation

$$
\begin{aligned}
r_{y_{S2}y_{S2}}(t,u) &= \mathrm{E}\left\{y_{S2}(t)\,y_{S2}(t+u)\right\} \\
&= \frac{(A^2 G_T A_S G_L)^2}{4}\mathrm{E}\left\{\Delta\varphi_S(t)\frac{1}{2j}\left(e^{j(2\pi f_{BS}t+\Phi_S)} - e^{-j(2\pi f_{BS}t+\Phi_S)}\right)\right. \\
&\qquad \left.\Delta\varphi_S(t+u)\frac{1}{2j}\left(e^{j(2\pi f_{BS}(t+u)+\Phi_S)} - e^{-j(2\pi f_{BS}(t+u)+\Phi_S)}\right)\right\} \\
&= \frac{(A^2 G_T A_S G_L)^2}{16j^2}\mathrm{E}\{\Delta\varphi_S(t)\,\Delta\varphi_S(t+u)\}\left[-\left(e^{j2\pi f_{BS}u} + e^{-j2\pi f_{BS}u}\right)\right. \\
&\qquad \left.+ \left(e^{j(2\pi f_{BS}(2t+u)+2\Phi_S)} + e^{-j(2\pi f_{BS}(2t+u)+2\Phi_S)}\right)\right] \\
&= \frac{(A^2 G_T A_S G_L)^2}{16j^2}c_{\Delta\varphi_S\Delta\varphi_S}(u)\left[-2\cos(2\pi f_{BS}u)\right. \\
&\qquad \left.+ 2\cos(2\pi f_{BS}(2t+u) + 2\Phi_S)\right]. \tag{9}
\end{aligned}
$$

From Fig. 3 and (9) it can be observed that $y_{S2}(t)$ is not a stationary process. Due to the chosen parameters for a chirp duration of $T = 100\,\mu\mathrm{s}$ the beat frequency signal of the SR leakage is evaluated over a single period in our example. The signal $y_{S2}(t)$ can be considered as one period of a cyclostationary process with the average auto-correlation as

$$\bar{r}_{y_{S2}y_{S2}}(u) = \frac{(A^2 G_T A_S G_L)^2}{8}c_{\Delta\varphi_S\Delta\varphi_S}(u)\cos(2\pi f_{BS}u), \tag{10}$$

since the last term in (9) vanishes due to the averaging process. Further, with $S_{\Delta\varphi_S\Delta\varphi_S}(f)$ from (8) the average PSD evaluates to

$$\bar{S}_{y_{S2}y_{S2}}(f) = \frac{(A^2 G_T A_S G_L)^2}{8} \left[S_{\varphi\varphi}(f - f_{BS}) \left(1 - \cos(2\pi(f - f_{BS})\tau_S)\right) \right.$$
$$\left. + S_{\varphi\varphi}(f + f_{BS}) \left(1 - \cos(2\pi(f + f_{BS})\tau_S)\right) \right]. \tag{11}$$

Finally, the beat frequency f_{BS} is comparably small, that is $10\,\mathrm{kHz}$ in our example. Thus, the average PSD from (11) can be approximated well as

$$\bar{S}_{y_{S2}y_{S2}}(f) \approx \frac{(A^2 G_T A_S G_L)^2}{4} S_{\varphi\varphi}(f) \left(1 - \cos(2\pi f \tau_S)\right). \tag{12}$$

We use (11) to investigate the sensitivity degradation caused by the SR leakage. For that, the same system parameters as in Sect. 3.1 are used. The resulting average PSD of $y_{S2}(t)$ is depicted in Fig. 3. It can be observed that the DPN's power contribution exceeds that of the AWGN from the channel for frequency offsets larger than $200\,\mathrm{kHz}$, which is the actual IF frequency range of interest. Consequently, the overall noise floor of the system is increased and the target detection sensitivity degraded.

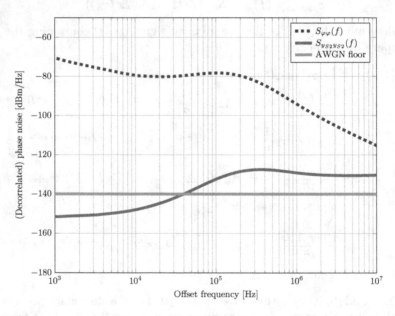

Fig. 3. Power spectral density of the PN and the DPN caused by the SR leakage for $d_S = 15\,\mathrm{cm}$. It exceeds the AWGN noise floor from the channel for frequency offsets larger than $50\,\mathrm{kHz}$, therewith degrading sensitivity of the FMCW radar.

4   Simulation Results

In this section we carry out a full FMCW radar system simulation based on Fig. 1 to evidence our analytical derivations. We consider a typical automotive radar application scenario where the bumper is a few centimeters distant from the radar antennas. The PLL has an output power of 0 dBm and ramps from 6 to 7 GHz, thus $B = 1$ GHz. Note that state of the art automotive radars operate at 77 GHz, however the reduced frequency is used solely for computational reasons and does not affect the results as the SR leakage is analyzed purely in the IF domain.

The on-chip leakage is assumed with an isolation of $A_L = -40$ dB and a delay $\tau_L = 10$ ps, while the SR leakage has a reflection factor of $A_S = -8$ dB and a delay of $\tau_S = 1$ ns (distance $d_S \approx 15$ cm). Further, a single target is considered within the channel at approximately 50 m distance. The transmission power amplifier and the LNA have a gain of $G_T = 10$ dB and $G_L = 20$ dB, respectively.

As derived analytically in Sect. 3, the SR leakage's DPN exceeds the channel noise floor at -140 dBm/Hz in the IF domain. Consequently the target at 3.3 MHz cannot be resolved in the presence of the SR leakage. Also, cancelation of the beat frequency signal only, that is $y_{S1}(t)$ in (6), does not improve the sensitivity as the high-frequent noise remains in the IF signal.

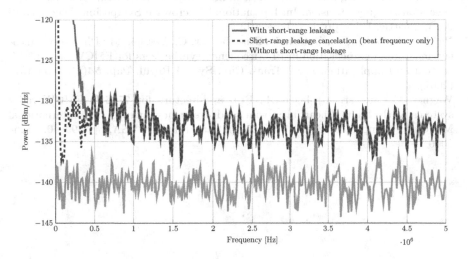

Fig. 4. Estimated power spectral density of the lowpass filtered IF signal. With the SR leakage the noise floor is increased and thus the target at 3.3 MHz is covered in noise.

Conclusion

In this work we investigated the sensitivity degradation caused by an SR leakage in an automotive FMCW radar transceiver. The decorrelated phase noise raises the total noise floor of the system and consequently limits the sensitivity of the radar. A full FMCW radar system simulation is employed to evidence the analytical derivations. For future work cancelation of the unwanted SR signal reflection is aspired, however, for that the instantaneous PN or DPN in the time-domain would need to be known.

References

1. Lin, K., Wang, Y.E., Pao, C.-K., Shih, Y.-C.: A Ka-Band FMCW radar front-end with adaptive leakage cancellation. IEEE Trans. Microwave Theor. Tech. **54**(12), 4041–4048 (2006)
2. Lin, K., Wang, Y.: Transmitter noise cancellation in monostatic FMCW radar. In: The IEEE/MTT-S International Microwave Symposium Digest, vol. 2006, pp. 1406–1409 (2006)
3. Lee, J., et al.: A UHF mobile RFID reader IC with self-leakage canceller. In: Proceedings of the Radio Frequency Integrated Circuits Symposium (RFIC 2007), Honolulu, pp. 273–276, June 2007
4. Stove, A.G.: Linear FMCW radar techniques. In: The IEE Proceedings F, Radar and Signal Processing, vol. 139, no. 5, pp. 343–350, October 1992
5. Budge, M.C., Jr., Burt, M.P.: Range correlation effects in radars. In: Record of the 1993 IEEE National Radar Conference, Lynnfield, USA, pp. 212–216 (1993)
6. Thurn, K., Ebelt, R., Vossiek, M.: Noise in homodyne FMCW radar systems and its effects on ranging precision. In: International Microwave Symposium Digest (IMS 2013), Seattle, USA, pp. 1–3, June 2013
7. Pichler, M., Stelzer, A., Gulden, P., Seisenberger, C., Vossiek, M.: Phase-error measurement and compensation in PLL frequency synthesizers for FMCW sensors – I: context and application. IEEE Trans. Circ. Syst. I Regul. Pap. **54**(5), 1006–1017 (2007)
8. Wagner, C., Stelzer, A., Jäger, H.: PLL architecture for 77-GHz FMCW radar systems with highly-linear ultra-wideband frequency sweeps. In: International Microwave Symposium Digest (IMS 2006), San Francisco, USA, pp. 399–402, June 2006

Parameter Optimization for Step-Adaptive Approximate Least Squares

M. Lunglmayr$^{(\boxtimes)}$ and M. Huemer

Institute of Signal Processing, Johannes Kepler University Linz, Linz, Austria
Michael.Lunglmayr@jku.at

Abstract. We discuss possible approaches for the adaption of the step width of Step-Adaptive Approximate Least Squares. We present and compare two low complexity and practically feasible adaptation functions whose parameters have been optimized based on computer simulations. We show that by applying these approaches the performance deviation of Step-Adaptive Approximate Least Squares lies within the single percentage range compared to the optimal least squares solution.

Keywords: Estimation · Least squares · Approximate least squares · Implementation

1 Introduction

The linear least squares (LS) estimation approach is an important concept in electrical engineering, especially in digital signal processing. Example applications range from localization [1] and positioning [2], over robotics [3], power and battery applications [4], biomedical applications [5], as well as image processing [6].

For LS estimation we assume the following system model:

$$\mathbf{y} = \mathbf{H}\mathbf{x} + \mathbf{n} \tag{1}$$

where $\mathbf{y}$ is a measured vector, $\mathbf{H}$ is a known system matrix of dimension $m \times p$, $\mathbf{n}$ is a noise vector and $\mathbf{x}$ is the parameter vector that we want to estimate.

The linear least squares solution to this estimation problem is well known as

$$\hat{\mathbf{x}}_{LS} = \mathbf{H}^\dagger \mathbf{y}. \tag{2}$$

with the pseudoinverse $\mathbf{H}^\dagger = (\mathbf{H}^T\mathbf{H})^{-1}\mathbf{H}^T$. Such a direct calculation of the solution as is often called *batch solution* in literature [7].

For many realtime applications a low complexity implementation is preferred over an exact solution. For this reason the calculation of the batch solution is usually avoided for such applications, due to its computational complexity and its large memory requirements. To provide a low complexity approximate approach for the LS estimation problem we developed a method that we call *Approximate*

© Springer International Publishing Switzerland 2015
R. Moreno-Díaz et al. (Eds.): EUROCAST 2015, LNCS 9520, pp. 521–528, 2015.
DOI: 10.1007/978-3-319-27340-2_65

Least Squares (ALS) [8]. It can be seen as a variant of the Kaczmarz algorithm [9] for overdetermined and inconsistent linear equation systems.

ALS is based on the iterative least squares (ILS) approach that iteratively calculates

$$\hat{\mathbf{x}}^{(k)} = \hat{\mathbf{x}}^{(k-1)} - \mu \mathbf{d}(\hat{\mathbf{x}}^{(k-1)}). \tag{3}$$

Here $\mathbf{h}_i^T$ is the ith row of $\mathbf{H}$. The function

$$\mathbf{d}(\mathbf{x}^{(k-1)}) = \sum_{i=1}^{m} 2\mathbf{h}_i(\mathbf{h}_i^T \hat{\mathbf{x}}^{(k-1)} - y_i) \tag{4}$$

is the gradient of the least squares cost function

$$J(\hat{\mathbf{x}}) = \sum_{i=1}^{m} (y_i - \mathbf{h}_i^T \hat{\mathbf{x}})^2 \tag{5}$$

that has its minimum at $\hat{\mathbf{x}}_{LS}$. It can be shown that for $k \to \infty$, $\hat{\mathbf{x}}^{(k)}$ converges to $\hat{\mathbf{x}}_{LS}$ given that the iteration step width μ fulfills $0 < \mu < 1/(2s_1^2(\mathbf{H}))$ [12], with $s_1(\mathbf{H})$ as the largest singular value of $\mathbf{H}$. Figure 1 schematically shows one iteration of ILS. The gradient $\mathbf{d}(\mathbf{x}^{(k-1)})$ can be seen as a sum of partial gradients

$$d_i(\hat{\mathbf{x}}^{(k-1)}) = 2\mathbf{h}_i(\mathbf{h}_i^T \hat{\mathbf{x}}^{(k-1)} - y_i). \tag{6}$$

2   Approximate Least Squares

To reduce the complexity of this approach we proposed to use only one of these partial gradients per iteration, leading to the ALS iteration:

$$\hat{\mathbf{x}}^{(k)} = \hat{\mathbf{x}}^{(k-1)} + 2\mu \mathbf{h}_{k\urcorner}(y_{k\urcorner} - \mathbf{h}_{k\urcorner}^T \hat{\mathbf{x}}^{(k-1)}). \tag{7}$$

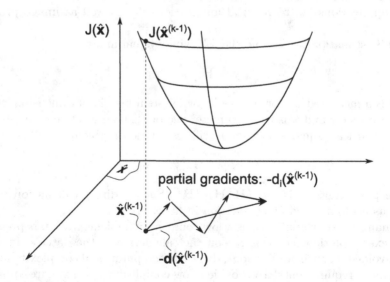

Fig. 1. Schematical drawing of the gradient and partial gradients.

In the above equation the operator " $\urcorner$ " is defined as: $k^\urcorner = ((k-1) \bmod m) + 1$ for a positive natural number k. For better readability we don't write the dependence of this operator on m in the operator's symbol. For ALS m is always the number of rows of the matrix $\mathbf{H}$. Using this operator naturally allows to have more iterations than the number of rows of $\mathbf{H}$, which is typically required for ALS to obtain a good performance.

As we described in [8], the error $\mathbf{e}^{(k)} = \hat{\mathbf{x}}^{(k)} - \mathbf{x}$ of the above iteration can be split into two parts

$$\mathbf{e}^{(k)} = \mathbf{e}_0^{(k)} + \mathbf{e}_\Delta^{(k)}, \tag{8}$$

with $\mathbf{e}_0^{(k)}$ as the error depending on the initial value $\hat{\mathbf{x}}^{(0)}$ of the algorithm before the first iteration, and $\mathbf{e}_\Delta^{(k)}$ as the error depending on the noise vector $\mathbf{n}$. As we showed in [8], the error $\mathbf{e}_0^{(k)}$ goes to zero as the number of iterations goes to infinity, while the noise dependent error $\mathbf{e}_\Delta^{(k)}$ persists even if $k \to \infty$. Due to the cyclic re-use of the rows of $\mathbf{H}$ as well as the measurement values in $\mathbf{y}$, the errors $\mathbf{e}^{(k)}$ converge to m different values for $k \to \infty$:

$$\mathbf{e}^{(mk+i)} = \mathbf{e}_\Delta^{(mk+i)} = \mathbf{e}_{\Delta_\infty}^{(i)} \text{ for } i = 1, \ldots, m \tag{9}$$

In Fig. 2 we plotted a typical case of the error norm of $\hat{\mathbf{x}}^{(k)}$ for an example 100×10 matrix $\mathbf{H}$ over the iterations k as well as the error norm of the algorithm's output $\hat{\mathbf{x}}_{ALS}$, as described below. For better visibility, the error norm of $\hat{\mathbf{x}}_{ALS}$ has been depicted has a horizontal line, although it is available only at the end of the algorithm. When analyzing the norm of the error $\mathbf{e}^{(k)}$ over the iterations, one can see an oscillatory behavior. This comes from the fact that for large k the ALS algorithm produces approximately the same m recurring error vectors (up to the vanishing deviation $\mathbf{e}_0^{(k)}$). To reduce the final error norm of the vector output by the ALS algorithm, we introduced an averaging step in the final m iterations of the algorithm.

The basic ALS algorithm is summarized in the following pseudocode (Algorithm: ALS).

Algorithm: ALS

$\hat{\mathbf{x}}_{ALS} = \mathbf{0}$
$\hat{\mathbf{x}}^{(0)} = \mathbf{0}$
for $k = 1, \ldots, N$ **do**
    $\hat{\mathbf{x}}^{(k)} = \hat{\mathbf{x}}^{(k-1)} + \mu 2 \mathbf{h}_{k^\urcorner}(y_{k^\urcorner} - \mathbf{h}_{k^\urcorner}^T \hat{\mathbf{x}}^{(k-1)})$
    if $k > N - m$ **then**
        $\hat{\mathbf{x}}_{ALS} = \hat{\mathbf{x}}_{ALS} + \hat{\mathbf{x}}^{(k)}$
    end if
end for
$\hat{\mathbf{x}}_{ALS} = \frac{1}{m} \hat{\mathbf{x}}_{ALS}$

Here N denotes the number of iterations of the algorithm and $\hat{\mathbf{x}}_{ALS}$ is the approximation of $\hat{\mathbf{x}}_{LS}$ that is output by the algorithm. $\mathbf{0}$ denotes the zero vector.

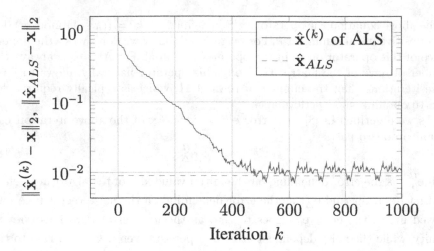

Fig. 2. ALS error norms.

As one can see from the algorithm's description the averaging only has to be done *once*, it therefore presents only a minor complexity increase (overall only pm additions and p multiplications with the constant $1/m$ have to be performed additionally).

As one can see in the above algorithm, if k reaches m, then for the following iterations the first rows of $\mathbf{H}$ and the first elements of $\mathbf{y}$ are re-used again in a cyclic manner. This approach has the advantage, that compared to ILS, about m times less multiplications per iteration are required.

But ALS also has the drawback – as we show in [8] and as discussed above – that for a constant step width μ, a persistent oscillating error $\mathbf{e}^{(k)} = \hat{\mathbf{x}}^{(k)} - \mathbf{x}_{LS}$ exists, even if $k \to \infty$. This error depends on the noise as well as on the parameter μ of the algorithm. While a large value of μ leads to a fast decrease of the error $\mathbf{e}_0^{(k)}$ at early iterations it leads to a higher error $\mathbf{e}_\Delta^{(k)}$ and thus to a high final error. Choosing small values leads to small final errors but requires a large number of iterations because the error $\mathbf{e}_0^{(k)}$ is decreasing more slowly. Supporting these findings, in [10] it has been shown that the ALS iteration converges to the LS solution, if $\mu \to 0$ and $k \to \infty$. However, for a practical application of the algorithm, one is interested in a reduction method providing a fast convergence close to $\mathbf{x}_{LS}$.

For this reason we proposed to adjust the step width μ of the algorithm during the iterations. We call this approach Step-Adaptive Approximate Least Squares (SALS) [11].

3   Step-Adaptive Approximate Least Squares (SALS)

In [11] we proposed to adjust the step width $\mu = \mu_k$ at every iteration. For this we divide the overall ALS iteration process into two phases, the *reduction phase* and the *oscillation phase*. In the reduction phase the error norm $\|\mathbf{e}^{(k)}\|_2$ decreases while in the oscillation phase the error norm is approximately cyclically repeating as described above. In Fig. 2 the reduction phase lasts the first 500 iterations. During the reduction phase, the error part $\mathbf{e}_0^{(k)}$ (due to the initial value $\mathbf{x}^{(0)}$) contributes most to $\mathbf{e}^{(k)}$ in (8), thus a high value of μ_k should be used to decrease the overall error. In the oscillation phase, the error $\mathbf{e}_\Delta^{(k)}$ contributes most to $\mathbf{e}^{(k)}$. Here a high value of μ would prevent a further decrease of the error, thus a low value of μ_k is beneficial in this phase. For the reduction phase we propose, to use

$$\mu_k = \frac{1}{2\|\mathbf{h}_{k\urcorner}^T\|_2^2}. \tag{10}$$

As one can show [11], this is the largest value of μ for which $\mathbf{e}_0^{(k)} \to \mathbf{0}$ as $k \to \infty$. To detect whether or not the algorithm is already in the oscillation phase we used the following method. The oscillation phase is characterized by the occurrence of approximately the same error vectors, every m iterations. When inspecting (7) one can see that the error vector is only influenced by the term $(y_{k\urcorner} - \mathbf{h}_{k\urcorner}^T\hat{\mathbf{x}}^{(k-1)})$. By comparing this value with the value m iterations before one can detect the oscillation phase if the difference is below a predefined threshold. After the oscillation phase is detected, the idea for SALS is to reduce

---

Algorithm: SALS

$\hat{\mathbf{x}}_{SALS} \leftarrow \mathbf{0}$
$\hat{\mathbf{x}}^{(0)} \leftarrow \mathbf{0}$
$v_k \leftarrow 0$
$v_{k-m} \leftarrow 1$
DontReduceMu $\leftarrow$ True
for $k = 1 \ldots N$ **do**
    $v_k \leftarrow y_{k\urcorner} - \mathbf{h}_{k\urcorner}^T\hat{\mathbf{x}}^{(k-1)}$
    if DontReduceMu **then**
        $\mu \leftarrow \mu_{k\urcorner}$ according to (10)
        if $k^\urcorner = 1$ **then**
            if $|v_k - v_{k-m}| < v_{th}$ **then**
                DontReduceMu $\leftarrow$ False
                $\mu \leftarrow \dfrac{1}{2\max\limits_{i=1\ldots m}\|\mathbf{h}_i^T\|_2^2}$
            end if
            $v_{k-m} \leftarrow v_k$
        end if
    else
        $\mu \leftarrow f(\mu)$
    end if
    $\hat{\mathbf{x}}^{(k)} \leftarrow \hat{\mathbf{x}}^{(k-1)} + \mu 2\mathbf{h}_{k\urcorner}v_k$
    if $k > N - m$ **then**
        $\hat{\mathbf{x}}_{SALS} \leftarrow \hat{\mathbf{x}}_{SALS} + \hat{\mathbf{x}}^{(k)}$
    end if
end for
$\hat{\mathbf{x}}_{SALS} \leftarrow \frac{1}{m}\hat{\mathbf{x}}_{SALS}$

---

the step width μ to as well reduce the final error of the ALS solution. The overall SALS algorithm is presented in the following pseudocode (Algorithm: SALS). The function $f(\mu)$ is used to reduce μ once the oscillation phase is detected. The first reduction is done by setting μ to the minimum of the m values used in the iterations before. In every following iteration μ is furthermore reduced via a reduction function $f(\mu)$. In the following section we present and compare two low complexity variants of $f(\mu)$.

4   Simulation Results

The aim of Approximate Least Squares is to provide a low complexity approximate solution of the linear least squares problem. For this reason we restrict ourselves to reduction functions causing only a negligible complexity overhead compared to the basic ALS algorithm. We specifically compare the two reduction functions

$$\mu_k = \mu_{k-1} - s = f_1(\mu_{k-1}) \tag{11}$$

as well as

$$\mu_k = (1 - 2^{-c})\mu_k = f_2(\mu_{k-1}), \tag{12}$$

with a positive fractional s and a positive integer c. For (11) only one subtraction per iteration is required, while for (12) only one shift operation and a subtraction is required per iteration. Figure 3 shows simulation results for random $\mathbf{H}$ matrices for ALS and SALS using these reduction functions, respectively. The entries of these matrices have been sampled from a uniform distribution out of $[0,1]$. Every simulation has been done for white Gaussian noise with zero mean and standard deviation $\sigma \in S = \{10^{-4}, 10^{-3}, 10^{-2}, 10^{-1}, 1\}$, respectively. In the SALS algorithms v_{th} was set to 10^{-6}.

For (11), we used $s = \mu_i/(N-i)$, with i as the iteration when the oscillation phase was detected and μ_i as the corresponding step width, respectively. For (12), c was set to $\lfloor log_2(N) \rfloor$. These values of s and c have been found and optimized by extensive simulations, respectively.

The figure shows the relative error of ALS and SALS, respectively, compared to the optimum least squares solution. It shows the maximum relative increase of the error norms of ALS and SALS, respectively, over the averaged error norms of LS. The maximization has been done over the elements of S: $r_{ALS} = \max\limits_{S}\left(\frac{||\hat{\mathbf{x}}_{ALS}-\mathbf{x}||_2}{||\hat{\mathbf{x}}_{LS}-\mathbf{x}||_2} - 1\right)$ and $r_{SALS} = \max\limits_{S}\left(\frac{||\hat{\mathbf{x}}_{SALS}-\mathbf{x}||_2}{||\hat{\mathbf{x}}_{LS}-\mathbf{x}||_2} - 1\right)$, respectively. As one can see from these results, SALS performs significantly better than the basic ALS algorithm. Its deviation to the least squares error norm is within the single percentage range. For large $\mathbf{H}$ matrices f_1 performs significantly better than f_2. For the simulated matrices with 1000 rows, the average error norm deviation r_{SALS} was below 2%. For a practical application, especially when thinking of an implementation in fixed point precision, such an error deviation is typically considered negligible.

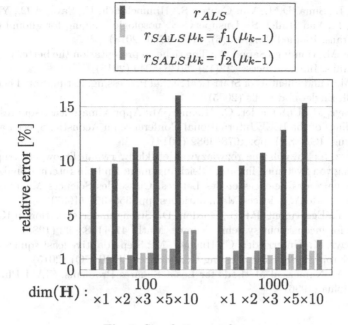

Fig. 3. Simulation results.

5 Conclusion

We present and compare different low complexity approaches for reducing the step width of Step-Adaptive Approximate Least Squares. We show that with Step-Adaptive Approximate Least Squares an error norm performance can be achieved that is within the single percentage range compared to the optimal least squares error performance. For many applications such an error norm can be considered practically equivalent to the optimum least squares solution that is obtainable only with a much higher computational effort.

References

1. Choi, K.H., Ra, W.-S., Park, S.-Y., Park, J.B.: Robust least squares approach to passive target localization using ultrasonic receiver array. IEEE Trans. Ind. Electron. **61**(4), 1993–2002 (2014)
2. Thomas, R.R., Maharaj, B.T., Zayen, B., Knopp, R.: Multiband time-of-arrival positioning technique using an ultra-high-frequency bandwidth availability model for cognitive radio. IET Radar Sonar Navig. **7**(5), 544–552 (2013)
3. Gautier, M., Janot, A., Vandanjon, P.-O.: A new closed-loop output error method for parameter identification of robot dynamics. IEEE Trans. Control Syst. Technol. **21**(2), 428–444 (2013)
4. Unterrieder, C., Zhang, C., Lunglmayr, M., Priewasser, R., Marsili, S., Huemer, M.: Battery state-of-charge estimation using approximate least squares. J. Power Sources **278**, 274–286 (2015)

5. Yuqian, L., Sima, D.M., Van Cauter, S., Himmelreich, U., Sava, A.C., Yiming, P., Yipeng, L., Van Huffel, S.: Unsupervised nosologic imaging for glioma diagnosis. IEEE Trans. Biomed. Eng. **60**(6), 1760–1763 (2013)
6. Rouhani, M., Domingo Sappa, A.: The richer representation the better registration. IEEE Trans. Image Process. **22**(12), 5036–5049 (2013)
7. Kay, S.M.: Fundamentals of Statistical Signal Processing: Estimation Theory. Prentice Hall, Englewood Cliffs (2005)
8. Lunglmayr, M., Unterrieder, C., Huemer, M.: Approximate least squares. In: 2014 Proceedings of the IEEE International Conference on Acoustic, Speech and Signal Processing (ICASSP), pp. 4678–4682 (2014)
9. Kaczmarz, S.: Przyblizone rozwiazywanie ukladw rwnan liniowych. Angenäherte Auflösung von Systemen linearer Gleichungen. In: Bulletin International de lAcadmie Polonaise des Sciences et des Lettres. Classe des Sciences Mathmatiques et Naturelles, Srie A, Sciences Mathmatiques, pp. 355–357 (1937)
10. Censor, Y., Eggermont, P.P.B., Gordon, D.: Strong underrelaxation in Kaczmarz's method for inconsistent systems. Numer. Math. **41**(1), 83–92 (1983)
11. Lunglmayr, M., Unterrieder, C., Huemer, M.: Step-adaptive least squares. Submitted to European Signal Processing Conference (EUSIPCO) (2015)
12. Björck, A.: Numerical Methods for Least Squares Problems. SIAM Philadelphia, Philadelphia (1996)

Extrinsic LLR Computation by the SISO LMMSE Detector: Four Different Approaches

Werner Haselmayr[(⊠)] and Andreas Springer

Institute for Communications Engineering and RF-Systems,
Johannes Kepler University Linz, Linz, Austria
{werner.haselmayr,andreas.springer}@jku.at

Abstract. In this paper we present four different approaches for the computation of the *extrinsic* information by a soft-input soft-output LMMSE detector used in a turbo equalization system. Moreover, we show the equivalence of the four approaches. All methods apply a Gaussian approximation, but at different stages, e.g. Gaussian approximation on the LMMSE filter output. Each approach offers different strategies for reducing the computational complexity, where the factor graph approach is the most promising solution.

Keywords: Extrinsic information · Factor graph · Gaussian message passing · LLR · SISO LMMSE detector · Turbo equalization

1 Introduction

Turbo equalization is an important receiver concept for coded communication systems, achieving impressive performance gains [1]. It consists of a soft-input soft-output (SISO) decoder and a SISO detector, which iteratively exchange reliability (soft) information of the code bits. The soft information passed between the two components is referred to as *extrinsic* information, since *a priori* information is excluded. Usually, *extrinsic* information is represented in the form of log-likelihood ratios (LLRs). In this paper we present four different approaches for the *extrinsic* LLR computation by a SISO linear minimum mean square error (LMMSE) detector. All methods apply a Gaussian approximation, but at different stages. The first approach, referred to as Tuechler approach [2], applies LMMSE filtering for data symbol estimation, where *a priori* information of the concerned symbols is excluded in the filter coefficient computation. *Extrinsic* LLRs of the code bits are computed based on the Gaussian approximation of the LMMSE filter output. In the second approach, referred to as joint Gaussian (JG) approach [3], the *extrinsic* LLRs of the code bits are derived based on the Gaussian approximation of the noise-plus-interference component with respect to a particular data symbol. The third method, referred to as Gaussian model approach [4], temporarily assumes that the data symbols are Gaussian distributed[1]. Then, a conventional

---

[1] Usually, data symbols are drawn from a discrete symbol alphabet (e.g., binary phase shift keying (BPSK)).

© Springer International Publishing Switzerland 2015
R. Moreno-Díaz et al. (Eds.): EUROCAST 2015, LNCS 9520, pp. 529–536, 2015.
DOI: 10.1007/978-3-319-27340-2_66

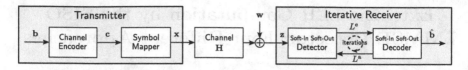

Fig. 1. Block diagram of a coded communication system with iterative receiver (turbo equalization). Note that for simplicity (de)interleaving is omitted.

MMSE estimation is performed resulting in *a posteriori* mean and variance of each data symbol. By excluding the *a priori* means and variances of the symbols results in *extrinsic* means and variances, which are used to compute the *extrinsic* LLRs. In the fourth approach, referred to as factor graph (FG) approach, Gaussian message passing on a factor graph results in output messages, characterized by their means and variances, that coincide with the *extrinsic* means and variances derived in the Gaussian model approach.

For BPSK it was shown in [5] that the Tuechler, the JG and the Gaussian model approach are equivalent. Moreover, for higher order modulation schemes the equivalence between the Tuechler and the Gaussian model approach was proven in [4]. The main contributions of this paper can be summarized as follows:

- We show the equivalence between the JG and the Gaussian model approach for higher order modulation schemes. Hence, we can conclude that the Tuechler, the JG and the Gaussian model approach are equivalent.
- We propose a fourth approach for computing the *extrinsic* LLRs by applying Gaussian message passing on a factor graph and show its equivalence to the aforementioned methods.

The paper is organized as follows: In Sect. 2 we introduce the system model. Section 3 discusses the four approaches for computing the *extrinsic* LLRs and in Sect. 4 the equivalence between the approaches is shown. Finally, Sect. 5 concludes the paper.

Notation: We use lower-case bold face variables ($\mathbf{a}$, $\mathbf{b}$, ...) to indicate vectors and upper-case bold face variables ($\mathbf{A}$, $\mathbf{B}$, ...) to indicate matrices. The identity matrix is defined by $\mathbf{I}$, a zero-vector of size M is given by $\mathbf{0}_M$ and $\mathbb{I}(\cdot)$ denotes the indicator function. To indicate a diagonal matrix with the elements of the vector $\mathbf{a}$ on its diagonal we use diag($\mathbf{a}$). The transposition or conjugate transposition of a vector/matrix is denoted by $(\cdot)^{\mathrm{T}}$ and $(\cdot)^{\mathrm{H}}$, respectively. A complex multivariate Gaussian probability density function (pdf) is denoted by $\mathcal{CN}(\mathbf{m}, \mathbf{V})$, with $\mathbf{m}$ as its mean vector and $\mathbf{V}$ as its covariance matrix.

2   System Model

We consider a coded communication system with turbo equalization at the receiver as depicted in Fig. 1. At the transmitter a sequence of information bits $\mathbf{b}$ is encoded and interleaved yielding the codeword $\mathbf{c}$. The codeword is divided into

N blocks of length Q, i.e. $\mathbf{c} = [\mathbf{c}_1, \ldots, \mathbf{c}_N]^T$ with $\mathbf{c}_n = [c_{n,1}, \ldots, c_{n,Q}]^T$. Each bit vector $\mathbf{c}_n$ is mapped to a (complex-valued) symbol $x_n \in \mathcal{X} = \{\alpha_1, \ldots, \alpha_M\}$. The finite symbol alphabet $\mathcal{X}$ contains $M = |\mathcal{X}| = 2^Q$ symbols, and each symbol α_i corresponds to a certain bit pattern. The symbol sequence $\boldsymbol{x} = [x_1, \ldots, x_N]^T$ is transmitted over a channel (e.g., intersymbol interference (ISI) channel) represented by the matrix $\mathbf{H} \in \mathbb{C}^{M \times N}$ and is distorted by additive complex white Gaussian noise given by $\mathbf{w} \sim \mathcal{CN}(\mathbf{0}_M, \sigma_w^2 \mathbf{I})$. Hence, the received signal vector $\mathbf{z}$ is given by

$$\mathbf{z} = \mathbf{H}\boldsymbol{x} + \mathbf{w}. \tag{1}$$

At the receiver the SISO detector computes the *extrinsic* LLRs L^e of the code bits. This is accomplished on the basis of the received vector $\mathbf{z}$, the channel state information ($\mathbf{H}$ and σ_w^2) and the *a priori* LLRs L^a obtained from the SISO decoder. The *extrinsic* information is passed to the decoder which computes new *extrinsic* LLRs that are fed back to the detector and are interpreted as new *a priori* LLR L^a. A cycle of feed back information from the decoder to the detector, followed by detection and decoding, is referred to as one iteration. If a maximum number of iterations is reached the channel decoder provides a hard-output estimate of the transmitted information bit stream $\hat{\mathbf{b}}$.

3   Extrinsic LLR Computation

The *extrinsic* LLR of the code bit $c_{n,q}$ is computed by the SISO detector according to [4]:

$$L^e(c_{n,q}|\mathbf{z}) = \ln \frac{P(c_{n,q} = 0|\mathbf{z})}{P(c_{n,q} = 1|\mathbf{z})} - \ln \frac{P(c_{n,q} = 0)}{P(c_{n,q} = 1)}, \tag{2}$$

where the first and the second term in (2) correspond to the *a posteriori* LLR L^p and the *a priori* LLR L^a, respectively. Applying Bayes' theorem gives

$$L^e(c_{n,q}|\mathbf{z}) = \ln \frac{\displaystyle\sum_{\alpha_i \in \mathcal{X}_q^0} p(\mathbf{z}|x_n = \alpha_i) \prod_{q'=1; q' \neq q}^{Q} P(c_{n,q'})}{\displaystyle\sum_{\alpha_i \in \mathcal{X}_q^1} p(\mathbf{z}|x_n = \alpha_i) \prod_{q'=1; q' \neq q}^{Q} P(c_{n,q'})}, \tag{3}$$

with $\mathcal{X}_q^b$ being a subset of $\mathcal{X}$ including symbols mapped with $c_{n,q} = b \in \{0,1\}$. Moreover, $p(\mathbf{z}|x_n)$ denotes the likelihood function and $P(c_{n,q})$ corresponds to the *a priori* probability of the code bit $c_{n,q}$. It can be observed from (3) that the complexity for computing $L^e(c_{n,q}|\mathbf{z})$ is mainly determined by calculating the likelihood function $p(\mathbf{z}|x_n)$. Thus, the task of the SISO detector is the efficient computation of $p(\mathbf{z}|x_n)$. In the following we will present four different approaches fulfilling this task. For each approach the main steps are briefly summarized. Please refer to the reference related to a particular method for more details (e.g., Tuechler approach $\Rightarrow$ [2]).

3.1   Approach 1 - Tuechler Approach

1. Determine the linear MMSE estimate of x_n by

$$m_n^{\mathrm{p}} = m_n^{\mathrm{a}} + v_n^{\mathrm{a}} \mathbf{h}_n^{\mathrm{H}} (\mathbf{H} \mathbf{V}^{\mathrm{a}} \mathbf{H}^{\mathrm{H}} + \sigma_w^2 \mathbf{I})^{-1} (\mathbf{z} - \mathbf{H} \mathbf{m}^{\mathrm{a}}),$$

where m_n^{p}, m_n^{a} and v_n^{a} denote the *a posteriori* mean and the *a priori* mean and variance of the nth symbol, respectively. The *a priori* covariance matrix is defined by $\mathbf{V}^{\mathrm{a}} = \mathrm{diag}([v_1^{\mathrm{a}}, \dots, v_N^{\mathrm{a}}])$ and $\mathbf{h}_n$ corresponds to the nth column of $\mathbf{H}$.

1a. Exclude the *a priori* information in m_n^{p}, i.e. $m_n^{\mathrm{a}} = 0$ and $v_n^{\mathrm{a}} = 1$

2. Apply a Gaussian approximation to m_n^{p}, i.e. $m_n^{\mathrm{p}} \sim \mathcal{CN}(\mu_{n,i}, \sigma_{n,i}^2)$

3. Compute the *extrinsic* LLR by replacing $p(\mathbf{z}|x_n = \alpha_i)$ with

$$p(m_n^{\mathrm{p}}|x_n = \alpha_i) \propto \exp\left(-\frac{|m_n^{\mathrm{p}} - \mu_{n,i}|^2}{\sigma_{n,i}^2}\right).$$

3.2   Approach 2 - Joint Gaussian Approach

1. Rewrite the system model in (1) as

$$\mathbf{z} = \mathbf{H}\mathbf{x} + \mathbf{w} = \mathbf{h}_n x_n + \sum_{j=1; j \neq n}^{N} \mathbf{h}_j x_j + \mathbf{w} = \mathbf{h}_n x_n + \mathbf{e}_n,$$

where $\mathbf{e}_n$ denotes the noise-plus-interference component.

2. Apply a Gaussian approximation to $\mathbf{e}_n$, i.e. $\mathbf{e}_n \sim \mathcal{CN}(\mathbf{m}_{e_n}, \mathbf{V}_{e_n})$

3. Compute the *extrinsic* LLR

$$p(\mathbf{z}|x_n = \alpha_i) \propto \exp\left(-\|\mathbf{z} - \mathbf{h}_n \alpha_i - \mathbf{m}_{e_n}\|_{\mathbf{V}_{e_n}}^2\right),$$

with $\| \cdot \|_{\mathbf{V}}^2 = (\cdot)^{\mathrm{H}} \mathbf{V}^{-1} (\cdot)$.

3.3   Approach 3 - Gaussian Model Approach

1. Apply a Gaussian assumption on the symbols x_n, i.e. $x_n \sim \mathcal{CN}(m_n^{\mathrm{a}}, v_n^{\mathrm{a}})$

2. Compute the *a posteriori* pdf of x_n

$$p(x_n|\mathbf{z}) = \mathcal{CN}(m_n^{\mathrm{p}}, v_n^{\mathrm{p}}),$$

where m_n^{p} denotes the *a posteriori* mean as defined in the Tuechler approach and v_n^{p} corresponds to the diagonal elements of $\mathbf{V}^{\mathrm{p}} = \mathbf{V}^{\mathrm{a}} - \mathbf{V}^{\mathrm{a}} \mathbf{H}^{\mathrm{H}} (\mathbf{H} \mathbf{V}^{\mathrm{a}} \mathbf{H}^{\mathrm{H}} + \sigma_w^2 \mathbf{I})^{-1} \mathbf{H} \mathbf{V}^{\mathrm{a}}$.

3. Compute the *extrinsic* LLR

$$p(\mathbf{z}|x_n = \alpha_i) \propto \exp\left(-\frac{|\alpha_i - m_n^{\mathrm{e}}|^2}{v_n^{\mathrm{e}}}\right),$$

with

$$v_n^{\mathrm{e}} = (1/v_n^{\mathrm{p}} - 1/v_n^{\mathrm{a}})^{-1}$$
$$m_n^{\mathrm{e}} = v_n^{\mathrm{e}}(m_n^{\mathrm{p}}/v_n^{\mathrm{p}} - m_n^{\mathrm{a}}/v_n^{\mathrm{a}}).$$

3.4   Approach 4 - Factor Graph Approach

The iterative receiver depicted in Fig. 1 can be represented as a factor graph (cf. Fig. 2). The messages in the FG are computed and exchanged according to the sum-product algorithm[2] (SPA). We will show in the following that the messages towards the SISO decoder correspond to the *extrinsic* LLRs defined in (3). According to the SPA the message from the demapper to the decoder is given by

$$m_{\text{dem}\rightarrow\text{dec}}(c_{n,q}) = \sum_{\sim\{c_{n,q}\}} p(x_n|\mathbf{c}_n)m_{\text{det}\rightarrow\text{dem}}(x_n) \prod_{q'\neq q} m_{\text{dec}\rightarrow\text{dem}}(c_{n,q'}),$$

with

$$p(x_n|\mathbf{c}_n) = \mathbb{I}\{x_n = f_x(\mathbf{c}_n)\}$$

$$m_{\text{det}\rightarrow\text{dem}}(x_n) = \sum_{\sim\{x_n\}} p(\mathbf{z}|\mathbf{x}) \prod_{j\neq n} m_{\text{dem}\rightarrow\text{det}}(x_j) \propto p(\mathbf{z}|x_n)$$

$$m_{\text{dec}\rightarrow\text{dem}}(c_{n,q}) = P(c_{n,q}),$$

where the deterministic function $f_x(\cdot)$ denotes the mapping of $\mathbf{c}_n$ to x_n. Hence, the message $m_{\text{dem}\rightarrow\text{dec}}(c_{n,q})$ can be written as

$$m_{\text{dem}\rightarrow\text{dec}}(c_{n,q} = b) = \sum_{\alpha_i\in\mathcal{X}_q^b} p(\mathbf{z}|x_n = \alpha_i) \prod_{q'=1;q'\neq q}^{Q} P(c_{n,q'}).$$

Defining the *extrinsic* LLR by

$$L^e(c_{n,q}|\mathbf{z}) = \ln\frac{m_{\text{dem}\rightarrow\text{dec}}(c_{n,q} = 0)}{m_{\text{dem}\rightarrow\text{dec}}(c_{n,q} = 1)},$$

and substituting the messages derived above gives the *extrinsic* LLR in (3). However, the task for efficiently computing the likelihood function $p(\mathbf{z}|x_n = \alpha_i)$, corresponding to the message $m_{\text{det}\rightarrow\text{dem}}(x_n = \alpha_i)$, remains.

Similar to the Gaussian model approach presented in Sect. 3.3, we temporarily assume that the symbol x_n are Gaussian distributed, i.e. $x_n \sim \mathcal{CN}(m_n^a, v_n^a)$. Thus all messages in the FG are Gaussian pdfs, characterized by their mean values and variances. Gaussian message passing on the FG according to the SPA gives m_n^e and v_n^e which describe the message as follows

$$m_{\text{det}\rightarrow\text{dem}}(x_n = \alpha_i) \propto p(\mathbf{z}|x_n = \alpha_i) \propto \exp\left(-\frac{|\alpha_i - m_n^e|^2}{v_n^e}\right).$$

Note that m_n^e and v_n^e are similar to the Gaussian model approach. Gaussian message passing on FGs offers many degrees of freedom in the implementation, leading to computational efficient solutions (see e.g., [5]). Thus, the factor graph approach is the most promising solution for an efficient *extrinsic* LLR computation.

---

[2] For more information on FGs and the sum-product algorithm please refer to [6].

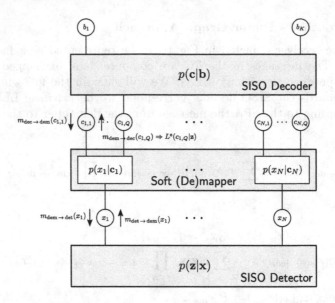

Fig. 2. Factor graph representation of an iterative receiver.

4   Equivalence of the Approaches

For BPSK it was shown in [5] that the Tuechler, the JG and the Gaussian model approach are equivalent and for higher order modulation schemes the equivalence between the Tuechler and the Gaussian model approach was proven in [4]. These relations are illustrated in Fig. 3. However, the equivalence between the JG and the Gaussian model approach for higher order modulation schemes has not been shown yet, which we will proof in the following.

According to the JG approach (cf. Sect. 3.2) the noise-plus interference component is approximated as Gaussian distribution $\mathbf{e}_n \sim \mathcal{CN}_{e_n}(\mathbf{m}_{e_n}, \mathbf{V}_{e_n})$ with

$$\mathbf{m}_{e_n} = \mathbf{Hm}^a - \mathbf{h}_n m_n^a$$
$$\mathbf{V}_{e_n} = \mathbf{HV}_{x(n)}^a \mathbf{H}^H + \sigma_w^2 \mathbf{I},$$

and $\mathbf{V}_{x(n)}^a = \text{diag}([v_1^a, \ldots, v_{n-1}^a, 0, v_{n+1}^a, \ldots, v_N^a]^T)$. With the Gaussian approximation of $\mathbf{e}_n$ the likelihood function is given by

$$p(\mathbf{z}|x_n) \propto \exp\left(-\|\mathbf{z} - \mathbf{m}_{e_n} - \mathbf{h}_n x_n\|_{\mathbf{V}_{e_n}}^2\right),$$

$$\propto \exp\left(-\|\overbrace{\mathbf{z} - \mathbf{Hm}^a + \mathbf{h}_n m_n^a}^{A} - \mathbf{h}_n x_n\|_{\mathbf{V}_{e_n}}^2\right)$$

$$\propto \exp\left((A - \mathbf{h}_n x_n)^H \mathbf{V}_{e_n}^{-1}(A - \mathbf{h}_n x_n)\right).$$

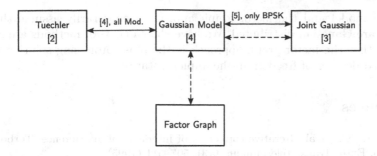

Fig. 3. Equivalence between the presented approaches, including the references of the corresponding proofs. Dashed line connections correspond to not proven relations.

Writing the likelihood function as a function of x_n and applying straightforward mathematical manipulation gives[3]

$$p(\mathbf{z}|x_n) \propto \exp(-x_n^* \underbrace{\mathbf{h}_n^H \mathbf{V}_{e_n}^{-1} \mathbf{h}_n}_{1/v_{x_n}} x_n + 2\mathrm{Re}\{x_n^* \underbrace{\mathbf{h}_n^H \mathbf{V}_{e_n}^{-1} A}_{m_{x_n}/v_{x_n}}\})$$

$$\propto \mathcal{CN}_{x_n}\left(\underbrace{\frac{\mathbf{h}_n^H \mathbf{V}_z^{-1}(\mathbf{z} - \mathbf{H}\mathbf{m}^a + \mathbf{h}_n \mathbf{m}_n^a)}{\mathbf{h}_n^H \mathbf{V}_z^{-1} \mathbf{h}_n}}_{m_{x_n}}, \underbrace{\frac{1}{\mathbf{h}_n^H \mathbf{V}_z^{-1} \mathbf{h}_n} - v_n^a}_{v_{x_n}} \right),$$

with $\mathbf{V}_z = \mathbf{H}\mathbf{V}^a\mathbf{H}^H + \sigma_w^2 \mathbf{I}$. This results in

$$p(\mathbf{z}|x_n = \alpha_i) \propto \exp\left(\frac{|\alpha_i - m_{x_n}|^2}{v_{x_n}} \right).$$

The mean m_n^e and the variance v_n^e of the Gaussian model, defined in (21) and (22) in [4], are similar to m_{x_n} and v_{x_n} and therefore we can conclude that the JG and the Gaussian model approach are equivalent.

The similarity between the Gaussian model and the factor graph approach follows from the fact that both methods temporarily assume that the symbols are Gaussian distributed. Hence, we conclude that all presented approaches are equivalent.

5   Conclusion

We have presented four different approaches for the computation of *extrinsic* LLRs by a SISO LMMSE detector used in a turbo equalization system. All approaches apply a Gaussian approximation, but at different stages. The Tuechler and the joint Gaussian approach apply a Gaussian assumption to the LMMSE filter output and to the noise-plus-interference component, respectively. The

---

[3] Note that terms that are independent of x_n can be neglected.

Gaussian model and the factor graph approach temporarily assume that the symbols are Gaussian distributed. We have shown that all methods are equivalent and that the factor graph approach is the most promising solution due to the offered degrees of freedom in the implementations.

References

1. Douillard, C., et al.: Iterative correction of intersymbol interference: Turbo equalization. Euro. Trans. Telecommun. **6**(3), 507–511 (1995)
2. Tuechler, M., et al.: Minimum mean squared error equalization using a priori information. IEEE Trans. Signal Process. **50**(3), 673–683 (2002)
3. Liu, L., et al.: Simple iterative chip-by-chip multiuser detection for CDMA systems. In: Proceedings of the 57th Vehicular Technology Conference, vol. 3, pp. 2157–2161, April 2003
4. Guo, Q., et al.: A concise representation for the soft-in soft-out LMMSE detector. IEEE Commun. Lett. **15**(5), 566–568 (2011)
5. Guo, Q., Ping, L.: LMMSE turbo equalization based on factor graphs. IEEE J. Select Areas in Commun. **26**(2), 311–319 (2008)
6. Wymeersch, H.: Iterative Receiver Design. Cambridge University Press, New York (2007)

CWCU LMMSE Estimation Under Linear Model Assumptions

Oliver Lang$^{(\boxtimes)}$ and Mario Huemer

Institute of Signal Processing, Johannes Kepler University Linz, Linz, Austria
{oliver.lang,mario.huemer}@jku.at

Abstract. The classical unbiasedness condition utilized e.g. by the best linear unbiased estimator (BLUE) is very stringent. By softening the "global" unbiasedness condition and introducing component-wise conditional unbiasedness conditions instead, the number of constraints limiting the estimator's performance can in many cases significantly be reduced. In this paper we extend the findings on the component-wise conditionally unbiased linear minimum mean square error (CWCU LMMSE) estimator under linear model assumptions. We discuss the CWCU LMMSE estimator for complex proper Gaussian parameter vectors, and for mutually independent (and otherwise arbitrarily distributed) parameters. Finally, the beneficial properties of the CWCU LMMSE estimator are demonstrated in two applications.

1 Introduction

Usually, when we talk about unbiased estimation of a parameter vector $\mathbf{x} \in \mathbb{C}^{n \times 1}$ out of a measurement vector $\mathbf{y} \in \mathbb{C}^{m \times 1}$, then the estimation problem is treated in the classical framework [1]. Letting $\hat{\mathbf{x}} = \mathbf{g}(\mathbf{y})$ be an estimator of $\mathbf{x}$, then the classical unbiased constraint asserts that

$$E_{\mathbf{y}}[\hat{\mathbf{x}}] = \int \mathbf{g}(\mathbf{y}) p(\mathbf{y}; \mathbf{x}) d\mathbf{y} = \mathbf{x} \quad \text{for all possible } \mathbf{x}, \tag{1}$$

where $p(\mathbf{y}; \mathbf{x})$ is the probability density function (PDF) of vector $\mathbf{y}$ parametrized by the unknown parameter vector $\mathbf{x}$. The index of the expectation operator shall indicate the PDF over which the averaging is performed. Equation (1) can also be formulated in the Bayesian framework, where the parameter vector $\mathbf{x}$ is treated as random, and whose realization is to be estimated. Here, the corresponding problem arises by demanding global conditional unbiasedness, i.e.

$$E_{\mathbf{y}|\mathbf{x}}[\hat{\mathbf{x}}|\mathbf{x}] = \int \mathbf{g}(\mathbf{y}) p(\mathbf{y}|\mathbf{x}) d\mathbf{y} = \mathbf{x} \quad \text{for all possible } \mathbf{x}. \tag{2}$$

The attribute *global* indicates that the condition is made on the whole parameter vector $\mathbf{x}$. However, the constricting requirement in (2) prevents the exploitation

---

This work was supported by the Austrian Science Fund (FWF): I683-N13.

R. Moreno-Díaz et al. (Eds.): EUROCAST 2015, LNCS 9520, pp. 537–545, 2015.
DOI: 10.1007/978-3-319-27340-2_67

of prior knowledge about the parameters, and hence leads to a significant reduction in the benefits brought about by the Bayesian framework.

In component-wise conditionally unbiased (CWCU) Bayesian parameter estimation [2–5], instead of constraining the estimator to be globally unbiased, we aim for achieving conditional unbiasedness on one parameter component at a time. Let x_i be the ith element of $\mathbf{x}$, and $\hat{x}_i = g_i(\mathbf{y})$ be an estimator of x_i. Then the CWCU constraints are

$$E_{\mathbf{y}|x_i}[\hat{x}_i|x_i] = \int g_i(\mathbf{y})p(\mathbf{y}|x_i)d\mathbf{y} = x_i, \tag{3}$$

for all possible x_i (and all $i = 1, 2, ..., n$). The CWCU constraints are less stringent than the global conditional unbiasedness condition in (2), and it turns out that a CWCU estimator in many cases allows the incorporation of prior knowledge about the statistical properties of the parameter vector.

The paper is organized as follows: In Sect. 2 we discuss the CWCU linear minimum mean square error (LMMSE) estimator under different linear model assumptions, and we extend the findings of [2]. We particularly distinguish between complex proper jointly Gaussian (cf. [6]), and mutually independent (and otherwise arbitrarily distributed) parameters. Then, in Sect. 3 the CWCU LMMSE estimator is compared against the best linear unbiased estimator (BLUE) and the LMMSE estimator in two different applications.

2   CWCU LMMSE Estimation

We assume that a complex vector parameter $\mathbf{x} \in \mathbb{C}^{n \times 1}$ is to be estimated based on a measurement vector $\mathbf{y} \in \mathbb{C}^{m \times 1}$. Additionally, we assume that $\mathbf{x}$ and $\mathbf{y}$ are connected via a linear model

$$\mathbf{y} = \mathbf{Hx} + \mathbf{n}, \tag{4}$$

where $\mathbf{H} \in \mathbb{C}^{m \times n}$ is a known observation matrix, $\mathbf{x}$ has mean $E_{\mathbf{x}}[\mathbf{x}]$ and covariance matrix $\mathbf{C_{xx}}$, and $\mathbf{n} \in \mathbb{C}^{m \times 1}$ is a zero mean noise vector with covariance matrix $\mathbf{C_{nn}}$ and independent of $\mathbf{x}$. Additional assumptions on $\mathbf{x}$ will vary in the following. We note that the CWCU LMMSE estimator for the linear model under the assumption of complex proper Gaussian $\mathbf{x}$ and complex and proper white Gaussian noise with covariance matrix $\mathbf{C_{nn}} = \sigma_n^2 \mathbf{I}$ has already been derived in [2].

As in LMMSE estimation we constrain the estimator to be linear (or actually affine), such that

$$\hat{\mathbf{x}} = \mathbf{Ey} + \mathbf{c}, \tag{5}$$

with $\mathbf{E} \in \mathbb{C}^{n \times m}$ and $\mathbf{c} \in \mathbb{C}^{n \times 1}$. Note that in LMMSE estimation no assumptions on the specific form of the PDF $p(\mathbf{x})$ have to be made. However, the situation is different in CWCU LMMSE estimation as will be shown shortly. Let us consider the ith component of the estimator

$$\hat{x}_i = \mathbf{e}_i^H \mathbf{y} + c_i, \tag{6}$$

where $\mathbf{e}_i^H$ denotes the ith row of the estimator matrix $\mathbf{E}$. Furthermore, let $\mathbf{h}_i \in \mathbb{C}^{m \times 1}$ be the ith column of $\mathbf{H}$, $\bar{\mathbf{H}}_i \in \mathbb{C}^{m \times (n-1)}$ the matrix resulting from $\mathbf{H}$ by deleting $\mathbf{h}_i$, x_i be the ith element of $\mathbf{x}$, and $\bar{\mathbf{x}}_i \in \mathbb{C}^{(n-1) \times 1}$ the vector resulting from $\mathbf{x}$ after deleting x_i. Then we can write $\mathbf{y} = \mathbf{h}_i x_i + \bar{\mathbf{H}}_i \bar{\mathbf{x}}_i + \mathbf{n}$, and (6) becomes

$$\hat{x}_i = \mathbf{e}_i^H (\mathbf{h}_i x_i + \bar{\mathbf{H}}_i \bar{\mathbf{x}}_i + \mathbf{n}) + c_i. \tag{7}$$

The conditional mean of $\hat{x}_i$ therefore is

$$E_{\mathbf{y}|x_i}[\hat{x}_i|x_i] = \mathbf{e}_i^H \mathbf{h}_i x_i + \mathbf{e}_i^H \bar{\mathbf{H}}_i E_{\bar{\mathbf{x}}_i|x_i}[\bar{\mathbf{x}}_i|x_i] + c_i. \tag{8}$$

From (8) we can derive conditions that guarantee that the CWCU constraints (3) are fulfilled. There are at least the following possibilities:

1. (3) can be fulfilled for all possible x_i if the conditional mean $E_{\bar{\mathbf{x}}_i|x_i}[\bar{\mathbf{x}}_i|x_i]$ is a linear function of x_i. For complex proper Gaussian $\mathbf{x}$ this condition holds (for all $i = 1, 2, ..., n$).
2. (3) can be fulfilled for all possible x_i (and all $i = 1, 2, ..., n$) if $E_{\bar{\mathbf{x}}_i|x_i}[\bar{\mathbf{x}}_i|x_i] = E_{\bar{\mathbf{x}}_i}[\bar{\mathbf{x}}_i]$ for all possible x_i (and all $i = 1, 2, ..., n$), which is true if the elements x_i of $\mathbf{x}$ are mutually independent.
3. (3) is fulfilled for all possible x_i (and all $i = 1, 2, ..., n$) if $\mathbf{e}_i^H \mathbf{h}_i = 1$, $\mathbf{e}_i^H \bar{\mathbf{H}}_i = \mathbf{0}^T$, and $c_i = 0$ for $i = 1, 2, \cdots, n$. These constraints and settings correspond to the ones of the BLUE.

2.1   Complex Proper Gaussian Parameter Vectors

We start with the first case from above, assume a complex proper Gaussian parameter vector, i.e. $\mathbf{x} \sim \mathcal{CN}(E_{\mathbf{x}}[\mathbf{x}], \mathbf{C}_{\mathbf{xx}})$, and start with the derivation of the ith component $\hat{x}_i$ of the estimator. Because of the Gaussian assumption we have $E_{\bar{\mathbf{x}}_i|x_i}[\bar{\mathbf{x}}_i|x_i] = E_{\bar{\mathbf{x}}_i}[\bar{\mathbf{x}}_i] + (\sigma_{x_i}^2)^{-1} \mathbf{C}_{\bar{\mathbf{x}}_i x_i}(x_i - E_{x_i}[x_i])$, where $\mathbf{C}_{\bar{\mathbf{x}}_i x_i} = E_{\mathbf{x}}[(\bar{\mathbf{x}}_i - E_{\bar{\mathbf{x}}_i}[\bar{\mathbf{x}}_i])(x_i - E_{x_i}[x_i])^H]$, and $\sigma_{x_i}^2$ is the variance of x_i. Consequently (8) becomes

$$E_{\mathbf{y}|x_i}[\hat{x}_i|x_i] = \mathbf{e}_i^H \mathbf{h}_i x_i + \mathbf{e}_i^H \bar{\mathbf{H}}_i \left(E_{\bar{\mathbf{x}}_i}[\bar{\mathbf{x}}_i] + (\sigma_{x_i}^2)^{-1} \mathbf{C}_{\bar{\mathbf{x}}_i x_i}(x_i - E_{x_i}[x_i]) \right) + c_i. \tag{9}$$

Note that the only requirement on the noise vector so far was its independence on $\mathbf{x}$. From (9) we see that $E_{\mathbf{y}|x_i}[\hat{x}_i|x_i] = x_i$ is fulfilled if

$$\mathbf{e}_i^H \mathbf{h}_i + \mathbf{e}_i^H \bar{\mathbf{H}}_i (\sigma_{x_i}^2)^{-1} \mathbf{C}_{\bar{\mathbf{x}}_i x_i} = 1 \tag{10}$$

and

$$c_i = \mathbf{e}_i^H \bar{\mathbf{H}}_i (\sigma_{x_i}^2)^{-1} \mathbf{C}_{\bar{\mathbf{x}}_i x_i} E_{x_i}[x_i] - \mathbf{e}_i^H \bar{\mathbf{H}}_i E_{\bar{\mathbf{x}}_i}[\bar{\mathbf{x}}_i]. \tag{11}$$

With (10) and (11) can be reformulated according to

$$\begin{aligned} c_i &= E_{x_i}[x_i] - \mathbf{e}_i^H \mathbf{h}_i E_{x_i}[x_i] - \mathbf{e}_i^H \bar{\mathbf{H}}_i E_{\bar{\mathbf{x}}_i}[\bar{\mathbf{x}}_i] \\ &= E_{x_i}[x_i] - \mathbf{e}_i^H \mathbf{H} E_{\mathbf{x}}[\mathbf{x}]. \end{aligned} \tag{12}$$

Furthermore, (10) can be simplified to obtain the constraint

$$\mathbf{e}_i^H \mathbf{H} \mathbf{C}_{\mathbf{x}x_i} = \sigma_{x_i}^2. \tag{13}$$

Inserting (6), (12) and (13) into the Bayesian MSE cost function $E_{\mathbf{y},\mathbf{x}}[|\hat{x}_i - x_i|^2]$ immediately leads to the constrained optimization problem

$$\mathbf{e}_{\mathrm{CL},i} = \arg\min_{\mathbf{e}_i} \; (\mathbf{e}_i^H (\mathbf{H} \mathbf{C}_{\mathbf{xx}} \mathbf{H}^H + \mathbf{C}_{\mathbf{nn}}) \mathbf{e}_i - \sigma_{x_i}^2) \quad \text{s.t. } \mathbf{e}_i^H \mathbf{H} \mathbf{C}_{\mathbf{x}x_i} = \sigma_{x_i}^2, \tag{14}$$

where "CL" shall stand for CWCU LMMSE. The solution can be found with the Lagrange multiplier method and is given by

$$\mathbf{e}_{\mathrm{CL},i}^H = \frac{\sigma_{x_i}^2}{\mathbf{C}_{x_i \mathbf{x}} \mathbf{H}^H (\mathbf{H} \mathbf{C}_{\mathbf{xx}} \mathbf{H}^H + \mathbf{C}_{\mathbf{nn}})^{-1} \mathbf{H} \mathbf{C}_{\mathbf{x}x_i}} \mathbf{C}_{x_i \mathbf{x}} \mathbf{H}^H (\mathbf{H} \mathbf{C}_{\mathbf{xx}} \mathbf{H}^H + \mathbf{C}_{\mathbf{nn}})^{-1}. \tag{15}$$

Introducing the estimator matrix $\mathbf{E}_{\mathrm{CL}} = [\mathbf{e}_{\mathrm{CL},1}, \mathbf{e}_{\mathrm{CL},2}, \ldots, \mathbf{e}_{\mathrm{CL},n}]^H$ together with (12) and (15) immediately leads us to the first part of the

Proposition 1. *If the observed data* $\mathbf{y}$ *follow the linear model in* (4), *where* $\mathbf{y} \in \mathbb{C}^{m \times 1}$ *is the data vector,* $\mathbf{H} \in \mathbb{C}^{m \times n}$ *is a known observation matrix,* $\mathbf{x} \in \mathbb{C}^{n \times 1}$ *is a parameter vector with prior complex proper Gaussian PDF* $\mathcal{CN}(E_{\mathbf{x}}[\mathbf{x}], \mathbf{C}_{\mathbf{xx}})$, *and* $\mathbf{n} \in \mathbb{C}^{m \times 1}$ *is a zero mean noise vector with covariance matrix* $\mathbf{C}_{\mathbf{nn}}$ *and independent of* $\mathbf{x}$ *(the PDF of* $\mathbf{n}$ *is otherwise arbitrary), then the CWCU LMMSE estimator minimizing the Bayesian MSEs* $E_{\mathbf{y},\mathbf{x}}[|\hat{x}_i - x_i|^2]$ *under the constraints* $E_{\mathbf{y}|x_i}[\hat{x}_i|x_i] = x_i$ *for* $i = 1, 2, \cdots, n$ *is given by*

$$\hat{\mathbf{x}}_{\mathrm{CL}} = E_{\mathbf{x}}[\mathbf{x}] + \mathbf{E}_{\mathrm{CL}}(\mathbf{y} - \mathbf{H} E_{\mathbf{x}}[\mathbf{x}]), \tag{16}$$

with

$$\mathbf{E}_{\mathrm{CL}} = \mathbf{D} \mathbf{C}_{\mathbf{xx}} \mathbf{H}^H (\mathbf{H} \mathbf{C}_{\mathbf{xx}} \mathbf{H}^H + \mathbf{C}_{\mathbf{nn}})^{-1}, \tag{17}$$

where the elements of the real diagonal matrix $\mathbf{D}$ *are*

$$[\mathbf{D}]_{i,i} = \frac{\sigma_{x_i}^2}{\mathbf{C}_{x_i \mathbf{x}} \mathbf{H}^H (\mathbf{H} \mathbf{C}_{\mathbf{xx}} \mathbf{H}^H + \mathbf{C}_{\mathbf{nn}})^{-1} \mathbf{H} \mathbf{C}_{\mathbf{x}x_i}}. \tag{18}$$

The mean of the error $\mathbf{e} = \mathbf{x} - \hat{\mathbf{x}}_{\mathrm{CL}}$ *(in the Bayesian sense) is zero, and the error covariance matrix* $\mathbf{C}_{\mathbf{ee},\mathrm{CL}}$ *which is also the minimum Bayesian MSE matrix* $\mathbf{M}_{\hat{\mathbf{x}}_{\mathrm{CL}}}$ *is*

$$\mathbf{C}_{\mathbf{ee},\mathrm{CL}} = \mathbf{M}_{\hat{\mathbf{x}}_{\mathrm{CL}}} = \mathbf{C}_{\mathbf{xx}} - \mathbf{A} \mathbf{D} - \mathbf{D} \mathbf{A} + \mathbf{D} \mathbf{A} \mathbf{D}, \tag{19}$$

with $\mathbf{A} = \mathbf{C}_{\mathbf{xx}} \mathbf{H}^H (\mathbf{H} \mathbf{C}_{\mathbf{xx}} \mathbf{H}^H + \mathbf{C}_{\mathbf{nn}})^{-1} \mathbf{H} \mathbf{C}_{\mathbf{xx}}$. *The minimum Bayesian MSEs are* $\mathrm{Bmse}(\hat{x}_{\mathrm{CL},i}) = [\mathbf{M}_{\hat{\mathbf{x}}_{\mathrm{CL}}}]_{i,i}$.

The part on the error performance can simply be proved by inserting in the definition of $\mathbf{e}$ and $\mathbf{C}_{\mathbf{ee}}$, respectively. From (17) it can be seen that the CWCU LMMSE estimator matrix can be derived as the product of the diagonal matrix $\mathbf{D}$ with the LMMSE estimator matrix $\mathbf{E}_{\mathrm{L}} = \mathbf{C}_{\mathbf{xy}} \mathbf{C}_{\mathbf{yy}}^{-1} = \mathbf{C}_{\mathbf{xx}} \mathbf{H}^H (\mathbf{H} \mathbf{C}_{\mathbf{xx}} \mathbf{H}^H + \mathbf{C}_{\mathbf{nn}})^{-1}$. Furthermore, we have $E_{\mathbf{y}|x_i}[\hat{x}_{\mathrm{L},i}|x_i] = [\mathbf{D}]_{i,i}^{-1} x_i + (1 - [\mathbf{D}]_{i,i}^{-1}) E_{x_i}[x_i]$ for the LMMSE estimator. From (18) it also follows that

$$\mathbf{D} = \mathrm{diag}\{\mathbf{C_{xx}}\}\,(\mathrm{diag}\{\mathbf{A}\})^{-1}. \tag{20}$$

The CWCU LMMSE estimator will in general not commute over linear transformations, an exception is the transformation over a diagonal matrix as partly discussed in [5].

2.2 Complex Parameter Vectors with Mutually Independent Elements

In case the elements of the parameter vector are mutually independent (8) becomes

$$E_{\mathbf{y}|x_i}[\hat{x}_i|x_i] = \mathbf{e}_i^H \mathbf{h}_i x_i + \mathbf{e}_i^H \bar{\mathbf{H}}_i E_{\bar{\mathbf{x}}_i}[\bar{\mathbf{x}}_i] + c_i. \tag{21}$$

$E_{\mathbf{y}|x_i}[\hat{x}_i|x_i] = x_i$ is fulfilled if $\mathbf{e}_i^H \mathbf{h}_i = 1$ and $c_i = -\mathbf{e}_i^H \bar{\mathbf{H}}_i E_{\bar{\mathbf{x}}_i}[\bar{\mathbf{x}}_i]$. No further assumptions on the PDF of $\mathbf{x}$ are required. Following similar arguments as above again leads to a constrained optimization problem [5]. Solving it leads to

Proposition 2. *If the observed data* $\mathbf{y}$ *follow the linear model in* (4), *where* $\mathbf{y} \in \mathbb{C}^{m \times 1}$ *is the data vector,* $\mathbf{H} \in \mathbb{C}^{m \times n}$ *is a known observation matrix,* $\mathbf{x} \in \mathbb{C}^{n \times 1}$ *is a parameter vector with mean* $E_{\mathbf{x}}[\mathbf{x}]$, *mutually independent elements and covariance matrix* $\mathbf{C_{xx}} = \mathrm{diag}\{\sigma_{x_1}^2, \sigma_{x_2}^2, \cdots, \sigma_{x_n}^2\}$, $\mathbf{n} \in \mathbb{C}^{m \times 1}$ *is a zero mean noise vector with covariance matrix* $\mathbf{C_{nn}}$ *and independent of* $\mathbf{x}$ *(the PDF of* $\mathbf{n}$ *is otherwise arbitrary), then the CWCU LMMSE estimator minimizing the Bayesian MSEs* $E_{\mathbf{y},\mathbf{x}}[|\hat{x}_i - x_i|^2]$ *under the constraints* $E_{\mathbf{y}|x_i}[\hat{x}_i|x_i] = x_i$ *for* $i = 1, 2, \cdots, n$ *is given by* (16) *and* (17), *where the elements of the real diagonal matrix* $\mathbf{D}$ *are*

$$[\mathbf{D}]_{i,i} = \frac{1}{\sigma_{x_i}^2 \, \mathbf{h}_i^H (\mathbf{H C_{xx} H}^H + \mathbf{C_{nn}})^{-1} \mathbf{h}_i}. \tag{22}$$

Since for mutually independent parameters the ith row of the LMMSE estimator is $\mathbf{e}_{\mathrm{L},i}^H = \sigma_{x_i}^2 \mathbf{h}_i^H (\mathbf{H C_{xx} H}^H + \mathbf{C_{nn}})^{-1}$ it follows from (22) that

$$[\mathbf{D}]_{i,i} = (\mathbf{e}_{\mathrm{L},i}^H \mathbf{h}_i)^{-1}. \tag{23}$$

It therefore holds that $\mathrm{diag}\{\mathbf{E}_{\mathrm{CL}}\mathbf{H}\} = \mathbf{1}$. Furthermore, in [5] we showed that for mutually independent parameters $\mathbf{e}_{\mathrm{CL},i}$ does not depend on $\sigma_{x_i}^2$ and is also given by $\mathbf{e}_{\mathrm{CL},i} = (\mathbf{h}_i^H \mathbf{C}_i^{-1} \mathbf{h}_i)^{-1} \mathbf{C}_i^{-1} \mathbf{h}_i$, where $\mathbf{C}_i = \bar{\mathbf{H}}_i \mathbf{C}_{\bar{\mathbf{x}}_i \bar{\mathbf{x}}_i} \bar{\mathbf{H}}_i^H + \mathbf{C_{nn}}$.

2.3 Other Cases

If $\mathbf{x}$ is whether complex proper Gaussian nor a vector with mutually independent parameters, then we have the following possibilities: If $E_{\mathbf{y}|x_i}[\hat{x}_i|x_i]$ is a linear function of x_i for all $i = 1, 2, \cdots, n$ then we can derive the CWCU LMMSE estimator similar as in Sect. 2.1. In the remaining cases still an estimator can be found that fulfills the CWCU constraints. As discussed above the choice $\mathbf{e}_i^H \mathbf{h}_i = 1$, $\mathbf{e}_i^H \bar{\mathbf{H}}_i = \mathbf{0}^T$ together with $c_i = 0$ for all $i = 1, 2, \cdots, n$ ensures that (3) holds. Inserting these constraints into the Bayesian MSE cost functions and solving the constrained optimization problems leads to

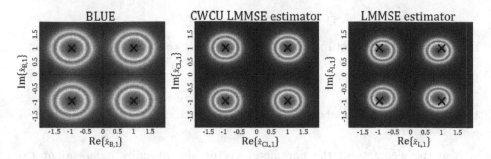

Fig. 1. Visualization of the relative frequencies of the estimates $\hat{x}_{B,1}$, $\hat{x}_{CL,1}$, and $\hat{x}_{L,1}$, respectively. The black crosses mark the ideal 4-QAM constellation points (Color figure online).

$$\hat{\mathbf{x}}_B = \mathbf{E}_B \mathbf{y} = (\mathbf{H}^H \mathbf{C}_{nn}^{-1} \mathbf{H})^{-1} \mathbf{H}^H \mathbf{C}_{nn}^{-1} \mathbf{y}, \qquad (24)$$

with $\mathbf{C}_{ee,B} = (\mathbf{H}^H \mathbf{C}_{nn}^{-1} \mathbf{H})^{-1}$ as the Bayesian error covariance matrix. $\mathbf{e}_i^H \mathbf{h}_i = 1$ & $\mathbf{e}_i^H \bar{\mathbf{H}}_i = \mathbf{0}$ for all $i = 1, 2, \cdots, n$ is equivalent to $\mathbf{EH} = \mathbf{I}$. This implies $\hat{\mathbf{x}}_B = \mathbf{E}_B \mathbf{y} = \mathbf{x} + \mathbf{E}_B \mathbf{n}$. It follows that the estimator in (24) also fulfills the global unbiasedness condition $E_{\mathbf{y}|\mathbf{x}}[\hat{\mathbf{x}}_B|\mathbf{x}] = \mathbf{x}$ for every $\mathbf{x} \in \mathbb{C}^{n \times 1}$. This estimator which is the BLUE is not able to exploit any prior knowledge about $\mathbf{x}$. Usually the BLUE is treated in the classical instead of the Bayesian framework.

3   Applications

3.1   QPSK Data Estimation

An example that exhibits the properties of the CWCU LMMSE concept most demonstrative is the estimation of channel distorted and noisy received quadrature amplitude modulated (QAM) data symbols. We assume an underlying linear model as in (4), with a parameter vector $\mathbf{x}$ consisting of 4 mutually independent 4-QAM symbols, each out of $\{\pm 1 \pm j\}$, complex proper additive white Gaussian noise (AWGN) with variance σ_n^2, and a 4×4 channel matrix $\mathbf{H}$. Due to the mutually independence of the 4-QAM data symbols we use the CWCU LMMSE estimator from Proposition 2. The experiment is repeated a large number of times for a fixed σ_n^2 and for a particularly chosen channel matrix $\mathbf{H}$. Figure 1 visualizes the relative frequencies of the estimates $\hat{x}_{B,1} = [\hat{\mathbf{x}}_B]_1$ (BLUE), $\hat{x}_{CL,1} = [\hat{\mathbf{x}}_{CL}]_1$ (CWCU LMMSE), $\hat{x}_{L,1} = [\hat{\mathbf{x}}_L]_1$ (LMMSE) in the complex plane. The estimates of both $\hat{x}_{B,1}$ and $\hat{x}_{CL,1}$ are centered around the true constellation points since these estimators fulfill the CWCU constraints. The Bayesian MSE of $\hat{x}_{CL,1}$ is clearly below the one of $\hat{x}_{B,1}$ since the former is able to incorporate the prior knowledge inherent in $\mathbf{C}_{\mathbf{xx}} = \sigma_{\mathbf{x}}^2 \mathbf{I}$. $\hat{x}_{L,1}$ is conditionally biased towards the prior mean which is 0. While the LMMSE estimator exhibits the lowest Bayesian MSE it can be shown that the LMMSE and CWCU LMMSE estimator lead to the same bit error ratio (BER) when the decision boundaries are adapted properly. However, the BLUE shows a worse performance in the MSE and in the BER.

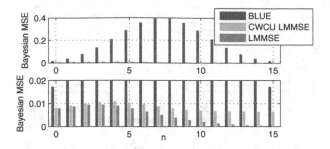

Fig. 2. Top: Bayesian MSEs of the estimated CIR coefficients; Bottom: zoomed version (Color figure online).

3.2   Channel Estimation

As a second example to demonstrate the properties of the CWCU LMMSE estimator we choose the well-known channel estimation problem for IEEE 802.11a/n WLAN standards [7], which extends our investigations in [5]. The standards define two identical length $N = 64$ preamble symbols designed such that their discrete Fourier transformed (DFT) versions show ± 1 at 52 subcarrier positions (indexes $\{1, ..., 26, 38, ...63\}$) and zeros at the remaining ones (indexes $\{0, 27, ..., 37\}$). The channel impulse response (CIR) is modeled as a zero mean complex proper Gaussian vector, i.e. $\mathbf{h} \sim \mathcal{CN}(\mathbf{0}, \mathbf{C_{hh}})$, with $\mathbf{C_{hh}} = \text{diag}\{\sigma_0^2, \sigma_1^2, ..., \sigma_{l_h-1}^2\}$ and exponentially decaying power delay profile with $\sigma_i^2 = \left(1 - e^{-T_s/\tau_{rms}}\right) e^{-iT_s/\tau_{rms}}$ for $i = 0, 1, ..., l_h - 1$. T_s and τ_{rms} are the sampling time and the channel delay spread, respectively, and l_h is the channel length which can be assumed to be considerably smaller than N. In our setup we chose $T_s = 50$ns, $\tau_{rms} = 100$ns, and $l_h = 16$. The transmission of the training symbols over the channel can again be written as a linear model with complex proper AWGN noise, and with $\mathbf{h}$ as the vector parameter whose realization is to be estimated, cf. [5]. Figure 2 shows the Bayesian MSEs of the BLUE ($\hat{\mathbf{h}}_B$), the LMMSE estimator ($\hat{\mathbf{h}}_L$), and the CWCU LMMSE estimator ($\hat{\mathbf{h}}_{CL}$) for a time domain noise variance of $\sigma_n^2 = 0.01$. Proposition 2 has been used to derive $\hat{\mathbf{h}}_{CL}$ since the elements of $\mathbf{h}$ are mutually independent. $\hat{\mathbf{h}}_{CL}$ almost reaches the performance of $\hat{\mathbf{h}}_L$, and in contrast to the latter it additionally shows the property of conditional unbiasedness. Both estimators incorporate the prior knowledge inherent in $\mathbf{C_{hh}}$ which results in a huge performance gain over $\hat{\mathbf{h}}_B$. We now turn to frequency response estimators and note that the vector of frequency response coefficients $\tilde{\mathbf{h}} \in \mathbb{C}^{64 \times 1}$ (which corresponds to the DFT of the zero-padded impulse response $[\mathbf{h}^T\ \mathbf{0}^T]^T$) consists of proper Gaussian elements, but the PDF of $\tilde{\mathbf{h}}$ cannot be written in the form of a multivariate proper Gaussian PDF. The LMMSE estimator $\hat{\tilde{\mathbf{h}}}_L$ is simply obtained by the DFT of $[\hat{\mathbf{h}}_L^T\ \mathbf{0}^T]^T$ (since it commutes over linear transformations). As discussed in [5], the BLUE $\hat{\tilde{\mathbf{h}}}_B$ can be derived correspondingly. The CWCU LMMSE estimator $\hat{\tilde{\mathbf{h}}}_{CL}$ cannot be derived in this way since it does

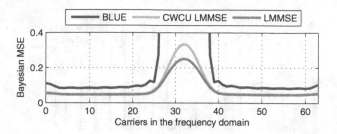

Fig. 3. Bayesian MSEs for the elements of $\hat{\tilde{\mathbf{h}}}_{\mathrm{B}}$, $\hat{\tilde{\mathbf{h}}}_{\mathrm{L}}$, and $\hat{\tilde{\mathbf{h}}}_{\mathrm{CL}}$, respectively.

not commute over general linear transformations. However, although $\tilde{\mathbf{h}}$ is not a proper Gaussian vector, $E_{\tilde{\mathbf{h}}_i|\tilde{h}_i}[\hat{\tilde{\mathbf{h}}}_i|\tilde{h}_i]$ is linear in $\tilde{h}_i$ (for all $i = 0, 1, \cdots, N-1$), and one can easily show that (16)–(18) can be applied to determine the CWCU LMMSE estimator. The frequency domain version of the prior covariance matrix $\mathbf{C_{hh}}$ is required for its derivation. Figure 3 shows the Bayesian MSEs of $\hat{\tilde{\mathbf{h}}}_{\mathrm{B}}$, $\hat{\tilde{\mathbf{h}}}_{\mathrm{L}}$, and $\hat{\tilde{\mathbf{h}}}_{\mathrm{CL}}$, respectively. $\hat{\tilde{\mathbf{h}}}_{\mathrm{B}}$ is outperformed by $\hat{\tilde{\mathbf{h}}}_{\mathrm{L}}$ and $\hat{\tilde{\mathbf{h}}}_{\mathrm{CL}}$ at all frequencies, but the performance loss is significant at the large gap from subcarrier 27 to 37, where no training information is available. In contrast, $\hat{\tilde{\mathbf{h}}}_{\mathrm{L}}$ and $\hat{\tilde{\mathbf{h}}}_{\mathrm{CL}}$ show excellent interpolation properties along this gap. Large estimation errors of $\hat{\tilde{\mathbf{h}}}_{\mathrm{B}}$ in this spectral region are spread over all time domain samples which explains the poor performance of $\hat{\mathbf{h}}_{\mathrm{B}}$. Note that in practice this is only critical if $\hat{\mathbf{h}}_{\mathrm{B}}$ is incorporated in the receiver processing, however, pure frequency domain receivers only require estimates at the occupied 52 subcarrier positions.

4   Conclusion

In this work we investigated the CWCU LMMSE estimator for the linear model. First, we derived the estimator for complex proper Gaussian parameter vectors, and for the case of mutually independent (and otherwise arbitrarily distributed) parameters. For the remaining cases the CWCU LMMSE estimator may correspond to a globally unbiased estimator. The implications of the CWCU constraints have been demonstrated in a data estimation example using a discrete alphabet, and in a channel estimation application. In both applications the CWCU LMMSE estimator considerably outperforms the globally unbiased BLUE.

References

1. Kay, S.M.: Fundamentals of Statistical Signal Processing: Estimation Theory, 1st edn. Prentice-Hall PTR, Upper Saddle River (2010)
2. Triki, M., Slock, D.T.M.: Component-wise conditionally unbiased bayesian parameter estimation: general concept and applications to kalman filtering and LMMSE channel estimation. In: Proceedings of the Asilomar Conference on Signals, Systems and Computers, Pacific Grove, USA, pp. 670–674, November 2005

3. Triki, M., Salah, A., Slock, D.T.M.: Interference cancellation with Bayesian channel models and application to TDOA/IPDL mobile positioning. In: Proceedings of the International Symposium on Signal Processing and its Applications, pp. 299–302, August 2005
4. Triki, M., Slock, D.T.M.: Investigation of some bias and MSE issues in block-component-wise conditionally unbiased LMMSE. In: Proceedings of the Asilomar Conference on Signals, Systems and Computers, Pacific Grove, USA, pp. 1420–1424, November 2006
5. Huemer, M., Lang, O.: On component-wise conditionally unbiased linear bayesian estimation. In: Proceedings of the Asilomar Conference on Signals, Systems, and Computers, Pacific Grove, USA, pp. 879–885, November 2014
6. Adali, T., Schreier, P.J., Scharf, L.L.: Complex-valued signal processing: the proper way to deal with impropriety. IEEE Trans. Sig. Process. **59**(11), 5101–5125 (2011)
7. IEEE Std 802.11a-1999, Part 11: Wireless LAN Medium Access Control (MAC) and Physical Layer (PHY) specifications: High-Speed Physical Layer in the 5 GHz Band (1999)

Model Based Design of Inductive Components - A Comparision Between Measurement and Simulation

Mario Jungwirth[1], Daniel Hofinger[1]([✉]), Alexander Eder[2],
and Günter Ritzberger[2]

[1] University of Applied Sciences Upper Austria,
Campus Wels, Stelzhamerstrasse 23, 4600 Wels, Austria
{mario.jungwirth,daniel.hofinger}@fh-wels.at
http://www.fh-ooe.at
[2] Research and Development, Fronius International GmbH,
Günter Fronius Strasse 1, 4600 Wels-Thalheim, Austria
{eder.alexander,ritzberger.guenter}@fronius.com
http://www.fronius.at

1 Introduction

Inductors are one of the main components in power electronic systems. In order to reduce the time to market of such systems, a computer aided tool for inductor design has been developed. This easy to use tool is able to predict the physical behaviour of inductors in operation and enables the designer to optimize all significant design parameters in a short time. As a best practice design example a PFC-inductor in a three-phase photovoltaic inverter is investigated. The principle design process and the relevant results are presented. To emphasis the usability of the tool, the optimized PFC-inductor is compared to calorimeter measurements regarding losses resulting in deviations less than 10 %.

2 Application Description

PFC-inductors are needed in switching mode power supplies to filter high frequency harmonics from the 50 Hz line current. A PFC-inductor is the simplest but bulkiest way for EMI filtration. The design of chokes is a trade-off between performance, costs and size. A good relation between those three aspects contributes to a proper design. The PFC-inductor under investigation is used in a 20 kW grid-connected inverter for photovoltaic systems. High efficiency of the inductors over the whole power range plays an important role in designing grid connected transformerless inverters. The customer requires as much energy output of the system as possible. Another goal is to be as cost effective as possible at a high quality level. Therefore several materials for cores and wires as well as different geometries have to be compared and analysed in terms of quality and cost. An easy handling of the inverter needs less weight of the electronic components and small parts - to be as compact as possible. An example of a photovoltaic inverter of this category can be seen in Fig. 1. In order to validate the simulation results measurements are made at different load states.

© Springer International Publishing Switzerland 2015
R. Moreno-Díaz et al. (Eds.): EUROCAST 2015, LNCS 9520, pp. 546–551, 2015.
DOI: 10.1007/978-3-319-27340-2_68

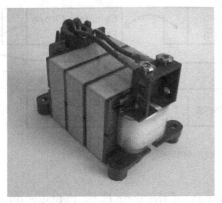
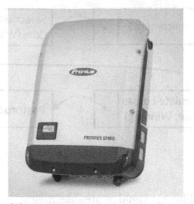

(a) PFC inductor example

(b) Modern grid connected inverter for photovoltaic systems

Fig. 1. Analyzed power electronic system (© Fronius International GmbH)

3   Modelling Process

Various contradictory design requirements and a comprehensive variety of assembly componentes make inductor design an extensive process. Existing design guide lines often remain unused, because of their complexity or simply the lack of awareness. Therefore the usual design procedure often results in trial and error method, which is time consuming and expensive. In previous publications an easy-to-use program is presented to determine proper component parameters for optimal inductor designs [1]. Main features of the program are a comprehensive database of all inductor assembly parts, a detailed calculation routine for the determination of core and winding losses, including a finite element algorithm to simulate eddy current losses in massive and litze wire windings and an extensive post processing package [2]. The design flow, depicted in Fig. 2, starts with the determination of the electric application requirement, which is followed by the choice of appropriate inductor components and ends with the calculation of all electromagnetic parameters including the prediction of powerloss and temperature rise.

The design of the PFC-choke has to fulfill the required inductance L_{nom} at a nominal current I_{nom} without saturating the magnetic core. Furthermore the temperature rise caused by the occuring power loss has to be limited to a magnitude so it doesn't exceed the parts thermal limits. After the determination of the specification, the minimum volume of the magnetic core V_{emin} and the air gap length S are selected by applying the I^2L-method. It compares the required magnetic energy E_{max} which has to be stored according to the specification with the storage capability of a certain minimal core volume V_{emin}:

$$E_{max} = \frac{1}{2}I_{nom}^2 L_{nom} = B_{sat}^2 \frac{V_{emin}}{\mu_0 \mu_e} \tag{1}$$

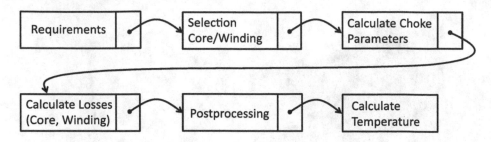

Fig. 2. Workflow and princip of the tool

The maximal storeable magnetic energy of the core E_{max} depends on the volume of the core V_{emin}, the staturation flux density B_{sat} and the effective permeability μ_e which is a function of air gap length S, core geometry and permeability of the magnetic material μ_r. In this example three C-core pairs were stacked using an amorphous material, which has high saturation flux density and reasonable power loss at the occuring switching frequency. After the core size and the air gap length are fixed, the required winding number N_{min} can be calculated from the AL-value:

$$N_{min} = ceil\left(\sqrt{\frac{L_{nom}}{AL}}\right) = ceil\left(\sqrt{\frac{L_{nom}}{\mu_e \frac{A_e}{l_e}}}\right) \tag{2}$$

For power inductors two main types of electric wires can be selected. Solid wires in round or rectangular shape are considerable cheap, but induce eddy current losses at higher frequencies and therefore smaller skin depths. Litze wires reduce eddy current losses but are more expensive. In chokes the effect of eddy current losses mainly depend on the fringing flux at the airgaps. To estimate the quantity of the effect the magnetic field destribution in the winding structure must be known. The magnetic field is described by maxwell's equations. For harmonic excitation of the magnetic field, the equations can be written into the Helmholtz equation, a linear elliptic partial differential equation (PDE):

$$\left(j\omega\sigma - \omega^2\epsilon\right)\boldsymbol{A} + \nabla \times \left(\mu^{-1}\nabla \times \boldsymbol{A} - \boldsymbol{M}\right) - \sigma\boldsymbol{v} \times \left(\nabla \times \boldsymbol{A}\right) = \boldsymbol{J}^e + j\omega\boldsymbol{P} \tag{3}$$

All magnetic quantities of interest, like the distribution of current density and power density can be derived from the magnetic vector potential $\boldsymbol{A}$, the unknown variable. The vector potential $\boldsymbol{A}$ can be solved numerical using the methode of finite elements. To model litze wire a frequency dependent complex permeability is used as described in [4]. The resulting eddy current losses for a certain type of wire offer clues on which wire is most suitable for the application. For PFC-chokes the ratio between the low frequency 50 Hz components and the high frequency components of the currents spectrum, essentially decide, if a litze wire is required. For this PFC-choke a solid rectangular copper wire was used. Simulations of four different load stages were performed. The results for the nominal load stage shows $P_{cu}/P_{total} = 75.58\,\%$ of copper losses, at which $P_{dc}/P_{total} = 31.14\,\%$

can be assigned to conventional rms power losses and $P_{ac}/P_{total} = 44.44\%$ to eddy current losses. The core losses result in $P_{core}/P_{total} = 24.42\%$. They are calculated by using a modiefied Steinmetz equation which takes into account for non-sinusoidal current waveforms [5].

4 Measurement Setup

Measuring power loss accurately is of great importance for power electronics systems designs. In general power loss can be determined by measuring electric or thermal quantities. The occurrence of high di/dt and dv/dt in switching mode power supplies introduce serious EMI problems at the measurement of electric quantities. The measurement of thermal quantities and calculating the power loss using the calorimetric method therefore is more convenient, but has other drawbacks [3]. To measure the power loss of the inductive components in power electronics applications an open type calorimeter was realized. Equation 4 is used to calculate the power loss of the device under test (DUT).

$$P_{total} = \dot{m}c_p \Delta T = \dot{m}c_p(T_{out} - T_{in}) \qquad (4)$$

Where P_{total} is the total powerloss of the DUT, $\dot{m}$ is the mass flow, c_p is the heat capacity and T the temperature of the cooling medium . The final measurement setup is shown in Fig. 3b.

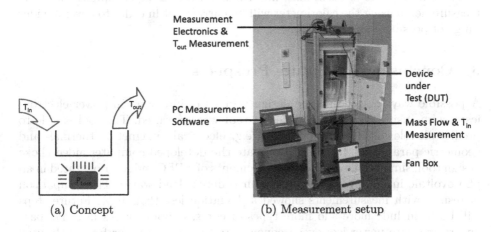

(a) Concept   (b) Measurement setup

Fig. 3. Concept and setup of an open type calorimeter

The inflow is generated by a radial fan and heated to serveral degrees above ambient temperature to prevent temperature fluctuation of the air stream. The mass flow rate and the temperature of the air stream are measured by sensors at the inlet. The DUT is operated in a thermally insulated box. To minimise thermal conduction through the box walls active heat flux compensation is done by heating the outer walls of the insulation to the temperature of the inner walls. The temperature of the airstream is then measured again at the outlet. The accuracy of the measurement setup relies on the one hand on the precision of the sensors and on the other hand on the actual amount of heat, which is transfered into the air stream and is not lost by thermal conduction through the box walls or connectors of the DUT. For DUTs producing low power losses the relative measurement error is around 10 % of the true value. The accuracy is better at higher power losses resulting in higher mass flow rates, where the measurement error is below 5 %. The detectable power loss of the DUT ranges from $10W$ to $150W$. The measurement of the PFC-choke at the same load conditions resulted in a measured power of $P_{measure}/P_{total} = 92.72\%$ of simulated total power loss.

5 Comparison Between Measurement and Simulation

In order to take advantage of the computer aided tool for inductor design confidence in simulation results has to be established. Therefore, the simulation results were verified using an open type calorimeter as described in Chap. 4. An overall deviation less than 10 % was identified. Depending on the point of operation the deviation is below 5 %. This can be explained by simplifications made in the finite element simulation or by the fact, that a certain amount of the measured total heat is not dissipated through the cooling medium, but by thermal conduction through the test chamber housing which is comparatively lower for high power losses or mass flow rates. Further design examples including measurements using the calorimeter will be carried out in order to cover a wider range of possible inductor designs.

6 Conclusion and Future Prospects

A possible way to speed-up the design process of inductors in power electronics systems using an automated design tool was presented. The tool is able to predict all relevant design parameters, e.g. electrical-, magnetic-, thermal- and geometric parameters. In order to validate the developed computer aided choke design tool, simulations and loss-measurements of a PFC-inductor operated in an photovoltaic inverter where made at four different load states. The comparison of results with measurements showed a deviation less than 10 %. Future steps will be to include more and more types of cores, bobbins, wires in a database and to measure power-loss over frequency and temperature for frequently used core-materials.

References

1. Weinzierl, H., Hofinger, D., Jungwirth, M.: Automated modeling of inductive power electronic components. In: Computer Aided Systems Theory – EUROCAST 2013 (2013)
2. Rossmanith, H., Manfred, A., Janina, P., Alexander, S.: Improved characterization of the magnetic properties of hexagonally packed wires. In: Proceedings of the 2011–14th European Conference on Power Electronics and Applications (EPE 2011) (2011)
3. Xiao, C., Chen, G., Odendaal, W.G.H.: Overview of power loss measurement techniques in power electronics systems. IEEE Trans. Ind. Appl. **43**(3), 657–664 (2007)
4. Stadler, A., Gulden, C.: Copper losses of litz-wire windings due to an air gap. In: 15th European Conference on Power Electronics and Applications, EPE 2013 ECCE Europe (2013)
5. Reinert, J., Brockmeyer, A., De Doncker, R.W.: Calculation of losses in ferro- and ferrimagnetic materials based on the modified Steinmetz equation. IEEE Trans. Ind. Appl. **37**, 1055–106 (2001)

Model-Based System Design, Verification and Simulation

Dynamic Validation of Contracts in Concurrent Code

Jan Fiedor[1]([✉]), Zdeněk Letko[1], João Lourenço[2], and Tomáš Vojnar[1]

[1] FIT, IT4Innovations Centre of Excellence,
Brno University of Technology, Brno, Czech Republic
{ifiedor,iletko,vojnar}@fit.vutbr.cz
[2] NOVA LINCS, Department de Informática,
FCT – Universidade Nova de Lisboa, Almada, Portugal
joao.lourenco@fct.unl.pt

Abstract. Multi-threaded programs allow one to achieve better performance by doing a lot of work in parallel using multiple threads. Such parallel programs often contain code blocks that a thread must execute atomically, i.e., with no interference from the other threads of the program. Failing to execute these code blocks atomically leads to errors known as atomicity violations. However, frequently it not obvious to tell when a piece of code should be executed atomically, especially when that piece of code contains calls to some third-party library functions, about which the programmer has little or no knowledge at all. One solution to this problem is to associate a contract with such a library, telling the programmer how the library functions should be used, and then check whether the contract is indeed respected. For contract validation, static approaches have been proposed, with known limitations on precision and scalability. In this paper, we propose a dynamic method for contract validation, which is more precise and scalable than static approaches.

1 Introduction

With multi-core processors present in all the newest computers, multi-threaded programs are becoming increasingly common. However, multi-threaded programs require proper synchronisation to restrict the thread interleavings and make the program produce correct results. Failing to do so often leads to various critical errors, which occur under some very specific timing scenarios only, and standard testing and debugging techniques are less effective or even useless for their detection.

Atomicity violations are a class of errors which result from an incorrect definition of the scope of an atomic region. Such errors are usually hard to localise and diagnose, which becomes even harder when using (third-party) software libraries where it is unknown to the programmer how to form the atomic regions correctly when accessing the library. Even new synchronisation techniques, such as transactional memories, designed to ease the process of writing concurrent programs, do not entirely avoid this problem and suffer from atomicity violations as well [3].

© Springer International Publishing Switzerland 2015
R. Moreno-Díaz et al. (Eds.): EUROCAST 2015, LNCS 9520, pp. 555–564, 2015.
DOI: 10.1007/978-3-319-27340-2_69

One way to address the problem of proper atomicity is to associate a *contract* with each program module/library and then check whether the contract is indeed respected. In fact, the notion of contract is, in general, not restricted to concurrent programs. In the general case, a contract [8] regulates the use of methods of an object by specifying a set of pre-conditions the program must meet before calling the object methods. For the particular case of concurrent programs, Sousa et al. proposed in [10] the concept of the so-called *contracts for concurrency*. A contract for concurrency contains a set of clauses where each clause defines a (finite) set of sequences of method calls that must be executed atomically whenever they are executed on the same object. Contract clauses may be written by the software module/library developer or inferred automatically from the program (based on its typical usage patterns) [10].

In this paper, assuming that the appropriate contracts for concurrency have been obtained, we propose a method for dynamically verifying that such contracts are respected at program run time. In particular, our method belongs among the so-called *lockset-based* dynamic analyses whose classic example is the Eraser algorithm for data race detection [9] and whose common feature is that they track sets of locks that are held by various threads and used for various synchronization purposes. The tracked lock sets are used to extrapolate the synchronization behaviour seen in the witnessed test runs, allowing one to warn about possible errors even when they do not directly appear in the witnessed test runs. We have implemented our approach in a prototype tool, and we present some encouraging experimental results obtained with our implementation.

2   Related Work

A notion of *contract* was first introduced by Meyer [8] in 1992 as a sequence of tasks (commands) with defined pre- and post-conditions. If this sequence was executed without meeting these conditions, the contract was violated. Contracts in the form of regular expressions were used to specify protocols for accessing objects in sequential [1] as well as concurrent scenarios [2,7,10]. Hurlin in [7] proposes a technique to validate the correctness of contracts by checking contracts on a set of artificially generated programs that use a particular object. Both Demeyer in [2] and Sousa in [10] propose to use a static approach to address the contract validation.

The static approaches of [2,10] can formally prove that no contract violation is possible. For that, however, they assume that properly handled contracts must appear in code blocks declared as atomic (with the atomicity assured by the runtime support). If a different way of guarding the contracts is used, a false alarm is issued. Moreover, the approaches scale to relatively small programs only. For more complex programs, one has to restrict the analysis to program fragments, e.g., individual methods, in order to achieve a reasonable performance. This leads to a loss of precision as contracts may span across several methods and thus be missed by the analysis.

Another problem with the static approach is related to the fact that contracts for concurrency are required to operate atomically only when all the involved method calls operate on the same object. This is a natural requirement since the atomic execution is critical only when working with data elements that are mutually related, which is assumed to be reflected in that they are stored within one object. However, static validation does not have precise information on which objects the methods are called on. Hence, calls of methods on different objects are mixed together, leading to possible false alarms. Classic alias and escape analyses can be used to infer this information from the source code of the program, but these analyses provide only approximate information and may still lead to false alarms.

Our dynamic approach of contract validation avoids the above false alarms since it has precise run-time information about the objects that particular methods are executed on. Moreover, it also scales quite well. On the other hand, despite the lockset-based method that we use extrapolates to some degree the behaviour of the witnessed test runs, our approach can miss some contract violations that do not happen in the witnessed test runs nor they can be deduced from the locking patterns used in these traces. In order to minimize the number of possibly missed contract violations, one can combine our approach with *noise injection* techniques [6] that maximize the number of thread interleavings witnessed in a set of test runs.

3   Contracts for Concurrency

A *contract for concurrency* [10] (or simply *contract* herein) is a protocol for accessing the public services of a module, i.e., the methods of its public API, in a concurrent setting. Each module shall have its own contract, which contains one or more sequences of tasks (methods). The condition to be met here is that the sequences of methods must be executed atomically whenever executed on the same object.

Formally, let Σ_c be a set of all public method names (API) of a module (or library). A *contract* is a set S of *clauses* where each clause $s \in S$ is a star-free regular expression over Σ_c. A contract is violated if any of the sequences represented by the contract is not executed atomically when executed on the same object o, meaning that it is interleaved with an execution of some method from Σ_c on the object o.

4   Dynamic Validation of Contracts

In order to detect atomicity violations in more complex programs and to reduce the number of false alarms, we propose a dynamic approach to check whether a contract is violated or not. Our dynamic validation looks for contract violations based on concrete program executions. Possible violations not witnessed during the execution of the program may be missed, but all of the methods encountered during the execution are taken into account, and so contract violations caused by method calls from all over the program are detected. Since all of the threads are running and all objects are known when the program is executing, we know precisely whether all of the methods called in a sequence use the same object, and we do not report any false alarms due to mixing calls on different objects as is common in static analysis.

Since we look for contract violations based on concrete executions, we can avoid some false alarms, but on the other hand, we can miss some errors. In order to minimise this possibility, we employ one of the dynamic analysis techniques—namely, the *lock sets* [9]—to extrapolate the actually witnessed behaviour and hence detect possible contract violations even when they were not actually witnessed. Moreover, we utilise noise injection techniques [6] to enforce synchronisation scenarios, which normally appear only rarely, leading to behaviours (and possibly contract violations) that would not be covered by extrapolation of the common synchronisation scenarios only.

4.1 Detection of Contracts

In order to validate a contract, we first need to detect the sequences it contains in the execution of a program. To do that, we encode each contract, i.e., all of its sequences, as a single finite state automaton. As each clause of the contract represents a regular expression, we use standard methods for transforming (star-free) regular expressions[1] into finite automata to perform the conversion and then merge all these automata into a single one. The transitions of the automaton represent method calls and the accepting states represent situations where a contract sequence was detected.

Each thread manages a list of finite state automata instances which represent the currently encountered incomplete contract sequences. Whenever a method $m \in \Sigma_c$ is encountered, we try to advance each of these instances using the method m. If we cannot advance the instance, the contract sequence is invalid and we discard it. If we successfully advanced the instance to the next state, call it q, we check if q is an accepting state. If yes, a contract sequence is detected; if not, we leave the instance in q and go on. Moreover, we check if we can advance any of the finite state automata from their starting state using the method m. If yes, then the beginning of another contract sequence was detected and we create a new instance of the automaton which will monitor the execution of this contract sequence to check if it can be accepted or not.

4.2 Checking the Atomicity Condition

When a contract sequence is detected, the next step is to check if the atomicity condition is met, i.e., if the program ensures that all methods of this contract sequence are executed atomically. The static approach does this by checking if all of the methods of the detected contract sequence are enclosed in code blocks declared as atomic, which can be done by analysing the source code of the program.

---

[1] Star-free regular expressions are used in the static contract validation approach [10]. We can, however, easily generalize our approach to general regular expressions.

We propose a lockset-based method, inspired by [9], to perform these checks which is more suited for dynamic analysis. This method checks if at least one lock is held during the execution of a contract sequence by monitoring the lock acquisitions and releases during the execution of a contract sequence. If this condition is not satisfied, i.e., no locks are held throughout the execution, then the contract is being violated.

The method works online, i.e., it performs the contract validation during the execution of a program, and is based on the analysis state $\sigma = (A, H, R)$ where:

- $A : T \to 2^L$ records the set of locks acquired by a thread.
- $H : T \times S \to 2^L$ records the set of locks held by a thread when a contract sequence starts.
- $R : T \times S \to 2^L$ records the set of locks released by a thread during the execution of a contract sequence.

In the initial analysis state, all sets of locks are empty, reflecting that at the beginning of the execution, no locks are held by any thread, i.e., $\sigma_0 = (\emptyset, \emptyset, \emptyset)$. Figure 1 shows rules according to which the analysis state is updated for each operation of the target program.

The rule [CONTRACT SEQUENCE START] records that a thread t is starting an execution of a contract sequence s by remembering the locks which are currently held by the thread. It also clears the set of locks released by the thread as no locks could have been released yet.

The rule [CONTRACT SEQUENCE END] records that a contract sequence s was detected in a thread t and checks the atomicity condition by comparing the set of locks held when the contract sequence started its execution with the set of locks released during its execution. If at least one lock was held all the time the contract sequence was executed, the contract is valid, and no error is issued. If all locks held at the beginning of the execution of the contract sequence were released before its execution finished, a contract violation is reported.

The rule [LOCK ACQUIRED] records that a thread t acquired a lock m, and it updates the set of locks currently acquired by this thread. Finally, the rule [LOCK RELEASED] records that a thread t released a lock m, and it updates the set of locks released by the thread for each contract sequence currently executed by this thread.

[CONTRACT SEQUENCE START]
$$H' := H_t[s := A_t]$$
$$R' := R_t[s := \emptyset]$$
$$\frac{}{(A, H, R) \Rightarrow^{seq\_start(t,s)} (A, H', R')}$$

[CONTRACT SEQUENCE END]
$$\mathbf{if}\ H_t(s) \setminus R_t(s) = \emptyset\ \mathbf{then}\ \text{ERROR}$$
$$\frac{}{(A, H, R) \Rightarrow^{seq\_end(t,s)} (A, H, R)}$$

[LOCK ACQUIRED]
$$A' := A[t := A_t \cup \{m\}]$$
$$\frac{}{(A, H, R) \Rightarrow^{acq(t,m)} (A', H, R)}$$

[LOCK RELEASED]
$$\forall s \in S : R' := R_t[s := R_t(s) \cup \{m\}]$$
$$\frac{}{(A, H, R) \Rightarrow^{rel(t,m)} (A, H, R')}$$

Fig. 1. Analysis rules.

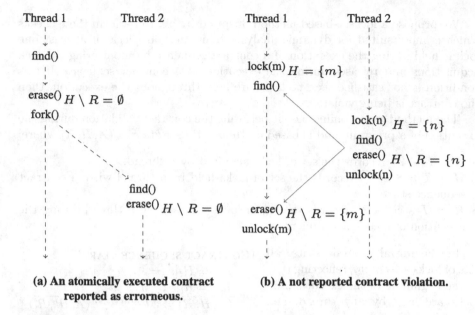

(a) An atomically executed contract
    reported as errorneous.

(b) A not reported contract violation.

Fig. 2. Examples of situations where the contract validation fails.

4.3 Discussion of the Proposed Approach

The above method may produce both false positives (i.e., false alarms) as well
as false negatives. False positives may be caused by the fact that not guarding
an execution of a contract sequence with a single lock throughout its entire
duration does not mean that it will not be executed atomically. Take the situation
shown in Fig. 2(a) as an example. Not a single one of the contract sequences is
guarded by a lock, yet there is no contract violation as the synchronisation
ensures that the contract sequence in Thread 1 is always executed before the
contract sequence in Thread 2. Therefore there is no interference between these
two contract sequences, and hence no contract violation. Yet the method reports
both of the contract sequences being violated.

False negatives may happen since holding a lock when executing a contract
sequence does not always ensure that no other thread interferes with it. Take the
situation in Fig. 2(b) as an example. The executions of the contract sequence in
both Thread 1 and Thread 2 are guarded by a lock. However, these locks are
different and thus the execution of the contract sequence in Thread 1 may be
interleaved with the execution of the contract sequence in Thread 2, violating
the contract sequence in Thread 1. Yet the method does not report any error.

To solve the above problems, we need to take into account thread interleavings. When guarding the same contract sequence with two different locks in two
different threads, we should issue an error only when these two threads may inter-
leave each other. Conversely, when a contract sequence is not guarded by a lock,
we should report an error only when this thread may be interleaved by another

thread executing the same contract sequence. When using the static approach, this information is hard to obtain as one would need to infer it from the source code of the program where the scheduling of threads is unknown. On the other hand, the dynamic approach actually sees the concrete thread interleavings, and so it is easier to get the needed information. Unfortunately, the lockset method does not work with it in any way. Moreover, incorporating this information into the lockset method would be counterproductive as it would kill the extrapolation which increases chances to detect errors. A way to go here seems to be a use of dynamic analysis based on the *happens-before relation* as used, e.g., in the GoldiLock data race detector [5], which is a part of our future work.

5   Experiments

This section presents an experimental comparison of the proposed dynamic validation of contracts with the static approach of [10]. To compare the approaches, we implemented the method described in Sect. 4 as a plug-in for the IBM Concurrency Testing Tool (ConTest) [4]. The ConTest infrastructure provides a fully automatic Java byte-code instrumentation and a listeners architecture that facilitated the implementation of the proposed method as well as execution and dynamic analysis of the benchmarks.

The comparison of the static and dynamic approaches is done using a subset of the small benchmark programs which were previously used to evaluate the static approach [10], namely, the Account, Allocate Vector, Arithmetic DB, Jigsaw, Store, and Vector fail test cases. All these benchmark programs had to be slightly modified in order to allow us to execute them and use ConTest to analyse their runs. Namely, we did the following modifications by hand: (1) test arguments were provided if missing; (2) infinite loops (which are not a problem for the static approach, but cannot be present during a dynamic analysis) were transformed to finite loops with a small number of iterations to avoid infinite executions; (3) exceptions generation and handling (commented out due to limits of the static approach) were uncommented; (4) the `Atomic` annotations preferred by the static approach were turned back to `synchronized` blocks; and (5) all assertions and correctness checks already present in the test cases were extended to send notifications to our ConTest plug-in. The dynamic analysis tests were executed on a Linux machine with an i5-4200M CPU (i.e., comparable with the machine used to evaluate the static approach in [10]), running Linux 3.16, and OpenJDK 1.6 JVM.

Table 1 summarises results of the comparison between our dynamic approach and the static approach of [10]. The table is divided into three sections. In the leftmost part, basic characteristics of the benchmark programs are provided. In particular, the test case name, the number of effective lines of the original Java code (without our modifications, which added only a few extra lines of code), and the number of contract clauses for the benchmark program as manually identified by the authors of the static approach.

Table 1. An experimental comparison of static and dynamic contract validation.

Program			Static analysis			Dynamic analysis		
Benchmark	LOC	Contract clauses	Duration (sec.)	CFG nodes	Detected violations	Duration (sec.)	Detected violations	Failed assertions
Account	68	2	0,041	158	2	0,011	2	0,96
Allocate vector	167	1	0,120	882	1	0,099	1	0,00
Arithmetic DB	325	2	0,272	2256	2	0,010	2	0,06
Jigsaw	147	1	0,044	125	1	0,009	1	0,44
Store	769	1	0,090	559	1	0,303	1	1,00
VectorFail	100	2	0,048	244	2	0,009	2	0,09

The middle part of Table 1 characterizes results of the static analysis obtained in [10]. Namely, the average analysis duration in seconds is provided with the number of control flow graph (CFG) nodes generated and processed. Finally, the number of detected violations of contract clauses for each benchmark program is shown.

The rightmost part of the table shows the average results (from 1000 test executions) obtained with our dynamic approach. In particular, the average execution time of the instrumented test in seconds is provided, followed by the average number of detected violations of contract clauses. Finally, the average ratio of failed assertions (usually implemented as conditions checking memory consistency) provided by the authors of the tests is reported. The standard deviations of the execution times as well as failed assertions were quite low. The standard deviation of the number of violated contract was zero (i.e., the algorithm always detected all the violations).

Concerning both the considered static as well as dynamic approach, there are two interesting aspects we would like to emphasize: (i) the ability of both approaches to detect contract violations; and (ii) the very low execution time taken by both approaches (of course, a further evaluation on larger test cases remains to be done).

In both approaches, all violations were *always* correctly reported. Such a good result of the dynamic approach depends on the quality of the test that executes the problematic part of the code and on the ability of the lockset approach to extrapolate other behaviours from the witnessed execution, and therefore to detect possible violations even from executions where the problem did not occur. This can, in particular, be demonstrated on the Allocate Vector, Arithmetic DB, and VectorFail benchmark programs where the assertion-based detection reported the problem in less than 10 % of executions while the dynamic approach always detected a possible violation.

Let us now get back to the time consumed by the analyses. In both cases, the analysis itself took less than one second for the considered simple test programs. However, there was a significant difference in the overhead of the underlying infrastructures. The initialisation of the static approach within the Soot analysis environment [10] took nearly 40 s for each benchmark. The dynamic approach was much faster. The bytecode instrumentation took about 0.5 s. The slowdown of the test execution was within 5 % because only the *method entry* and *lock operation* events were instrumented (i.e., most of the code was executed with no instrumentation and hence no overhead).

6 Conclusion

We presented a method for dynamic validation of contracts in concurrent code. When compared with previously proposed static approaches, our approach can suppress some of the false alarms produced by these approaches, and it is also more scalable. Since we build on observing concrete runs, our approach can miss some errors that would not be missed by static analysis. To detect as many contract violations as possible, our approach employs a lockset-based extrapolation of the synchronization behaviour observed in performed test runs, which allows the method to warn about possible contract violations even when they were not seen in a concrete execution. Moreover, noise injection may be used to increase the number of observed thread interleavings, and hence chances to see interleavings containing a contract violation or at least symptoms that such a violation is possible.

The extrapolation we use can suffer from both false positives and negatives due to the fact that the lockset method used does not utilise any information about thread interleavings. In order to solve this problem, we plan to use extrapolation methods based on the happens-before relations, which do reflect thread interleavings. Another interesting subject for future work is then generalization of the notion of contracts (e.g., by considering full regular expressions), exploiting the fact that such generalizations seem to be much easier in the context of dynamic analysis.

Acknowledgements. This work was supported by the ESF COST Action IC1001 (Euro-TM), the COST project LD14001 and the Kontakt II project LH13265 of the Czech ministry of education, the BUT project FIT-S-14-2486, the EU/Czech IT4Innovations Centre of Excellence project CZ.1.05/1.1.00/02.0070, the EU/Czech Interdisciplinary Excellence Research Teams Establishment project CZ.1.07/2.3.00/30.0005, and the Portuguese National Science Foundation in the strategic project FCT/MEC NOVA LINCS PEst UID/CEC/04516/2013.

References

1. Cheon, Y., Perumandla, A.: Specifying and checking method call sequences of java programs. Softw. Qual. Control **15**(1), 7–25 (2007)
2. Demeyer, R., Vanhoof, W.: Static application-level race detection in STM haskell using contracts. In: Proceedings of PLACCES. Open Publishing Association (2013)
3. Dias, R.J., Pessanha, V., Lourenço, J.M.: Precise detection of atomicity violations. In: Biere, A., Nahir, A., Vos, T. (eds.) HVC. LNCS, vol. 7857, pp. 8–23. Springer, Heidelberg (2013)

4. Edelstein, O., Farchi, E., Goldin, E., Nir, Y., Ratsaby, G., Ur, S.: Framework for testing multi-threaded java programs. Concurrency Comput. Pract. Experience **15**(3–5), 485–499 (2003)
5. Elmas, T., Qadeer, S., Tasiran, S.: Goldilocks: a race and transaction-aware java runtime. In: Proceedings of PLDI 2007. ACM (2007)
6. Fiedor, J., Hrubá, V., Křena, B., Letko, Z., Ur, S., Vojnar, T.: Advances in noise-based testing. STVR **24**(7), 1–38 (2014)
7. Hurlin, C.: Specifying and checking protocols of multithreaded classes. In: Proceedings of SAC 2009, pp. 587–592. ACM (2009)
8. Meyer, B.: Applying "design by contract". Computer **25**(10), 40–51 (1992)
9. Savage, S., Burrows, M., Nelson, G., Sobalvarro, P., Anderson, T.: Eraser: a dynamic data race detector for multi-threaded programs. In: Proceedings of SOSP 1997. ACM (1997)
10. Sousa, D.G., Dias, R.J., Ferreira, C., Lourenço, J.M.: Preventing atomicity violations with contracts. eprint arXiv:1505.02951, May 2015

Formal Modeling of a Client-Middleware Interaction System Regarding Content and Layout Adaptation

Roxana-Maria Holom(✉)

Christian-Doppler Laboratory for Client-Centric Cloud Computing Hagenberg,
Johannes Kepler University Linz, Linz, Austria
r.holom@cdcc.faw.jku.at

Abstract. In the context of Cloud services, a typical architecture of a Cloud system presumes the interaction with various end-devices. A well founded Cloud system should guarantee that its clients are able to access the same Cloud service from any kind of device (s)he is using, and that (s)he will receive the same output independently of the used device. Due to this problem and to the lack of formal modeling in Cloud Computing and Web development we decided to use ASMs for the specification and analysis of a client-Cloud interaction system to prove that the device information discovery is reliable and correct.

1 Introduction

Mobile cloud computing is emerging as an important trend in the software computing domain. In this context, a cloud service can be invoked by distinct devices having different characteristics; therefore, the content should be adapted to each device profile. Our solution proposes a Web application as an access point for the cloud services. Only content delivery without layout and content adaptation will not be a solution for mobile devices, because most of the web content is designed for desktop computers. To manage this problem, we present the formal model and analysis of an *adaptivity component* as part of a middleware application, that deals with the collection of device data necessary for the on-the-fly adaptation of cloud services. We focus on the simulation and verification as to ensure that the discovery of the device information is reliable and correct.

In [7] we initially proposed a rigorous model of the middleware based on *Abstract State Machines (ASMs)* [4] and we continued this work in [3] by fully exploiting the capabilities of ASMs as formal rigorous system engineering approach to develop correct distributed applications. We started with ASMs high-level models and produced detailed models in *ASMETA (ASM mETAmodeling)* framework[1] [2] by using the ASM refinement method. The proposed system tackles the adaptation problem by detecting the device properties, which are afterwards used on the server-side to modify the answers coming from cloud.

---

[1] http://asmeta.sourceforge.net/.

© Springer International Publishing Switzerland 2015
R. Moreno-Díaz et al. (Eds.): EUROCAST 2015, LNCS 9520, pp. 565–572, 2015.
DOI: 10.1007/978-3-319-27340-2_70

Each web page is parsed and modified corresponding to the device properties before displaying. The detection of properties is done using the *Modernizr* framework[2]. JavaScript tests are executed on client-side and the result is used by the *adaptivity* component on server-side to create a *device profile*. Such profile is used to adapt the content coming from the cloud that finally can be forwarded to the client. Our main motivation is to be able to automatically validate and verify the described framework.

The reminder of this paper is organized as follows: Sect. 2 discusses briefly about ASMs and the tools used for model checking the ASM models, Sect. 3 presents the Client-Cloud Adaptivity Component, from requirements to ASM models and ending with their validation and verification, and Sect. 4 concludes this paper and mentions some future work ideas.

2   Background

The ASM method [4] is a system engineering technique that leads the development process from requirements capture to implementation by using *stepwise-refinement* in an incremental design. We use *control state ASMs*, which are an extended form of finite state machines, to create the *ground models* of our specification, because they provide synchronous and asynchronous parallelism, which makes them suitable for the design of distributed systems. We take advantage of the validation and verification capabilities that ASMs offer by translating the control states ASMs to ASMETA framework and use its tools to automatically simulate and model check the specification.

ASM model validation is possible by means of the model simulator `AsmetaS` [8] (as shown in Subsect. 3.3). Further validation techniques are: building and executing scenarios of expected system behaviors with the validator `AsmetaV` [6] and by using *model review* validation technique to determine if a model has sufficient quality attributes. Validation precedes the formal analysis of the requirements and the verification of properties, which is possible by employing the model checker `AsmetaSMV` [1] (see Subsect. 3.4).

3   Client-Cloud Adaptivity Component

To deal with the lack of client-orientation and the lack of formal specifications of the Cloud software solutions, our research group came up with a *Client-Cloud Interaction Middleware (CCIM)* [5] that manages the interaction between the clients and the Cloud services owners. The CCIM contains various components, that are designed in a loosely coupled way. The *adaptivity component* [3,5] provides on-the-fly adaptivity of Cloud applications to different devices (e.g., smartphones, tablets, laptops) and environment. The following key objectives have been defined by the problem of making Cloud services usable to different end-devices, in presence of device fragmentation and variety of operating systems:

---

[2] http://modernizr.com/.

develop a prototype where Cloud services are adapted on-the-fly to various channels and end-devices without the need to install any extra tool (without providing different solutions for each type of device), describe the client-Cloud interaction by using a formal modeling approach, analyze the process of collection of device data necessary for the content and layout adaptation of cloud services, and prove (model checking of application's dependent and independent properties) that the high-level specifications are correct w.r.t. the requirements.

In this paper we focus on the formal specification of the *adaptivity* component and its communication with the clients, particularly on the formal validation and verification of the process of collection device data necessary for the content and layout adaptation of Cloud services.

3.1   Requirements Elicitation

The first step to be done in a development process is the requirements specification, which is also the starting point for our work. They are afterwards captured by the ASM ground models, in this way simplifying the transition from informal (natural-language) to formal (mathematical) representations. The requirements for the device information discovery were defined based on the key objectives mentioned previously and are displayed below:

1. A client initiates the communication with the Cloud by sending a request from its device.
2. The middleware intercepts the request and searches for the device information locally on the server.
3. If the necessary information is not available, the middleware sends a request to the device asking for the needed information.
4. If the device profile exists locally, the middleware still sends a request to the device asking for the information of the properties that are possible to change over time (e.g.: with a system update).
5. The client executes the code received from the middleware and sends back a response.
6. The middleware forwards the client's request to the Cloud and saves the *device profile* (a device profile contains information about the properties of the device, e.g., screen's width, audio/video format support, touch, etc.) in the local database.
7. The answer coming from the Cloud is intercepted by the middleware and processed.
8. The content and layout of the Cloud's answer are adapted by the middleware in accordance with the device profile.
9. The middleware sends the Cloud's answer (after processing it) to the client's device.
10. The client's device displays the message.

3.2   Formal Specification Using ASMs and ASMETA

This subsection introduces the *(control state) ASM ground model* of one of the ASM agents complying the requirements presented in Subsect. 3.1. To offer the possibility to automatically validate and verify the specification, the ASM ground models were translated into *Asmeta Language (AsmetaL)* models.

ASM Ground Models. The initial version published in [7] was later on improved in [3] by correcting the mistakes found and the models were refined into more detailed ones. The client-middleware-Cloud interaction is best designed by a multi-agent ASM composed of a family of agents of type *device*, owned by the clients, an agent of type *middleware*, and a family of runtime created agents of type *request handler*, one for each new client request. As in the previous work, the specification of Cloud-side is left abstract. In the current work we show a refined version of the *request handler* agent presented in Fig. 1 and its behavior is explained below. The (control state) ASM ground models of the client and of the middleware and their explanation are available in [3].

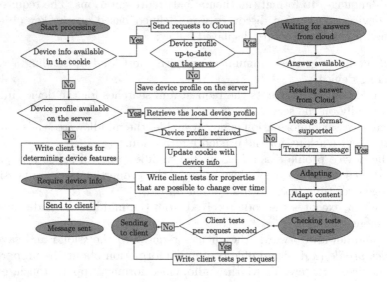

Fig. 1. Request handler - control state ASM ground model

The client initiates the communication process by selecting a Cloud service from the list filtered based on its credentials. The *adaptivity component* intervenes in the client-Cloud communication (without the awareness of the client) to gather information about client's device and to create a *device profile* stored in a local database. To discover the value of the device properties Modernizr framework is used, i.e. JavaScript tests are created. These tests are sent to the device to be executed and their result is sent back to the *adaptivity* component using the cookie. Only after the device information is available on the server-side, the *adaptivity* component forwards the client's request to the Cloud. The device profile is used to adapt the content of the answer coming from the Cloud, which is afterwards sent to the client. For generating different image and video formats third party tools are used. Only one communication round for each device was model checked (the process finishes when the client receives the adapted answer and displays it), because the device information gathering happens in the initial phase of the communication.

The control state ASM ground model in Fig. 1 describes the behavior of the *request handler* agent. This model relates what happens with a client's request on the server and how it is used by the adaptivity component to produce the device profile. The agent goes through various states from the initial state *Start processing* until it reaches the final state *Message sent*. Two guards are used to verify if the device information is either available in the cookie or on the server. If the information is not available, Modernizr tests are created in JavaScript, and the state of the request handler is updated to *Require device info*. The request containing the tests is returned to the client (the agent reaches the final state) for executing the JavaScript code and updating the device information in the cookie. The actions happening after the device profile is retrieved from the local database are part of the refinement applied to this control state. While the extracted device information is copied in the cookie, Modernizr is used to create JavaScript tests for the device properties that are possible to change over time (performing a system update could change the values of some device properties or new features could be included: e.g., new image/video formats or new location detection capabilities could be supported), which are afterwards sent to the device to be executed and the cookie will be in this way also updated. If the information is not available in the local database, then it is copied from the cookie. By sending the request to the Cloud the agent also reaches the state *Waiting for answers from cloud*. For each answer that returns from the Cloud, the handler agent verifies whether the device accepts the format and transforms it if necessary. After adapting the content, the agent checks if "tests per request" are necessary. If so, the corresponding JavaScript tests are generated and the agent goes to the *Sending to client* state. The message is sent and the *request handler* reaches the final state.

ASM Models in AsmetaL. To be able to validate and verify the specification, the graphical notation of the control state ASM is translated to the textual notation used in ASMETA, called AsmetaL. Each action, reported with a rectangle in Fig. 1, becomes a rule in the AsmetaL code. The AsmetaL encoding of a multi-agent ASMs requires the definition of at least one *main ASM* that imports all the *ASM modules* and, in its main rule, schedules all the other agents. For the client-adaptivity component interaction resulted five modules and one main ASM. Two modules represent the description and the actions of the *device* agents and another two the description and the actions of the *middleware* agent and of the *request handler* agents. One module contains the signature to model the process of message exchange between clients and adaptivity component. The main ASM of the multi-agent AsmetaL model is called `Mediator` and it is responsible for delivering messages among the other agents. We describe below the modules that represent the control state ASMs of the *middleware* and of the *request handler* shown in Fig. 1.

```
module IServer
signature:
    domain Middleware subsetof Agent
    dynamic domain ReqHandler subsetof Agent
    static middleware: Middleware
```

Code 1.1. IServer module

`IServer` module shown in Code 1.1 contains only the part of the signature that is accessed by other modules. We have two declarations of agent domains on the server-side, because there are two different types of agents: `Middleware` and `ReqHandler`. The agents of type `ReqHandler` are generated at runtime (inside the `Server` module as shown in Code 1.2) by the unique `middleware` agent.

```
module Server
import IServer
    ...
signature:
    enum domain MiddlewareState = {WAITING_REQUESTS}
    enum domain RequestHandlerState = {START_PROCESSING | REQ_DEVICE_INFO |
        WAITING_FROM_CLOUD | READING_ANSW_FROM_CLOUD | ADAPTING |
        CHECKING_CLIENT_TESTS_REQ | SENDING_TO_CLIENT | MSG_SENT}
    controlled mState: Middleware −> MiddlewareState
    controlled reqHandlerState: ReqHandler −> RequestHandlerState
    ...
definitions:
    ...
    rule r_WriteClientTests ($rh in ReqHandler) =
        extend Message with $ct do
            clientTests($rh) := $ct
    rule r_Send($d in Device, $mt in MessageType, $initReq in Message, $ans in Message) =
        outboxServer($d) := ($mt, $initReq, $ans)
    rule r_ProcessRequest = //Behavior of the request handler agent
    rule r ReceiveRequest = //Behavior of the middleware agent
        ...
        forall $d in Device do
            choose $dr in deviceRequests($d) with true do
                if isUndef(second($dr)) then
                    extend ReqHandler with $reqH do
                        ...
                endif
        forall $rh in ReqHandler with reqHandlerState($rh) != MSG_SENT do program($rh)
```

Code 1.2. Server module

Because of lack of space module `Server` is only partially shown in Code 1.2. Inside the signature part, the declared domains represent the states of the *middleware* agent and, respectively, of a *request handler* agent. The signature continues by specifying all the functions necessary for the flow of the two agents. The definitions part contains the body of the functions and of the rules. Rule `r_ReceiveRequest` describes the behavior of the *middleware* agent: for each new request a *request handler* agent is created and the existing *request handler* agents are awaken to finish their job. Rule `r_ProcessRequest` represents the behavior of the *request handler* agent and it invokes all the other rules available in the definitions part.

3.3   Validation

To prove that the specification correctly captured the intended behavior we used AsmetaS simulator to automatically validate the ASM models. Figure 2 shows an excerpt of a simulation's result. We can observe that in state 3 a *request handler* is created for the request sent by device1. By using the result of the simulation we can follow the execution flow and check if the desired actions were executed correctly. Moreover, the simulator performs *consistent updates checking* to examine that all the updates are consistent. When an *inconsistent update* is discovered, the simulation stops with the message saying which location was updated to two different values at the same time.

```
<State 1 (controlled)>
Device={device1}
Message={Message!1}
deviceRequests(device1)={}
...
</State 1 (controlled)>
...
<State 3 (controlled)>
...
Message={Message!1}
ReqHandler={ReqHandler!1}
deviceRequests(device1)={(Message!1,ReqHandler!1,undef)}
...
</State 3 (controlled)>
...
```

Fig. 2. Example of simulation trace

3.4   Verification

Model checking application specific properties was possible by using the AsmetaSMV tool, which translates ASM specifications into models of the NuSMV model checker. The *Computation Tree Logic (CTL)* properties written inside the ASMETA code are automatically translated to Promcla code and afterwards verified by the NuSMV model checker. In addition to the properties proved in [3], we have verified the refinement applied to the control state of the *request handler* shown in Fig. 1.

When the request handler starts processing the request, if the device profile is not available in the cookie, then the request handler will eventually send a request (containing the JavaScript tests) to the device.

```
ag(reqHandlerState(RQ1) = START_PROCESSING and
                    cookieInfoAvailable(device1) = false
    implies ef(reqHandlerState(RQ1) = REQ_DEVICE_INFO))
```

By verifying these type of temporal properties we wanted to guarantee the correctness and the reliability of the client-adaptivity component interaction w.r.t. device information detection.

4   Conclusions

The scope of this work is to prove that the creation of the device profile is correct, the communication is reliable, and that all device properties necessary for the processing of the cloud content are available on the server-side. We achieved this by refining the initial ASM ground models using ASMETA framework. We were able to perform the model simulation in both an interactive and automatic way by utilizing the simulator AsmetaS. Model checking of properties has been performed to guarantee application independent properties, as consistency and minimality, and application dependent properties (derived from the system requirements), as correctness and reliability. The properties to be verified were declared using CTL formulae directly in the AsmetaL model. Each agent was verified separately using AsmetaSMV tool. As future work, we plan to add the details regarding the *Document Object Model (DOM)* analysis, the content and layout adaptation of the web pages.

References

1. Arcaini, P., Gargantini, A., Riccobene, E.: AsmetaSMV: a way to link high-level ASM models to low-level NuSMV specifications. In: Frappier, M., Glässer, U., Khurshid, S., Laleau, R., Reeves, S. (eds.) ABZ 2010. LNCS, vol. 5977, pp. 61–74. Springer, Heidelberg (2010)
2. Arcaini, P., Gargantini, A., Riccobene, E., Scandurra, P.: A model-driven process for engineering a toolset for a formal method. Softw. Pract. Experience **41**, 155–166 (2011). http://dx.doi.org/10.1002/spe.1019
3. Arcaini, P., Holom, R.M., Riccobene, E.: Modeling and formal analysis of a client-server application for cloud services. In: 11th International Workshop on Web Services and Formal Methods: Formal Aspects of Service-Oriented and Cloud Computing (2014, to appear)
4. Börger, E., Stärk, R.: Abstract State Machines: A Method for High-Level System Design and Analysis. Springer, Heidelberg (2003)
5. Bósa, K., Holom, R.M., Vleju, M.B.: A formal model of client-cloud interaction. In: Thalheim, B., Schewe, K.D., Prinz, A., Buchberger, B. (eds.) Correct Web Applications, pp. 1–61. Springer, Heidelberg (2014)
6. Carioni, A., Gargantini, A., Riccobene, E., Scandurra, P.: A scenario-based validation language for ASMs. In: Börger, E., Butler, M., Bowen, J.P., Boca, P. (eds.) ABZ 2008. LNCS, vol. 5238, pp. 71–84. Springer, Heidelberg (2008)
7. Chelemen, R.M.: Modeling a web application for cloud content adaptation with ASMs. In: 2013 International Conference on Cloud Computing and Big Data (CloudCom-Asia), pp. 44–51 (2013)
8. Gargantini, A., Riccobene, E., Scandurra, P.: A metamodel-based language and a simulation engine for abstract state machines. J. Univers. Comput. Sci. **14**(12), 1949–1983 (2008)

Modeling Accuracy of Indoor Localization Systems

Tomasz Jankowski, Marek Bawiec, and Maciej Nikodem[✉]

Department of Computer Engineering,
Wrocław University of Technology, Wybrzeże Wyspiańskiego 27,
50-370 Wrocław, Poland
maciej.nikodem@pwr.edu.pl

Abstract. In recent years indoor localization systems and localization-based services gain more attention and become ubiquitous. Despite this, planning, development and deployment of localization systems and services is still an issue, that consumes a lot of effort and time. Situation may improve if efficient and accurate computer tools are available to support above mentioned tasks. This, on the other hand, requires modeling software that can numerically predict behavior of the system, recommend improvements and/or preform some optimization. This paper presents methods and preliminary results in the development of simplified, yet accurate, modeling tool that can support design and deployment of indoor localization system. Approaches presented were evaluated in real-life experiments.

1 Introduction

In recent years different indoor localization technologies gain lots of attention as number of practical applications emerge almost every day. At the same time, localization techniques are mature enough to provide accurate enough localization information with satisfying update frequency coverage and capacity (i.e. number of objects that can be simultaneously localized). Although the spectrum of technologies is very broad, a lot of attention is put on low-cost radio technologies. This is mainly due to the fact, that radio devices allow for fast and wireless data transmission while simultaneously being able to estimate distance between communicating devices. Knowing distances to reference points (called anchors), that have known positions, enables calculation of unknown location of mobile node. Simultaneously current development of low-cost radio transceivers gives low-power operation in unlicensed ISM bands over the distances of several and dozen of meters. This makes low-power radios a perfect solution for WSN/IoT applications – just to mention home/building automation, control and monitoring applications and for marketing/advertisement purposes.

Among radio technologies several techniques to determine mobile node location are possible. Received signal strength indicator (RSSI) is a measure reported by almost every radio transceiver. RSSI provides information on how strong is the radio signal received by the radio node. This information is used internally by

R. Moreno-Díaz et al. (Eds.): EUROCAST 2015, LNCS 9520, pp. 573–580, 2015.
DOI: 10.1007/978-3-319-27340-2_71

transceiver for clear channel assessment (and decision if and when to transmit) as well as for detection of incoming radio packets (to decide when to receive). Since RSSI drops with distance its value can be used to assess the distance between the receiver and transmitter. Unfortunately, the relation between distance and RSSI depends on number of different things, e.g. the localization area (shape, dimensions, construction materials), presence and location of obstacles. Consequently, the relation is never accurate and thus estimated distance is biased with errors that are often difficult to deal with. The other approach does not calculate distances from RSSI, but use raw RSSI measurements in order to decide where mobile node is located. Typical approach is to prepare a map of the localization area that provides RSSI values measured in each point of the map. While mobile node moves across the area measured RSSI values are refereed to the map in order to estimate node position. This technique is often used with WiFi and Bluetooth Low Energy (BLE) networks.

Another approach for localization is based on accurate measurements of time when radio packets were send and received. Ability to time-stamp packets allows to measure the time radio signal travels from transmitter to receiver and thus calculate the distance between them. Time of flight (ToF) measurements are possible even when clocks of communicating nodes are not synchronized. If synchronization of anchors' clocks is possible then position can be calculated based on the information when each anchor received the radio packet broadcasted by mobile node. This method, time difference of arrival (TDoA), reduces the communication overhead compared to ToF as single, one-way communication is enough to determine the unknown position of a mobile node.

Although current radio transceivers allow for highly accurate distance measurements and ToF/TDoA localization they are susceptible to errors resulting from imperfections of electronic circuits and radio propagation phenomena – mainly multipath and non line of sight (LoS) propagation. Despite the fact that nature and theory of the above mentioned phenomena is well known, its impact on real life localization systems is difficult to predict in real life applications. This is mostly due to the complexity of propagation that depends on several parameters that are difficult to be measured accurately (e.g. geometry of the localization area) and are difficult to be controlled (e.g. mobile node's antenna direction and location).

Accurate modeling of radio propagation is difficult and impractical for development of a software tool that is intended to support localization system development, deployment and configuration. Therefore, we propose to take different approach and construct a high level model of localization system directly. The model is developed based on real-life measurements of radio devices that provide localization functionality through time-based measurements. Model is focused on localization but also takes into account relevant aspects of radio propagation and phenomena. The idea for this approach is to model the localization system directly, reducing complexity of the model, improving modeling performance and ensuring ease of use (e.g. to release from the need to provide detailed area information) while keeping the model accurate enough for practical applications.

2   Related Work

Use of short-range radio communication (e.g. WiFi, Bluetooth) for indoor localization is not new and is quite popular in large number of practical implementations. However, existing systems determine position of mobile node based on
RSSI values measured to anchor nodes (e.g. WiFi access points) of known localization. For such systems number of numerical models relating RSSI with distance between nodes and modeling tools were developed.

Cisco Systems Inc. [1] provides wireless location appliance that, among other
things, allows to analyze the floor plan of the area of interest and recommend
deployment of access points. The tool takes into account number of different
information, including type of the access point, type of the services that need to
be provided in the network and parameters of the area including area type (e.g.
cubicles, rooms), construction material used (e.g. thin/thick wall, glass, door)
and propagation models. The tool outputs information on how access points
should be deployed and estimates quality of the service that will be provided –
this includes signal power, throughput and expected localization accuracy.

Recently several papers addressing modeling of time-based localization systems showed up. For example paper by Montorsi et al. [6] propose map-aware
models for indoor localization using either RSSI or time measurements (ToF or
TDoA). The model proposed takes into account information about area floor
plan (map) and attempts to relate the localization error to LOS and non-LOS
propagation that may affect ranging measurements. Authors propose simplified
model as they assume multipath propagation is not a case, time selectivity issues
can be ignored and bias in distance measurements only results from non-LoS
propagation through obstacles. Consequently the applicability of the model is
limited.

Yang et al. [7] addressed modeling of ToF ranging error in indoor environments. Based on real-life experiments they were able to present that normal
distribution is not an accurate model for ranging measurements error. They proposed different statistical models that take into account skewness of the error
distribution and reflect reality much better. Although ranging modeling appears
very promising, it cannot explain localization errors measured in indoor environments. Paper [7] suggests that geometry between nodes and area needs to be
taken into account but leaves this as future work.

Taking into account geometry of the area and locations of the communicating
nodes requires tools that ray trace the important signals traveling from transmitter to receiver. Laaraiedh et al. [4] analyzed application of ray tracing (RT)
to localization systems in order to support fingerprinting and to model location
dependent parameters of ranging/localization systems. The solution proposed is
based on accurate modeling of radio propagation that requires detailed information about the area of interest (usually provided in form of CAD files), parameters of construction materials used, as well as models of human behavior/moves
within the area. For fingerprint-based localization the RT simulation prove to
fairly accurate approximate the error of real localization systems. Consequently,

RT appears to be a tool that can be also used to model and later design/develop localization systems for given area.

Although RT is sound the accurate modeling of all the rays of interest for whole area is time-consuming, inefficient and impractical as large number of detailed information needs to be provided. As presented in [3] this issue can be alleviated if simplified yet accurate enough RT tools are used. Paper by Laaraiedh et al. propose a graph based RT tool that takes into account area floor plan and simulates propagation of radio rays. The output of the simulation is then post-processed in order to get information such as RSSI and ToF. Evaluation for UWB signals in real environments shows a good match of the model.

Our research focus on modeling of indoor environments for time-based localization modeling and algorithms for efficient planning of localization systems. Similar to previous work we take into account geometry of the area and model radio propagation. In contrast to what was done so far we keep the propagation modeling as simple as possible (in terms of number of parameters required, complexity of floor-plan information, lack of human behavior model, etc.) and take into account significant phenomena of radio propagation (non-LoS and multipath propagation, direct path attenuation, time-selectivity of radio devices, etc.).

3   Challenges in Accuracy Modeling

Localization error strongly depends on two factors: ranging error and localization algorithm that computes position given several distance measurements.

We first focused on ranging errors and proposed a numerical model to approximate the error defined as a difference between the measured and real distance. Prior to modeling errors were processed: first outliers were filtered out, then root mean square error (RMSE) was calculated. This allowed to clear the data from incorrect values (e.g. resulting from temporary interferences) and take into account both positive and negative values of error.

We have evaluated two modeling techniques often used in literature: polynomial and kernel regression. In the former technique error values were approximated with polynomial function of given degree in order to find the best fit. The kernel regression method does not take any assumptions regarding the form of resulting model. Instead it creates the model by traversing input data with sliding window and processing subsets of data points (that fit into window). The width of the window is a parameter to kernel regression and processing is realized by applying kernel function to data points inside the window. Resulting model is an array of estimated distance errors.

We have evaluated the models using real-life measurements that were conducted in the corridor at our faculty (over 100 m long, 2.8 m wide corridor with a square cross-section). In the experiment DiZiC [2] radio modules were used. Eight anchor nodes were placed at fixed positions along the corridor. Mobile node was moved to selected reference points along the corridor where distance measurements were taken. Afterward the root mean square error (RMSE) of

Table 1. Summary of error model evaluation. Models were created using different parameters: degree 2, 9, 16, 19 for polynomial model and window size of 2, 16 for kernel regression. All values reported are in meters.

Model (S_1)	Eval. (S_2)	Polynomial model				Kernel model	
		2	9	16	19	2	16
A2	A5	1.7375	1.7762	1.5577	1.6330	1.6604	1.8000
	A7	7.5252	7.4200	7.4153	7.4300	7.3003	7.3475
	Avg.	3.2603	3.1433	2.9877	3.0061	2.9929	3.2579
	Std.	2.1711	2.2525	2.3305	2.3448	2.2641	2.1052
A5	A2	1.5544	1.5371	1.4726	1.4814	1.5102	1.5657
	A7	8.0154	7.9806	8.1007	8.0876	8.0599	7.7715
	Avg.	3.2955	3.2625	3.1993	3.1875	3.1705	3.2655
	Std.	2.3930	2.4343	2.5523	2.5537	2.4935	2.3021
A7	A2	7.6997	7.6467	7.5421	7.4319	7.5492	7.4510
	A5	8.0126	8.0595	8.2262	8.1289	8.1355	7.5943
	Avg.	6.8804	6.8208	6.6929	6.6579	6.6768	6.6941
	Std.	2.5900	2.7150	2.8120	2.8424	2.8467	2.3749
All anchors	A2	2.8704	2.6303	2.3392	2.3977	2.5551	2.9616
	A5	3.0508	2.9251	2.6854	2.7188	2.8952	3.0652
	Avg.	3.8330	3.6875	3.3945	3.3978	3.5070	3.9017
	Std.	1.2958	1.2883	1.3485	1.3384	1.2695	1.2954

measurements for each reference point was calculated and used for model development and evaluation. Evaluation was conducted for different degree and window size of polynomial and kernel models. Since 8 anchors were used in tests the data available was split into two sets – S_1 used for model construction, and S_2 for model evaluation. Table 1 presents some of the results for models where S_1 contained measurements to anchors A2, A5, A7 as well as all the anchors (A1–A8). Resulting models were evaluated against data in S_2. By default S_2 contained RMSE errors for each anchor individually. The value reported in the table is an average absolute error between the model and RMSE from S_2. Results show that polynomial model works best for degrees of around 19 – this is relatively large value. Additionally, no model exists that can approximate all the measurements accurately – models created using measurements for single anchor yield small error values (below 2 m) for this anchor and large errors for the measurements to other anchors (even above 8 m). The average error and standard deviations for such models are also high – above 3 and 2 m respectively. The model created using all measurements gives the best results regardless of whether polynomial or kernel regression is used. The average error is around 3.7 m and standard deviation equals 1.3.

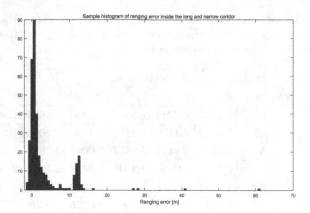

Fig. 1. Histogram of ranging error for corridor area. Two peaks of the distribution reflect situation when direct path is correctly received (peak at 1 m), and when it is attenuated and reflected ray is measured (peak at 12 m).

Both modeling approaches do not allow for accurate enough approximation of the ranging errors. This shows that statistical modeling of the ranging measurements must take into account additional parameters in order to more accurately reflect real life systems. This can be also seen on Fig. 1 that presents a cumulative histogram of error for 8 anchors deployed along the corridor and over 120 measurement points. The distribution of error is two-modal with clear peaks at 1 and 12 m errors. Closer analysis showed that peak at 12 m is due to two anchors that were located approximately 6 m from the end of the corridor. For those anchors large number of distance measurements were biased with 12 m error due to attenuation of direct path and reception of the reflected ray. Based on the above observation we propose to model the ranging error with a multi-modal probability distribution, with modes determined by geometry of the area, relative location of anchors and possible ranging errors due to multi-path propagation phenomena. The intensity of each peak in the distribution depends on the estimated relative powers of the signals. Power estimation takes into account both length, time spread, phase shift and resulting attenuation of each propagation path. Experiments also revealed that ranging error does not depend on the distance, which is quite common assumption in literature. In fact, the devices were able to measure the distance of 500 m with error below 5 m, which was largerly due to imperfect measurement of the ground truth distance.

The other aspect for modeling localization systems is to model the localization algorithm itself. The reason for that is the fact, that there is no single lateration algorithm that can be used in order to determine the node position given distance measurements. Moreover, all lateration algorithms output inaccurate location when given inaccurate distance measurements and the error in position depends heavily on the algorithm used.

In our research we have taken two approaches to lateration algorithm modeling: partial derivatives and absolute distance. First approach works if the

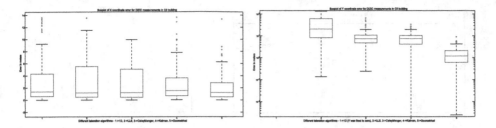

Fig. 2. Localization error along X and Y coordinates for 5 different lateration algorithms.

lateration algorithm is given as a differentiable function. In such case accuracy of the position can be represented as function of partial derivatives and ranging errors. This approach works for algorithms that use linear least square method ([5]) and was the one used in our experiments. If lateration cannot be represent as a differentiable function then error is calculated as a distance between real and estimated position.

The error in linear least square lateration algorithms grows quickly with ranging error but also strongly depends on the geometry of anchors. The best results are achieved when anchors are deployed in a square grid. When anchors are deployed in rectangular grid, with one side significantly longer then the other (which is the case for corridor area), then the error magnifies. This effect is clearly seen if we compare localization error along different coordinates (Fig. 2). Error along the corridor length (X coordinate) is in most case below 2.5 m. On the other hand the error across the corridor (Y coordinate) is large, even up to dozens of meters. This is a direct consequence of linearization that propagates and magnifies Y coordinate errors.

4   Conclusions

Real-life measurements confirmed that the localization error strongly depends on the geometry of the area and relative position of ranging nodes. They have also revealed that the error does not depend on the distance. Consequently, in order to model the error one needs to take into account area geometry and radio propagation phenomena, and use this information to build statistical model of ranging/localization error. Therefore we model:

- ranging error with multi-modal distribution where each mode represents the most likely propagation path between communicating nodes,
- localization error as a function of ranging error and the procedure used for localization (e.g. selection of reference points, filtering and statistical analysis of raw data) and using partial derivatives if possible.

By now we have developed a tool for evaluation of localization algorithms and for numerical simulation of radio propagation within the area of interest

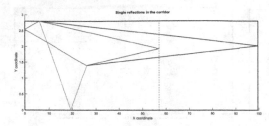
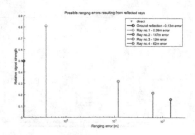

Fig. 3. Single reflections for the corridor area and nodes located at (6, 2.8) and (26, 1.8) points. Right figure presents possible ranging errors resulting from the reflections. The height of the peak gives relative power of the signal wrt. to direct ray.

(Fig. 3). Although the tool now offers only simple propagation modeling it can already explain some of the real-life measurements. Simplifications implemented in the model are all due to real-life experiments that disclose that in most case single or double reflections affect the radio propagation in the most significant way. This allows to simplify the model and reduce overhead while searching for possible explanations of real-life measurements.

Acknowledgement. Research funded by Foundation for Polish Science, agreement no. 41/UD/SKILLS/ 2015, as part of SKILLS-IMPULS initiative co-funded from European Social Fund.

References

1. Wi-Fi location-based services 4.1 design guide. Technical report, Cisco Systems Inc., May 2008
2. DiZiC DZ-TN-Gx ranging module - data sheet. Technical report, DiZiC Co., Ltd. (2011)
3. Laaraiedh, M., Amiot, N., Uguen, B.: Efficient ray tracing tool for UWB propagation and localization modeling. In: 2013 7th European Conference on Antennas and Propagation (EuCAP), pp. 2307–2311, April 2013
4. Laaraiedh, M., Uguen, B., Stephan, J., Corre, Y., Lostanlen, Y., Raspopoulos, M., Stavrou, S.: Ray tracing-based radio propagation modeling for indoor localization purposes. In: 2012 IEEE 17th International Workshop on Computer Aided Modeling and Design of Communication Links and Networks (CAMAD), pp. 276–280, September 2012
5. Liu, Y., Yang, Z.: Location, Localization, and Localizability, Location-awareness Technology for Wireless Networks. Springer, New York (2011)
6. Montorsi, F., Pancaldi, F., Vitetta, G.M.: Map-aware models for indoor wireless localization systems: an experimental study. CoRR abs/1402.3783 (2014). http://arxiv.org/abs/1402.3783
7. Yang, Y., Zhao, Y., Kyas, M.: A non-parametric modeling of time-of-flight ranging error for indoor network localization. In: 2013 IEEE Global Communications Conference, GLOBECOM 2013, Atlanta, GA, USA, 9–13 December 2013, pp. 189–194. IEEE (2013). http://ieeexplore.ieee.org/xpl/articleDetails.jsp?arnumber=6831069

Request Driven Generation of RFLP Elements at Product Definition

László Horváth[(⊠)] and Imre J. Rudas

Institute of Applied Mathematics, John Von Neumann Faculty of Informatics,
Óbuda University, Budapest, Hungary
horvath.laszlo@nik.uni-obuda.hu, rudas@uni-obuda.hu

Abstract. Recent achievements in product modeling emphasize self adaptive instancing of generic models, active intelligent property (IP) representations, and multidisciplinary product concept definitions. Although current leading product lifecycle management models (PLM) are in possession of these advanced capabilities, new complexity related problems arise at definition of active knowledge and higher level abstraction model entities. As contribution to solution for the above problems, this paper introduces new request driven behavior centered method for the generation of requirements, functional, logical, and physical (RFLP) structure elements and active knowledge features in PLM model. The requirements, functional, and logical elements provide high level abstraction for representation of multidisciplinary product concept design while knowledge features assist generation of product features on the physical level. The proposed method is aimed to be suitable for intelligent application purposed extension of PLM modeling systems.

1 Introduction

Representation of product information in order to achieve better engineering activities and support design, analysis, and manufacturing automation started to develop at engineering areas where conventional drawing and documentation failed. Examples for these areas were representation of three dimensional surfaces (CAD), finite element analysis (CAE) and computer aided programming of manufacturing equipment (CAM). These isolated solutions were gradually integrated into product model where new aim was to support all engineering activities during the lifecycle of product from the first idea to legal recycling. Development of model for product lifecycle management (PLM) system included more or less integration of models from various engineering areas. However, real integration of mechanical, electrical, electronic, software and hardware representations in a single model was possible only on the conceptual design of multidisciplinary product. In order to realize this, well proven model structure was introduced from systems engineering (SE). This is the requirements, functional, logical, and physical (RFLP) structure.

The above changes were associated with new solutions for handling changes in the growing model structures during the development of products in order to fulfill demands for well engineered products and shortened innovation cycle. These demands enforced advanced generic, feature driven, knowledge controlled, contextual, and self

© Springer International Publishing Switzerland 2015
R. Moreno-Díaz et al. (Eds.): EUROCAST 2015, LNCS 9520, pp. 581–588, 2015.
DOI: 10.1007/978-3-319-27340-2_72

adaptive characteristics of PLM model. The Laboratory of Intelligent Engineering Systems (LIES) at the Óbuda University joined to these efforts in research for model representations which give better handling of high level abstraction and human request driven self instantiation in PLM models. This chapter introduces one of recent results at the LIES. This result is a new model structure to assist human request originated content driven generation of elements in RFLP structured PLM models.

2   Knowledge Driven Self Adaptive Product Model

Engineering activities for lifecycle of increasingly complex products have been concentrated in highly integrated product lifecycle management (PLM) modeling systems [6]. This integrated modeling methodology was grounded by the Integrated Product Information Model (IPIM) which became international standard. In order to achieve capability of PLM model for self modification in case of changed situation and new event, active intellectual property (IP) driven generic product model constitutes key area of PLM research. As result, recent PLM models are capable of self modification through chains of contextually connected product features [1]. Model modifies itself for changed situation and new events through chains of contextually connected feature parameters. PLM model demands feature definition for lifecycle of product [9].

Recent developments of product model system completed the pure physical level product model with request, functional, and logical representations in RFLP structure. In this multidisciplinary model, R, F, and L levels provide representation of integrated product concept for mechanical, electrical, electronic and other area specific product units in a single model [2]. F and L levels are capable of behavior representation providing virtually executable PLM model. The way is open for intensive application of active intelligent content in product model [1].

The request driven behavior centered generation of RFLP structure elements which is the main contribution in this chapter assists development of product lifecycle management (PLM) model in a modeling environment which is outlined in Fig. 1. First of all, the most important change is that modeling is multidisciplinary in order to achieve really integrated representation of multidisciplinary product. The previous efforts for interdisciplinary group work engineers resulted connected or integrated individual results while multidisciplinary group work provides results which are built on each other. Organic integration of mechanical, electrical, electronic, hardware and software units in a single common model is done only on the conception level of product design.

In the new scenario of engineering, human contributes to product development by RFLP structure based product definition. The request driven behavior centered generation of RFLP structure elements applies content which is suitable to replace direct human decisions on these elements. Following this, the model definition is continued on two branches. Separation of physical level development gives the possibility for direct physical level product definition. At the same, time, product concept definition on the other branch makes integration of R, F, and L level abstraction entity generation with the physical level definition possible. On the physical branch, physical (P) level definitions initiate active knowledge feature generation and product feature generation. Generic model is developed which is capable of self adaptive instancing [8].

The request driven behavior centered generation of RFLP structure elements was motivated by the problem with R, F, and L structure element dialogues. Capturing complex contextual knowledge in the course of these dialogues is a new challenge for engineers. The proposed method is aimed to develop representations for collected active knowledge content in product model. This content drives RFLP element generation. At full application of the proposed method, multidisciplinary product concept is defined prior to physically existing parts.

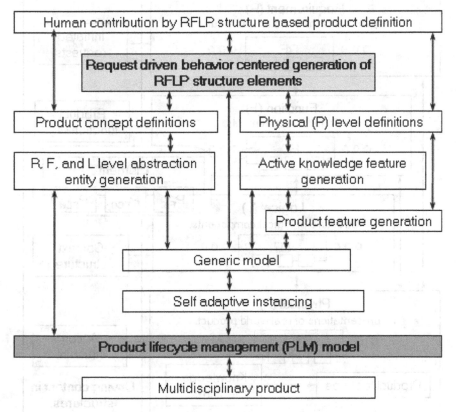

Fig. 1. Modeling environment of the proposed product definition

Because the proposed modeling is dedicated for RFLP structure element generation, it is planned to integrate in a PLM system with RFLP structure development capabilities. At the same time, these capabilities can be utilized at the request driven behavior centered model. In order to realize this advantage, configuration and open system capabilities should be applied. This implementation is not a subject of this chapter.

The main RFLP structure and the proposed driving content for each level are shown in Fig. 2. RE, FE, LE, and PE elements are placed in level structures for requirements the product has to fulfill (R), function (F) to fulfill requirements, logical structure of product (L), and physical (P) representations of real world product, respectively. Because level of RFLP structure is a structure of elements, the proposed model for driving content consists of levels and element structures on levels. Content for the R, F, L, and P level elements is available in relevant elements on levels of initiated requests, product functionality, context structure, and action structure, respectively.

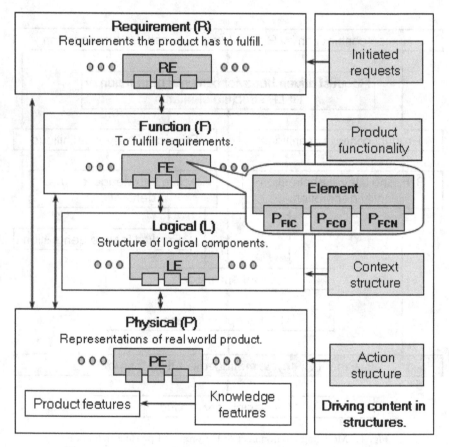

Fig. 2. RFLP structure elements and the proposed driving content

The RFLP and the proposed content structure elements are connected by ports (Fig. 2) for inter-element communication (P_{FIC}, control of element (P_{FCO}, and for exchange of content information (P_{FCN}). Driving content consists of coordinated human request representations and their processing into lower level entities such as behaviors, contextual connections, and physical level object parameters. Formerly applied knowledge, experience, and expertise entities are represented in content elements and applied as consistent intellectual property (IP) in product model. In order to achieve this, the abstraction method in the proposed modeling is based on the five level abstractions in [4].

3   Request Driven Element and Feature Definition

Structure of content for the request driven behavior centered generation of RFLP structure elements is summarized in Fig. 3. Encircled letter *C* means driving connection in the direction of arrow. Engineer submit request in the form of content. Request may be initiated or already decided. Authorization is controlled by relevant PLM procedures using allowed context for each interacting human. Initiated requests are recorded and placed in structured request (SR) as organized initiatives. SR organizes requests from all engineers who are in appropriate context. Decided requests are included in actual product definition. Content is mapped to organized initiatives. Structured request (SR) includes initiatives for product functions, specifications, objects, processes, and entity generation methods. Definition and decision [7] activities enhance and complete this structure during the lifecycle of product.

Because behavior representations in F and L level elements of RFLP structure enhance product model into virtually executable one, content for behavior has key importance on the way of development of the proposed modeling. Requests are converted into product behavior (PB) definition considering their structural connections in SR structure. Product behavior (PB) content definition is controlled by product functionality and product characteristics. Behavior related content is placed in structured behaviors. In PB, structured behaviors can cover all of the product functionality and characteristics using a previously published generalized definition of behavior [5].

In this stage of content definition, product structure is available in the form of awaited and decided product behavior definitions. Behavior controls generation action (GA). GA is a structure which backed up by content in the form of constructor and active knowledge product features for the P level of RFLP structure. GA structure also can be configured for direct drive of product and knowledge features in conventional P level product models under the coordination of CD structure.

P level object contexts are organized logically in context definition (CD) structure. This can be defined prior to physical object definition and includes content for logical structure of product. This content drives L level element generation in the RFLP structure. Direct context drives logical connection for product objects while indirect contents drives logical connections of driving knowledge objects and driven product objects in the product model. In the indirect case, logical connections are established between object which change knowledge objects parameter values and results firing of knowledge objects.

As it can be followed in Fig. 3, the proposed modeling is composed by contextual chain of SR, PB, GA, and CD structures. Elements in these structures have driving connections to relevant contextual RFLP structure elements as it is summarized in Fig. 4. Driving contexts in Fig. 4 were mentioned above. Content background and driven RFLP structure level driving connections include SR-R for requests, SR-F for functions, PB-F and PB-L for behaviors, GA-P for physical object generation, and

CD-L for connections in logical model of product. In the course of definition of content structure and its driving connections, arbitrary connection of elements within and between content driving content background and product RFLP structure can be established in accordance with the context of engineer who defines the connection.

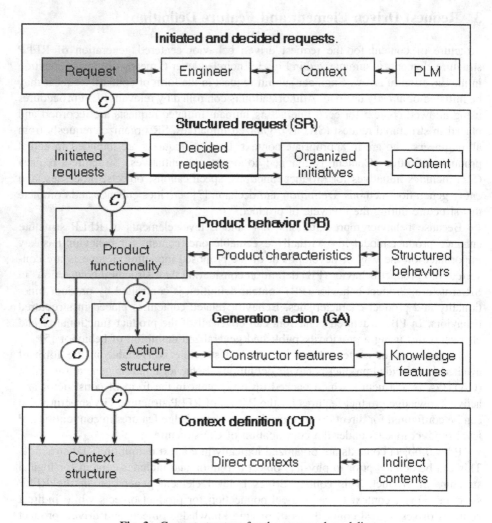

Fig. 3. Content structure for the proposed modeling

Driving connections and the connected content between levels of the content background (Fig. 3) implies complex content representation structure on each level. For the inside structure of levels, content type based substructures were proposed (Fig. 4). Substructure is a structure of elements on a level. RFLP structure management of known PLM solutions allows for establish structure within level of RFLP structure. This practice is planned to apply also on content levels. Because content elements and connections may be very complex, generic modeling must be applied for the greatest extent possible. On the level of structured request (SR), substructures are proposed for request specification (RS), requested product function (RF), requested objects (RO), requested definition method (RM), and requested definition process (RP). RS specifies human defined request which includes specified objects and their specified parameters and drives relevant RF, RM, and RP element definition. In other words, specification initiates content for product function, as well as product entity definition method and process. Sometimes sets or patterns of product objects are mapped to function. Along the contextual chain in Fig. 4, product object may be specified along with its definition method or process. Finally, definition process may be driven by method. The SR structure is extended and improved during the lifecycle of product. Driving RFLP structure elements by SR elements can be restricted to critical engineering activities.

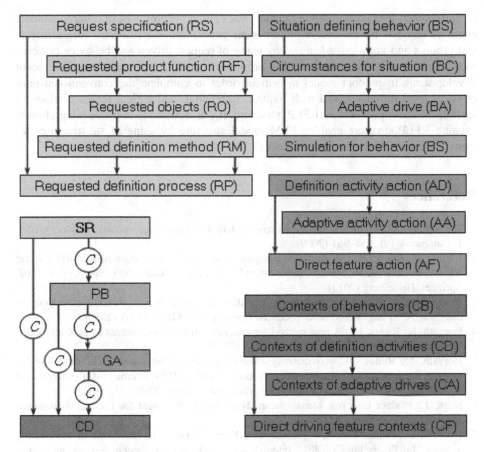

Fig. 4. Substructures on levels of content structure

On the level of product behavior (PB), substructures are proposed for situation which includes content for defining behavior (BS), circumstances (BC) in the form of set of parameter definitions in the background of situation, adaptive drive (BA) which includes content for the drive of product objects, and simulation (BS) which is for analyses in order to assure defined behavior. Elements in this level are defined in the context of structured request (SR) substructure elements. While contextual connections are established between elements, content transfer is done by object parameter values and relationships.

On the level of generation action (GA) definition activity action (AD), adaptive activity action (AA) substructures organize product feature, and knowledge feature generation content. Direct feature action (AF) substructure is record of direct human feature definitions. Context definition (CD) level includes substructures for the four main types of logically connected model entities as it can be seen on Fig. 4.

4 Conclusions

In this chapter, four leveled driving content background is proposed in order to connect engineer requests for product definition with generation of RFLP structure elements and product and knowledge features by using of request driven and behavior centered method and model representation. The proposed modeling is a contribution to recent developments in product model system in order to complete the conventional pure physical level product model with request, functional, and logical representations of multidisciplinary products in (RFLP) structure. It was devoted to improve integration in existing RFLP structure enabled PLM model structure by using of substructure elements and their ports of advanced host PLM systems.

References

1. Horváth, L., Rudas, I.J.: Human intent representation in knowledge intensive product model. J. Comput. **4**(10), 954–961 (2009)
2. Kleiner, S., Kramer, C.: Model based design with systems engineering based on RFLP using V6. In: Abramovici, M., Stark, R. (eds.) Smart Product Engineering. LNPE, vol. 5, pp. 93–102. Springer, Heidelberg (2013)
3. Brière-Côté, A., Rivest, L., Desrochers, A.: Adaptive generic product structure modelling for design reuse in engineer-to-order products. Comput. Ind. **61**(1), 53–65 (2010)
4. Horváth, L., Rudas, I.J.: A new method for enhanced information content in product model. WSEAS Trans. Inf. Sci. Appl. **5**(3), 277–285 (2008)
5. Horváth, L., Rudas, I.J.: Associativity, adaptivity and behavior aspects in modeling for manufacturing related robot systems. In: Proceedings of the IEEE International Conference on Robotics and Automation, pp. 3006–3011, Barcelona, Spain (2005)
6. Stark, J.: Product Lifecycle Management: 21st Century Paradigm for Product Realisation. Birkhäuser, Heidelberg (2004)
7. Horváth, L., Rudas, I.J.: New product model representation for decisions in engineering systems. In: Proceedings of 2011 International Conference on System Science and Engineering (ICSSE 2011), pp. 546–551, Macau, China (2011)
8. Horváth, L., Rudas, I.J.: Active knowledge for the situation-driven control of product definition. Acta Polytech. Hung. **10**(2), 217–234 (2013)
9. Sy, M., Mascle, C.: Product design analysis based on life cycle features. J. Eng. Des. **22**(6), 387–406 (2011)

Modeling of a High Voltage Ignition Coil with Nonlinear Magnetic Behavior

Klaus Stadlbauer[1]([✉]), Georg Meyer[2], Florian Poltschak[1],
and Wolfgang Amrhein[1]

[1] JKU HOERBIGER Research Institute for Smart Actuators, Johannes Kepler
University Linz, Altenbergerstr. 69, 4040 Linz, Austria
{Klaus.Stadlbauer,Florian.Poltschak,Wolfgang.Amrhein}@jku.at
[2] Institute for Fluid Mechanics and Heat Transfer, Vienna University of Technology,
Karlsplatz 13, 1040 Vienna, Austria
Georg.Meyer@tuwien.ac.at

Abstract. Ignition systems are wide spread in common life and industry. Cars for example are part of everybody's daily life, gas motors are
common in industry. The heart of the system, the prt which both have
in common, the premise for the functionality, is the ignition of the fuel
with a spark. Problems occur when the fuel is not ignited correctly. Misfire and more exhaustion than necessary result from sparks which are to
small in power for proper ignition. Sparks can be blown out like a candle
in wind and therefore don't ignite the fuel at all.

A multi-exciting system not only improves the power of the spark,
it can even prolong the duration to assure proper ignition and therefore
combustion.

To cope with industry demands like the design of components or
improving efficiency the system is described in a mathematical model
comprising the non linear behavior of the ignition coil. Optimization of
parts like the ignition coil for higher efficiency is the next logical step.

Keywords: Capacitive high voltage ignition system · Nonlinear magnetic behavior · Multi-excitation ignition

1 Introduction

An everyday issue not receding in importance in science is the reduction of
exhaust emissions due to the environmental and ecological impact. The combustion engine is one of the biggest players in producing exhaust emissions such as
oxides of nitrogen, total hydrocarbons and carbon monoxide. To reduce these
exhaust emissions a good combustion of the fuel is a prerequisite which is directly
dependent on the quality of the ignition [1].

The process of ignition is a complex issue. It starts with the electronic system
for storing a certain amount of energy that is transfered to a combustible fuel
via a spark. After the breakdown the process continuous with the propagation of
the spark between the two electrodes (i.e. spark plug) and the dynamic behavior

© Springer International Publishing Switzerland 2015
R. Moreno-Díaz et al. (Eds.): EUROCAST 2015, LNCS 9520, pp. 589–596, 2015.
DOI: 10.1007/978-3-319-27340-2_73

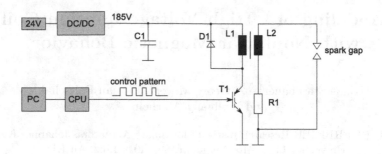

Fig. 1. A high voltage ignition system.

within the gas flow during ignition, especially in the first phase. Last but not least the ignition itself and the following combustion of the expanding gas is part of it. The ignition coil consists of a primary and a secondary winding and an iron core. Latter is preferably made of SMC in order to reduce eddy currents.

This work deals with the mathematical model of the high voltage ignition coil [2] and its surrounding system (see Fig. 1) which is used in a recently developed capacitive discharge ignition system [3–5]. Hereby, main focus in system modeling lies on the fast time-transient behavior of the ignition coil. The development of the mathematical model is highly important for better understanding and ongoing system design. The basis is a differential equation system in state space

$$\dot{x} = Ax + bu. \tag{1}$$

The number of ODEs varies due to the corresponding level of simplification. A system consisting of 6 states is superior to the computational time and the quality of the results.

The resistance of the spark gap is preliminary modeled regarding the law of Paschen without taking fluid dynamics into account. Since no prolongation of the spark and therefore no considerable change of the gap resistance is anticipated this is seen as justified. For simulating spark ignition in a fluid dynamic environment this simple model of a spark gap can be replaced by another more sophisticated model. In that case the calculation requires a Finite Element software (e.g. FLUENT) yielding corresponding mathematical parameters.

2   Simulation

For gaining a compact and fast model the degrees of freedom shall be minimized as much as possible. Furthermore, due to the stiffness of the problem (some capacitors are very small whereas for example the resistance of the spark gap can be as high as several mega-ohm) using a model with too many degrees of freedom the calculation time could explode or the calculation itself even breaks down. For further optimization of the whole system or parts of it like the ignition coil genetic optimization tools like MagOpt can be used. Such a software uses a

computer cluster for parallelized calculation where at each computer one model
is sent for calculation [6]. Using a model which consists of a minimum number
of degrees of freedom one calculation becomes fast enough to produce results for
the whole optimization in an acceptable time span.

As important variables which cannot be neglected the following ones are
identified

$$x = (u_B, i_p, i_\mu, i'_s, u_{CT}, u_{SP}) \tag{2}$$

and consist of the voltage u_B over the energy storing capacitance C_B, the primary current i_p flowing through the primary windings, i_μ the current is flowing
through the main inductance L_h, to the primary side transformed secondary current i'_s flowing through the secondary windings, the voltage u_{CT} which applies
to the ignition cables capacitance C_{CT} and u_{SP} which matches the voltage over
the spark gap.

The scheme of the corresponding model can be seen in Fig. 2. Further parameters are the resistance R_B, the energy storing capacitor C_B, the resistor R_x
and diode D_1 in the free wheeling circuit on the primary side of the ignition coil.
R_p, $L_{\sigma,1}$ and R_s, $L_{\sigma,2}$ are the resistances and leakage inductances of the primary
side and secondary side respectively of the ignition coil, the resistances R_{cl1}, R_{cl2}
of the ignition cable and a corresponding capacitance C_{CT} and a shunt resistor
R_{100} for measuring the current through the spark gap.

Furthermore, the spark gap is modeled with a resistance R_{SP} and a parallel
capacitance C_{SP}.

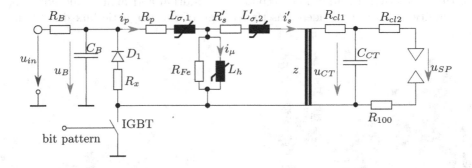

Fig. 2. Electrical circuit of the high voltage ignition system.

For the case where the IGBT is switched on following equations are given

$$\dot{u}_B = -\frac{u_B}{R_B C_B} - \frac{i_p}{C_B} + \frac{u_{in}}{R_B C_B}, \tag{3}$$

$$\dot{i}_p = -\frac{R_p + R_{Fe}}{L_{\sigma,1}(i_p, i'_s)} i_p + \frac{R_{Fe}}{L_{\sigma,1}(i_p, i'_s)} i_\mu + \frac{R_{Fe}}{L_{\sigma,1}(i_p, i'_s)z} i_s + \frac{u_{Cbatt}}{L_{\sigma,1}(i_p, i'_s)}, \tag{4}$$

$$\dot{i}_\mu = \frac{R_{Fe}}{L_h(i_p, i_s)} i_p - \frac{R_{Fe}}{L_h(i_p, i_s)} i_\mu - \frac{R_{Fe}}{L_h(i_p, i_s)z} i_s, \tag{5}$$

$$\dot{i}_s = -\frac{R_{Fe}+R_s'+R_{cl,1}z^2}{L_{\sigma,2}'(i_p,i_s')}i_s+\frac{zR_{Fe}}{L_{\sigma,2}'(i_p,i_s')}i_p-\frac{zR_{Fe}}{L_{\sigma,2}'(i_p,i_s')}i_\mu-\frac{u_{CT}z^2}{L_{\sigma,2}'(i_p,i_s')}, \quad (6)$$

$$\dot{u}_{CT} = \frac{1}{C_{CT}}i_s - \frac{u_{CT}-u_{SP}}{(R_{cl,2}+R_{100})C_{CT}} \quad and \quad (7)$$

$$\dot{u}_{SP} = \frac{u_{CT}-u_{SP}}{(R_{cl,2}+R_{100})C_{SP}} - \frac{u_{SP}}{R_{SP}C_{SP}}. \quad (8)$$

In the case where the IGBT is switched off Eqs. 3 and 4 have to be replaced by following two equations

$$\dot{u}_B = -\frac{u_B}{R_B C_B} + \frac{u_{in}}{R_B C_B} \quad and \quad (9)$$

$$\dot{i}_p = -\frac{R_p+R_{Fe}}{L_{\sigma,1}(i_p,i_s')}i_p+\frac{R_{Fe}}{L_{\sigma,1}(i_p,i_s')}i_\mu+\frac{R_{Fe}}{L_{\sigma,1}(i_p,i_s')z}i_s. \quad (10)$$

Switching back and forth between latter two equations and the corresponding original ones (Eqs. 3 and 4) it is possible to simulate a multi exciting ignition. Furthermore, the resistance R_{SP} depends on the state whether a spark is existent or not. If there exist a spark the resistance drops very low due to the flow of electrons. Whereas the lack of a spark creates a very high value for the corresponding resistance.

By using the Finite Element software *FEMM* the inductivities of the ignition coil are pre-calculated and therefore it is possible to take the nonlinear behavior of the magnetic saturation into account. The mutual and main inductivities of the ignition coil are considered as the change of the magnetic flux due to the

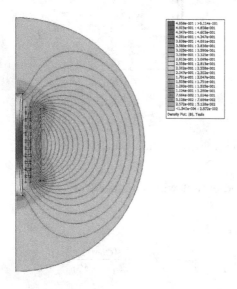

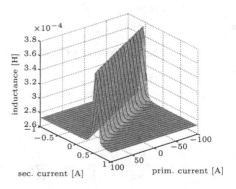

Fig. 3. Magnetic field of ignition coil.   **Fig. 4.** Main inductance L_{11}.

change of the primary and secondary current between two quasi static states with reasonably small margins. The main inductances L_{11} and L_{22} and the mutual inductances L_{12} and L_{21} are calculated this way. As an example the result of the main inductance L_{11} is plotted in Fig. 4. It can be seen that there is a significant difference between the non-saturated and the saturated states. Please note, that only the second and fourth quadrant of this result (i.e. different signs of the primary and secondary current) are used due to Lenz's law.

3   Test Rig and Measurement

A test rig was developed and installed at Johannes Kepler University Linz as depicted in Fig. 5. Hence, it is possible to test the development of a spark under pressure or under a certain gas flow. For pressurizing the iron tube two lids close each side of the iron tube enabling a pressure up to 40 bars.

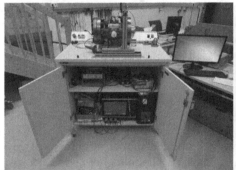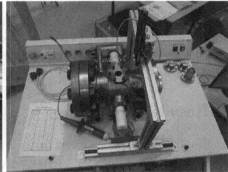

Fig. 5. Test rig of the ignition system.

Removing the two lids a wind channel can be connected to the iron tube allowing a test environment with a laminar air flow. In front of the electrodes lattices with different size of holes can be installed at a specified distance. Hence, a specified turbulent gas flow can be created depending on the size of the holes of the grid.

A high speed camera which is mounted above the test rig captures the development of the spark which can be visualized at a speed of 10 kHz. A drawback is the use of only one camera which is why the three dimensional proliferation of the spark under turbulent flow is difficult to determine. Nevertheless, the distortion of the spark due to a wind flow is clearly detectable and useful for ongoing studies concerning the development of a spark in the environment of a real combustion chamber.

For data acquisition and control several instruments are used (Fig. 6). Using a data acquisition unit one can measure the temperature and the pressure inside

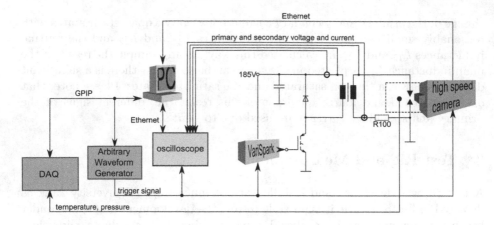

Fig. 6. Scheme of the data acquisition of the test rig.

the iron tube. These measurements can be used to calculate the break down voltage of the spark. The arbitrary waveform generator is used to trigger the ignition at the control electronics (*VariSpark*) and the measurement at the same time started from a Matlab-script running on a PC. This enables the user to visualize primary and secondary current and voltage on a high resolution oscilloscope.

4   Results

The simulations are performed with a very simplified model of the spark gap (consisting of a resistor and a parallel capacitance). The model of the spark gap switches either to a high value (this means there is no spark existent) or to a low value for the resistance (this means a spark is existent and therefore electrons can flow through the gas).

Test results are measured in a static environment and compared to the model. Even for this simple model of a spark gap a very good accordance between measurement and simulation can be seen in Figs. 7, 8, 9 and 10 - lines in red show the measurements acquired with the oscilloscope whereas the lines in blue show the simulation results of the system.

In Fig. 7 the primary voltage of the ignition coil is depicted. A multi-excitation of four pulses can be seen occurring at $20\,\mu s$, $157\,\mu s$, $294\,\mu s$ and $431\,\mu s$ for the duration of $38\,\mu s$. The simulation and the measurement accord over the whole time. After the peaks of the pulses when the IGBT is closed the discharging of the capacitance can be seen. The voltage declines steadily down during the multi-ignition. Between the peaks, while opening the IGBT the voltage drops below zero due to the flow of current through R_x and D_1 originating of the collapsing magnetic field of the primary windings.

Figure 8 shows the primary current which rises with each excitement pulse. A deviation can be found at the slope after the last impulse where the blue line (which depicts the simulations result) is slower dropping than the measurements result. The origin of this inaccuracy has to be determined.

The secondary voltage can be seen in Fig. 9. Immediately after the first pulse the voltage is rising very high (more than 14 kV) until the breakdown of the spark occurs. Afterwards, the voltage drops to a certain level and rests there regulated like the voltage in a glow lamp. When the current drops below a certain level the voltage breaks down (at 670 μs).

Figure 10 shows the corresponding secondary current. Immediately after the first excitement pulse (at 27 μs) the current rises very high due to the dropping resistance of the spark gap and the high secondary voltage before the breakdown. After the breakdown it drops very fast again and then behaves according to the primary current.

All in all the simulated results relate to the measured ones very well. Further measurements with different exciting pulses (differing in duration and number) were repeated and compared with simulation results. Again, the results show good accordance between measurement and simulation.

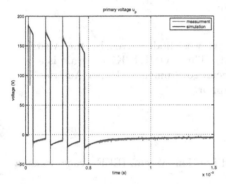

Fig. 7. Primary voltage u_P (Color figure online).

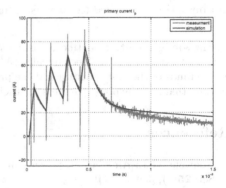

Fig. 8. Primary current i_P (Color figure online).

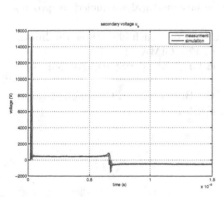

Fig. 9. Secondary voltage u_S (Color figure online).

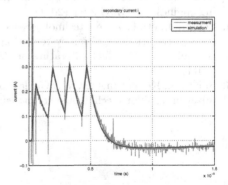

Fig. 10. Secondary current i_S (Color figure online).

5   Conclusion and Outlook

Concludingly it can be said that with the presented spark excitation it is possible to prolong the duration and amplify the power of the spark which guarantees a stable ignition while reducing misfire.

By using a minimum number of states it is possible to create a mathematical model which is fast and accurate. The results show a very good accordance between measurement and simulation even for the model with the simple spark gap. The model was converted into a C-code s-function which makes it flexible to be used in different software systems like Matlab/Simulink or FLUENT. Even a microprocessor could be programmed with it for current and/or voltage control of the spark. Thus, the mathematical model not only allows optimizing the system parameters for a better fuel combustion. Furthermore, it opens the possibility for system designers to create customized ignition coils.

Latter is the aim of ongoing studies in order to predefine the characteristics of the voltage and current of the spark.

Hence, with a better understanding of the system the combustion process can be optimized to reduce exhaust emissions.

Acknowledgement. Scientific advisory support was kindly given by the Austrian Center of Competence in Mechatronics (ACCM). This COMET/K2 program is aided by the funds of the state Austria and the provincial government of Upper Austria. The authors thank all involved partners for their support.

References

1. Rohwein, G.J.: An efficient, power-enhanced ignition system. IEEE Trans. Plasma Sci. **25**(2), 306–310 (1997)
2. Maier, M.: Untersuchung und Entwicklung von Netzwerkmodellen fuer belastete KFZ-Zuendsysteme. Cuvillier Verlag, Goettingen (2006)
3. Bell, D.E., Lepley, J.M., Lepley, D.T., Pirko, S.B.: Validation and performance analysis of a directed energy ignition system on large natural gas-fueled reciprocating engines. In: GMC 2011 (2011)
4. Lepley, J., et al.: A new technology electronic ignition which eliminates the limitations of traditional ignition systems. Paper No. 173, CIMAC (2011)
5. Altronic LLC, Product Literature on Altronic CPU XL VariSpark, Altronic LLC (2011)
6. Silber, S., Koppelstaetter, W., Weidenholzer, G., Bramerdorfer, G.: MagOpt - optimization tool for mechatronic components. In: ISMB14 (2014)

Simple Models of Central Heating System with Heat Exchangers in the Quasi-static Conditions

Anna Czemplik[✉]

Faculty of Electronics, Wroclaw University of Technology, Wroclaw, Poland
anna.czemplik@pwr.edu.pl

Abstract. A characteristic element of heating systems is heat exchanger dedicated to efficient heat transfer from one medium to another. The paper presents simple models of a heating system with heat exchangers designed for studies of control systems based on a control of heat carriers flow. Presented studies are necessary for a development of new control strategies in heating, ventilating, air conditioning and refrigeration systems. Three variants of heat exchangers models were examined – a typical model containing the logarithmic mean of temperatures, a model including assumptions about the arithmetic mean of temperatures and a model with an assumption of perfect mixing of medium in an exchanger. Usefulness of the models in designing of control systems was verified under quasi-static conditions.

Keywords: Heat exchanger · Central heating system · Control system

1 Introduction

Heat exchangers are widely used in various kinds of industrial and domestic installations especially in heating, ventilating, air conditioning and refrigeration systems (HVAC&R). The exchangers have different structures but their main purpose is to separate heat carriers and efficient heat transfer between them. This paper focuses on the use of heat exchangers in district heating systems (DHS) including district heating networks, heating substations and radiator systems in buildings with water as a heat carrier. However, the purpose of the analysis is not designing of DHS but designing of a control for these systems.

There exist various solutions for a control of DHS but generally they are based on controlling either a temperature of heat carrier flowing into an exchanger or a flow rate through an exchanger. The flow control is widely used in practice but an obtained control system is nonlinear what makes it difficult to analyze. Furthermore, heating systems are spatially extensive and contain many exchangers, thus studies of multi-loop control systems are necessary. As to deal with these difficulties, in order to obtain a reliable control system, simple models of plant dynamics are required.

Models of heat exchangers found in the literature can be divided into three categories. The most accurate ones are based on partial differential equations (PDE) and generally are dedicated to design and to build virtual prototypes of exchangers [1–3].

© Springer International Publishing Switzerland 2015
R. Moreno-Díaz et al. (Eds.): EUROCAST 2015, LNCS 9520, pp. 597–604, 2015.
DOI: 10.1007/978-3-319-27340-2_74

Dynamics of a heat exchanger described by partial differential equations makes difficult application of theories and control design techniques developed for lumped systems [4, 5]. The simplest models of heat exchangers used while examining a dynamics of plants or control systems have the form of transmittance [6]. However, these models are too simple since the transmittance is, by definition, a linear model while flow control is non-linear. The most popular models used for designing systems with exchangers (needed for exchangers' selection) have a form of balance equations with a function called the logarithmic mean temperature difference (LMTD) [7]. These models are the reference point for models studied in the paper.

The content of the paper is organized as follows. In Sects. 2 and 3 basic types and simple models of heat exchangers are presented. Simulation tests are described in Sect. 4 followed by analytical studies given in Sect. 5. Section 6 concludes the paper.

2 The Basic Heat Exchangers

In presented studies three types of heat exchangers were taken into account: parallel-flow exchanger (PFE), counter-flow exchanger (CFE) and capacitive exchanger (CE), as depicted in Fig. 1.

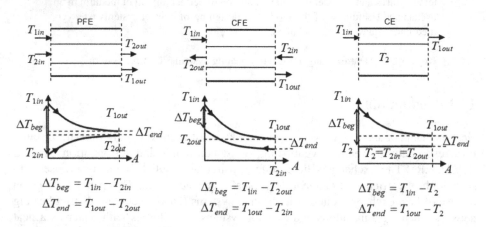

Fig. 1. Three types of heat exchangers (a description of variables see in text).

In the quasi-static conditions this types of exchangers can be described by equations in a form of a general energy balance

$$m_1(T_{1in}-T_{1out}) = k\Delta T = m_2(T_{2out}-T_{2in}) \quad \text{(for PFE/CFE)} \tag{1}$$

$$m_1(T_{1in}-T_{1out}) = k\Delta T \quad \text{(for CE)}$$

where: m_1 and m_2 are functions of flow rate f_1, f_2 ($m_1 = c_p\rho f_1$, $m_2 = c_p\rho f_2$), T_{1in}, T_{1out} – inlet and outlet temperatures of primary heat carrier, T_{2in}, T_{2out} – temperatures of secondary heat carrier, k – thermal conductivity coefficient, ΔT – the mean temperature difference between both media, ΔT_{beg} - the temperature difference at the "beginning" of a heat exchanger, ΔT_{end} – the temperature difference at the "end" of a heat exchanger, A – a heat exchange surface. In the most popular model used to design of heating systems, difference ΔT originates from a solution of partial differential equations describing an exchanger. In the primary solution of the integrated equations difference ΔT depends on flows of heat carriers and is given by

$$\Delta T = \Delta T_{beg}\left(1-e^{km}\right)/(km) \tag{2}$$

where $m = m_{lp} = 1/m_1 + 1/m_2$ for PFE, $m = m_{lc} = 1/m_1-1/m_2$ for CFE, and $m = m_l = 1/m_1$ for CE. After eliminating of flow rates from (2) the logarithmic mean temperature difference is obtained

$$\Delta T = \left(\Delta T_{end}-\Delta T_{beg}\right)/\ln\left(\Delta T_{end}/\Delta T_{beg}\right) \tag{3}$$

Equations (1) and (3) are typically used to determine nominal flow rates of heat carriers and the thermal coefficient k (and hence a size of a heat exchanger) on the base of inlet and outlet temperatures of an exchanger and heat demand of a system. However, during a testing of a control system the coefficient k, inlet temperatures and flow rates are known and the model is used to determine the outlet temperatures. Therefore, for study of systems with changes of flows Eqs. (1) and (2) are more suitable.

3   The Simple Models of Heat Exchangers

In this paper, three kinds of models of heat exchangers are analyzed. The first model (L) using LMTD (3) is the reference point. In the second model (M) the simplest assumption about the ideal mixing of heat carriers is used, thus ΔT is calculated as

$$\Delta T = T_{1out}-T_{2out} \tag{4}$$

This is a very strong assumption and a common opinion is that such simple model is not appropriate for exchangers modelling. However, presented later on studies show that the model is sufficient. The third model (A) is based on an arithmetical mean of temperatures

$$\Delta T = T_{1in}-T_{1out}/2 - (T_{2in}-T_{2out})/2 \tag{5}$$

and seems to be more accurate than the second one. These simple models do not describe temperature distribution along a heat exchange surface. Only model L is derived from partial equations which take into account a distribution of temperature. Models M and A are very simplified, especially model M.

On the base of Eqs. (1–5) following formulas for output variables (T_{1out}, T_{2out}) depending on input variables of exchanger (T_{1in}, T_{2in}, m_1, m_2) can be derived

$$T_{1out} = a_{11}T_{1in} + a_{11}T_{2in}, T_{2out} = a_{21}T_{1in} + a_{22}T_{2in} \quad \text{(for PFE/CFE)} \qquad (6)$$

$$T_{1out} = a_{11}T_{1in} + a_{11}T_2 \quad \text{(for CE)}.$$

Coefficients a_{11}, a_{12}, a_{21}, a_{22} for all models are collected in Table 1.

Table 1. Coefficients a in formulas (6) for models L, M, A.

	Model L		Model M	Model A
	PFE	CFE	PFE/CFE	PFE/CFE
a_{11}	$\dfrac{m_2 e^{-km_{lp}} + m_1}{m_1 + m_2}$	$\dfrac{(m_1-m_2)e^{-km_{lc}}}{m_1 e^{-km_{lc}} - m_2}$	$\dfrac{m_1(m_2+k)}{m_1 m_2 + k(m_1+m_2)}$	$\dfrac{4m_1 m_2 + 2k(m_1-m_2)}{4m_1 m_2 + 2k(m_1+m_2)}$
a_{12}	$\dfrac{-m_2 e^{-km_{pw}} + m_2}{m_1 + m_2}$	$\dfrac{m_2 e^{-km_{lc}} - m_2}{m_1 e^{-km_{lc}} - m_2}$	$\dfrac{m_2 k}{m_1 m_2 + k(m_1+m_2)}$	$\dfrac{4m_2 k}{4m_1 m_2 + 2k(m_1+m_2)}$
a_{21}	$\dfrac{-m_1 e^{-km_{lp}} + m_1}{m_1 + m_2}$	$\dfrac{m_1 e^{-km_{lc}} - m_1}{m_1 e^{-km_{lc}} - m_2}$	$\dfrac{m_1 k}{m_1 m_2 + k(m_1+m_2)}$	$\dfrac{4m_1 k}{4m_1 m_2 + 2k(m_1+m_2)}$
a_{22}	$\dfrac{m_1 e^{-km_{lp}} + m_2}{m_1 + m_2}$	$\dfrac{m_1 - m_2}{m_1 e^{-km_{lc}} - m_2}$	$\dfrac{m_2(m_1+k)}{m_1 m_2 + k(m_1+m_2)}$	$\dfrac{4m_1 m_2 + 2k(m_2-m_1)}{4m_1 m_2 + 2k(m_1+m_2)}$
	CE		CE	CE
a_{11}	e^{-km_l}		$\dfrac{m_1}{m_1+k}$	$\dfrac{2m_1-k}{2m_1+k}$
a_{12}	$1 - e^{-km_l}$		$\dfrac{k}{m_1+k}$	$\dfrac{2k}{2m_1+k}$

4 The Simulation Studies

Models L, M and A were used for simulation studies of a domestic central heating system. The test plant depicted in Fig. 2 consists of a substation with the heat exchanger PFE or CFE and a radiator system represented by the exchanger CE.

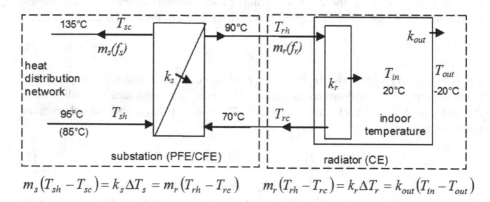

$$m_s\left(T_{sh} - T_{sc}\right) = k_s \Delta T_s = m_r\left(T_{rh} - T_{rc}\right) \qquad m_r\left(T_{rh} - T_{rc}\right) = k_r \Delta T_r = k_{out}\left(T_{in} - T_{out}\right)$$

Fig. 2. Model of a domestic central heating system

The heat balance of the plant in nominal (design) conditions is given by

$$q_N = m_{sN}(T_{shN} - T_{scN}) = k_s \Delta T_{sN} = m_{rN}(T_{rhN} - T_{rcN}) = k_r \Delta T_{rN} = k_{out}(T_{inN} - T_{outN}).$$
$$(7)$$

Parameters of the model were evaluated according to (7) and taking following nominal values: $T_{outN} = -20°C$, $T_{inN} = 20°C$, $q_N = 500$ kW, $T_{shN} = 135°C$, $T_{scN} = 95°C$ for PFE (85°C for CFE), $T_{rhN} = 90°C$, $T_{rcN} = 70°C$. Results are presented in Table 2.

Table 2. Values of parameters of the model (7) with PFE and CFE

$q_N = 500$ kW	Substation PFE + radiator $T_{shN}/T_{scN}/T_{rhN}/T_{rcN}$ 135/95/90/70 °C			Substation CFE + radiator $T_{shN}/T_{scN}/T_{rhN}/T_{rcN}$ 135/85/90/70°C		
model	L	M	A	L	M	A
ΔT_{sN}, °C	23.4	5.0	35.0	27.3	−5.0	30.0
ΔT_{rN}, °C	59.4	50.0	60.0	59.4	50.0	60.0
k_s, W/°C	21 376	100 000	14 286	18 310	−100 000	16 667
k_r, W/°C	8 412	10 000	8 333	8 412	10 000	8 333
k_{out}, W/°C	12 500					
m_{sN}, W/°C	12 500			10 000		
m_{rN}, W/°C	25 000					

It can be noticed large differences between values of models L and M, and even negative value of coefficient k_s for a plant with CFE. However, model M is not used to design of a heat exchanger. The following relationship between the parameters of models L, M, and A could be obtained which allows for scaling parameters from one model to another

$$k_{s(L)}\Delta T_{sN(L)} = k_{s(M)}\Delta T_{sN(M)} = k_{s(A)}\Delta T_{sN(A)} = q_N \qquad (8)$$

$$k_{r(L)}\Delta T_{rN(L)} = k_{r(M)}\Delta T_{rN(M)} = k_{s(A)}\Delta T_{rN(A)} = q_N.$$

Simulation studies of the system will be carried out in two steps. First, the substation and the radiator are examined separately and then the system is examined as a whole.

Characteristics of output variables of the substation (PFE/CFE) and the radiator (CE) treated separately were determined on the base of Eq. (6)

$$T_{sc} = a_{1sh}T_{sh} + a_{1rc}T_{rc}, \quad T_{rh} = a_{2sh}T_{sh} + a_{2rc}T_{rc} \quad \text{(for PFE/CFE)} \qquad (9)$$

$$T_{rc} = a_{3rh}T_{rh} + a_{3out}T_{out}, \quad T_{in} = a_{4rh}T_{rh} + a_{4out}T_{out} \quad \text{(for CE)}.$$

Coefficients a are calculated according to Table 1, therefore they depend on variants of the model, a type of heat exchanger and the functions of flow m_s and m_r. For the nominal values of flow rates given in Table 2, values of coefficients a for each model L, M, A are the same. Thus, characteristics of output variables depending on inlet temperatures (input variables) are linear and are the same for all models L, M, A.

The most interesting are non-linear characteristics of the output variables as the function of flow rates. Characteristics for all exchangers (PFE, CFE, CE) are very similar. Exemplary plots for PFE are presented in Fig. 3. It can be noticed that models M and L exhibit very similar behavior while model A is definitely different.

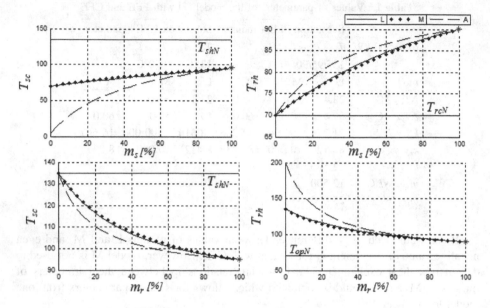

Fig. 3. The non-linear characteristics of PFE

For the system examined as a whole, i.e. the substation PFE/CFE in co-operation with the radiator CE, input variables are temperatures T_{sh} and T_{out}, and functions of flows m_s and m_r. The output variables (the same as above) were calculated as

$$T_{sc} = b_{1sh}T_{sh} + b_{1out}T_{out}, T_{rh} = b_{2sh}T_{sh} + b_{2out}T_{out} \qquad (10)$$

$$T_{rc} = b_{3sh}T_{sh} + b_{3out}T_{out}, \ T_{in} = b_{4sh}T_{rh} + b_{4out}T_{out}.$$

Coefficients b of (10) are presented in Table 3.

Table 3. Coefficients b in formulas (10), $M = 1 - a_{2rc}a_{3rh}$

b_{1sh}	$\frac{a_{1sh}M + a_{1rc}a_{2rc}a_{2sh}}{M}$	b_{1out}	$\frac{a_{1rc}a_{3out}}{M}$
b_{2sh}	$\frac{a_{2sh}}{M}$	b_{2out}	$\frac{a_{2rc}a_{3out}}{M}$
b_{3sh}	$\frac{a_{3rh}a_{2sh}}{M}$	b_{3out}	$\frac{a_{3out}}{M}$
b_{4sh}	$\frac{a_{4rh}a_{2sh}}{M}$	b_{4out}	$\frac{a_{4rh}a_{2rc}a_{3out} - a_{4out}M}{M}$

Linear characteristics of dependences on the input temperatures are the same for all variants of the models (L, M, A), both for the system with PFE as well as with CFE. Nonlinear characteristics of dependences of temperatures on flow rates m_s and m_r for models L and M are very similar and differ for model A. Figure 4 shows dependences on variable m_s for the model with PFE. Similar characteristics are obtained for a changing flow rate m_r and for CFE model.

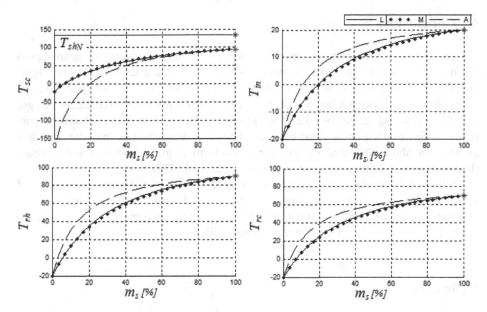

Fig. 4. The non-linear characteristics of the model with PFE (the dependence on m_s)

5 The Analytical Studies

Similarity of models M and L is quite surprising because the assumption of perfect mixing, taken into model M, from the definition ignores a temperature distribution along a heat exchange surface. Later on, it will be shown that model M is an approximation of model L. For this purpose two variants of approximation (linearization of type $e^x \approx 1 + x$ presented in Table 4) were applied to L models of PFE, CFE and CE.

Table 4. Two types of the applied approximation

A: Approximation of composite functions	B: Approximation of components of functions
$e^{-m_{lp}k} = \frac{1}{e^{m_{lp}k}} \approx \frac{1}{1+m_{lp}k} = \frac{1}{1+\left(\frac{1}{m_1}+\frac{1}{m_2}\right)k}$	$e^{-m_{lp}k} = \frac{1}{e^{k/m_1}e^{k/m_2}} \approx \frac{1}{\left(1+\frac{k}{m_1}\right)\left(1+\frac{k}{m_2}\right)}$
$e^{-m_{lc}k} = \frac{1}{e^{m_{lc}k}} \approx \frac{1}{1+m_{lc}k} = \frac{1}{1+\left(\frac{1}{m_1}-\frac{1}{m_2}\right)k}$	$e^{-m_{lc}k} = \frac{e^{k/m_2}}{e^{k/m_1}} \approx \frac{1+\frac{k}{m_2}}{1+\frac{k}{m_1}}$

After applying the approximation of a composite function (type A), model L of PFE gets the form of model M. In the model L of CFE the approximation of components of the function (type B) is necessary to obtain the same result. In the case of model L of CE both types of approximations give identical outcome and lead to model M. After approximation, models L have the form of models M but the models will be equivalent only after the scaling of the coefficients according to (8).

6 Conclusions

Presented studies demonstrated that the models containing an arithmetic mean should not be used to studies of control systems with variable flow rates because they differ significantly from models with LMTD. Whereas the simplest model based on the assumption of perfect mixing, which have too low accuracy for exchangers design, may be applied to studies of control strategies in circuits with heat exchangers, particularly for controlling a flow of heat carrier. It was shown, that the physical assumption about the ideal mixing corresponds to a mathematical approximation (linearization) of an exponential function included in LMTD model.

Although Computer Aided Control System Design (CACSD) allows for using of accurate models of HVAC&R systems, but there is still a need for very simple models of plants since such models facilitate the design of complex control systems and may be applied in model-based control algorithms (MBC) [4].

References

1. Bilirgen, H., Dunbar, S., Levy, E.: Numerical modelling of finned heat exchanger. Appl. Therm. Eng. **61**, 278–288 (2013)
2. Karmo, D., Ajib, S., Khateeb, A.: New method for design an effective finned heat exchanger. Appl. Therm. Eng. **51**, 539–550 (2013)
3. Léal, L., Topin, F., Lavieille, P., Tadrist, L., Miscevic, M.: Simultaneous integration, control and enhancement of both fluid flow and heat transfer in small scale heat exchangers: a numerical study. Int. Commun. Heat Mass Transf. **49**, 36–40 (2013)
4. Åström, K., Hägglund, T.: Advanced PID Control. ISA, Triangle Park (2006)
5. Tóth, L., Nagy, L., Szeifert, F.: Nonlinear inversion-based control of a distributed parameter heating system. Appl. Therm. Eng. **43**, 174–179 (2012)
6. Chmielnicki, W.: Energy Control in Buildings Connected to Urban Heating Sources. PAN, Warszawa (1996)
7. Recknagel, H., Spenger, E., Hönmann, W., Schramek, E.: Taschenbuch für Heizung und Klimatechnik 92/93. Oldenbourg Verlag GmbH, München (1994)

Microprocessor Hazard Analysis Via Formal Verification of Parameterized Systems

Lukáš Charvát[✉], Aleš Smrčka, and Tomáš Vojnar

FIT, IT4Innovations Centre of Excellence, Brno University of Technology,
Božetěchova 2, 612 66 Brno, Czech Republic
{icharvat,smrcka,vojnar}@fit.vutbr.cz

Abstract. The current stress on having a rapid development cycle for microprocessors featuring pipeline-based execution leads to a high demand of automated techniques supporting the design, including a support for its verification. We present an automated technique exploiting static analysis of data paths and formal verification of parameterized systems in order to discover flaws caused by improperly handled data hazards. In particular, as a complement of our previous work on read-after-write hazards, we focus on write-after-write and write-after-read hazards in microprocessors with a single pipeline.

1 Introduction

Implementation of pipeline-based execution of instructions in purpose-specific microprocessors is an error prone task, which implies a need of proper verification of the resulting designs. Therefore, our long-term goal is to develop a set of verification techniques with formal roots, each of them specialised in checking absence of a certain kind of errors in pipeline-based execution of such microprocessors. The main idea is that, this way, a high degree of automation and scalability can be achieved since only parts of a design related to a specific error are to be investigated. In our previous works [4,5], we proposed, with the above goal in mind, fully automated approaches for checking correctness of the implementation of instructions when executing in isolation and for verifying absence of read-after-write (RAW) hazards. In this paper, we extend our approach to handle also *write-after-write (WAW)* and *write-after-read (WAR)* hazards in microprocessors with a single pipeline. We have implemented our approach and present encouraging results from its experimental evaluations.

Related Work. Showing absence of data hazards is a native part of checking conformance between an RTL design and a formally encoded ISA description.

This work was supported by the Czech Science Foundation under the project 14-11384S, the EU/Czech IT4Innovations Centre of Excellence project CZ.1.05/ 1.1.00/02.0070, and the internal BUT project FIT-S-14-2486.

© Springer International Publishing Switzerland 2015
R. Moreno-Díaz et al. (Eds.): EUROCAST 2015, LNCS 9520, pp. 605–614, 2015.
DOI: 10.1007/978-3-319-27340-2_75

The perhaps most cited approach to such checking is the so-called flushing technique [3], which has been extended, e.g., in [7,9,13], to handle rather complicated designs with multi-cycle execution units, exceptions, and branch prediction. The main challenge of these works is to overcome the semantic gap between the different levels of a processor description. Dealing with this issue typically requires a significant user intervention in the form of providing various additional assertions about the design or transforming it to a purpose-specific description language.

In [8], the so-called self-consistency check that compares possible executions of each instruction in two scenarios is introduced. The comparison is made wrt. a property given by the user, e.g., a property concerning data hazards which deals with (i) executions of an instruction enclosed by any (random) instructions within the pipeline and (ii) executions of the same instruction surrounded by NOP instructions only. If the self-consistency check succeeds, conformance of the RTL and ISA descriptions of a processor can be established by separately showing conformance of the RTL/ISA descriptions of each individual instruction. The main drawback of the approach is that it requires the enclosing instructions from the first run not to violate a so-called consistent state of the microprocessor, which has to be manually defined by the user.

In [1], a formal model based on a notion of stages, parcels (instructions), and hazards has been introduced. Once the user defines predicates needed for describing the pipeline, the design can be automatically formally proven correct under a correctness criterion given in the work. Another, a bit similar approach has been proposed in [10]. The approach introduces an abstract formal model whose components are to be linked by the user with the concrete cycle-accurate implementation through a number of mappings. Afterwards, the validity of several properties based on the established mappings and together implying correctness of the pipeline behaviour is checked. Again, both of the above methods require a significant manual user intervention.

Compared with the above approaches, we do not aim at full conformance checking between RTL and ISA implementations. Instead, we address one specific property—namely, absence of problems caused by data hazards. On the other hand, our approach is almost fully automated—the only step required from the user is to identify the architectural resources (such as registers and memory ports) and the program counter.

2   Preliminaries

Our approach expects a processor to be described in the form of a so-called *processor structure graph* (PSG) which can be represented by a tuple $G = (V, E, s, t)$. Here, V is a finite set that is the union $V_s \cup V_f$ of a set V_s of *storages* and a set V_f of *Boolean circuits*, $V_s \cap V_f = \emptyset$. The set V_s further consists of a set V_a of *architectural* and a set V_p of *pipeline* storages, $V_a \cap V_p = \emptyset$. To simplify the explanation, we will not deal with micro-architectural registers, memories and their ports in this paper, however as we show in [5], designs including these entities can be easily verified by the proposed approach as well. Without a loss of generality, we can also expect all storages of the set V_s to have a unit write and zero read delay since longer access times can be modelled by introducing sequentially connected registers emulating the required delay. The set V_f of Boolean circuits is the union $V_{mx} \cup V_g$ of a set V_{mx} of circuits implementing *multiplexers* and a set V_g of the remaining (generic) circuits, $V_{mx} \cap V_g = \emptyset$.

Next, E denotes a finite set of *transfer edges*. Then, mappings $s, t : E \rightarrow V \times \mathbb{T}$ assign to each edge its source (resp., target) vertex where $\mathbb{T} = \{$d, q, en, st, cl, sel$\} \cup \{$a$_i$, c$_i$ $\mid i \in \mathbb{N}\}$ is a set of *connection types*. It is required that a PSG contains no cycle formed only by vertices representing Boolean circuits. The d, q, and en connection types represent commonly used input, output, and enable connections of flip-flop registers with their usual semantics. Pipeline registers do also have st (stall) and cl (clear) connections. In case of stalling, each stalled register keeps its current value to the next cycle. Clearing a register sets its value to zero. The a$_i$ connection types represent arguments of functional vertices $v_g \in V_g$. Further, sel and c$_i$ are connection types related to multiplexers only. The value transferred through the sel connection selects which of its c$_i$ inputs is propagated to the q output of a multiplexer. Since each vertex $v \in V$ can have at most one inbound edge for a single connection type, one can use a notation $v.$c to uniquely describe an edge $e \in E$ that satisfies $t(e) = (v, c)$.

In this paper, we will work with an annotated version of a PSG. The annotation can be given via a *stage* mapping $\varphi \colon V_s \rightarrow \mathbb{S}$, $\mathbb{S} = \{0, ..., n\}$, $n \in \mathbb{N}$, assigning storages to pipeline stages. The annotation can be given manually or techniques such as data-flow analysis [5] can be used to obtain one. From a stage mapping φ, we can easily get the *write stage* φ_{wr} (*read stage* φ_{rd}, respectively) mapping, $\varphi_{wr}, \varphi_{rd} \colon V_s \rightarrow 2^{\mathbb{S}}$, describing which stages directly influence (use) the content of the given storage.

Our approach further uses the common notion of a parameterized system operating on a linear topology where processes (i.e., executed instructions) may perform local transitions or universally/existentially guarded global transitions [2,6]. A parameterized system is a pair $P = (Q, \Delta)$ where Q is a finite set of states of a process and Δ is a set of transition rules over Q. A transition rule is of the form $\mathbb{Q}j \circ i \colon G \models q \rightarrow q'$ where $\mathbb{Q} \in \{\forall, \exists\}$, $\circ \in \{<, >, =\}$, $G \subseteq Q$, and $q, q' \in Q$. A parameterized system induces a transition system whose configurations are finite words over Q. A configuration $q_1...q_i...q_n$, $1 \leq i \leq n$, changes to $q_1...q_i'...q_n$ when the ith process goes from its state q_i to q_i' using some of the transition rules. The rule can be applied only if its guard is satisfied. For example, the meaning of the guard $\exists j < i \colon G$ is "there should be at least one process j to the left of i (in the linear topology) so that the jth process is in a state that belongs to the set G".

We will work with the reachability problem given by a parameterized system P, a regular set $I \subseteq Q^+$ of initial configurations, and a regular set $Bad \subseteq Q^+$ of bad configurations. In particular, we assume Bad to be given as the upward closure of a finite set $B \subseteq Q^+$ of minimal bad configurations, this is, $Bad = \{c \in Q^+ \mid \exists b \in B \colon b \sqsubseteq c\}$ where $\sqsubseteq$ is the usual sub-word relation (i.e.,

$u \sqsubseteq s_1...s_n \Leftrightarrow u = s_{i_1}...s_{i_k}$ for some $1 \leq i_1 \leq ... \leq i_k \leq n$, $0 \leq k \leq n$). Now, let $R \subseteq Q^*$ denote the set of all reachable configurations. We say that the system P is safe wrt. I and Bad iff no bad configuration is reachable, i.e., $R \cap Bad = \emptyset$.

3 Description of the Proposed Data Hazard Verification Method

We assume the processor under verification to be represented using a PSG, which can be easily obtained from a description of the processor on the register transfer level (RTL) written in common hardware description languages, such as VHDL or Verilog.

Our approach consists of the following steps: (i) a static detection of instructions that can potentially cause a data hazard, (ii) generation of a parameterized system modelling mutual interaction among the instructions, and (iii) an analysis of the constructed parameterized system identifying whether some unhandled data hazard may occur.

Example 1. Figure 1 shows a PSG describing a part of a simple microprocessor with an accumulator architecture with two architectural registers: X (a memory index register) and A (an accumulator). For the sake of brevity, the PSG exhibits only the parts of the microprocessor that are used during execution of arithmetic and instructions with an auto-increment. Moreover, it also omits control connections (en, st, and cl) of pipeline registers. In the CPU, an instruction fetched from the memory is stored into the storage id_ir representing the instruction register. The opcode part is sent to the decoder to determine the type of the ALU operation to be performed and to select its destination by activation of the appropriate enable (en) connection of the X or A register. An early auto-increment of register X can be performed in stage 3. Such a feature allows the CPU to execute sequences of instructions working with juxtaposed data in the

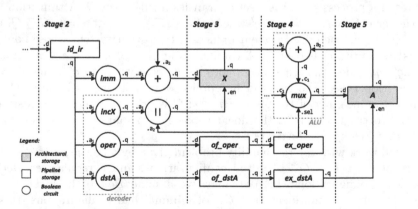

Fig. 1. A processor structure graph of a part of a CPU with an accumulator architecture.

memory without a penalty (brought, e.g., by unnecessary stalls of the pipeline) which would be present if the update of X was done in a later stage.   ◁

3.1 Static Detection of Data Hazards

A static hazard analysis examines the PSG and its annotation in the form of the pipeline stage mappings φ, φ_{wr}, and φ_{rd} to identify a finite set of so-called *hazard cases*, each of them describing one potential source of a data hazard. In order to construct the hazard cases, we will use a notion of an *influence path*.

We define an *influence path* as a path $\langle v_1, e_1, ..., v_k \rangle$ in a PSG where the value read from an architectural storage $v_1 \in V_a$ can influence a value stored to an architectural storage $v_a \in V_a$ by writing to a *target* storage $v_k \in V_s$. Each influence path must fulfill the following set of properties: (i) The target storage v_k must either be (a) an architectural register, i.e., the case when $v_k = v_a$, or (b) a pipeline register s.t. $t(e_{k-1}) = (v_k, \texttt{cl})$. Indeed, clearing of the pipeline register v_k will surely influence all programmer visible storages that belong to stages $s \geq \varphi(v_k)$. Next, (ii) the influence path must not traverse through stall connections of pipeline registers. Such paths cannot influence the value of any programmer visible register. Their only impact can be stalling a stage which does not influence a proper execution of instructions if one assumes correctness of in-order execution of instructions (that can be automatically checked by the method described in [11]). Finally, (iii) there must exist an *execution plan* $\tau: V \to \mathbb{S}$ which assigns elements of the path to stages from which they are accessed by an instruction that performs a computation over the given influence path.

The access stage of each element that is given by the execution plan has to conform to φ_{rd} and φ_{wr}, i.e., (a) $v_i \in V_s \Rightarrow \tau(v_i) + 1 \in \varphi_{rd}(v_i)$ for all $1 \leq i < k$ and (b) $v_j \in V_s \Rightarrow \tau(v_j) \in \varphi_{wr}(v_j)$ for all $1 < j \leq k$. Moreover, the stages of the execution plan must form a non-decreasing sequence, i.e., (c) $\tau(v_{i-1}) \leq \tau(v_i)$ which increases at each path element with a write delay, i.e., (d) $\tau(v_i) = \tau(v_{i-1}) + 1$ if $v_i \in V_s$. Otherwise, in the case that any of the rules (a–d) fails, there could not be any instruction capable of a data transfer along the influence path.

An incorrectly handled data hazard is manifested upon the first write of improper data into some programmer visible storage of the design. Therefore, it suffices to further deal with the minimal influence path which is an influence path where $v_i \notin V_a$ and $t(e_{i-1}) \notin V_p \times \{\texttt{cl}\}$ for all $1 < i < k$. A standard breadth-first

Table 1. The access stage mappings for architectural registers.

Register	Stage φ	Write stages φ_{wr}	Read stages φ_{rd}
X	3	$\{2,4\}$	$\{2,4\}$
A	5	$\{4\}$	$\{4\}$

search algorithm with rules (i–iii) and the minimality checked on-the-fly can be used to obtain the minimal influence paths in the given PSG.

A *WAR hazard case* is a tuple $(v_a, s_w, s_r, v_t, s_t, \pi)$ consisting of (i) an architectural storage $v_a \in V_a$, (ii) its write stage $s_w \in \varphi_{wr}(v_w)$, and (iv) read stage $s_r \in \varphi_{rd}(v_a)$ such that $s_w < s_r$ in order that the storage is written before it is read to evoke a WAR hazard, (v) a target storage v_t where the potentially incorrect value read from v_a is stored, (vi) a stage $s_t \in \varphi_{wr}(v_t)$, $s_r \leq s_t$, in which the incorrect value is stored, and (vii) a minimal influence path π describing how data are propagated from v_a to v_t between the stages s_r and s_t. Similarly, a *WAW hazard case* (v_a, s_{w_1}, s_{w_2}) consists of an architectural storage $v_a \in V_a$ and its two different write stages $s_{w_1}, s_{w_2} \in \varphi_{wr}(v_w)$, $s_{w_2} < s_{w_1}$ so the WAW hazard may occur. There is no need to include any influence path in this case since an error in WAW hazard case handling would be demonstrated instantly by writing an incorrect value to the storage v_a. Note that, since the definitions of a hazard cases speak about storages, their access stages, and the path along which the problematic data is transferred, it is not related to a single instruction only but to an entire class of instructions.

Example 2. Consider the PSG from Fig. 1 and the mappings shown in Table 1. One can see that there is a potential WAR hazard on register X because, for example, it can be written in stage 2 ($\varphi_{wr}(X) = \{2, 4\}$) and read in stage 4 ($\varphi_{rd}(X) = \{2, 4\}$). By the definition, to form a WAR hazard, there must also exist an influence path π in the PSG leading from X to some target storage. For instance, we can assume the register A (written in stage 4) as a target with $\pi = \langle X, +.\mathsf{a}_1, +, mux.\mathsf{c}_1, mux, A.\mathsf{d}, A \rangle$. This observation gives us a WAR hazard case $hc = (X, 2, 4, A, 4, \pi)$. A similar reasoning can applied to derive WAW hazard cases as well.   ◁

3.2   Construction of Parameterized Systems Modelling the Potential Hazards

As we have shown in [5], the behaviour of the instructions given by constraints of a hazard case can be modelled using a parameterized system $P = (Q, \Delta)$ which maps n instructions in the pipeline to n processes in a linear array. Initially, they are in a state saying that their execution has not started. Then, they proceed through individual stages of the pipeline during which they may interact with each other by means of the pipeline flow logic, e.g., an earlier instruction may force a later instruction to be stalled or cleared. Finally, the instructions end up in a state denoting that they left the pipeline. The structure of the generated parameterized system depends on the type of the hazard case. The system P models interactions among three classes of processes (and hence 3 types of instructions) for both WAR and WAW hazard case. For a WAR hazard case $(v_a, s_w, s_r, v_t, s_t, \pi)$, a w-class of processes is used to model every instruction that writes to the storage v_a in the stage s_w. An rw-class models instructions that read from the storage v_a in the stage s_r, perform a data computation that involves the data path π, and write to the storage v_t in the stage s_t. Finally, *any*-class instructions are used as pipeline fillers representing *any* other instructions. For a WAW hazard case (v_a, s_{w_1}, s_{w_2}), we use processes of the w_1-class (w_2-class, respectively) which model instructions writing to the storage v_a in the stage s_{w_1} (s_{w_2}). The purpose of the *any*-class instructions remains the same as in the previous case.

The set Q of states of a parameterized system P is then given by pairs (k, s) where k gives a class of an instruction and s gives the stage in which the instruction is currently executed. We will use the notation q_s^k to denote a state $(k, s) \in Q$. For a pipeline of length m, the sequence $q_1^k, ..., q_m^k$ records each step of a k-class instruction in the pipeline. Transition rules Δ of a system P are then constructed by reasoning over constraints given in the from of bit-vector logic formulae. These formulae describe behaviour in each state of the execution of a k-class instruction.

The required reasoning is done automatically by utilizing an SMT solver (for additional technical details regarding the construction of Δ, please see [5]). Such a system is then checked whether there exists some sequence of instructions that could reach hazardous conditions. In parameterized systems, hazard conditions can in particular be expressed by the regular set Bad of bad configurations. The most crucial part for the construction of the Bad set is determination of the so-called *commit* and *hazardous states*, which is discussed below.

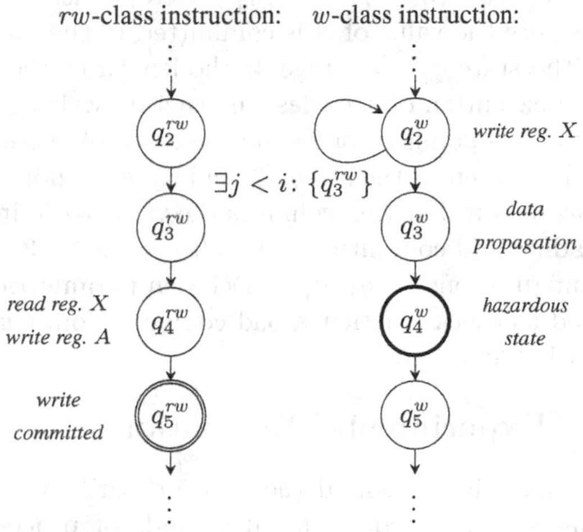

Fig. 2. A part of the control automata of processes representing rw/w-class instructions involved in the hazard case hc from Example 2.

Given a WAR hazard case $(v_a, s_w, s_r, v_t, s_t, \pi)$, $s_w < s_r \le s_t$, one can infer that the data supposed to be written to v_a are computed in the stage s_w, and the computed value is committed to v_a in the next cycle, thus in the stage $s_w + 1$. To ensure that the value read in stage the s_r is correct, no write to v_a can occur for $h = s_r - (s_w + 1)$ cycles which is the difference between reading and commitment of the value from/to v_a. Otherwise, an rw-class instruction would necessarily read and compute with incorrect data that were written too early (in stage s_w) by a later w-class instruction. The WAR hazard is exhibited only after commitment of the incorrectly fetched data from the register v_a in the stage s_r to the register v_t which happens in the stage $s_t + 1$. Such a data propagation lasts $p = (s_t + 1) - s_r$ cycles. Note that, if the rw-class instruction is canceled during the propagation period of p, there is no further write to v_t caused by the instruction. Thus, for a w-class instruction, we denote the states $\{q_{s_w+p+i}^w \mid 1 \le i \le h\}$ as hazardous. A configuration of the parameterized system P is then considered as bad if it includes an occurrence of a commit state $q_{s_t+1}^{rw}$ of an rw-class instruction followed by a hazard state.

An analogical reasoning can be performed also for a WAW hazard case (v_a, s_{w_1}, s_{w_2}), $s_{w_2} < s_{w_1}$. Here, no write to v_a can occur for $h = s_{w_2} - s_{w_1}$ cycles. Otherwise, the execution of an earlier w_1-class instruction would overwrite the value storage v_a that was already set by a later w_2-class instruction. Therefore, we tag the states $\{q_{s_{w_2}+i}^{w_2} \mid 1 \leq i \leq h\}$ as hazardous. Finally, we include a configuration into *Bad* if it contains a commit state $q_{s_{w_1}+1}^{w_1}$ of a w_1-class instruction followed by a hazard state.

Example 3. Consider the hazard case hc described in Example 2 and the inferred processes shown in Fig. 2. The execution of the rw-class instructions reading X and writing to A is passing through the sequence of states $q_0^{rw}, q_1^{rw}, q_2^{rw}, q_3^{rw}, q_4^{rw}, q_5^{rw}, q_6^{rw}$. Here, X is read and A written in the state q_4^{rw}. Because the value of A is committed in the state q_5^{rw} (in stage 5) and X is read in the state q_4^{rw} (in stage 4) the length of the data propagation p is $5 - 4 = 1$. The execution of a w-class instruction writing to the X register is described by a process going through the sequence of states $q_0^w, q_1^w, q_2^w, q_3^w, q_4^w, q_5^w, q_6^w$ where X is written in the state q_2^w and q_0, q_6 denote initial, resp. final, state. Because a w-class instruction commits the value to X in stage 3, the distance h (between reading and commitment from/to X) is $4 - 3 = 1$. Thus, the set of minimal bad configurations is $\{q_5^{rw} q_4^w\}$. A chosen parametric verification method can then be used to check whether a bad configuration, e.g., $q_6^{any} q_5^{rw} q_4^w q_3^{any} q_2^{any} q_1^{any} q_0^{any}$, is reachable.   ◁

4   Experimental Evaluation

We have implemented the above described method in a prototype tool called *Hades* and tested it on three kinds of processors: *TinyCPU* is a small 8-bit processor that we mainly use for testing of new verification methods. *CompAcc* is an 8-bit processor based on an accumulator architecture. Finally, *DLX5AI* is a 5-staged 32-bit processor able to execute a subset of the instruction set (without floating point instructions) of the DLX architecture which differs from commonly known implementation [12] by having an auto-increment logic. Some of the processors were in multiple variants that differ from each other, e.g., in the way how data hazards are avoided, yielding seven test cases in total.

We conducted a series of experiments on a PC with Intel Core i7-3770K @3.50 GHz and 16 GB RAM with results presented in Table 2. The columns give the verified processor, its variant, the time needed for

Table 2. Verification times.

Processor features		Static analysis [s]	Parametric model verification [s]	Total time [s]	Hazard cases [#]
TinyCPU	S	1	24	25	14
	SF	1	25	26	14
	B	1	38	39	24
CompAcc	SF	2	70	72	31
	BF	2	61	63	33
DLX5AI	S	5	418	423	69
	B	384	420	804	69

S - stalling logic, B - bypassing logic, F - flag reg.

the static analysis, and the time spent by verification of the parameterized systems that are created based on each hazard case, and the overall verification time. The last column represents the number of hazard cases that had to be verified during the model verification phase. Note that each hazard case represents a separate task so the part of model verification can be run in parallel. As can be seen, the results look promising in that the verification times are in minutes for all types of the presented microprocessors. The longer time of static analysis encountered for DLX is mainly due to the larger number of paths that have to be considered (by the BFS algorithm) during the computation of the sets of hazard cases.

5   Conclusion

We have presented an approach that harnesses methods for formal verification of parameterized systems in order to discover incorrectly handled data hazards in the RTL implementation of pipeline-based execution. The approach was developed with the aim to be highly automated, not requiring any additional efforts from the developers (apart from specifying the architectural registers). We have implemented the approach and successfully tested it on several non-trivial microprocessors.

In the future, we plan to further extend the approach presented in the paper by techniques suitable for verification of other processor features, such as control hazards. This is motivated by our general idea of trying to split processor verification into several simpler, more specialised tasks.

References

1. Aagaard, M.D.: A hazards-based correctness statement for pipelined circuits. In: Geist, D., Tronci, E. (eds.) CHARME 2003. LNCS, vol. 2860, pp. 66–80. Springer, Heidelberg (2003)
2. Abdulla, P.A., Haziza, F., Holík, L.: All for the price of few. In: Giacobazzi, R., Berdine, J., Mastroeni, I. (eds.) VMCAI 2013. LNCS, vol. 7737, pp. 476–495. Springer, Heidelberg (2013)
3. Burch, J.R., Dill, D.L.: Automatic verification of pipelined microprocessor control. In: Dill, D.L. (ed.) CAV 1994. LNCS, vol. 818, pp. 68–80. Springer, Heidelberg (1994)
4. Charvat, L., Smrcka, A., Vojnar, T.: Automatic formal correspondence checking of ISA and RTL microprocessor description. In: Proceedings of MTV 2012, pp. 6–12. IEEE (2012)
5. Charvat, L., Smrcka, A., Vojnar, T.: Using formal verification of parameterized systems in RAW hazard analysis in microprocessors. In: Proceedings of MTV 2014, pp. 83–89. IEEE (2014)
6. Clarke, E., Talupur, M., Veith, H.: Environment abstraction for parameterized verification. In: Emerson, E.A., Namjoshi, K.S. (eds.) VMCAI 2006. LNCS, vol. 3855, pp. 126–141. Springer, Heidelberg (2006)
7. Hao, K., Ray, S., Xie, F.: Equivalence checking for function pipelining in behavioral synthesis. In: Proceedings of DATE 2014, pp. 1–6. IEEE (2014)
8. Jones, R.B., Seger, C.H., Dill, D.L.: Self-consistency checking. In: Srivas, M., Camilleri, A. (eds.) FMCAD 1996. LNCS, vol. 1166, pp. 159–171. Springer, Heidelberg (1996)

9. Koelbl, A., Jacoby, R., Jain, H., Pixley, C.: Solver technology for system-level to RTL equivalence checking. In: Proceedings of DATE 2009, pp. 196–201. IEEE (2009)

10. Kuhne, U., Beyer, S., Bormann, J., Barstow, J.: Automated formal verification of processors based on architectural models. In: Proceedings of FMCAD 2010, pp. 129–136. IEEE (2010)

11. Mishra, P., Tomiyama, H., Dutt, N., Nicolau, A.: Automatic verification of in-order execution in microprocessors with fragmented pipelines and multicycle functional units. In: Proceedings of DATE 2002, pp. 36–43. IEEE (2002)

12. Patterson, D.A., Hennessy, J.L.: Computer Organization and Design: The Hardware/Software Interface, 4th edn. Morgan Kaufmann, Boston (2012)

13. Velev, M.N., Gao, P.: Automatic formal verification of multithreaded pipelined microprocessors. In: Proceedings of ICCAD 2011, pp. 679–686. IEEE (2011)

Digital Signal Processing Methods
and Applications

Evaluation and Optimization of GPU Based Unate Covering Algorithms

Bernd Steinbach[1]([✉]) and Christian Posthoff[2]

[1] Institute of Computer Science, Freiberg University of Mining and Technology,
Bernhard-von-Cotta-Str. 2, 09596 Freiberg, Germany
steinb@informatik.tu-freiberg.de
[2] The University of The West Indies,
St. Augustine Campus, St. Augustine, Trinidad and Tobago
christian@posthoff.de

Abstract. The calculation of an exact minimal cover of a Boolean function is an NP-complete problem which has important applications in circuit design. We could reduce the required time for the calculation by a factor of more than $3.5 * 10^7$ in [9], more than $8 * 10^8$ in [8], and even $9 * 10^9$ using a single CPU-core. Using a GPU, we achieved in [7] even a factor of improvement of $1.2 * 10^{11}$ [7].

In this paper we compare our so far best approach with a powerful algorithm for the same problem recently published by other authors [1]. The second aim of this paper is the optimization of our so far fastest algorithm which solves the Unate Covering Problem on a GPU. An extended abstract of this paper was published in [6].

Keywords: Unate covering problem · Evaluation · Optimization · GPU · CUDA · Warp vote function

1 Introduction

The *Unate Covering Problem* UCP [3] must be solved to find minimal sets of prime conjunctions which completely cover the required Boolean function of a circuit. Consequently, the required circuit space can be reduced, and less power will be consumed.

Figure 1 shows the results of our previous work to solve the UCP. We used in our previous papers [7–9] Algorithm 1 (ABS(DIST($P(\mathbf{p})$))) of [7] for simple direct comparisons. This algorithm is already 10^4 times faster than the trivial UCP-algorithm. Figure 1 uses a logarithmic scale for the factor of improvements because the needed time to solve a UCP could be drastically shortened by utilization of properties of the application domain, the small number of CPU cores together with MPI, as well as several hundreds of GPU cores and CUDA.

Here we compare our so far fastest approach that utilizes a GPU with a new optimized algorithm which has been published in [1].

© Springer International Publishing Switzerland 2015
R. Moreno-Díaz et al. (Eds.): EUROCAST 2015, LNCS 9520, pp. 617–624, 2015.
DOI: 10.1007/978-3-319-27340-2_76

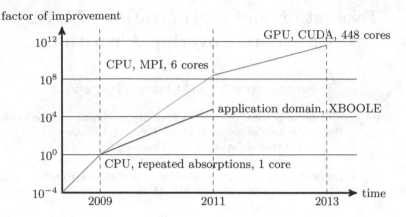

Fig. 1. Improvements of solving the UCP in the last years.

2 Unate Covering - the Problem

We consider a special SAT-problem without negated variables. Such functions are called *Petrick functions* $P(\mathbf{p})$. The Petrick function defined by (1) depends on 8 variables and is given by 9 clauses:

$$(p_4 \vee p_5 \vee p_6 \vee p_8) \wedge (p_2 \vee p_3 \vee p_4 \vee p_7 \vee p_8) \wedge (p_1 \vee p_3 \vee p_4 \vee p_7 \vee p_8) \wedge$$
$$(p_1 \vee p_4 \vee p_5 \vee p_7 \vee p_8) \wedge (p_1 \vee p_2 \vee p_5 \vee p_6) \wedge (p_4 \vee p_5 \vee p_6 \vee p_7 \vee p_8) \wedge \quad (1)$$
$$(p_1 \vee p_4 \vee p_5 \vee p_6 \vee p_7 \vee p_8) \wedge (p_4 \vee p_6 \vee p_7) \wedge (p_1 \vee p_2 \vee p_4 \vee p_8) = 1.$$

The classical approach to solve the unate covering problem applies the distributive law [4] to the clauses, simplifies the created conjunctions using the idempotence law [4], and reduces the found disjunctive form [5] using the absorption law [4]. A remarkable speedup of more than 10^4 is reached by the IT(DIST/ABS)-algorithm which applies the distributive law for the next clause and reduces the found conjunction immediately using the absorption law. We use this approach as basis for comparison of improved algorithms.

3 Evaluation of UCP-Algorithms

We represent each clause of $P(\mathbf{p})$ by a binary vector; a value 1 in these vectors indicates that the associated variable p_i appears in the clause. In this way, the *Petrick functions* $P(\mathbf{p})$ is modeled by a clause vector cv.

The necessary and sufficient condition that the binary vector $f_j^{S_i}(\mathbf{p})$ satisfies $P(\mathbf{p}) = \bigvee_{ic=1}^{cv.elements} C_{ic}(\mathbf{p})$ is:

$$\forall\, ic \in \{1, \ldots, cv.elements\} \quad f_j^{S_i}(\mathbf{p}) \wedge C_{ic}(\mathbf{p}) \neq 0 \quad (2)$$

where S_i indicates an elementary symmetric function with i values 1 in the binary vectors. All binary vectors $f_j^{S_i}(\mathbf{p})$ are represented by the permutation vector pv.

Algorithm 1. $sv = $ BDIF_kernel(pv, cv) for the GPU

1: **for** $ic \leftarrow 0, ic < cv.elements, ic \leftarrow ic + 1$ **do**
2:   **if** $pv.vector[ip] \wedge cv.vector[ic] = 0$ **then**
3:     **break**
4:   **end if**
5: **end for**
6: **if** $ic = cv.elements$ **then**
7:   $sv.vector[is] \leftarrow pv.vector[ip]$
8:   $is \leftarrow is + 1$
9: **end if**

Algorithm 1 shows the **binary difference** algorithm (BDIF) useable as kernel for a GPU to evaluate (2).

We call this approach *Restricted Complete Evaluation* on a GPU (RCE-GPU). The benefits of RCE-GPU are:

– the ordered evaluation of $f^{S_i}(\mathbf{p})$ with growing values of i to avoid all evaluations of binary vectors $f_j^{S_i}(\mathbf{p})$ which contain more than the wanted exact minimal number of values 1, and
– the immediate break of the evaluation in line 3 of Algorithm 1 when an orthogonal clause $C_{ic}(\mathbf{p})$ is detected.

Borowik and Łuba recently published an improved algorithm [1] that solves the UCP using a tree-based complement algorithm which was basically suggested in [2]. They used this algorithm in the area of data mining.

Algorithm 2. Minimal Disjunctive Form using a Decision Tree (MDF-DT)

1: $n_{\min} \leftarrow n$
2: **for all** orders of the variables x_i **do**
3:   $n_{smallest}^{dec} \leftarrow$ recursively decompose $f(\mathbf{x})$ given in conjunctive form
4:   **if** $n_{smallest}^{dec} < n_{\min}$ **then**
5:     merge decision variables to a disjunctive form of $f(\mathbf{x})$
6:   **end if**
7: **end for**

The sources of improvements of Algorithm 2 are:

– Subsets of ordered variables must not repeatedly evaluated.
– A decomposition branch k can be truncated if $f_k(\mathbf{x}) = 0$ or if $f_k(\mathbf{x})$ consists of a single clause.
– The decomposition in the tree is truncated if $n_{smallest}^{dec} \geq n_{\min}$.
– Heuristic rules to select a preferred variable order help to find a small value of $n_{smallest}^{dec}$.

In order to exclude all side effects we used the original programs

- `sobve_g_55.exe` for RCE-GPU programmed by Bernd Steinbach and
- `exact_reduct_calculator.exe` for MDF-DT programmed by Grzegorz Borowik.

We executed these programs on the same computer (CPU: Intel® Xenon® X5650@2.67 GHz and GPU: NVIDIA Tesla C2070 with 448 cores) for both the so far used largest `petInput`-benchmarks and the data mining benchmarks not prepared by ourselves. Table 1 shows the ratio based on the measured run-times of these programs.

Table 1. Comparison of the algorithms RCE-GPU and MDF-DT

Benchmark			Solution		Time in milliseconds		Ratio
Name	#v	#c	#v	#s	RCE-GPU	MDF-DT	MDF-DT/RCE-GPU
petInput_32 × 64	32	64	4	398	0.695	140.0	201.55
petInput_32 × 128	32	128	4	22	0.761	93.0	122.14
petInput_32 × 256	32	256	5	38	2.924	171.0	58.49
petInput_32 × 512	32	512	5	2	3.304	468.0	141.66
petInput_32 × 1024	32	1,024	6	1271	20.849	2,902.0	139.19
breast-cancer-wisconsin	9	81	5	24	0.324	1,014.0	3,129.63
house	16	1,900	8	1	2.031	219.0	107.83
kaz	21	220	5	35	0.716	31.0	43.30
agaricus-lepiota-mushroom	22	158	4	3	0.389	369,377.0	949,555.27

Our program `sobve_g_55.exe` runs for both benchmark sets faster. The improvements range from 58 to more than 200 for the `petInput` benchmarks of 32 variable. For the data mining benchmarks of 9 to 22 variables which contain 81 to 1,900 clauses runs our program `sobve_g_55.exe` on the same computer 43 to 949,555 times faster. The wide spreading form about 40 to nearly one million in the ratio for the data mining benchmark set indicates the impact of the heuristic in the MDF-DT approach.

4 Optimization of the Fastest GPU-Algorithm

Despite the much shorter run-times of our so far fasted approach to solve the UCP we tried to improve the RCE-GPU approach even more. The drawback of Algorithm 1 is that the execution of the kernel BDIF_kernel(pv, cv) will be finished not before all threads of one warp executed in parallel have detected an orthogonal clause $C_{ic}(\mathbf{p})$ or a solution vector. Figure 2(a) illustrates this property which is caused the *single instruction multiple thread* (SIMT) paradigm of CUDA. In this approach 512 binary vectors $pv.vector[ip]$ are evaluated in parallel for the same clause $cv.vector[ic]$.

The key to conquer this drawback is the utilization of a warp vote function provided by CUDA. A warp is a group of 32 threads within a block. A warp

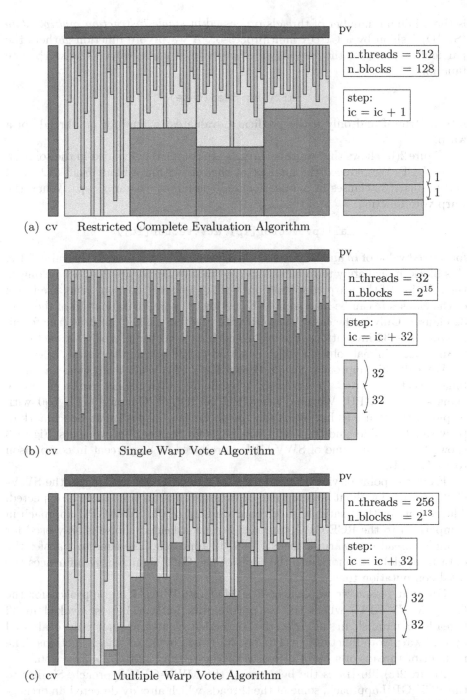

Fig. 2. Alternative parallel algorithms to solve the UCP on a GPU: (a) restricted complete evaluation (RCE-GPU), (b) single warp vote (SWV-GPU), (c) multiple warp vote (MWV-GPU).

is the minimum number of threads processed in *single instruction multiple data* (SIMD) fashion by a CUDA multiprocessor. A warp vote function gathers the particular results of the threads in a warp to a single value. The warp vote function

```
__all(int predicate)
```

returns true if and only if the predicate evaluates to true for all threads of a warp.

Figure 2(b) shows that waiting threads are completely avoided in the solution of the UCP. We reduced the number of threads within a block from 512 to 32 and evaluate 32 clauses in parallel for a single binary vector $f_j^{S_i}(\mathbf{p})$. When the warp vote function

```
__all(pv.vector[ip] &cv.vector[ic])
```

for a fixed value of *ip* and 32 selected clauses *cv.vector*[*ic*] returns the value false, this block immediately terminates knowing that *pv.vector*[*ip*] does not belong to the solution. If the warp vote function __all() returns the value true, the index of the clauses *ic* can be incremented by 32 for the parallel evaluation of the next 32 clauses. Only in the case that warp vote function __all() returns true for all *cv.elements*/32 invocations, the evaluated binary vector $f_j^{S_i}(\mathbf{p}) = pv.vector[ip]$ is an exact minimal solution which is added to the solution vector *sv*.

We call this approach *Single Warp Vote* (SWV-GPU) because a single binary vector $f_j^{S_i}(\mathbf{p}) = pv.vector[ip]$ is evaluated with regard to the necessary clauses on the GPU. We used one GPU NVIDIA® GeForce GTX 690 with Kepler architecture as hardware and the so far largest petInput benchmark of [7] with 32 variables and 1024 clauses as basis for further improvements. Figure 3 shows that the run-time of SWV-GPU is reduced to 81 percent in comparison to RCE-GPU.

From the point of view that all cores of the GPU are working in the SWV-GPU approach without interruption, an even shorter run-time could be expected. The reason for the relatively small improvement of the SWV-GPU approach in comparison to the RCE-GPU approach is that a loaded clause is only used for a single thread in a warp of the SWV-GPU approach. The time to transfer the data from global memory into the cores of the GPU significantly influences the total computation time.

For that reason we implemented a *Multiple Warp Vote* approach for the GPU (MWV-GPU) where the warp vote function __all() is invoked in 32 threads in parallel. In this way, the 32 loaded clauses are not only evaluated by one warp vote function __all() but 32 times by 32 of these functions. The number of threads of a block increases therefore from 32 to $32 \times 32 = 256$.

Figure 2(c) illustrates the behavior of the MWV-GPU approach. Similar to the RCE-GPU approach, some of the threads which already detected an orthogonal clause $C_{ic}(\mathbf{p})$ must wait for a final decision of the other threads in the warp. However, this share is reduced by a factor of $512/32 = 8$ because only 32 binary vectors $f_j^{S_i}(\mathbf{p}) = pv.vector[ip]$ are evaluated in one warp in parallel by the

MWV-GPU approach instead of 512 such vectors in the case of the RCE-GPU approach. Accepting a certain amount of passive threads, but extending the number of threads within the blocks to an optimal number, we could again reduce the calculation time. Figure 3 shows that the benefit of multiple use of once loaded clauses predominates the loss of waiting threads such that the run-time of the MWV-GPU approach is reduced to about 33 percent of the RCE-GPU approach.

5   Experimental Results

Here we summarize our experimental results.

Using the same computer, we compared our best algorithm RCE-GPU with the MDF-DT algorithm based on both the so far largest `petInput` benchmarks and data-mining benchmarks for which the MDF-DT algorithm was optimized:

– RCE-GPU is 58 to 201 times faster than the MDF-DT for the `petInput` benchmarks with 32 variables.
– RCE-GPU is 43 to almost one million times faster than the MDF-DT for the data-mining benchmarks with 9 to 22 variables.

Figure 3 shows the reached improvements of the new approaches SWV-GPU and MWV-GPU in comparison to the so fare fastest approach REC-GPU. We used the largest `petInput` benchmark with 32 variables p_i and 1024 clauses for this comparison.

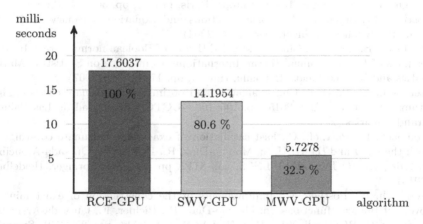

Fig. 3. Time to calculate the solution for the UCP `petInput_32x1024.txt` on the GPU.

6   Conclusion

The comparison of our so far fastest approach RCE-GPU [7] to solve the UCP with an optimized and recently published implementation MDF-DT [1] confirms that our approach is in the range of 40 to almost one million times faster.

Despite this good performance of our algorithm, we explored two more approaches which reduces the run-time even more. Using the CUDA warp vote function `__all(int predicate)` and exchanging pv and cv in the parallel algorithm we could reduce the time to solve the largest `petInput` UCP down to 33 percent. The analysis of these approaches shows that it is not enough to utilize as much as possible GPU cores, but the data loaded once from the global memory also must be reused as much as possible. May be a compromise is necessary between different aims.

Acknowledgment. We thank Grzegorz Borowik for providing us his executable program that solves the UCP using the algorithm presented in [1].

References

1. Borowik, G., Łuba, T.: Fast algorithm of attribute reduction based on the complementation of Boolean function. In: Klempous, R., Nikodem, J., Jacak, W., Chaczko, Z. (eds.) Advanced Methods and Applications in Computational Intelligence, pp. 25–40. Springer, Heidelberg (2014)
2. Brayton, R.K., Hachtel, G.D., McMullen, C.T., Sangiovanni-Vincentelli, A.: Logic Minimization Algorithms for VLSI Synthesis. Kluwer Academic Publishers, Dordrecht (1984)
3. Cordone, R., Ferrandi, F., Sciuto, D., Wolfler Calvo, R.: An efficient heuristic approach to solve the unate covering problem. In: Proceedings of the Conference on Design, Automation and Test in Europe, Paris, France, pp. 364–371 (2000)
4. Posthoff, C., Steinbach, B.: Logic Functions and Equations - Binary Models for Computer Science. Springer, Dordrecht (2004)
5. Steinbach, B., Posthoff, Ch.: An extended theory of Boolean normal forms. In: Proceedings of the 6th Annual Hawaii International Conference on Statistics, Mathematics and Related Fields, Honolulu, Hawaii, pp. 1124–1139 (2007)
6. Steinbach, B., Posthoff, Ch.: Evaluation and optimization of unate covering algorithms. In: EUROCAST 2015, pp. 195–196. IUCTC Universidad de Las Palmas, Grand Canaries (2015)
7. Steinbach, B., Posthoff, C.: Fast calculation of exact minimal unate coverings on both the CPU and the GPU. In: Moreno-Díaz, R., Pichler, F., Quesada-Arencibia, A. (eds.) EUROCAST 2013. LNCS, vol. 8112, pp. 234–241. Springer, Heidelberg (2013)
8. Steinbach, B., Posthoff, C.: Improvements of the construction of exact minimal covers of Boolean functions. In: Moreno-Díaz, R., Pichler, F., Quesada-Arencibia, A. (eds.) EUROCAST 2011, Part II. LNCS, vol. 6928, pp. 272–279. Springer, Heidelberg (2012)
9. Steinbach, B., Posthoff, C.: Parallel solution of covering problems super-linear speedup on a small set of cores. GSTF Int. J. Comput. Singap. 1(2), 113–122 (2011). Global Science and Technology Forum (GSTF), Singapore

On the Complexity of Rules
for the Classification of Patterns

Claudio Moraga[1,2(✉)]

[1] European Centre for Soft Computing, 33600 Mieres, Asturias, Spain
rules@claudio-moraga.eu
[2] Department of Computer Science,
TU Dortmund University, 44227 Dortmund, Germany

Abstract. The paper introduces a Pattern Classification problem in an archeological scenario. Basic assumptions to work with this class of problem are addressed: close-worlds, feature extraction, generation of classification rules, non-monotonic reasoning. A Chaitin-Kolmogorov type of complexity measure for the classification rules is introduced and compared with a handling complexity based on the usage of the rules.

1 Introduction

There are different approaches to Pattern Recognition and Classification. Among the most important ones, Statistical (see e.g. [6]), Syntactical [3], multi-classifiers based [7] and rules based (see e.g. [5]) should be mentioned. In the latter case the rules may be expressed in a formal language representing statements in a given logic, where the truth values *true* and *false* are associated to two classes to be distinguished, respectively. The rules may also be expressed in a natural language, for which complexity measures will be introduced and their meaning analyzed. It will be argued that the complexity of a given set of rules may be evaluated differently depending on the context and the purpose, ranging from Information Theory to the tractability by human users.

2 Scenarios

2.1 Introductory Remark

Whenever visiting an archeological site or a museum, people will be presented with reproductions of paintings found on the walls of caves, and possibly with artifacts of daily life like tools, hunting weapons, pottery and pieces of ornament. As a possible exception, brick-type clay tablets with Sumerian writings (dated 2,500 B.C.) may be mentioned and, more recently discovered small triangular clay plates (of about 10 cm per side) in the "*cueva pintada*" (painted cave), in Gáldar [4], Gran Canaria, insular Spain, with recursive geometric carvings, reminiscent of the Sierpinsky's triangles [10].

Work leading to this paper was partially supported by the Foundation for the Advance of Soft Computing, Mieres, Asturias, Spain.

© Springer International Publishing Switzerland 2015
R. Moreno-Díaz et al. (Eds.): EUROCAST 2015, LNCS 9520, pp. 625–631, 2015.
DOI: 10.1007/978-3-319-27340-2_77

2.2   Gedanken Experiment

Let it be assumed that a new archeological search was initiated in Tassili, Najjer, Algeria, where a large number of paleolithic paintings and carvings in different styles on cliff faces have already been found (see e.g. [11] pages 6–7), however comparatively less paintings on walls of caves. All these testimonies of late paleolithic art have been dated form 8,000 to 2,000 B.C. Let it further be assumed that the archeological studies focused on two recently discovered Tassili caves, distant about 50 km from each other. In what follows they will simply be called cave north and cave south, respectively.

The team exploring the north cave found, as expected, some wall paintings representing hunting scenes and also every-day-life scenes, what is not unusual for the Tassilian paleolithic art. The team working at the south cave, found no paintings, but carvings on the cliffs leading to the cave. However in a small chamber in the cave they found a set of five small clay tiles with geometric carvings, comprising "squares" of up to five different sizes, as shown in Fig. 1.

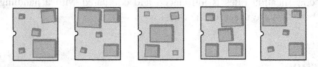

Fig. 1. Tiles found in the south cave.

Before starting any efforts to try and understand the *meaning* of the five tiles, the south team made use of satellite based smart-phones to contact the north team, report about the finding and send a picture of the five clay tiles. The archeologists and anthropologists of the north team were very much impressed, and at the same time, they were strongly motivated to continue examining "their" cave, paying special attention to possible chambers. The latter was effective: on the next day the north archeologists discovered a hidden chamber, where they (also) found five small clay tiles with geometric carvings, comprising "squares" of up to five different sizes, as shown in Fig. 2. A comparison with the picture of the tiles found in the south cave lead to the conclusion that the new tiles were similar, but different. This discovery gave rise to several conjectures and hypotheses. The strongest one, accepted by both teams, was the assumption of the early existence of a large tribe, which for reasons of survival – (food, water, shelter)– had to split. The sets of tiles suggested the development of (at least) two new tribes, which would migrate in different directions, and that would preserve some possibly cultic traditions of their ancestors, as indicated by the tiles sharing the shape, type of representation, an "alphabet" of four symbols of the same

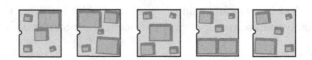

Fig. 2. Tiles found in the north cave

kind, and a common unusual "technology" otherwise only found in archaeologic searches in the Sumer area in southern Mesopotamia. It seemed a reasonable strategy to start exploring available paths between the two caves, hoping to find new evidences of possible migration of the new tribes or traces of the ancestors. However, considering the possibility of finding new tiles, or eventually related paintings or carvings in some cliff faces, it became apparent the need for a simple but effective method to determine whether a new fund could be associated to the north cave or to the south cave. This is a typical Pattern Recognition/Classification problem. Without further information, some basic assumptions to keep the problem tractable were needed. The most basic one refers to Occam's Razor [9]: *manage a problem with as much complexity as needed, but as little as possible.* Tiles were considered as abstract patterns with geometrical symbols *called* squares (even though the largest were of rectangular rather than square shape). Moreover not all squares had their sides parallel to the borders of the tiles, which might well be a way of representing *nuances* of the meaning of whatever concept represented a tile. This however would fall under the scope of interpretation, not of (simple) classification. The rather unusual kind of objects the teams were dealing with: clay-brick tiles, allowed to consider the Closed Worlds Assumption model (CWA) [8]: In the particular case under consideration this would mean that any tile not belonging to the north cave, would be assigned to the south cave, and vice versa. Finally, instead of comparing millions of pixels of a HD picture to assign the classification of a tile, a classification based on features is a valid choice. In the case of the patterns of the tiles, with geometric symbols, frequently the number of the symbols are already effective features. (See Table 1).

Table 1. Elementary features (symbols count)

	south cave					north cave			
	t	s	m	l		t	s	m	l
S1	2	1	1	1	N1	1	2	1	1
S2	2	0	2	1	N2	1	1	1	2
S3	2	1	1	1	N3	1	2	1	1
S4	0	1	3	1	N4	1	1	1	2
S5	2	0	2	1	N5	1	2	1	1
	t: tiny; s: small; m: medium; l: large								

From the (shaded) data in Table 1, the following simple rules could be deduced:
    R1: *If a tile has two tiny or three medium size squares, it is a tile from the south cave.*
    R2: *If a tile has only one tiny square, it is a tile of the north cave.*
    It is agreed that e.g. "a tile has two tiny squares" means that a tile has *exactly* two tiny squares. This constitutes a metarule to avoid misinterpretations.

It is simple to see that the tiles shown in Figs. 1 and 2 satisfy the rules and no tile would be given a wrong classification.

As agreed, the teams started to move towards each other paying special attention to wall paintings, engravings on cliff faces and possible cave entries. Not far from the cave the north team discovered a glen going down, where some menhirs and dolmens could be seen.

Under the central dolmen they discovered rests of destroyed tiles, but after careful additional search the team discovered one tile that had remained preserved along the centuries (see Fig. 3).

Fig. 3. The dolmen tile

The team noticed that this tile was different than the tiles found in the north cave, moreover, since the tile had two *tiny* squares, according to the Rule 1, it should be a tile from the south cave, in spite of having been found near the north one!

A message and a picture were sent immediately to the south team. The south team realized that the new tile was also different to the ones of the south cave. The fact that this new tile falsified the rule 1, meant that the original CWA was wrong, and that the rules had to be re-designed. A typical situation of non-monotonic reasoning [1]. The CWA could however be extended to three classes: {north cave, dolmen, south cave}. *A tile not belonging to any two classes, belongs to the third one* (see Fig. 4).

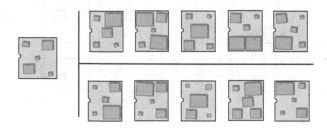

Fig. 4. The three classes of tiles. Top: the north cave, bottom: the south cave, left: the dolmen.

To resolve the conflict produced by the dolmen tile with respect to Rule 1, new rules would be needed, and for this, "second level" features combining size and relative position of the elementary symbols were used. Since with four of them was already possible to distinguish the three classes, as shown in Table 2, no other possibilities were tried. (Notice that for the class north, the former Rule 2 could have been pre-served, since that rule had no conflict with the dolmen tile.)

Table 2. Second level features (symbols count and position)

	south cave					north cave			
	UL	LR	UL	B		UL	LR	UL	B
	t	*m*	*m*	*s*		*t*	*m*	*m*	*s*
S1	1	0	0	0	N1	0	0	0	1
S2	0	1	0	0	N2	0	0	0	1
S3	1	0	0	0	N3	0	0	0	1
S4	0	1	0	0	N4	0	0	1	0
S5	0	1	0	0	N5	0	0	1	1
The *dolmen* class hat 0-entries over all four columns									
UL: upper left; LR: lower right; B: bottom row									

Based on Table 2, the new rules would be:

R1': *If a tile has a tiny square at the left upper corner or a middle size square at the right lower corner, then it is a tile of the south cave.*

R2': *If a tile has a middle size square at the left upper corner or a small square at the bottom row, then it is a tile of the north cave.*

From Table 2 it would be possible to obtain the following rule R3': *If a tile has neither a tiny nor a middle size square at the left upper corner, nor a middle size square at the lower right corner, nor a small square at the bottom row, then it is a tile of the dolmen class.* Later it will be discussed why this rule would not be convenient. From Fig. 3, however, the following rule may be obtained:

R3': *If a tile has a middle size square both at the upper right and at the lower left corners, then it is a tile of the dolmen class.*

3   Analysis of Complexity

One of the most well known approaches to the complexity of a *string* of symbols (i.e. a text) is the Algorithmic Complexity of Chaitin [2], expressed as the shortest program running on a Universal Turing Machine, that generates the string.

For the problem under consideration an adaptation of the Chaitin-Kolmogorov complexity may be used: *The complexity of a set of rules will be given by the length of the shortest non-ambiguous text in a natural language, effectively expressing the rules.*

Comparing the rules R1 and R2 with the rules R1' and R2' it is simple to see that R1 and R2 have a much lower Chaitin-Kolmogorov (adapted) algorithmic complexity than R1' and R2', respectively, just by counting the words used to express the corresponding rules (19 + 16 against 31 + 30).

From a totally different point of view, it is possible to define a user oriented *handling complexity*, representing the number of elementary handling-steps needed by a user, in the worst case, to reach a correct classification. For the working problem, the elementary handling steps could be: "per default check the symbols from top to bottom, from left to right", "determine the size of a symbol", "move to the next symbol", "count positive partial results", and "determine the final result obtained with the rule".

If Rule 1 is considered, ("*If a tile has (exactly) two tiny or three medium size squares, it is a tile from the south cave.*"), in any case the user has to check first all five symbols to be sure that two (and only two) tiny squares are available or not, and (in the worst case) the user has to check again all five symbols to find out by counting, whether (precisely) three medium size squares are available.

In the case of Rule 1', ("*If a tile has a tiny square at the left upper corner or a middle size square at the right lower corner, then it is a tile of the south cave.*"), the user does not start from a default condition. The rule tells her/him to check the symbol at the left upper corner, and (in the worst case) to go to the right lower corner and check that symbol. No searching is needed, no counting is needed: just three elementary handling steps: two for checking, and one to determine the final result.

Similarly for rules 2 and 2'. Notice that Rule 2, ("*If a tile has only one tiny square, it is a tile of the north cave*") has the lowest Chaitin-Kolmogorov complexity of all four rules under consideration, but the user is required to check *in any case* all five symbols before knowing whether the rule gives a positive result (if a single tiny square is found) or a negative result (otherwise). On the other hand, with Rule 2' ("*If a tile has a middle size square at the left upper corner or a small square at the bottom row, then it is a tile of the north cave*") the user is guided to start at the left upper corner and then move to the bottom row, checking only three symbols in the worst case.

Finally, Rules 1' and 2' have an additional user-friendly feature: *both* start checking the symbol at the left upper corner.

A similar analysis done for the rule R3' obtained from Table 2 shows that this rule has a Chaitin-Kolmogorov complexity of 44 and the user has to check all four conditions; meanwhile the rule R3' obtained from Fig. 3 has a Chaitin-Kolmogorov complexity of 28 and the user has to check only two positions.

This illustrates that the adapted Chaitin-Kolmogorov complexity and the handling complexity of a set of classification rules are not necessarily similar. The additional content of rules R1' and R2' was the result of working with "second level" features, which however turned up to give complementary handling instructions to the user *as part of the rules*. The price was a higher Chaitin-Kolmogorov complexity, but leading to a lower handling complexity.

4   Conclusions

A simple Pattern Classification problem was introduced, and basic aspects as the Closed Worlds Assumption, features extraction, nonmonotonic reasoning, and the formulation of classification rules were addressed. The complexity of the rules was particularly analyzed. The algorithmic complexity of Chaitin-Kolmogorov was adapted to measure the complexity of the classification rules as strings of text-symbols. Additionally the concept of *handling complexity*, from the perspective of the user (of the rules) was introduced and measured in terms of the number of elementary steps required to apply a given rule. It was shown that rules with a high Chaitin-Kolmogorov complexity may however have a low handling complexity if besides the satisfiability conditions –(*what* to check)– the rules contain some implicit indications on *how* to check whether a rule is satisfied or not.

References

1. Brewka, G.: Nonmonotonic Reasoning: Logical Foundations of Commonsense. Cambridge University Press, Cambridge (1991)
2. Chaitin, G.J.: Algorithmic Information Theory. Cambridge University Press, Cambridge (1987)
3. Fu, K.S.: Syntactical Pattern Recognition, Applications. Communications and Cybernetic, vol. 14. Springer, Heidelberg (1977)
4. Galdar. http://www.spain-grancanaria.com/uk/places/galdar.html
5. Giakoumakis, E., Papaconstantinou, G., Skordalakis, E.: Rule-based systems and pattern recognition. Pattern Recogn. Lett. **5**(4), 267–272 (1987)
6. Jain, A.K., Duin, R.P.W., Mao, J.: Statistical pattern recognition: a review. IEEE Trans. Pattern Anal. Mach. Intell. **22**(1), 4–37 (2000)
7. Kuncheva, L.: Combining Pattern Classifiers: Methods and Algorithms. Wiley, New York (2004)
8. Reiter, R.: On closed world data bases. In: Gallaire, H., Minker, J. (eds.) Logic and Data Bases, pp. 119–140. Plenum Press, New York (1978)
9. Rodríguez-Fernández, J.L.: Ockham's Razor. Endeavour **23**(3), 121–125 (1999)
10. Sierpinski. http://de.wikipedia.org/wiki/Sierpinski-Dreieck
11. Tassili. http://www.cvsanten.net/ (Select Tassili from the panel Pictorial Accounts)

Remarks on Characterization of Bent Functions in Terms of Gibbs Dyadic Derivatives

Radomir S. Stanković[1(✉)], Jaakko T. Astola[2], Claudio Moraga[3,4],
Milena Stanković[1], and Dušan Gajić[1]

[1] Department of Computer Science, Faculty of Electronics,
University of Niš, Niš, Serbia
radomir.stankovic@gmail.com
[2] Department of Signal Processing,
Tampere University of Technology, Tampere, Finland
[3] European Center for Soft Computing, 33600 Mieres, Spain
[4] Technical University of Dortmund, 44221 Dortmund, Germany

Keywords: Bent functions · Walsh functions · Dyadic derivatives · GPU

1 Introduction

The term dyadic derivative was coined by F. Pichler [9] for a differential operator introduced by J.E. Gibbs in 1967 [3] which was initially called the logic derivative since being acting on the set of binary n-tuples. Both names, the logic derivative and the dyadic derivative, are related with the property that this set equipped with the addition modulo 2 (EXOR) expresses the structure of a group C_2^n called the finite dyadic group, which is viewed as a natural domain to define binary-valued switching functions.

The dyadic Gibbs derivative is defined as an operator having the discrete Walsh functions as eigenfunctions with eigenvalues being the elements of the set $G = \{0, 1, \ldots, 2^n - 1\}$.

Bent functions are a class of switching functions with important applications in cryptography [11,12]. They are defined as switching functions farthest from affine switching functions [2]. It has been shown that the Hamming distance of a bent function to affine functions is $2^{n-1} - 2^{n/2-1}$, (see for example [8]).

In the spectral domain, bent functions are characterized as functions with a flat Walsh spectrum meaning that the Walsh coefficients have the same absolute value equal to $2^{n/2}$ where n is the number of variables [1].

In this paper, we give a characterization of bent functions in terms of the dyadic Gibbs derivative by showing that the values of the dyadic Gibbs derivative of bent functions are equal to elements of the set G of eigenvalues of this operator with permutations and sign changes allowed under certain restrictions. This characterization of bent functions in terms of the dyadic Gibbs derivative can be useful in checking if a function is bent. Experimental results confirm that computing the dyadic Gibbs derivative is faster than performing Fast Walsh

© Springer International Publishing Switzerland 2015
R. Moreno-Díaz et al. (Eds.): EUROCAST 2015, LNCS 9520, pp. 632–639, 2015.
DOI: 10.1007/978-3-319-27340-2_78

Transform (FWT) providing resources to perform computations of partial derivatives in parallel as specified by the corresponding fast algorithm.

2   Background Theory

Binary switching functions are defined as mappings $f : \{0,1\}^n \to \{0,1\}$, where n is the number of variables. They can be viewed as functions on the finite group C_2^n, where C_2 is the cyclic group of order 2.

The elements of C_2^n are the n-tuples $x = (x_0, x_1, \ldots, x_{n-1})$ with $x_i \in \{0,1\}$. The group operation $\oplus$ is coordinatewise addition modulo 2.

The space of all bounded complex-valued functions f on C_2^n will be denoted by L, and it involves binary-valued switching functions assuming that the function values 0 and 1 are interpreted as the corresponding integers.

When switching functions are viewed as functions on C_2^n, they can be processed in the spectral domain defined in terms of the Walsh transform.

Definition 1. *For a function of n variables $f(x_1, x_2, \ldots, x_n)$ specified by the function-vector $\mathbf{F} = [f(0), f(1), \ldots, f(2^n - 1)]^T$, the Walsh spectrum can be represented by a vector $\mathbf{S}_f = [S_f(0), S_f(1), \ldots, S_f(2^n - 1)]^T$ determined as*

$$\mathbf{S}_f = \mathbf{W}(n)\mathbf{F},$$

where the Walsh transformation matrix is defined as

$$\mathbf{W}(n) = \bigotimes_{i=1}^{n} \mathbf{W}(1), \quad \mathbf{W}(1) = \begin{bmatrix} 1 & 1 \\ 1 & -1 \end{bmatrix}.$$

The function f is reconstructed from its Walsh spectrum as

$$\mathbf{F} = 2^{-n}\mathbf{W}(n)\mathbf{S}_f.$$

When the Walsh transform is applied to binary switching functions it is good to use the encoding $(0, 1) \to (1, -1)$, which results from the mapping $x \to (-1)^x$ with $x \in \{0, 1\}$. This makes the functions to be processed more close to the basis functions used in the transform, resulting in some useful properties of the Walsh spectrum [4,5]. Some of these features, will be used in this paper. For example, with the encoding $(0, 1) \to (1, -1)$, Walsh coefficients of switching functions are even numbers, and further, not all combinations of even integers are allowed as spectral coefficients of switching functions. In this paper, we will further assume that the functions, when written in matrix notation as function vectors are in the $(1, -1)$ encoding. We keep the Boolean notation for analytic expressions.

Example 1. *Consider the function $f(x_1, x_2) = x_1 x_2$, $x_1, x_2 \in \{0, 1\}$, with multiplication defined modulo 2, i.e., as Boolean AND. The encoded function-vector is $\mathbf{F} = [1, 1, 1, -1]^T$ and the Walsh spectrum is $\mathbf{S}_f = \mathbf{W}(2)\mathbf{F} = [2, 2, 2, -2]^T$.*

2.1 Bent Functions

Bent functions are defined as switching functions encoded in $(1, -1)$ that have flat Walsh spectra. It follows that the Walsh coefficients of a bent function must take either the value $2^{n/2}$ or $-2^{n/2}$. Therefore, bent functions can be viewed as a subset of functions representing solutions of the generalized eigenfunctions problem for the Walsh transform since they must satisfy

$$\mathbf{WF} = \pm 2^{n/2}\mathbf{PF},$$

where $\mathbf{P}$ is a generalized permutation matrix. The generalization means that some of the non-zero elements in $\mathbf{P}$ may have negative sign, i.e., are equal to -1.

Notice that this property is certainly satisfied for the generalized permutation matrices derived from the permutation matrices allowed by the spectral invariant operations [4,5].

Example 2. *The function $f = x_1 x_3 \oplus x_2 x_3 \oplus x_2 x_4$, whose function vector is $\mathbf{F} = [1,1,1,1,1,-1,-1,1,1,1,-1,-1,1,-1,1,-1]^T$, is bent, since its Walsh spectrum is $\mathbf{S}_f = [4,4,4,4,4,-4,4,-4,4,-4,-4,4,4,4,-4,-4]^T$.*

3 Dyadic Gibbs Derivative

Gibbs derivatives are a broad class of differential operators on groups [10]. In the case of functions on C_2^n, the dyadic Gibbs derivative, is used.

Definition 2. *To each function $f \in L$ we assign a function $f^{[1]} \in L$ defined by*

$$f^{[1]}(x) = -\frac{1}{2}\sum_{r=0}^{n-1}(f(x \oplus 2^r) - f(x))2^r, \quad (x \in B_n). \tag{1}$$

We call $f^{[1]}$ the (first-order) dyadic Gibbs derivative of f. The corresponding operator $D : L \to L$, defined by $Df = f^{[1]}$, $(f \in L)$, will be called the dyadic Gibbs differentiator.

3.1 Matrix Interpretation of the Dyadic Gibbs Derivative

Formulation of the Gibbs derivative in matrix form is useful for its computation, since the fast computation algorithms for the Walsh transform can be used [10].

In matrix notation, the value-vector of $f^{[1]}(x)$ of an n-variable function $f(x)$ specified by the function vector $\mathbf{F}$ is determined as

$$\mathbf{F}^{[1]} = \mathbf{D}(n)\mathbf{F}, \tag{2}$$

where the $(2^n \times 2^n)$ matrix of the Gibbs derivative $\mathbf{D}(n)$, called the Gibbs matrix, is defined as a matrix whose typical element is

$$d_{\xi,\eta} = \frac{1}{2}\left((2^n - 1)\delta(\xi \oplus \eta, 0) - \sum_{r=0}^{n-1}2^r\delta(\xi \oplus \eta, 2^r)\right),$$

where δ is the Kronecker delta.

The matrix $\mathbf{D}(n)$ can be factorized as

$$\mathbf{D}(n) = 2^{-n}\mathbf{W}(n)\mathbf{G}(n)\mathbf{W}(n), \tag{3}$$

where $\mathbf{W}(n)$ is the Walsh matrix of order n and $\mathbf{G}(n) \overset{def}{=} diag(0, 1, 2, \ldots, 2^n - 1)$. Thus, $\mathbf{D}$ is the similarity transformation of $\mathbf{G}$ with respect to the Walsh matrix. The matrix $\mathbf{D}$ is diagonalizable, since it is similar to the diagonal matrix $\mathbf{G}$. From (3), we can see that the eigenvalues of $\mathbf{D}(n)$ are $0, 1, 2, \ldots, 2^n - 1$, and that the Walsh functions are the corresponding eigenvectors.

Another way to define the dyadic derivative on C_2^n is in terms of the partial dyadic Gibbs derivatives, i.e., as a linear combination of partial dyadic Gibbs derivatives on C_2.

Definition 3. *The partial Gibbs dyadic derivative of a function* $f(x_1, x_2, \ldots, x_n)$ *with respect to the i-th variable* x_i, $i = 1, 2, \ldots, n$, *is defined as*

$$(D_i f)((x_1, \ldots, x_n)) = f((x_1, \ldots, x_i \oplus 1, \ldots, x_n)) - f((x_1, \ldots, x_n)). \tag{4}$$

The dyadic Gibbs derivative is expressed in terms of partial dyadic Gibbs derivatives as

$$f^{[1]}(x_1, \ldots, x_n) = -\frac{1}{2}\sum_{i=1}^{n} 2^{n-i}(D_i f)((x_1, \ldots, x_n)). \tag{5}$$

In matrix notation, the partial Gibbs dyadic derivative can be expressed as

$$\mathbf{D}_i = \bigotimes_{j=1}^{n} \mathbf{A}_j, \quad \mathbf{A}_j = \begin{cases} \mathbf{A}(1) = \begin{bmatrix} -1 & 1 \\ 1 & -1 \end{bmatrix}, \text{ for } j = i, \\ \mathbf{I}(1) = \begin{bmatrix} 1 & 0 \\ 0 & 1 \end{bmatrix}, \quad \text{ for } j \neq i. \end{cases} \tag{6}$$

The Gibbs dyadic derivative can be expressed as

$$\mathbf{D} = -\frac{1}{2}\sum_{i=1}^{n} 2^{n-i}\mathbf{D}_i. \tag{7}$$

3.2   Computing the Dyadic Gibbs Derivative

The relation (3) shows that the dyadic Gibbs derivative can be computed by a convolution-like algorithm with complexity equal to that of two times performing the Fast Walsh Transform (FWT) [6,10].

The definition of the Gibbs dyadic derivative in terms of partial derivatives appears to be very convenient for parallel computations since partial derivatives can be computed simultaneously. Further, even a brief inspection of the matrix interpretation of partial derivatives shows a strong resemblance with steps in

FWT-like algorithms for various spectral transforms on finite dyadic groups. Therefore, computing the partial derivative with respect to the variable x_i can be performed by a step of the FWT-like algorithm with the basic butterfly operation defined by the matrix $\mathbf{A}_i = \mathbf{A}(1) = \begin{bmatrix} -1 & 1 \\ 1 & -1 \end{bmatrix}$. As in all FFT-like algorithms, butterfly operations are performed in parallel over different sets of data, which ensures the efficiency of the algorithm.

Example 3. *Figure 1 shows steps of the FWT-like algorithm for computing Gibbs dyadic derivatives for functions of $n = 4$ binary variables. The outputs of these steps $\mathbf{D}_1$, $\mathbf{D}_2$, $\mathbf{D}_3$, and $\mathbf{D}_4$ are used to compute the Gibbs dyadic derivative by (7). The scaling factor $-1/2$ is omitted.*

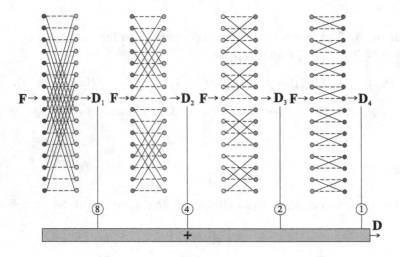

Fig. 1. FFT-like algorithm for computing the dyadic Gibbs derivative for $n = 4$.

4   Dyadic Derivative and Bent Functions

The definition of bent functions in terms of flat Walsh spectrum and definition of the dyadic Gibbs derivative as an operator having Walsh functions as eigenfunctions suggest that it could be interesting to formulate a characterization of bent functions in terms of this differential operator.

Statement 1. *A switching function f of n-variables, where n is an even natural number, is bent if the absolute values of elements of the vector $\mathbf{D}_f$ representing its dyadic Gibbs derivative $f^{[1]}(x)$, are mutually distinct and equal to the elements of the set $G = \{0, 1, 2, \ldots, 2^n - 1\}$. In other words, f is bent if its dyadic Gibbs derivative by the absolute values is equal to the eigenvalues of the derivative, permutations allowed.*

For any function $f \in L$, the sum of values of the dyadic Gibbs derivative is equal to 0. Thus, this holds also for bent functions. Moreover, for bent functions, the values of the dyadic Gibbs derivative have the negative values at the same positions where the bent function f in the $(1, -1)$ encoding has the value -1. Thus, $\mathbf{F}^{[1]} = (\mathbf{PG})(n) \odot \mathbf{F}$, where $\mathbf{P}$ is a permutation matrix, and $\odot$ is the componentwise multiplication (Hadamard product). For each bent function f, the permutation matrix $\mathbf{P}$ is different. For a given n, the set of permutation matrices used in this characterization of bent functions can be derived form spectral invariant operations for the Walsh transform [4].

It follows that in $\mathbf{F}^{[1]}$ signs are assigned to elements of $\mathbf{D}_f$ such that the sums of elements with the positive and the negative values are equal to $(2^n - 1)(2^{(n-2)})$, since the sum of values of elements in $\mathbf{G}(n)$ is $(2^n - 1)(2^{(n-1)})$.

The dyadic Gibbs derivative preserves the same sign at each position as in the function vector for a bent function, and 0 in $\mathbf{G}(n)$ can multiply either $+1$ or -1 in the function vector for f.

Example 4. *The dyadic Gibbs derivative for the function f in Example 2 with the function vector $\mathbf{F} = [1,1,1,1,1,-1,-1,1,1,1,-1,-1,1,-1,1,-1]^T$, is given by the vector $\mathbf{D}_f = [0,4,12,8,3,-7,-15,11,2,6,-14,-10,1,-5,13,-9]^T$. Notice that in these two vectors, $\mathbf{F}$ and $\mathbf{D}_f$, elements with negative signs appears at the same positions. Thus, the dyadic Gibbs derivative preserves the sign of bent functions. For $n = 4$, the sum of positive and negative values in the vector of the dyadic Gibbs derivative of a bent function is $4 \times 15 = 60$ and -60, respectively.*

In the case of non-bent functions, the values of the dyadic Gibbs derivatives can be sets of integers different from eigenvalues of this operator, the same values can repeated, and the sum of positive and negative values will be different from $(2^n - 1)(2^{(n-2)})$.

4.1   Checking if a Function Is Bent

A straightforward way to check if a switching function is bent is to compute its Walsh spectrum and see if it is flat. The WFT algorithm ensures that this can be done efficiently in terms of time. Computing the dyadic Gibbs derivative can be performed faster than computing the Walsh spectrum if the algorithm in terms of partial dyadic Gibbs derivatives is used, since partial derivatives can be computed in parallel provided sufficient computing resources are available. This algorithm is suitable for implementation on Graphics Processing Units (GPU) based systems.

To check if a function is bent, we need to check if the values of its dyadic Gibbs derivative are all distinct and by the absolute values are in the set $\{0, 1, 2, \ldots, 2^n - 1\}$. In programming implementation this can be done as follows. We define an auxiliary vector $\mathbf{V} = [V(0), V(1), \ldots, V(2^n - 1)]^T$, with initial values $V(i) = 0$. Then, when computed, values of the dyadic Gibbs derivative are stored in the positions $V(|D(i)|) = D(i)$. If $|D(i)| > 2^n - 1$, an error occurs, which means that the function is not bent. After the computing is done, we check if $V(i) \neq 0$

for $i = 1, \ldots, 2^n - 1$. Notice that 0 is saved in the position $V(0)$. In this way, we avoid ordering of values of the dyadic Gibbs derivative and complexity of the procedure is comparable to checking if the absolute values of elements of the Walsh spectrum are equal to $2^{n/2}$.

We compared the computing times for calculating the Walsh spectrum and the dyadic Gibbs derivative on the GPU Nvidia GTX 560 Ti that has 8 streaming multiprocessors with 48 streaming processors each which makes 384 in total, with 1 GB GDDR5 RAM and 128 GB/s memory bandwidth with the CPU Intel i7-920 running at 2.8 GHz.

For this hardware platform, the computations were done in the following way

1. For $n < 8$, all partial derivatives are computed in parallel.
2. For $n = 8, 9, 10$, up to 7 partial derivatives are computed in parallel on the hardware level.
3. For $n = 11, 12$, up to 4 partial derivatives are computed in parallel.
4. For $n = 13$, two partial derivatives are computed in parallel.
5. For $n \geq 14$, partial derivatives are computed sequentially.

Table 1 shows the computing times for the Walsh spectrum and the dyadic Gibbs derivative and the time for necessary memory transfers which is equal in both cases. When partial derivatives can be computed in parallel, the corresponding algorithm is faster. For $n = 17$ and larger, the computation of the Walsh spectrum becomes faster on the used hardware, since the partial dyadic Gibbs derivatives are computed sequentially with the so-called atomic operations used in to ensure correctness of the computations in (7).

Table 1. Times [msec] for computing the Walsh spectrum and the Gibbs derivative for binary functions with n variables.

n	Walsh coefficients	Gibbs derivative	Memory transfers	Task parallelism
6	11.0	2.8	3.0	All partial derivatives
7	11.8	3.1	3.1	
8	13.3	3.8	3.1	Up to 7 partial derivatives
9	15.7	4.6	3.3	
10	19.8	6.0	3.7	
11	30.1	10.5	5.0	Up to 4 partial derivatives
12	32.6	10.6	7.4	
13	34.7	17.3	15.2	2 partial derivatives
14	38.0	31.8	25.8	Partial derivatives computed sequentially
15	69.4	64.7	47.5	
16	132.8	127.8	91.2	
17	266.6	303.9	178.2	

It follows that the characterization of bent functions in terms of the dyadic Gibbs derivative can be useful in checking if a given switching function is bent or otherwise. It is assumed that the underlying hardware platform allows parallel computing of partial dyadic Gibbs derivatives.

5 Concluding Remarks

The characterization of bent functions in terms of the Walsh spectrum suggests that another characterization in terms of the dyadic Gibbs derivative is possible, since this is a differential operator whose eigenvectors are the Walsh functions. Such a characterization can be useful in checking if a given switching function is bent or otherwise, since the computation of the dyadic Gibbs derivative can be performed in parallel by using both data and task parallelism with sufficient hardware resources provided. Notice that in the case of the Fast Walsh transform algorithm, the data parallelism is used, while steps of the algorithm are performed sequentially.

References

1. Butler, J.T.: Bent function discovery by reconfigurable computer. In: Proceedings of 9th International Workshop on Boolean Problems, Freiberg, Germany, 16–17 September, pp. 1–12 (2010)
2. Carlet, C., Ding, C.: Highly non-linear mappings. J. Complex. **20**(2–3), 205–244 (2004)
3. Gibbs, J.E.: Walsh spectrometry, a form of spectral analysis well suited to binary digital computation. Nat. Phys. Lab., 24 pp. (1967)
4. Hurst, S.L.: Logical Processing of Digital Signals. Crane Russak and Edward Arnold, London and Basel (1978)
5. Hurst, S.L., Miller, D.M., Muzio, J.C.: Spectral Techniques in Digital Logic. Academic Press, Bristol (1985)
6. Karpovsky, M.G., Stanković, R.S., Astola, J.T.: Spectral Logic and Its Application in the Design of Digital Devices. Wiley, Hoboken (2008)
7. Meier, W., Staffelbach, O.: Nonlineairty criteria for cryptographic applications. In: Quisquater, J.-J., Vandewalle, J. (eds.) EUROCRYPT 1989. LNCS, vol. 434, pp. 549–562. Springer, Heidelberg (1990)
8. Nyberg, K.: Constructions of bent functions and difference sets. In: Damgård, I.B. (ed.) EUROCRYPT 1990. LNCS, vol. 473, pp. 151–160. Springer, Heidelberg (1991)
9. Pichler, F.: Walsh functions and linear system theory. Technical Research Report, T-70-05, Dept. of Electrical Engineering, University of Maryland, College Park, Maryland 20742, April 1970, ii+46
10. Stanković, R.S., Moraga, C., Astola, J.T.: Applications of Fourier Analysis on Finite Non-Abelian Groups in Signal Processing and System Design. IEEE Press/Wiley (2005)
11. Tokareva, N.: Generalizations of bent functions. Diskretn. Anal. Issled. Oper. **17**(1), 34–64 (2010). A Survey, translated from Discrete Analysis and Operation Research
12. Tokareva, N.: On the number of bent funcitons from interative constructions - lower bounds and hypotheses. Adv. Math. Commun. **5**(4), 609–621 (2011)

The Extended 1-D (One-Dimensional) Discrete Phase Retrieval Problem

Corneliu Rusu[1]([✉]) and Jaakko Astola[2]

[1] Faculty of Electronics, Telecommunications and Information Technology,
Technical University of Cluj-Napoca, Cluj-Napoca, Romania
corneliu.rusu@ieee.org
http://sp.utcluj.ro
[2] Tampere International Center for Signal Processing,
Tampere University of Technology, Tampere, Finland

Abstract. In this work we discuss some difficulties that can be encountered when one uses iterative methods for finding a solution of a one-dimensional discrete phase retrieval problem. Iterative methods are widely used but, unfortunately, they often stagnate. We shall show that by using an extended form of the one-dimensional discrete phase retrieval problem, we can find a solution to the problem.

Keywords: Signal reconstruction · Phase retrieval

1 Introduction

Signal reconstruction from Fourier transform magnitude is also called phase retrieval [3]. The term comes from the fact that often we can measure only the Fourier magnitude and to reconstruct the signal the phase must be estimated (retrieved). The phase retrieval problem has attracted considerable interest because of its importance in a variety of applications, including optical astronomy, microscopy, Fourier-transform spectroscopy, x-ray crystallography, particle scattering, speckle interferometry, lens testing, single-sideband communication, and design of radar signals [4].

Although certain constraints may be added according to application, the basic one-dimensional discrete phase retrieval (1-D DPhR) problem can be stated as follows:

Let $\tilde{X}(k)$ a sequence of positive numbers, which will be called the input magnitude data. To solve the 1-D DPhR problem means to find a discrete signal $x(n)$ of length N for which its N-point Discrete Fourier Transform (DFT):

$$X(k) = \sum_{n=0}^{N-1} x(n)e^{-j\frac{2\pi kn}{N}}, \quad k = 0, 1, \ldots, N-1. \tag{1}$$

satisfies

$$|X(k)| = \tilde{X}(k) \tag{2}$$

© Springer International Publishing Switzerland 2015
R. Moreno-Díaz et al. (Eds.): EUROCAST 2015, LNCS 9520, pp. 640–647, 2015.
DOI: 10.1007/978-3-319-27340-2_79

for all $k = 0, 1, \ldots, N - 1$.

There are several methods to solve the 1-D DPhR problem: Hilbert transform [6], computation of cepstral coefficients [12] or solving linear systems of equations [11]. Another way to obtain a solution to 1-D DPhR problem is by finding the zeros of z-transform of autocorrelation, also called as root finding approach or direct method. This may provide the minimum-phase solution, however such method behaves poorly numerically and can be recommended only for rather short length [1]. Perhaps the most common approaches are iterative transform algorithms [7], which alternate between time and frequency domains. This type of algorithms can implement very easily time-domain constraints like compactness of the support. It has been observed that these algorithms fail to converge to a solution as they usually stagnate [5].

The goal of this work is to show that the stagnation of the iterative methods can be overpassed by using the extended formulation of the 1-D DPhR problem. In Sect. 2 we present the iterative algorithm for 1-D DPhR problem, then we illustrate this method by using a couple of examples (Sect. 3). In Sect. 4 the extended one dimensional discrete phase retrieval is stated and experimental results are provided.

2   The Iterative Algorithm for 1-D DPhR Problem

The iterative transform algorithm or 1-D DPhR problem is a standard iterative technique in which the estimate of $x(n)$ is improved in each iteration [2]. The iterative technique to reconstruct the sequence $x(n)$ or its DFT $X(k)$ from the DFT input magnitude data $\tilde{X}(k)$, $k = 0, 1, \ldots, N - 1$ is described as follows.

1. We begin with $\angle X_1(k)$, an initial guess of the unknown DFT phase, and form the first estimate $X_1(k)$ of $X(k)$, using the specified magnitude function, i.e.

$$X_1(k) = \tilde{X}(k)e^{j\angle \tilde{X}_1(k)}.$$

   Computing the inverse DFT of $X_1(k)$ provides the first estimate $x_1(n)$ of $x(n)$. Since an N-point DFT is used, $x_1(n)$ is an N-point sequence which is, in general, nonzero for $M \leq n \leq N - 1$.

2. From $x_1(n)$, another sequence $\tilde{x}_2(n)$ is defined by

$$\tilde{x}_2(n) = \begin{cases} x_1(n), & 0 \leq n \leq M - 1, \\ 0, & M \leq n \leq N - 1, \end{cases}$$

   where $M = N/2$ when N is even, and $M = (N + 1)/2$ when N is odd.

3. The phase $\angle \tilde{X}_2(k)$ of the $\tilde{X}_2(k)$ (the N-point DFT of $\tilde{x}_2(n)$) is then considered as a new estimate of $\angle X(k)$. A new estimate of $X(k)$ is formed by

$$X_2(k) = \tilde{X}(k)e^{j\angle \tilde{X}_2(k)}.$$

   From this, a new estimate $x_2(n)$ is obtained from the inverse DFT of $X_2(k)$.

Repetitive application of Steps 2 and 3 defines the standard iterative algorithm.

In this iterative procedure, an error function may be introduced:

$$E_p = \frac{1}{N} \sum_{k=0}^{N-1} \left| \tilde{X}(k) - |\tilde{X}_p(k)| \right|^2, \tag{3}$$

which is the mean-square difference between the known magnitude and the estimate on each iteration.

It has been shown that E_p is non increasing [8]. Since E_p has a lower bound of zero, then it must converge to a limit point, which may be zero or a positive nonzero number. If $\lim_{p \to \infty} E_p = 0$, then we get the correct solution, which may be affected by the certain ambiguities [11]. Unfortunately the iterative algorithm often stagnates [7].

3   Case Studies

In the following we shall consider two examples of input magnitude data and we shall present the results of the iterative method for these input magnitude data.

Let $N = 5$ [10] and

$$\tilde{X}(k) = \begin{cases} 2, \ k = 0; \\ 1, \ k = 1, 2, 3, 4. \end{cases} \tag{4}$$

Then 1-D DPhR problem has a correct solution by zeros allocation:

$$x(n) = \begin{cases} 1.0736, \ n = 0; \\ 0.3675, \ n = 1; \\ 0.5589, \ n = 2; \\ 0, \qquad \text{otherwise.} \end{cases}$$

We run the iterative phase-retrieval procedure and the variation of E_p is shown in Fig. 1. It can be seen that the error function is fast converging towards zero and finally we get the solution of 1-D DPhR problem mentioned above.

Alternatively, if we have [9]:

$$\tilde{X}(k) = \begin{cases} 3, \ k = 0; \\ 1, \ k = 1, 2, 3, 4, \end{cases} \tag{5}$$

then the Fourier transform of the folded of circular autocorrelation is not always positive. In such situation an attempt to solve 1-D DPhR problem by direct method is unsuccessful. We have implemented the iterative phase-retrieval algorithm for the input magnitude data given by (5). The mean-square difference between the known magnitude and the estimate on each iteration decreases and finally stagnates (Fig. 2). In this situation we cannot obtain the solution of 1-D DPhR problem using the iterative algorithm.

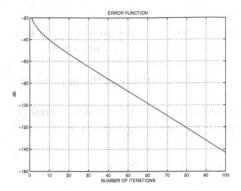 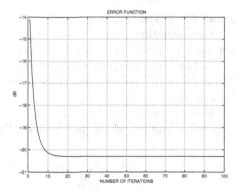

Fig. 1. The variation of E_p (dB) for input magnitude data given by (4).

Fig. 2. The variation of E_p (dB) for input magnitude data given by (5).

4   The Extended 1-D DPhR Problem

We have seen that the 1-D DPhR problem cannot be solved always by the iterative method. In case of similar problems like *Nearest autocorrelation* problem [1], the folded autocorrelation sequence is replaced with other sequence, and the new sequence has a nonnegative Fourier transform. Obviously, the DFT of the new sequence differs from the DFT of folded autocorrelation, i.e. it differs from $\tilde{X}(k)$. In such scenario, we have to accept measurement errors on input magnitude data.

In the following we shall consider that the measurements of input magnitude are free of errors, but the set of input magnitude data is not complete, i.e. some $\tilde{X}(k)$ are missing. Such situation may appear when the time domain sampling or the frequency domain sampling were not appropriate.

4.1   Statement of the Extended One Dimensional Discrete Phase Retrieval Problem

The extended one dimensional discrete phase retrieval problem (Ext. 1-D DPhR) can be formulated in three ways:

I. Let $\tilde{X}(k)$ a sequence of positive numbers, where $k = 0, 1, 2, \ldots, N - 1$. These input magnitude data came from the initial 1-D DPhR problem given by (1) and (2).

To solve the *First Ext. 1-D DPhR* means to find $x(n)$ a discrete signal of length $2N$ and for which its $2N$-point Discrete Fourier Transform (DFT):

$$X(k) = \sum_{n=0}^{2N-1} x(n)e^{-j\frac{2\pi kn}{2N}}, \quad k = 0, 1, \ldots, 2N - 1.$$

satisfies

$$|X(k)| = \tilde{X}(k) \tag{6}$$

for all $k = 0, 1, 2, \ldots, N - 1$.

Such situation happens when the sampling frequency of the analog signal has not been properly selected and we need to double the sampling frequency.

II. Let $\tilde{X}(k)$ a sequence of positive numbers, where $k = 0, 2, 4, \ldots, 2(N - 1)$. These input magnitude data came from the initial 1-D DPhR problem given by (1) and (2).

To solve the *Second Ext. 1-D DPhR* means to find $x(n)$ a discrete signal of length $2N$ and for which its $2N$-point Discrete Fourier Transform (DFT):

$$X(k) = \sum_{n=0}^{2N-1} x(n)e^{-j\frac{2\pi kn}{2N}}, \quad k = 0, 1, \ldots, 2N - 1.$$

satisfies

$$|X(k)| = \tilde{X}(k) \tag{7}$$

for all $k = 0, 2, 4, \ldots, 2(N - 1)$.

Such situation happens when the length of DFT has not been properly selected and we need to double the length of DFT.

III. Let $\tilde{X}(k)$ a sequence of positive numbers, where $k = 0, 2, 4, \ldots, 2(N-1)$. These input magnitude data came from the initial 1-D DPhR problem given by (1) and (2).

To solve the *Third Ext. 1-D DPhR* means to find $x(n)$ a discrete signal of length $4N$ and for which its $4N$-point Discrete Fourier Transform (DFT):

$$X(k) = \sum_{n=0}^{2N-1} x(n)e^{-j\frac{2\pi kn}{2N}}, \quad k = 0, 1, \ldots, 4N - 1.$$

satisfies

$$|X(k)| = \tilde{X}(k) \tag{8}$$

for all $k = 0, 2, 4, \ldots, 2(N - 1)$.

Such situation may happen when both the sampling frequency of analog signal and the length of the DFT have not been properly selected.

For all these three problems one can try to find solutions by implementing different approaches. In the following we suggest that the iterative technique may be used to reach this goal, since this algorithm can implement easily constraints of the support. Note that for all these three problems we have to modify (1) to only for those indexes k which are specified in the statements of the Ext. 1-D DPhR problem, i.e. to those k which appear in (6), (7), and (8). As in any iterative procedure we must have a way to decide whether the iterative algorithm should stop or not. One way to measure the error is to change the error function (3) to:

$$E_p^{\mathcal{K}} = \frac{1}{N} \sum_{k \in \mathcal{K}} \left| \tilde{X}(k) - |\tilde{X}_p(k)| \right|^2, \tag{9}$$

where $\mathcal{K} = \{0, 1, 2, \ldots, N - 1\}$ for the first Ext. 1-D DPhR problem and $\mathcal{K} = \{0, 2, 4, \ldots, 2(N - 1)\}$ for the second and the third Ext. 1-D DPhR problem.

4.2 Example Revisited

Let us consider the input magnitude data given by (5). It has been shown that no solution to 1-D DPhR problem can be found using the standard iterative method. However, for this set of input magnitude data the first form, the second form and the third form of Ext. 1-D DPhR problem give solution by using the iterative method.

The first form learning curve is shown in Fig. 3.

The sequence $x(n)$ obtained after convergence and its DFT magnitude $X(k)$ are:

$$x(n) = \begin{cases} 0.8364 + 0.2950j, \ n = 0; \\ 0.4128 + 0.3254j, \ n = 1; \\ 0.5308 - 0.1451j, \ n = 2; \\ 0.6373 + 0.0033j, \ n = 3; \\ 0.5812 - 0.3885j, \ n = 4; \\ 0 \qquad\qquad\qquad n = 5, 6, 7, 8, 9. \end{cases}$$

and

$$X(k) = \begin{cases} 3, & k = 0; \\ 1, & k = 1, 2, 3, 4; \\ 1.0624, & k = 5; \\ 0.3476, & k = 6; \\ 1.0537, & k = 7; \\ 0.4273, & k = 8; \\ 2.6579 & k = 9. \end{cases}$$

The second form learning curve is shown in Fig. 4.

The sequence $x(n)$ obtained after convergence and its DFT magnitude $X(k)$ are:

$$x(n) = \begin{cases} 1.4, \ n = 0; \\ 0.4, \ n = 1, 2, 3, 4; \\ 0 \quad n = 5, 6, 7, 8, 9. \end{cases}$$

and

$$X(k) = \begin{cases} 3, & k = 0; \\ 1, & k = 2, 4, 6, 8; \\ 1.8643, & k = 1; \\ 1.4298, & k = 3; \\ 1.4, & k = 5; \\ 1.4298, & k = 7; \\ 1.8643 & k = 9. \end{cases}$$

The third form learning curve is similar to Figs. 3 and 4.

The sequence $x(n)$ obtained after convergence and its DFT magnitude $X(k)$ are:

$$x(n) = \begin{cases} 0.7, & n = 0; \\ 0.3 + 0.3078j, & n = 1; \\ 0.2, & n = 2, 4, 6, 8, ; \\ 0.3 + 0.0727j, & n = 3; \\ 0.3, & n = 5; \\ 0.3 + 0.0727j & n = 7; \\ 0.3 - 0.3078j, & n = 9; \\ 0.7, & n = \overline{10, 19}; \end{cases}$$

and

$$X(k) = \begin{cases} 3, & k = 0; \\ 1, & k = 2, 4, 6, 8; \\ 1.1525, & k = 1; \\ 0.7587, & k = 3; \\ 0.7616, & k = 5; \\ 0.8317, & k = 7; \\ 1.2421, & k = 9 \\ 0, & k = 10, 12, 14, 16, 18; \\ 0.7678, & k = 11; \\ 0.7, & k = 13; \\ 0.7616, & k = 15; \\ 1.0184, & k = 17; \\ 2.3632, & k = 19. \end{cases}$$

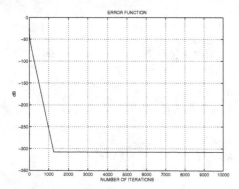

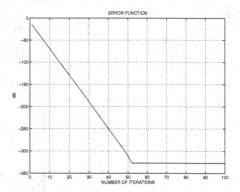

Fig. 3. The variation of $E_p^{\mathcal{K}}$ (dB) for input magnitude data given by (5) - form I.

Fig. 4. The variation of $E_p^{\mathcal{K}}$ (dB) for input magnitude data given by (5) - form II.

5   Conclusions

In this work we have presented some difficulties that can be encountered when one has to implement the iterative method for finding a solution of one-dimensional discrete phase retrieval problem. We have proven that we can find a solution to the one-dimensional discrete phase retrieval problem, by reformulating the one-dimensional discrete phase retrieval problem to an extended one-dimensional discrete phase retrieval problem. Although we have stated three forms of extended one-dimensional discrete phase retrieval problem, the second form seems to be the most appropriate, since it provides a real valued sequence.

Acknowledgments. The work of first author has been supported by Grant PAV3M PN-II-PT-PCCA-2013-4-1762.

References

1. Dumitrescu, B.: Positive Trigonometric Polynomials and Signal Processing Applications. Springer, Dordrecht, The Netherlands (2007)
2. Hayes, M.H., Lim, J.S., Oppenheim, A.V.: Signal reconstruction from phase or magnitude. IEEE Trans. Acoust. Speech Signal Process. ASSP **28**(6), 672–680 (1980)
3. Hurt, N.E.: Phase Retrieval and Zero Crossings. Kluwer Academic Publishers, Dordrecht/Boston/London (1989)
4. Izraelevitz, D., Lim, J.S.: A new direct algorithm for image reconstruction from Fourier transform magnitude. IEEE Trans. Acoust. Speech Signal Process. ASSP **35**(4), 511–518 (1987)
5. Oppenheim, A.V., Lim, J.S.: The importance of phase in signals. Proc. IEEE **69**(5), 529–541 (1981)
6. Oppenheim, A.V., Schafer, R.W., Buck, J.R.: Discrete-Time Signal Processing. Prentice-Hall, Upper Saddle River (1999)
7. Quatieri, T.F., Oppenheim, A.V.: Iterative techniques for minimum phase signal reconstruction from phase or magnitudes. IEEE Trans. Acoust. Speech Signal Process. ASSP **29**(6), 1187–1193 (1981)
8. Rusu, C., Astola, J.: Iterative one-dimensional phase. In: Proceedings of SMMSP 2006, Florence, pp. 95–100, 2–3 September 2006
9. Rusu, C., Astola, J.: About magnitude input data in 1-D discrete phase retrieval problem. In: Proceedings of EUSIPCO 2007, Poznan, 3–7 September 2007
10. Rusu, C., Astola, J.: About positive trigonometric polynomials and 1-D discrete phase retrieval problem. In: Proceedings of EUSIPCO 2012, Bucharest, 27–31 August 2012
11. Yagle, A.E., Bell, A.E.: One- and two-dimensional minimum and nonminimum phase retrieval by solving linear systems of equations. IEEE Trans. Sig. Process. **47**(11), 2978–2989 (1999)
12. Yegnanarayana, B., Saikia, D.K., Krishnan, T.R.: Significance of group delay functions in signal reconstruction from spectral magnitude and phase. IEEE Trans. Acoust. Speech Signal Process. ASSP **32**, 610–623 (1984)

Statistically Characterizing Void Density by Ultrasonic Speckles

Silvester Sadjina, Patrick Hölzl, and Bernhard G. Zagar(✉)

Johannes Kepler University, 4040 Linz, Austria
bernhard.zagar@jku.at
http://www.jku.at/emt/content

Abstract. We investigate the gradual emergence of so–called ultrasonic speckles as a hint to degradation processes deep in the volume of a specimen. These scatterers are caused by the combined action of thermal or electrical loads the specimen is subjected to during overload cycles it might experience as part of normal operation. These scatterers are typically too small to be directly imaged by ultrasound techniques. However, due to their spatial density evolving over time (over load cycles) they expose themselves by gradually forming these revealing US–speckles that increase in contrast over time. We can show that the speckle contrast is a good measure of the average total volume density of scattering voids and thus of the onset and evolution of delaminations via partially developed speckles.

Keywords: Ultrasound speckles · Non–destructive testing · Void density · Randomly distributed scatterers

1 Introduction

Several non–destructive methods do exist that allow to scan a specimen tomographically with the aim to detect delaminations, cracks or voids within the volume scanned. From coarse to fine resolution these are thermography techniques [1], scanning acoustic microscopy [2,3], micro computed tomography scans, acoustic near–field techniques (SNAM) [4], and X–ray diffraction methods. All techniques essentially are aiming for a spatial resolution sufficiently good to detect every single void (within their scope of resolution) and thus require a significant scanning and processing time to solve the inherent inverse problem associated with the method.

In our contribution we consider the problem of degradation detection as one that models the emerging voids as randomly scattered acoustic phase objects to be detected using techniques that were originally developed for analyzing laser speckles and are now applied to signals from an acoustic microscope. In the acoustic scanning microscopy technique [5] these sub–resolution random scatterers are causing ultrasound speckles [6]. These speckles and their emergence over mechanical or electrical stress cycles are analyzed with respect to the initial

© Springer International Publishing Switzerland 2015
R. Moreno-Díaz et al. (Eds.): EUROCAST 2015, LNCS 9520, pp. 648–654, 2015.
DOI: 10.1007/978-3-319-27340-2_80

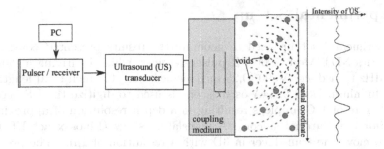

Fig. 1. Experimental setup. Voids in the specimen cause diffraction effects. The super-position of resulting waves cause speckles in the acoustic microscope image of Fig. 3.

state of the presumed homogeneous specimen. So they are compared to the zero phase deviations initially, over partly developed speckles for specimen in the void initiation phase, to fully developed speckles [7] for specimen experiencing sufficiently many randomly scattered voids [8,9].

Coherent imaging systems typically suffer from the effect known as speckles. They are experienced in synthetic aperture radar imaging, in laser illumination imaging systems [10–12] or also in ultrasonic imaging. Speckles are easily seen in the form of speckle noise overlaid onto the range image, the laser scan image or the echogenicity map in ultrasound images. Speckles themselves are a random but still deterministic interference pattern in an image that most of the time has a negative impact on the measurement problem at hand. They, however, convey sufficient information that can be put to good use in some other measurement problems. Those are related to laser applications where they act as fingerprints of an analyzed surface element whose load dependent motion can be tracked with a rather high spatial resolution [13].

In ultrasonic imaging speckles are typically reducing the ability to detect fine structures in a specimen by masking its echogenicity. Here also they are formed by isonifying a specimen presumably containing many sub–resolution scatterers with coherent radiation [14].

In some scientific fields the development over time of the density and average size of voids can be an indicator to the overall thermal or mechanical stress the specimen was to bear. The specimens might still be keeping its nominal operating performance even if it experiences a moderate density of cracks and voids with sizes below the typical detection limit of acoustic microscopes. The idea conveyed in this paper is to utilize the temporal development of spatial speckle noise overlaid onto an B–mode scan of a specimens structure to estimate the average density and possibly medium size of sub–resolution scatterers. It is organized as follows: in Sect. 2 the experimental set–up is described. Section 3 details the theory of speckle noise in US images and derives the speckle contrast as a measure of void density. Section 4 presents first results of an acoustic microscope adapted to the detection of voids and cracks.

2   Experimental Set–up

The experimental set–up used to generate the results presented consists of a Panametrics NDT Mod. 5900 PR pulser–receiver, which is driving a Panametrics 20 MHz transducer V390 (0.25 inch element size, 0.5 inch focal length). An Agilent Infiniium DSO 9254A oscilloscope is used to digitize the US–return at a sample rate of 1 Gsample/s resulting in a depth resolution of approximately 1.5 μm (for the material silicon). A translation stage (Linos x–act LT 100–1) allows to move the transducer in 3D with a resolution of 1 μm. The processing is done in Matlab as is the visualization. Volume data is rendered using the ParaView open source software. In Fig. 1 the schematics of our set–up is shown.

Figure 2 depicts the temporal impulse response of our transducer indicating a relative bandwidth of 70 % of the center frequency in the left panel and the spatial impulse response — the so–called point spread function — schematically in the right panel.

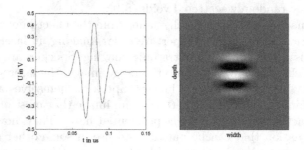

Fig. 2. (Left) temporal impulse response of a Panametrics 20 MHz transducer. (right) spatial impulse response of the same transducer in its focal plane.

3   Theory of US–Speckles

The modeling of the statistics of US–speckles is based upon some simplifying assumptions. (A) the carrier frequency ν (in our case 20 MHz) is sufficiently monochromatic to exhibit a coherence time that allows the constructive or destructive interference of contributions from scatterers located in the resolution cell of the set–up. For our case this can be interpreted in the temporal domain to have a pulse length of approximately 0.1 μs as can be seen from Fig. 2 left equating to approximately 120 μm in the depth dimension. (B) in the spatial domain the transducer focuses to approximately 10 μm (full width half maximum) as is depicted in Fig. 2 right. (C) The resolution cell is shaped as a prolate spheroid with said dimensions.

The sound pressure is modeled as a complex phasor

$$\underbrace{u(x,y,z,t)}_{\text{temporal\&spatial}} = \underbrace{A(x,y,z)}_{\text{spatial}} \cdot \underbrace{e^{j2\pi\nu t}}_{\text{temp.}}$$

with u representing spatial and temporal variations, A, the complex phasors magnitude, and ν the center frequency. The complex phasor A can be decomposed into its magnitude $|A|$ and phase term $e^{j\Theta(x,y,z)}$.

The complex phasor A results from the summation over all (indexed by n) contributions of single scatterers in the resolution cell with the following assumptions: (A) amplitude a_n and phase Θ_n of the n–th scatterer are statistically independent of each other and of all other scatterers in the resolution cell. (B) the phases of the scatterers are uniformly distributed in $[0, 2\pi)$, which means that their spatial distribution is such that many wavelength λ are in between them either in depth or lateral direction. Now further applying the central limit theorem allows to express A as the coherent sum of scaled contributions a_n, where the scale factor $\sqrt{N}$ takes the decreasing magnitude of single contributions into account if their number N increases.

$$A(x,y,z) = \frac{1}{\sqrt{N}} \sum_{n=1}^{N} |a_n| \cdot e^{\Theta_n}$$

Analyzing the probability density function (PDF) for A one can show [11], that a circular Gaussian PDF results.

Further assuming that in addition to the random weakly scattering scatterers there is a deterministic structure present that would result in a rather strong coherent contribution to A, it can be shown (again [8,11]) that a Riccian PDF will result.

$$p_A(a) = \frac{a}{\sigma^2} \cdot e^{\left(-\frac{a^2+s^2}{2\sigma^2}\right)} \cdot I_0\left(\frac{as}{\sigma^2}\right) ; \quad a \geq 0 \tag{1}$$

I_0 is the Bessel function of the first kind of order zero, σ is the standard deviation of the circular Gaussian PDF, and s is the strong coherent scattering of the deterministic structure. In analyzing Eq. 1 one can conclude that the image contrast as defined by the variation of intensity in a flat region of the image in relation to the mean brightness (caused by the deterministic structure) is a statistical parameter indicating the impact of density and average size of the scatterers sought.

4   Measurement Results

In order to demonstrate the applicability of the method one would have to resort to the acquisition of a rather lengthy experimental procedure. The necessary experimental equipment is currently under development and is thus not available yet to acquire real data. For that reason we did in fact acquire true US volume data which was demodulated (by Hilbert transform) to show in 3D the

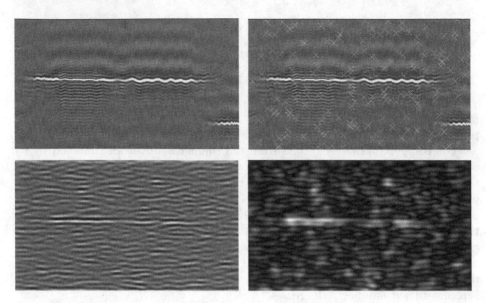

Fig. 3. Ultrasound image of the cross–section of a specimen with some pronounced structure top left; Top right: the same global structure with corresponding scattering function. This scattering function is derived from a randomly distributed population of sub–resolution scatterers (yellow ×'s). The scattering function is spatially convolved with the point spread function of the ultrasonic transducer (bottom left); Envelope demodulation of the RF–carrier results in strong speckles bottom right (Color figure online).

internal structure of the specimen. Subsequently randomly distributed scatterers of various echogenicity were added and the volume data convolved with the PSF shown in Fig. 2 to give the experienced US speckles. This process is described in more detail next. Speckles are present both in the RF data and the envelope – demodulated data as shown in Fig. 3. The top left panel shows the echogenicity map without random sub–resolution scatterers. The top right panel shows the scattering function by adding artificially sub–resolution scatterers. The bottom left panel shows the ultrasound RF data by scanning the echogenicity. The simulation is done by convolving in lateral dimension and in time (depth) with the PSF of the transducer as shown in Fig. 2.

The bottom right image is obtained by demodulating the RF data to yield the complex envelope which is imaged in gray–scale to yield a very obvious noisy (speckled) image of the original echogenicity (top left).

This data set was then statistically analyzed resulting in the image shown in Fig. 4. One clearly observes the increase in the variance σ_I^2 of the image intensity within the presumed flat area boxed, which is a measure of speckle contrast.

Figure 5 shows the complete data set in 3D.

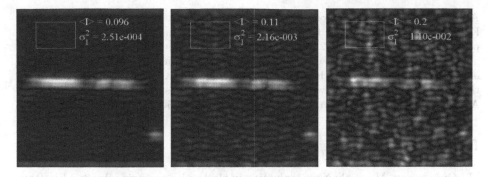

Fig. 4. Three B–mode scans exhibiting US speckles in increasing magnitude. All frames were generated adding 5000 sub–resolution scatterers (size $\approx \lambda/50$) each with relative scattering strength of -60 dB, -54 dB and -40 dB relative to the deterministic component (the bright horizontal bar) extending from left to right. One clearly observes the increase in the variance of the intensity σ_I^2.

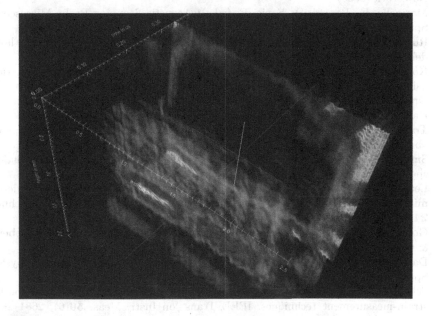

Fig. 5. Ultrasound volume data rendered using the ParaView software [15].

5   Conclusions

We have shown that ultrasound speckles that are usually considered a problem to be avoided can be exploited to indicate the gradual emergence of sub–resolution scatterers which might be caused by micro–cracks or small sized voids small enough still to not impair the nominal functionality of the specimen but possibly being indicative of an upcoming failure.

Acknowlegement. This work has been carried out at LCM GmbH as part of a K2 project. K2 projects are financed using funding from the Austrian COMET K2 programme. The COMET K2 projects at LCM are supported by the Austrian federal government, the federal state of Upper Austria, the Johannes Kepler University and all of the scientific partners which form part of the COMET K2 Consortium. Furthermore the authors gratefully acknowledge the partial financial support of this work by the Austrian Research Promotion Agency under grant 838515.

References

1. Oppermann, M., et al.: Nano evaluation in electronics packaging. In: 2nd Electronics Systemintegration Technology Conference, Greenwich UK (2008)
2. Every, A.G., Pluta, M., Grill, W.: Interference of non-aligned Airy diffraction patterns in transmission acoustic microscopy images of crystals. Proc. R. Soc. A **461**, 3847–3862 (2005)
3. Maev, R.G.: Acoustic Microscopy – Fundamentals and Applications. Wiley - VCH, New York (2008)
4. Marinello, F., Passeri, D., Savio, E. (eds.): Acoustic Scanning Probe Microscopy. Springer, Berlin (2013)
5. Rupitsch, S., Zagar, B.: Acoustic microscopy technique to precisely locate layer delamination. IEEE Trans. Instr. Meas. **56**(4), 1429–1434 (2007)
6. Kothbauer, R., Rupitsch, S.J., Zagar, B.G.: Characterization of micro-materials using laser speckles. In: Proceedings of the SPIE – The International Society for Optical Engineering, vol. 6371, pp. 63710Q- 1–9 (2006)
7. Halliwell, M. (ed.): Acoustical Imaging. Springer, Berlin (2013)
8. Trahey, G.E., Smith, S.W.: Properties of acoustical speckle in the presence of phase aberration part I: first order statistics. Ultrason. Imaging **10**, 12–28 (1988)
9. Smith, S.W., Trahey, G.E., Hubbard, S.M., Wagner, R.F.: Properties of acoustical speckle in the presence of phase. Ultrason Imaging **10**, 29–51 (1988)
10. Lettner, J., Zagar, B.: Two-wavelengths laser-speckle technique for thickness determination of transparent layers on rough surfaces. Measurement Sci. Technol. **24**(11), 115204 (2013)
11. Goodman, J.W.: Speckle Phenomena in Optics: Theory and Applications. Roberts & Co., Publ, Greenwood (2010)
12. Dainty, J.C.: Laser speckle and related phenomena. Topics in Applied Physics. Springer, Berlin (1984)
13. Schneider, S.C., Rupitsch, S.J., Zagar, B.G.: Signal processing for laser-speckle strain-measurement techniques. IEEE Trans. on Instr. Meas. **56**(6), 2681–2687 (2007)
14. Nadarajah, S.: Statistical distributions of potential interest in ultrasound speckle analysis. Phys. Med. Biol. **52**, N213–N227 aberration part II: correlation lengths. Ultrason. Imaging **10**(29–51), 1988 (2007)
15. Kitware open source software ParaView, Kitware Inc., Clifton Park, NY 12065 USA

The Quantization Effect on Audio Signals for Wildlife Intruder Detection Systems

Lacrimioara Grama and Corneliu Rusu$^{(\boxtimes)}$

Faculty of Electronics, Telecommunications and Information Technology,
Technical University of Cluj-Napoca, Cluj-Napoca, Romania
Lacrimioara.Grama@bel.utcluj.ro, corneliu.rusu@ieee.org
http://sp.utcluj.ro

Abstract. In this paper we present the influence of quantization of audio signals on D and S descriptors. These descriptors represent the number of samples between two consecutive real zeros and the number of points of local minima/maxima between two successive real zeros, respectively. It is shown that the number of the D/S pairs is almost constant and the behavior is almost the same till the number of bits is less than 6, in the proposed audio based wildlife intruder detection framework.

Keywords: Intruder detection · Zero crossings

1 Introduction

Humans play a significant role in ensuring the integrity of wild places. Nowadays there is a large interest in detecting illegal logging because damaging of rain forest is a leading contributor to climate change. Illegal logging alone is responsible for approximately 10% of all greenhouse gas emissions [1]. There are many natural reserves with flora, fauna, wildlife which are spread and practically impossible to be surveyed continuously. Even if most of these regions are protected by law, they are quite often the target of some people for hunting and forest cutting. While there is an international mandate to stop illegal deforestation, the hard part is enforcing it.

For these reasons monitoring systems like the video surveillance are popular and necessary these days, but they ask usually for expensive computational resources. Another attractive solution may be assimilated to an "acoustic eye", i.e. audio based wildlife intruder detection systems [2]. An ingenious way to convert used cell phones to solar powered listening devices was presented by Rainforest Connection. The devices can pick out the unmistakable sounds of chainsaws over a mile away, then transmit the information to a cloud API which sends an alarm to authorities on the ground instantly. Some pilot programs have been tested in regions with terrestrial wireless network [3].

Because a wildlife surveillance system requires the design of low complexity algorithms and the use of hardware with low power consumption, there is a need

© Springer International Publishing Switzerland 2015
R. Moreno-Díaz et al. (Eds.): EUROCAST 2015, LNCS 9520, pp. 655–662, 2015.
DOI: 10.1007/978-3-319-27340-2_81

to study the quantization effect on audio based wildlife intruder detection systems. The low complexity approach TESPAR (Time Encoded Signal Processing and Recognition) proved to be a fairly robust method for sound encoding and classification when various noisy environments were simulated and thus suitable for on site, real time signal processing applications. The bandwidth of received data can be significantly reduce and we are still able to detect the intruders [4].

The goal of this work is to study the quantization effect on two TESPAR method descriptors, namely the epoch duration D and the epoch shape S, in an audio based wildlife intruder framework. The paper is organized as follows: the theoretical backgrounds are briefly presented in Sect. 2 and the framework is illustrated in Sect. 3. Section 4 presents the quantization effect through experimental results and in Sect. 5 conclusions are drawn.

2　Theoretical Background

The time-domain digital language for coding "band-limited" signals, TESPAR, was first proposed by King and Glossing [5]. It needs few processing power and low memory requirements offering low-priced implementation costs. The features of the TESPAR model can be easily detected by visual inspection of the waveform, namely zero crossings and local extremal points [6].

A waveform contains both complex and real zeros. First attempts in the theory of zero-based analysis of the waveforms were made by Bond and Chan. They considered the representation and manipulation of signals by means of their real and complex zeros, and stated that natural information sources generate continuous band-limited functions that include complex zeros which are physically undetectable [7]. Real zeros can be easily determined by a simple visual inspection of the function (where the sign of a signal changes we have a zero crossing). Finding complex zeros is not such a trivial problem. Complex zeros are associated to the perturbations (points of minima/maxima) in the shape of the waveform, which appear between the well-defined real zeros [8].

Infinite clipping stays at the base of the TESPAR. It is a binary transformation which takes a waveform and transforms it in an array of numbers which contain information about the waveform's zeros. The intelligibility of the speech waveform based on the effects of infinite clipping was investigated by Licklidder and Pollack. They have removed all the amplitude information, keeping only the zero crossing information (this is infinite clipping). Even if a high amount of information was removed from the speech waveform, the result of the process shows that the mean random word intelligibility scores achieved were 97.9% [8]. It means that most of the useful information contained by the speech waveform can be found in zero crossing.

A TESPAR coder gives the following information [9]:

– epoch duration D between two real zeros; it represents the number of samples of the segment contained between two successive real zeros;

– epoch shape S between two real zeros; it represents the number of points of local minima/maxima between two consecutive real zeros (for the positive axis the points of minima are counted, while for the negative axis the points of maxima are counted).

After the array of D/S pairs are obtained they are coded using an alphabet which approximates the distribution of epochs in the D/S pairs plane by means of vector quantization. The TESPAR coder outputs an array of symbols. The resulting array can be converted in a series of descriptors: matrix $\mathbf{S}$ (Nx1) which counts the number of apparitions of each symbol of the alphabet in the symbol stream, and matrix $\mathbf{A}$ (NxN) which counts the number of apparitions of all the pairs of symbols, at a certain distance n (lag). As a classification mechanism the archetypes technique can be used. By adding together and then computing the average of the $\mathbf{A}$ and $\mathbf{S}$ matrices one can find the archetypes. After the archetypes are computed, they can be stored in databases and used later on for classification of unknown samples [2].

3   Framework

As we have already mentioned, in the context of a wildlife surveillance system which, by necessity, requires the design of low complexity algorithms and the use of low power consumption hardware [10], there is the need to study the quantization effect on audio based wildlife intruder detection systems. In our proposed framework the low complexity system only checks if a certain recorded event belongs to a human, a car or an engine, a gunshot or other possible sounds of interest that can be considered as intruders.

In the present paper we take into account two types of sound that can be considered as intruders in a wildlife area: sounds originate from chainsaws and sounds originate from gunshots. In the chainsaw sounds database we have 60 different audio samples corresponding to 10 different types of chainsaws [11], and in the gunshot sounds database we have 51 different audio samples corresponding to 25 different types of guns [12,13]. The sampling rate for all the considered signals is 16000 samples/second and 16-bit accuracy was used. All signals were recorded outside, thus they are not studio recordings.

4   Simulation Results – Quantization Effect

The influence of quantization of audio signals on D and S descriptors was tested using a collection of two types of audio recordings. We have perform simulations on signals available on the SPG (Signal Processing Group) Sound Database [11] and on some signals available online [12,13]. All initial signals were 16-bit accuracy. For simulations the signals were quantized using different number of bits (14, 12, 10, 8, 6, 4 and 2), in order to see the influence of number of bits used for quantization.

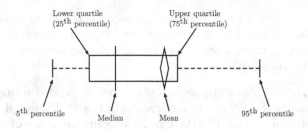

Fig. 1. Box and whisker definitions.

For illustrating the D and S vectors we have used histograms. For all of them on abscissa we have the number of bins and on the ordinate the probability density function estimate corresponding to the D and S descriptors. Above the histograms a box and whisker plot is used, it is detailed in Fig. 1.

For all signals tested, first, infinite clipping was performed (signal was scaled between -1 and 1). Then we have found zero crossings, we have counted the number of samples between two zero crossings (D - epoch duration) and then we have counted local minima/maxima (S - epoch shape).

The first signal used for exemplification corresponds to a chainsaw [11]. The duration of the signal is 7.498 s. In Figs. 2 and 3 the descriptors corresponding to the chainsaw sound are illustrated. By a visual inspection on the histograms it can be seen that quantization on 2 bits is not appropriate (for all chainsaw signals) in the case of D descriptor representation (see Fig. 2).

In order to better compare the influence of quantization, the D descriptor corresponding to the 2-bit accuracy signal was removed from the graph (Fig. 4).

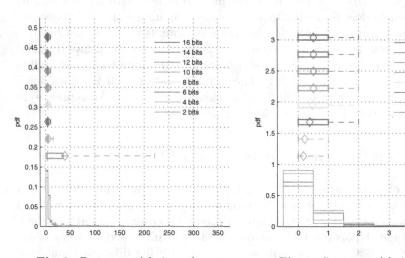

Fig. 2. D - vector (chainsaw).   **Fig. 3.** S - vector (chainsaw).

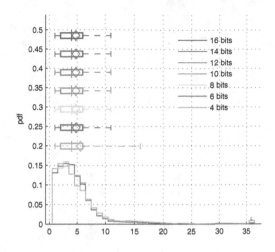

Fig. 4. D - vector (chainsaw) (without the signal quantized on 2 bits).

In the case of the D vector the $IQR = 4$ (interquartile range) when the signal is quantized on $16 \div 4$ bits, but the 95th percentile differs: when the signal is quantized on $16 \div 6$ bits it corresponds to the 11th bin, and when it is quantized on 4 bits it corresponds to the 15th bin. For the 2-bit quantization the $IQR = 35$ and the 95th percentile corresponds to the 222th bin. In the case of the S vector the $IQR = 1$ when the signal is quantized on $16 \div 6$ bits and the 95th percentile corresponds to the 3rd bin; when it is quantized on $4 \div 2$ bits the $IQR = 0$ and the 95th percentile corresponds to the 2nd bin.

In Table 1 the mean and standard deviation values for the chainsaw signal are presented. If the signal is quantized on 16, 14, 10 and 8 bits, respectively, the values for mean and standard deviation are almost the same. They differs a little bit when 6-bit quantization is used, and the difference is higher when 4-bit

Table 1. Mean and standard deviation values for the chainsaw signal.

Number of bits	D descriptor		S descriptor	
	Mean	Standard deviation	Mean	Standard deviation
16	4.77	4.31	0.51	0.96
14	4.77	4.31	0.51	0.96
12	4.77	4.32	0.51	0.96
10	4.77	4.33	0.51	0.95
8	4.77	4.32	0.48	0.91
6	4.81	4.42	0.39	0.79
4	5.57	6.37	0.22	0.67
2	39.90	79.61	0.18	0.68

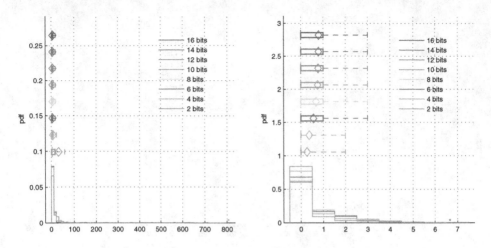

Fig. 5. D - vector (gunshot).   **Fig. 6.** S - vector (gunshot).

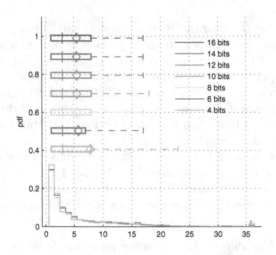

Fig. 7. D - vector (gunshot) (without the signal quantized on 2 bits).

or 2-bit quantization is performed (especially in the case of the D vector). Same behavior was observed for all 60 chainsaw signals tested.

The second signal used for exemplification corresponds to a gunshot [11]. The duration of the signal is 5.694 s. In Figs. 5 and 6 the descriptors corresponding to the gunshot sound are illustrated. As in the case of the chainsaw signal, it can be seen that 2-bit accuracy is not appropriate (for all gunshot signals) in the case of D descriptor representation (see Fig. 5).

In order to better compare the influence of quantization, the D descriptor corresponding to the 2-bit quantized signal was removed from the graph (Fig. 7).

Table 2. Mean and standard deviation values for the gunshot signal.

Number of bits	D descriptor		S descriptor	
	Mean	Standard deviation	Mean	Standard deviation
16	5.50	6.03	0.8	1.33
14	5.47	5.91	0.79	1.30
12	5.50	6.03	0.77	1.25
10	5.52	6.24	0.75	1.22
8	5.55	7.01	0.68	1.13
6	5.77	14.63	0.56	1.00
4	7.84	48.23	0.37	0.80
2	31.27	191.97	0.27	0.73

In the case of the D vector the $IQR = 7$ when the signal is quantized on $16 \div 8$ and 4 bits, $IQR = 6$ when is quantized on 6 bits and $IQR = 15$ when is quantized on 2 bits. For all of them the 5th percentile corresponds to the 1st bin, but the 95th percentile differs: when the signal is quantized on $16 \div 12$ and $8 \div 6$ bits it corresponds to the 17th bin, when is quantized on 10 bits it corresponds to the 18th bin, when is quantized on 4 bits it corresponds to the 23rd bin, and when is quantized on 2 bits it corresponds to the 58th bin. In the case of the S vector the $IQR = 1$ when the signal is quantized on $16 \div 6$ bits and the 95th percentile corresponds to the 4th bin; when it is quantized on $4 \div 2$ bits the $IQR = 0$ and the 95th percentile corresponds to the 3rd bin.

In Table 2 the mean and standard deviation values for the gunshot signal are presented. If 16, 14, 10 and 8-bit accuracy is used, the values for mean and standard deviation are almost the same. They differs a little bit when the quantization is performed on 6 bits and the difference is higher when the quantization is performed on 4 or 2 bits, especially in the case of D vector. Same behavior was observed for all 51 gunshot signals from the database.

5   Conclusions

We can say that for the given framework standalone systems must be utilized, low complexity algorithms and hardware with low power consumption. There must be an *apriori* knowledge of the system to be surveyed. Depending on the type of the intruders different type of approaches must be used.

In the present paper the experiments have been conducted for two classes of signals which can be considered as intruders in a wildlife area: sounds originate from chainsaws and sounds originate from gunshots. From the experimental results we can conclude that the D and S descriptors are robust when the number of bits are reduced (till the number of bits is less than 6).

Acknowledgments. This research is supported by the Human Resources Development Programme POSDRU/159/1.5/S/137516 financed by the European Social Fund and by the Romanian Government.

The work of second author has been supported by Grant PAV3M PN-II-PT-PCCA-2013-4-1762.

References

1. Bonadio, J.: Repurposed Phones Defend Rainforests (2015). http://billionsrising. org/repurposed-phones-defend-rainforests/
2. Ghiurcau, M.V., Rusu, C., Bilcu, R.C., Astola, J.: Audio based solutions for detecting intruders in wild areas. Signal Process. **92**(3), 829–840 (2012)
3. Ackerman, E.: Topher White: Repurposing Cellphones to Defend the Rain Forest (2015).   http://spectrum.ieee.org/geek-life/profiles/topher-white-repurposing-cellphones-to-defend-the-rain-forest
4. Ghiurcau, M.V., Rusu, C., Bilcu, R.C.: A modified TESPAR algorithm for wildlife sound classification. In: 2010 IEEE International Symposium on Circuits and Systems, pp. 2370–2373. IEEE Press, Paris (2010)
5. King, R.A., Glossing, W.: Electron. Lett. **14**(15), 456–457 (1978)
6. King, R.A., Phipps, T.C.: Shannon, TESPAR and approximation strategies. In: 9th International Conference on Signal Processing Applications and Technology, Toronto, Canada, vol. 2, pp. 445–453 (1998)
7. Bond, F.E., Cahn, C.R.: A relationship between zero crossings and Fourier coefficients for bandwidth-limited functions. IRE Trans. Inf. Theory **IT**–4, 110–113 (1958)
8. Licklidder, J.C.R., Pollack, I.: Effects of differentiation, integration and infinite peak clipping upon the intelligibility of speech. JASA **20**(1), 42–51 (1948)
9. Lupu, E., Feher, Z., Pop, P.G.: On the speaker verification using TESPAR coding method. In: International Symposium on Signals, Circuits & Systems, pp. 173–176. IEEE Press, Iasi (2003)
10. Popescu, M., Grama, L., Rusu, C., Sirbu, M.: Communication protocol for wireless sensor networks for energy consumption optimization. In: Workshop on Circuits, Systems and Information Technology (WCSIT). IEICE Press, Iasi (2014)
11. Todor, L., Zoicas, V., Grama, L., Rusu, C.: The SPG (signal processing group) sound database. Novice Insights Electron. Telecommun. Inf. Technol. **15**(1), 62–65 (2014)
12. FreeSFX: Gunshot sounds. http://www.freesfx.co.uk/sfx/gun
13. SoundBible: Free Sound Clips, Sound Bites, and Sound Effects. http://soundbible. com/

Combining Relational and NoSQL Database Systems for Processing Sensor Data in Disaster Management

Reinhard Stumptner[✉], Christian Lettner,
and Bernhard Freudenthaler

Software Competence Center Hagenberg, Data Analysis Systems,
Softwarepark 21, 4232 Hagenberg, Austria
{reinhard.stumptner,christian.lettner,
bernhard.freudenthaler}@scch.at

Abstract. In disaster and emergency management the integration of different kinds of sensor networks gains in importance and consequently more and more data becomes available. The upcoming NoSQL database systems are flexible and scalable data stores, but up to now lacking in connectivity to traditional data processing systems (data warehouses, business intelligence suites, etc.). Due to that in this work a combined relational and NoSQL data processing approach is proposed to reduce data volume and work load of the relational part and enable the integral solution to process huge amounts of data. In contrast to fully NoSQL-based data warehouse systems, this approach does not face compatibility and integrability issues.

1 Introduction and Motivation

Disaster or emergency management systems should implement a good action plan to handle effects of any emergencies. As time moves on in a disaster situation, and consequently more data becomes available – presuming that environmental sensors can be used and data from humans on site (helpers or inhabitants) can be collected – disaster managers get a good picture of the ongoing situation in the concerned area.

In order to reduce losses of any kind, property or human life, during an emergency situation, emergency managers should identify and/or anticipate potential risks in time, in order to reduce the probability of a disaster or to better react on it. It is essential to include procedures for determining whether and when an emergency situation would occur and at what point of time an emergency management plan should be activated.

In the frame of the research project "INDYCO" [1] a disaster management prototype was developed [10]. One aim was to have the possibility of easily integrating new data into the data base of the system and another one to process even huge sensor data streams near real-time. Using a net of various types of sensors, e.g. "multimedia sensors" or "social sensors", a heterogeneous sensor data set has developed. As this heterogeneous sensor network was growing, a wish arose to have a flexible data processing layer, which

---

[1] "Integrated Dynamic Decision Support System Component for Disaster Management Systems", ERA-NET EraSME program under the Austrian grant agreement No. 836684 (FFG).

© Springer International Publishing Switzerland 2015
R. Moreno-Díaz et al. (Eds.): EUROCAST 2015, LNCS 9520, pp. 663–670, 2015.
DOI: 10.1007/978-3-319-27340-2_82

can handle very high data volumes. At the same time there already were systems (e.g. control center systems) which one wanted to connect these data to. And these systems were very limited concerning their connectivity (to relational databases in general). Due to that, a combined NoSQL and relational data processing approach was developed.

2 Related Research

The database world currently is dominated by rational SQL systems, but NoSQL databases are becoming more and more relevant. These systems were built to handle large volumes of data which is not necessarily structured. Originally the development of these systems was motivated by Web 2.0 applications, being designed to scale to millions of users working in parallel, in contrast to the traditional DBMSs and data warehouses paradigms [1].

In the current literature NoSQL systems mainly were benchmarked using vast amounts of unstructured test data. Parker et al. [6] did that evaluation with "traditional" datasets – meaning moderate amounts of structured data. Results show that the NoSQL system performs equal or better than the relational database (except aggregations).

Veen et al. [9] show that an increasing variety of objects or structures which are monitored, lead to an increasing demand on platforms, where produced sensor data are stored. Virtualization and cloud platforms play a major role in this context. Traditional SQL systems have been used in this domain for a long time, but due to increasing availability and scalability of NoSQL systems, these gained in importance. A comparison shows that in future these new systems might be favored.

Krishnan [5] gives an introduction to data warehousing in times of Big Data. The author describes how Big Data approaches can fit into the data warehousing way of thinking and points out shortcomings, architecture options, and integration techniques for Big Data and the data warehouse.

Chai et al. [2] describe an approach on a fully document-oriented data warehouse, which shows better scalability, flexibility and efficiency compared to traditional data warehousing. But obviously, disadvantages of that approach are worse connectivity with or integrability into corporate system landscapes.

The approach presented in this contribution bases on some of these techniques (from [5] in particular). However, it incorporates NoSQL into traditional relational data warehousing as a pre-processing layer, which enables it to process very large amounts of data on the one hand and stay compatible with traditional data warehouse and business intelligence software on the other hand.

3 Combined Relational and NoSQL-Based Sensor Data Processing and Analysis

This contribution combines traditional relational with NoSQL-based approaches for sensor data processing. It aims to use the best of both worlds, to get a disaster management system with outstanding performance, throughput and response time. To achieve this, a method to close the gap between these approaches is proposed.

The main advantage of NoSQL systems over traditional ones is their simple scaling mechanism, which makes these systems attractive for processing Big (sensor-) Data [9]. This makes fast processing of vast data or data streams possible – if enough hardware can be made available. Nevertheless, the advantages of traditional information systems are for instance: connectivity and business intelligence (BI) tool support, which includes analytical models (OLAP), reporting, or data integration [4, 8].

Figure 1 gives an overview of the developed data processing architecture. For the NoSQL system a MongoDB [3] cluster is used, for the relational system a business intelligence layer operated by Microsoft SQL Server Business Intelligence in conjunction with several other data mining and machine learning tools (KNIME, Rapid-miner, R) is used. All sensor data details are stored in the NoSQL cluster. The big amount of fast growing data is handled by pre-processing them, which means building specified aggregates and making them available for the relational system. The interface between these two sub-systems is represented by the aggregate pool, which is located within the NoSQL system.

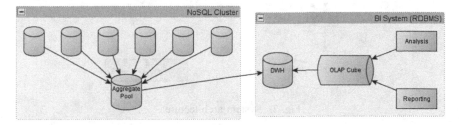

Fig. 1. Combination of NoSQL and relational based approach for data processing

The relational system is especially used for providing recurring reports, as well as for long-term learning tasks, like updating models or learning rules for the online monitoring system, the complex event processing (CEP) engine (see Fig. 2). To accomplish this, the required data is loaded from the aggregation pool into a data warehouse (DWH). Figure 2 shows the system architecture in detail. The middleware collects sensor data and performs a first evaluation and analysis in real-time using a CEP engine. Afterwards the detailed sensor data as well as the results from the first evaluation and analysis are stored in the NoSQL cluster (represented by the logical entities "Sensors", "Situations" and "Workflows" in Fig. 2). Using certain batch intervals, the aggregates for all logical entities stored in the aggregation pool are updated using a MapReduce job. Loading the data from the aggregation pool to the DWH is performed using an extract-transform-load (ETL) process. The DWH consists of two main layers, the staging and the DWH layer as shown in Fig. 4. The staging layer in principle represents a copy of the data source schemas, while the DWH layer represents a star schema. The staging copies are needed in some cases to be able to join with target tables for instance for efficient updates. The ETL processes are developed using the tool BIAccelerator [8], a template based approach for SQL Server Integration Services. Although there are many ETL processes at work within the system, they can be categorized into two types. The first type of ETL process is responsible for loading the data from the external data sources to the staging layer (ETL 1 in Fig. 4), while the second type is responsible for transforming the data from the staging area schemas into a star schema (ETL 2 in Fig. 4). Therefore only two ETL templates are needed for BIAccelerator to generate all needed ETL processes.

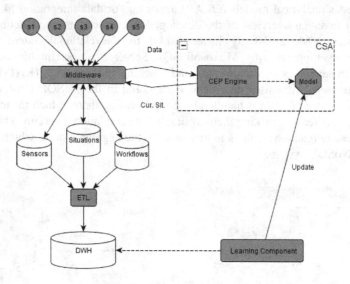

Fig. 2. System architecture

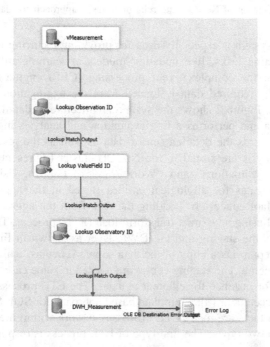

Fig. 3. ETL process "Staging-DWH" of entity "Measurement"

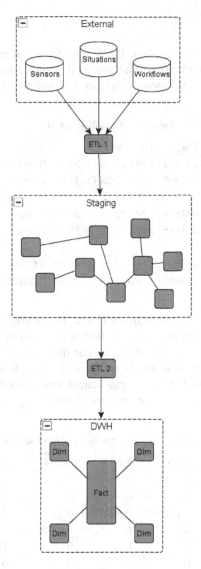

Fig. 4. ETL process

The key benefit of using a template based approach for ETL process design is when data from new sensors should be integrated into the system. After the database schemas are adapted to the new data (if necessary), the ETL processes can be generated automatically, without any further effort.

Figure 3 shows the generated ETL package which loads data from the staging layer into the DWH for the entity "Measurement". Overall 13 ETL packages were needed to implement the dataflow of the disaster management system.

4 Results

As explained in the previous section, RAW data from the environmental sensors is aggregated in the MongoDB cluster and provided to the relational layer through ETL packages. The following table shows a certain data sample (Table 1).

Table 1. Rainfall RAW data

Cnt	Timestamp	Value
494404	1999-12-28 08:30:00	0.0976
494405	1999-12-28 08:35:00	0.0958
...		
494534	1999-12-28 19:20:00	0.0889
494535	1999-12-28 19:25:00	0.0564
...		
494599	1999-12-29 00:45:00	0.0210
494600	1999-12-29 00:50:00	0.0012

These data are aggregated on different levels. The aggregation is done on multiple levels but it is not in a fully generic way. Rather it is customized for the certain data part or entity (like data from one rainfall sensor in the below table). But the aggregation on multiple levels (not all these levels are needed on application or data warehouse layer) should guarantee that the aggregate calculation procedures do not have to be redefined in any case of requirement changes (Table 2).

Table 2. Aggregates for a rainfall sensor

NG5	NG6	NG12	NG24	NG48
0	0	0	0	1.199219
0.09765625	0	0	0	1.101563
0	0.1015625	0.8007813	0	0
0	0	0	0.09765625	0
0	0	0	0	1.398438
0.4023438	0	0	0	0.9023438

These aggregates are transferred into the data warehouse. In the data warehouse further analysis of the data takes place (as described in the previous section); e.g. to calibrate the model of the online monitoring component. Furthermore, an OLAP cube based on Microsoft SQL Server Analysis Services was set up for traditionally browsing available data (simple aggregations on predefined measures; see Fig. 5).

In this example, using 1 h aggregates of sensors with a 5 min sampling rate, the amount of data in the data warehouse could be reduced by about 92 %, meaning detail data stays in the MongoDB cluster and about 8 % in the relational data warehouse which is a strong reduction of the load of the relational system.

As mentioned before, these data were integrated into a traditional data warehouse (see below figure) for further analysis.

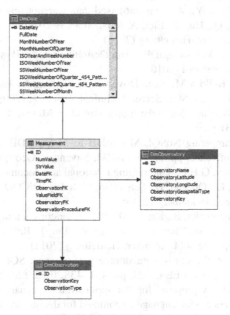

Fig. 5. SSAS OLAP cube

Moreover, data in the warehouse are accessed through data mining and machine learning tools (KINME, Rapidminer, R) to create or update flooding models for the online monitoring component.

5   Conclusion and Future Work

Although Business Intelligence Suits support the integration of data from NoSQL systems (to load data from these systems in particular), the advantage of scalability and flexible data structures would be lost [7]. Due to that the authors of this contribution propose an intermediate scalable NoSQL layer which performs pre-processing on RWA data and provides intermediate results to the BI system through an "aggregate pool". This approach reduces the load of the relational BI system drastically and enables the integral NoSQL/BI solution to process huge amounts of data but staying compatible with the corporate system landscape. The combination with the ETL generator suite automates the development of data flows to a large extent. Further investigations focus on accessing detail-data from the BI layer efficiently.

Acknowledgments. The research leading to these results has received funding from the ERA-NET EraSME program under the Austrian grant agreement No. 836684, project "INDYCO - Integrated Dynamic Decision Support System Component for Disaster Management Systems" and has been supported by the COMET program of the Austrian Research Promotion Agency (FFG).

References

1. Cattell, R.: Scalable SQL and NoSQL Data Stores. SIGMOD Rec. **39**(4), 12–27 (2011)
2. Chai, H., Wu, G., Zhao, Y.: A document-based data warehousing approach for large scale data mining. In: Zu, Q., Hu, B., Elçi, A. (eds.) ICPCA 2012 and SWS 2012. LNCS, vol. 7719, pp. 69–81. Springer, Heidelberg (2013)
3. Chodorow, K., Dirolf, M.: MongoDB - The Definitive Guide: Powerful and Scalable Data Storage. O'Reilly, Sebastopol (2010)
4. He, M. T. Gudyka: Build a Metadata-Driven ETL Platform by Extending Microsoft SQL Server Integration Services. SQL Server Technical Article. -, (2008)
5. Krishnan, K.: Data Warehousing in the Age of Big Data. Morgan Kaufmann Publishers Inc., San Francisco (2013)
6. Parker, Z. et al.: Comparing NoSQL MongoDB to an SQL DB. Proceedings of the 51st ACM Southeast Conference. pp. 5:1–5:6 ACM, Savannah, Georgia (2013)
7. Roijackers, J., Fletcher, G.H.L.: On bridging relational and document-centric data stores. In: Gottlob, G., Grasso, G., Olteanu, D., Schallhart, C. (eds.) BNCOD 2013. LNCS, vol. 7968, pp. 135–148. Springer, Heidelberg (2013)
8. Stumptner, R., Freudenthaler, B., Krenn, M.: BIAccelerator – a template-based approach for rapid ETL development. In: Chen, L., Felfernig, A., Liu, J., Raś, Z.W. (eds.) ISMIS 2012. LNCS, vol. 7661, pp. 435–444. Springer, Heidelberg (2012)
9. Veen, J.S., van der et al.: Sensor data storage performance: SQL or NoSQL, physical or virtual. In: Chang, R. (ed.) IEEE Cloud, pp. 431–438. IEEE (2012)
10. Ziebermayr, T. et al.: A proposal for the application of dynamic workflows in disaster management: a process model language customized for disaster management. In: Morvan, F. et al. (eds.) DEXA Workshops, pp. 284–288. IEEE Computer Society (2011)

Modelling and Control of Robots

An Almost Time Optimal Route Planning Method for Complex Manufacturing Topologies

Matthias Jörgl$^{(\boxtimes)}$, Hubert Gattringer, and Andreas Müller

Institute of Robotics, Johannes Kepler University Linz,
Altenbergerstr. 69, 4040 Linz, Austria
{matthias.joergl,hubert.gattringer,a.mueller}@jku.at
http://www.robotik.jku.at

Abstract. This paper focuses on time and distance optimal route planning for complex manufacturing topologies. The main idea of the proposed algorithm is to transform the manufacturing process into an undirected weighted graph, which can be treated as the well-known Traveling Salesman Problem (TSP). The optimal solution for the TSP is found with the help of Linear Integer Programming, which yields to Nondeterministic Polynomial-time (NP-hard). In order to overcome unpractical computation times for more complex tasks the optimal solution is approximated with the help of the Minimum Spanning Tree (MST) algorithm and alternatively with the Christofides algorithm. Simulation results and a comparison of the denoted methods are shown.

Keywords: Route planning · Integer linear programming · Traveling salesman problem · Christofides heuristic · Minimum spanning tree heuristic

1 Introduction

A main trend in today's automation industry is to reduce process time in order to increase production rate. In many applications like welding, punching and cutting, the execution sequence of the welds, holes etc. is crucial for the process time. Finding the optimal topology can be modeled as an undirected weighted graph and thereby treated in the same way as the well-known Traveling Salesman Problem (TSP). A main focus of this work is the choice of the weights of the graph, which have a strong influence on the quality of the solution.

The optimal solution of the TSP can be found with the help of Integer Linear Programming. While finding the optimal solution for the TSP is possible for small scaled problems, for more complex tasks the solution can only be approached. In this contribution the solution is approximated with the help of the Minimum Spanning Tree (MST) algorithm and with the help of the Christofides algorithm, which is an expansion of the MST. Both methods yield an approximation of the optimal solution in polynomial-time.

The considered paper is organized as follows: The problem formulation of a typically laser cutting process is dealt with in Sect. 2. Finding the optimal

© Springer International Publishing Switzerland 2015
R. Moreno-Díaz et al. (Eds.): EUROCAST 2015, LNCS 9520, pp. 673–680, 2015.
DOI: 10.1007/978-3-319-27340-2_83

topology with the help of Integer Linear Programming is shown in Sect. 3. In Sect. 4 the proposed heuristic methods will be discussed in more detail. Simulation results and a comparison to demonstrate the efficiency of all methods are shown in Sect. 5 and concluding remarks are given in Sect. 6.

2   Problem Formulation

The first part of finding an execution sequence is to transform the manufacturing process into an undirected weighted graph $G = (V, E)$, comprising a set V of vertices and a set E of edges with nonnegative edge costs $c\colon E \to \mathbb{R}^+$. Alternatively, a directed graph could also be used to manage that problem, but will lead to unpractical computation times. Now, finding an optimal route can be treated in the same way as the TSP. Figure 1 shows a typical layout for a laser cutting process (LCP) with the corresponding graph on the right side.

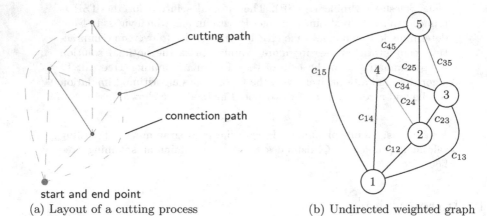

(a) Layout of a cutting process   (b) Undirected weighted graph

Fig. 1. Layout of a cutting process with all possible connections with corresponding weighted graph

The trajectories of individual manufacturing processes are defined as basis splines and are connected via straight lines. A trajectory using basis splines is generally computed to

$$\mathbf{p}(u) = \sum_{j=0}^{n} \mathbf{d}_j\, N_j^d(u), \tag{1}$$

with number of control points n, control points $\mathbf{d}$, basis spline degree d and basis functions $N_j^d(u)$, see [2] for further details.

Due to the large number of edges, the weighting must be kept as simple as possible. Assuming that the execution direction of a contour has no influence on the process time, each start and each end point is assigned to a node of the graph. Edges, which connect contours, are weighted in relation to the process time of the machine using the weighting function

$$c_{ij} = \frac{|x_i - x_j|}{V_{x,max}} + \frac{|y_i - y_j|}{V_{y,max}}, \tag{2}$$

with the maximum axis velocities $V_{x,max}$ and $V_{y,max}$ of a two axis linear robot (e.g. a laser cutting machine). The parameters x_i and y_i contain the position of each node of the graph. Contrary, the whole path length of the process can also be reduced with

$$c_{ij} = \sqrt{|x_i - x_j|^2 + |y_i - y_j|^2}, \tag{3}$$

which increases the life time of the machine by using only distances for weighting.

3   Integer Linear Program Formulation

To achieve an optimal route, the TSP can be formulated into an Integer Linear Program

$$\min_{\mathbf{x}} \sum_{i \in V} \sum_{j \in V \setminus \{i\}} c_{ij} \, x_{ij}$$

$$\text{s.t.} \quad \sum_{j \in V \setminus \{i\}} x_{ij} = 1$$

$$\sum_{i \in V \setminus \{j\}} x_{ji} = 1$$

$$u_i \in \mathbf{Z}$$

$$u_i - u_j + n \, x_{ij} \leq n - 1, \; 1 \leq i \neq j \leq n$$

$$0 \leq x_{ij} \leq 1, \; x_{ij} \text{ integer},$$

with the integer variables

$$x_{ij} = \begin{cases} 1 & \text{if } arc(i, i) \text{ is in the tour} \\ 0 & \text{otherwise.} \end{cases}$$

The first set of equalities guarantees that each node of the graph can be arrived from exactly one other node, and the second set of equalities guarantees that from each node only one departure to exactly one other node is possible. The last constraints enforce that there is only a single tour covering all nodes, see e.g. [1]. To ensure that every contour will be executed by the machine, the edge weights between start and end point of each contour have to be treated separately. A functional approach is to weight them negative in contrast to the contour connections. To obtain a solution, the Integer Linear Program was solved with a standard solver.

4   Heuristic Methods

There is a high computational burden when using Linear Programming for solving the TSP for complex tasks. Hence, in this section, two heuristic methods of finding an approximation of the optimal tour are shown. Beside the great number of heuristic methods, the MST - heuristic and the Christofides heuristic are outlined and compared in this paper.

4.1   MST - Heuristic

The first step of the MST - heuristic is to transform the manufacturing process into an undirected weighted graph introduced in Sect. 2 in order to get a graph $G = (V, E)$. The next step is to construct a minimum spanning tree T. A minimum spanning tree is a subgraph T of G, that contains all the vertices and is a tree with weight less than on equal to the weight of every other tree. In Fig. 2 the corresponding minimum spanning tree of the undirected weighted graph is pictured.

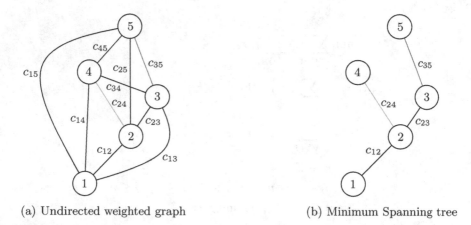

(a) Undirected weighted graph   (b) Minimum Spanning tree

Fig. 2. Minimum spanning tree of the undirected weighted graph

To achieve the minimum spanning tree of the graph G, the Prims's algorithm is used. The Prims's algorithm initialize the tree T with a single vertex, chosen arbitrarily from the graph G. After initialization, the algorithm grows the tree by one edge, which is not yet in the tree and which has minimum weight. After transforming it to the tree T, the algorithm repeats this step until all vertices are in the tree. For detailed information according this algorithm we refer to [5]. Finding a minimum spanning tree with the help of Prim's method yields to a time complexity of $\mathcal{O}(n^2 log_2(n))$, which is the most consuming one. To ensure that the tree T includes all cutting paths of the manufacturing process, the costs of these paths must be smaller than the smallest contour connection. Finally, our goal is to find an Eulerian tour in T, which proceeds to a Hamiltonian tour. A tour is said to be Eulerian in a graph G, if every edge of E is traversed exactly once. Whereupon a Hamiltonian tour is a tour containing each vertex exactly once.

In summary, the output of the whole algorithm provides an approximation of the optimal route for a complex distribution of contours (e.g. a cutting process), where each contour is processed exactly once.

4.2 Christofides Heuristic

The MST - heuristic can be extended with the help of perfect minimum matching, which yields to the Christofides algorithm. A perfect minimum matching M in G is a set of pairwise edges with odd degree, which matches all vertices of the graph with minimal total cost, see [6]. After calculating the perfect minimal matching M, the algorithm unite the minimal spanning tree T with the set M, see Fig. 3. Hence, impasses can be identified and are connected together in such a manner that the sum of these paths has minimal total process time (path length). This part is the most time consuming one, having a time complexity of $\mathcal{O}(n^3)$.

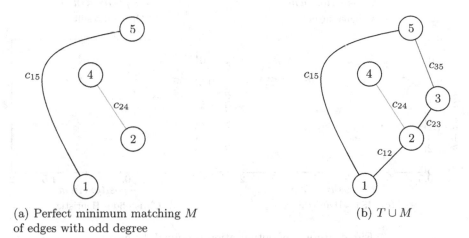

(a) Perfect minimum matching M of edges with odd degree

(b) $T \cup M$

Fig. 3. The perfect minimal matching M united with the minimal spanning tree T

Due to the fact, that the costs of the cutting paths are smaller than the smallest contour connection, the triangle inequality

$$c(u, v) \le c(u, w) + c(w, v), \forall u, v, w \in V, \tag{5}$$

of the graph G is not fulfilled. Thereby, in this case the benefit of the classical Christofides algorithm does not apply the estimation of the upper limit of the heuristic solution, which is at worst 50 % higher than the optimal ones (see [3,4] for more details). The last step of the Christofides algorithm is also to find a Hamiltonian tour as described in Sect. 4.1.

5   Results

In order to show the efficiency of the proposed algorithms, simulation results are given. Figure 4 pictures a comparison between the unsorted and sorted execution sequences of a typical laser cutting process, where the costs are in relation to the path lengths. Note, that the presented manufacturing process consists of 80 cutting paths. The solid profiles in Fig. 4 shows the corresponding control polygons of the cutting paths and the dashed lines represent the contour connections.

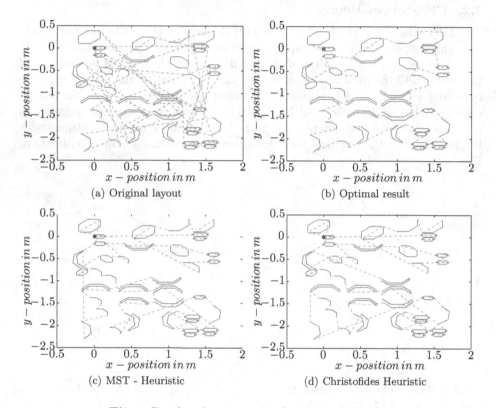

(a) Original layout

(b) Optimal result

(c) MST - Heuristic

(d) Christofides Heuristic

Fig. 4. Results of optimization (minimal distance)

Obviously, the whole path length of the process has been drastically reduced with the help of all algorithms. It turns out, that both heuristic methods produce similar results and reduce the whole path length by about 35 %, with a maximum computation time of 1.58 s on a standard PC. Whereat the optimal solution already leads to an unpractical computation time of 50.1 s. In this case, the Christofides algorithm has no advantages over the MST - heuristic. Instead the computation time is about 8 % higher. A summary of the results are presented in Table 1.

Contrary to the previous plots, Fig. 5 presents the results of the time optimal approach, where all edges are weighted in relation to the process time of the

Table 1. Results - distance optimization

Algorithm	Computation time	Process time	Total time	Process distance
Linear programming	50.10 s	72.66 s	122.76 s	34.03 m
MST	1.45 s	84.80 s	86.25 s	44.86 m
Christofides	1.58 s	83.69 s	85.27 s	44.06 m
Random layout	–	132.75 s	132.75 s	74.26 m

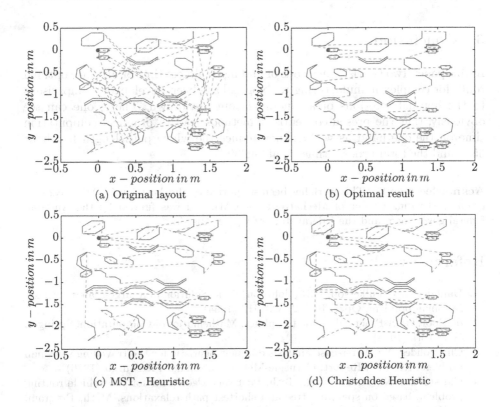

(a) Original layout   (b) Optimal result

(c) MST - Heuristic   (d) Christofides Heuristic

Fig. 5. Results of optimization (minimal time)

machine. In order to evaluate the effect of different axis velocities, $V_{x,max}$ is five times higher than $V_{y,max}$. Therefore, it is clearly evident that the main movement of all methods results along the x -axis. The results of the simulation are summarized in the Table 2.

An interesting observation is that both heuristic methods lead to the same approximation of the optimal route. This means, that the perfect minimum matching of the Christofides heuristic has no influence to the solution. Here, the heuristic methods reduce the total process time by about 59 %, whereat the optimal solution also leads to unpractical computation time.

Table 2. Results - time optimization

Algorithm	Computation time	Process time	Total time	Process distance
Linear programming	59.30 s	68.84 s	128.14 s	41.30 m
MST	1.47 s	79.07 s	80.54 s	49.05 m
Christofides	1.61 s	79.07 s	80.68 s	49.05 m
Random layout	–	132.75 s	132.75 s	74.26 m

6   Conclusion

In this paper, two heuristic methods of finding an almost time or distance optimal route for complex manufacturing topologies have been developed. Comparisons to the optimal solutions of a random layout are drawn. There, one can see obviously, that the presented heuristic methods lead to practical computation time on the one hand as well as they reduce the whole path length by about 35 % and the total process time by about 59 %.

Acknowledgments. This work has been supported by the Austrian COMET-K2 program of the Linz Center of Mechatronics (LCM), and was funded by the Austrian federal government and the federal state of Upper Austria.

References

1. Dantzig, G.B., Fulkerson, D.R., Johnson, S.M.: Solution of a large-scale traveling-salesman problem. Oper. Res. **2**, 393–410 (1954)
2. de Boor, C.: A Practical Guide to Splines. Mathematics of Computation. Springer, New York (1978)
3. Christofides, N.: Worst-case analysis of a new heuristic for the travelling salesman problem. Research Report, Carnegie-Mellon University, Pittsburgh (1976)
4. Christofides, N., Mingozzi, A., Toth, P.: Exact algorithms for the vehicle routing problem, based on spanning tree and shortest path relaxations. Math. Program. **20**(1), 255–282 (1981)
5. Prim, R.C.: Shortest connecting networks and some generalizations. Bell Syst. Tech. J. **36**, 1389–1401 (1957)
6. Gabow, H.N.: A scaling algorithm for weighted matching on general graphs. Ph.D. thesis, Stanford University (1974)

Serre-Frenet Frame in n-dimensions at Regular and Minimally Singular Points

Ignacy Duleba[✉] and Iwona Karcz-Duleba

Electronics Faculty, Wroclaw University of Technology,
Janiszewski St. 11/17, 50-372 Wroclaw, Poland
{ignacy.duleba,iwona.duleba}@pwr.edu.pl

Abstract. In contemporary robotics more and more complicated systems are considered. To plan their motions, well-known coordinate frames, living in natural, three-dimensional spaces, should be modified to cover multidimensional spaces as well. In this paper an algorithm is proposed to determine the Serre-Frenet frame in high dimensional spaces. The frame is examined at regular points where consecutive derivatives of a given curve, the robot moves along, are independent of each other. An interpolation procedure is provided when a minimally singular points appear and dimensionallity of the space spanned by the derivatives drops by one with respect to the regular, full dimensional space.

1 Introduction

With a smooth enough curve living in the real, n-dimensional space an orthonormal frame can be assigned. The construction known as the Serre-Frenet frame was described at the end of the nineteenth century (Jordan). At some point of the given curve, the frame is determined by n orthonormal vectors supplemented with $(n-1)$ generalized curvature parameters. For a long time, the frame attracted attention of mathematicians and physicists only. Recently, it is also exploited by roboticians. While designing a control strategy to move a robot along a prescribed trajectory, it is natural to define, at particular time point, an error between a current position of the robot and its desired location at that time point [1]. Then, a designed control law should dump the error either to the zero value (asymptotically, or even better exponentially) or to a small neighborhood of zero when small deviations are acceptable. The positions, mentioned above, are expressed at some frames. Here we have a choice, either to express all data in a global coordinate frame or to rely on local frames attached to a moving object and its desired phantom. The most natural approach is to associate with the tracked curve, along which the phantom robot is virtually moving, a frame (in which a desired behavior of the robot is specified) and another frame associated with a real robot. The control law should force the two frames to coincide. This approach was successfully exploited in three-dimensional Euclidean spaces [1]. In the nearest future, when more complex robots equipped with many effectors or a group of robots (described as a single, multidimensional system) will appear, also the Serre-Frenet frames of robotics are to be considered in dimensions exceeding the value of three.

© Springer International Publishing Switzerland 2015
R. Moreno-Díaz et al. (Eds.): EUROCAST 2015, LNCS 9520, pp. 681–688, 2015.
DOI: 10.1007/978-3-319-27340-2_84

In this paper, being extended and modified version of [2], a detailed algorithm will be presented to compute the Serre-Frenet frame in n dimensions where n denotes dimensionallity of the space a path of the robot is described. The contents of the paper is organized as follows: in Sect. 2 the theory of the n-dimensional Serre-Frenet frame, abbreviated later on as n-SF frame, will be presented. Based on the theory, an original algorithm to compute generalized curvatures and orthonormal versors associated with the n-SF frame are presented. The main topics of Sect. 3 is to determine what to do when along a curve (path) the singular n–SF frame appears. In Sect. 4 singularity passages are illustrated on examples. In Sect. 5 concluding remarks are collected.

2 n Dimensional Serre-Frenet Frame

Let be given a smooth enough curve $x(\cdot) \in \mathbb{C}^{n-1}$ describing a path for a robot to follow, i.e. there exist $(n-1)$ consecutive derivatives of the curve. Versors of the n-SF frame $(v_1, \ldots, v_n)$ and generalized curvatures $(k_1, \ldots, k_{n-1})$ should be derived at a particular point $x(s)$ along the curve. The data are coupled by the Frenet equations [3]

$$\dot{v}_1 = k_1 v_2, \tag{1}$$

$$\dot{v}_i = -k_{i-1} v_{i-1} + k_i v_{i+1}, \qquad i = 2, \ldots, n-1, \tag{2}$$

$$\dot{v}_n = -k_{n-1} v_n. \tag{3}$$

Unit-length versors v_i, $i = 1, \ldots, n$ form an orthonormal (and right-hand oriented) basis in R^n, i.e. $\langle v_i, v_j \rangle = \delta_{ij}$ and $\delta_{ij} = 0$, when $i \neq j$ or $\delta_{ij} = 1$ for $i = j$ and $\langle \cdot, \cdot \rangle$ denotes the inner product. Derivatives, with respect to the variable s parameterizing the curve, will be marked with dots ($\dot{x}$), slants (k'') or a natural number in brackets ($x^{(5)}$). Scalar values are written in a normal font, k_1, while vectors are bolded, x. The Euclidean norm, $\|x\|$, is used to get the length of the vector x.

An explicit formula for the n-SF frame would be obtained if versors and generalized curvatures depend directly on the derivatives of the curve $x(\cdot)$. In this paper a recursive formula will be exploited instead: v_1 is a function of $\dot{x}$, k_1 is a function of $\ddot{x}$. Then v_i, $i \geq 2$ depends on v_j and k_j, $j = 1, \ldots, i-1$. Finally, k_i, $i \geq 2$ depends on $x^{(i+1)}, v_{i+1}$ and previous k_j, $j = 1, \ldots, i-1$.

Without loosing generality, we can assume that

$$\|\dot{x}\| = \langle \dot{x}, \dot{x} \rangle = 1, \tag{4}$$

i.e. the motion along the curve is performed with a constant, unit-length velocity and the variable s describes the length of the curve started at $s = 0$. The versor v_1 is obtained immediately from Eq. (4)

$$v_1 = \dot{x}. \tag{5}$$

Equation (1) is obtained straightforward by deriving Eq. (4), using Eq. (5) and properties of the dot product

$$\overline{\langle v_1, v_1 \rangle} = \langle v_1, \dot{v}_1 \rangle = 0, \quad \Rightarrow \quad \dot{v}_1 = k_1 v_2,$$

where $v_2 \perp v_1$ and k_1 was introduced to preserve unit-length vector of v_2. In a similar fashion Eq. (2) can be derived. For example:

$$\overline{\langle v_1, v_2 \rangle} = \langle \dot{v}_1, v_2 \rangle + \langle v_1, \dot{v}_2 \rangle = \langle k_1 v_2, v_2 \rangle + \langle v_1, \dot{v}_2 \rangle = \langle v_1, k_1 v_1 \rangle + \langle v_1, \dot{v}_2 \rangle =$$
$$\langle v_1, k_1 v_1 + \dot{v}_2 \rangle = \langle v_1, k_2 v_3 \rangle = 0 \quad \Rightarrow \quad \dot{v}_2 = -k_1 v_1 + k_2 v_3.$$

Throughout this section, a regularity assumption will be respected, i.e. the set of vectors $\{x^{(i)}, i = 1, \ldots, n-1\}$ is linearly independent for any s and no singularities appear. From Eq. (1) we get immediately the second versor v_2 and the first curvature parameter k_1

$$\ddot{x} \overset{(5)}{=} \dot{v}_1 \overset{(1)}{=} k_1 v_2 \quad \Rightarrow \quad v_2 = \frac{\ddot{x}}{k_1}, \quad k_1 = \|\ddot{x}\| \tag{6}$$

In Eq. (6) and other equations, the number in parentheses placed over the equality symbol marks the equation the equality is based on. Now, Eq. (2) are processed. We start with a useful notation

$$K_i = \prod_{j=1}^{i} k_j \tag{7}$$

to inductively prove the following equality

$$L_i = K_i v_{i+1}, \tag{8}$$

where L_i collects all terms that do not depend on v_{i+1}. For $i = 1$, Eq. (8) is satisfied as from Eq. (6) we get

$$L_1 = \ddot{x} = K_1 \cdot v_2. \tag{9}$$

The i-th step of the induction procedure, $i = 2, \ldots, n-1$, is based on Eq. (2) and on Eq. (8)

$$-k_{i-1}v_{i-1} + k_i v_{i+1} \overset{(2)}{=} \dot{v}_i \overset{(8)}{=} \left(\frac{L_{i-1}}{K_{i-1}} \right)' = \frac{L'_{i-1} K_{i-1} - L_{i-1} K'_{i-1}}{(K_{i-1})^2} \overset{(8)}{=}$$
$$\frac{L'_{i-1} K_{i-1} - K_{i-1} v_i K'_{i-1}}{(K_{i-1})^2} = \frac{L'_{i-1} - K'_{i-1} v_i}{K_{i-1}}. \tag{10}$$

In order to get the required form (8), the first and the last expressions are equated, multiplied by K_{i-1}, and the definition (7) is applied

$$L_i \overset{def}{=} L'_{i-1} - K'_{i-1} v_i + k_{i-1} K_{i-1} v_{i-1} = K_i v_{i+1}, \tag{11}$$

which ends the proof of Eq. (8) and provides a recursive expression for L_i. Some remarks concerning L_i can be formulated:

- The term $\boldsymbol{x}^{(i+1)}$ in the expansion of $\boldsymbol{L}_i$, cf. Eqs. (15)–(17), always appears with a coefficient equal to 1. For $i = 1$, it comes from Eq. (9). From Eq. (11) we conclude that $\boldsymbol{x}^{(i+1)}$ results from $\boldsymbol{L}'_{i-1}$ only ($\frac{d}{ds}\boldsymbol{x}^{(i)} = \boldsymbol{x}^{(i+1)}$) as K_i depends explicitly on k_j, $j = 1, \ldots, i$, cf. Eq. (7).
- The term $\boldsymbol{x}^{(i+1)}$ is followed by a linear combination of $\boldsymbol{v}_j$, $j = 1, \ldots, i$ with coefficients depending on k_j, $j = 1, \ldots, i-1$ and possibly their derivatives. From Eqs. (9), (11) it is clear that $\boldsymbol{L}_i$ depends linearly on v_i, $i = 1, \ldots, i$. Coefficients of the combination depend on K_{i-1} and its derivative, so on k_i, $i = 1, \ldots, i-1$ and derivatives of k_i what ends the proof.
- The right equality in Eq. (11) is a straightforward consequence of the Gram-Schmidt orthogonalization procedure [4] where $\boldsymbol{x}^{(i+1)}$ can be expressed as a linear combination of vectors $\boldsymbol{v}_j$, $j = 1, \ldots, i+1$ and all versors must appear in the combination.

From Eq. (11) the next orthonormal vector $\boldsymbol{v}_{i+1}$ can be obtained

$$\boldsymbol{v}_{i+1} = \frac{\boldsymbol{L}_i}{\|\boldsymbol{L}_i\|} = \frac{\boldsymbol{L}_i}{K_i} \tag{12}$$

and also the next generalized curvature parameter

$$\|\boldsymbol{L}_i\| = K_i \quad \Rightarrow \quad k_i = \frac{\|\boldsymbol{L}_i\|}{K_{i-1}}. \tag{13}$$

Alternatively, k_i can be calculated based on Eq. (11) as it follows

$$k_i = \frac{\langle \boldsymbol{L}_i, \boldsymbol{v}_{i+1} \rangle}{K_{i-1}} = \frac{\langle \boldsymbol{x}^{(i+1)} + \sum_{j=1}^{i} \alpha_j(k_1, \ldots, k_{i-1})\boldsymbol{v}_j, \boldsymbol{v}_{i+1} \rangle}{K_{i-1}} = \frac{\langle \boldsymbol{x}^{(i+1)}, \boldsymbol{v}_{i+1} \rangle}{K_{i-1}} \tag{14}$$

because $\langle \boldsymbol{v}_i, \boldsymbol{v}_j \rangle = 0$ for $i \neq j$.

Eqations (11)–(14) with the initial condition (9) define the complete algorithm to compute the n-SF frame. The algorithm also uses Eqs. (1)–(3) because while computing $\boldsymbol{L}'_{i-1}$ derivatives of $\boldsymbol{v}_i$ should be substituted with term depending on $\boldsymbol{v}_{i-1}$ and $\boldsymbol{v}_{i+1}$. To illustrate the procedure, the proposed algorithm was run for $n = 5$. Because Eqs. (12)–(14) are straightforward, the whole computational effort is concentrated on consecutive values of $\boldsymbol{L}_i$ initialized with $\boldsymbol{L}_1 = \ddot{\boldsymbol{x}}$. Expressions for $\boldsymbol{L}_i$, $i = 2, 3, 4$, follow

$$\boldsymbol{L}_2 = \dddot{\boldsymbol{x}} + k_1^2 \boldsymbol{v}_1 - k_1' \boldsymbol{v}_2 (= k_1 k_2 \boldsymbol{v}_3). \tag{15}$$

$$\boldsymbol{L}_3 = \boldsymbol{x}^{(4)} + 3k_1 k_1' \boldsymbol{v}_1 + (k_1^3 - k_1'' + k_1 k_2^2)\boldsymbol{v}_2 - (2k_1' k_2 + k_1 k_2')\boldsymbol{v}_3 (= k_1 k_2 k_3 \boldsymbol{v}_4). \tag{16}$$

$$\begin{aligned}
\boldsymbol{L}_4 = &\boldsymbol{x}^{(5)} + (3(k_1')^2 + 4k_1 k_1'' - k_1^4 - k_1^2 k_2^2)\boldsymbol{v}_1 + (6k_1^2 k_1' - k_1''' + 3k_1' k_2^2 + 3k_1 k_2 k_2')\boldsymbol{v}_2 \\
&+ (k_1^3 k_2 - 3k_1' k_2 + k_1 k_2^3 - 3k_1' k_2' - k_1 k_2'' + k_1 k_2 k_3^2)\boldsymbol{v}_3 \\
&- (2k_1' k_2 k_3 + 2k_1 k_2' k_3 + k_1 k_2 k_3')\boldsymbol{v}_4 (= k_1 k_2 k_3 k_4 \boldsymbol{v}_5).
\end{aligned} \tag{17}$$

Expressions for L_i are more and more complicated as i increases, mainly due to taking derivative of L_{i-1} which includes many product-like terms. The expression for L_5 is the same as in the paper [5]. Obviously, a symbolic computation assistance in the determination of L_i is welcomed (for example Mathematica or Maple software).

It should be mention that the presented approach to determine the orthonormal frame composed of versors v_i, $i = 1,\dots,n$ is not the only possible. The alternative is to use the Gram-Schmidt orthogonalization procedure directly. The generalized curvature parameters would be retrieved from a set of identities obtained based on consecutive derivatives of Eq. (4), (the first two identities follow $\langle \dot{x},\ddot{x} \rangle = 0$, $\langle \dot{x},\dddot{x} \rangle + \langle \ddot{x},\ddot{x} \rangle = 0$)). However, this approach is much more difficult in constructing a simple and reliable algorithm.

3   n-SF Frame at Minimally Singular Points

The n-SF frame can not be determined uniquely at singular points. They appear when the set

$$X(s) = \{\dot{x}(s),\ddot{x}(s),\dddot{x}(s),\dots,x^{(n-1)}(s)\} \tag{18}$$

is not linearly independent for some (or one) point s, i.e. rank $X(s) = n - 1$. It is worth noticing that the n-th derivative is not required as the versor v_n corresponding to the derivative can be retrieved from the others to preserve right-oriented basis in $\mathbb{R}^n$. When the set is linearly independent, there is a regular point. Degree of degeneracy (singularity) is naturally measured by the number $\xi(s) = n - 1 - \dim(X(s))$. At regular points s, it takes the value of $\xi(s) = 0$. Later on, only minimally singular points will be considered, $\xi(s) = 1$, as the most frequently encountered in practice. A singular point can be isolated (in its neighborhood there are only regular points) or singular points can occupy an interval(s) in s.

In practical situations, it is desirable to preserve smoothness of varying of the n-SF frames as the variable s increases. When singular points occupy an interval in s domain, it is clearly possible (although when the interval is short, the amplitudes of versors' changes can be significant). Two types of the n-SF frame changes can be distinguished at isolated singular points. The first one, named the reflection-type, is characterized by only minor changes of the n-SF frames while passing through the singular point. The second, transversal-type, is described by large changes. Each particular type can be easily determined. Let versors of the regular frame placed just before and after the singularity point are

$$B = (b_1,\dots,b_{n-1}), \qquad \text{and} \qquad A = (a_1,\dots,a_{n-1}),$$

respectively. The distance between frames

$$\rho(B,A) = \max_i \|b_i - a_i\|$$

takes the value $\rho(B,A) \simeq 0$ at the reflection-type singularity and $\rho(B,A) \simeq 1$ at the transversal-type one. To illustrate the concepts three curves $x(\cdot)$ in $\mathbb{R}^3$ space will be considered in the vicinity of $s = 0$. For the first curve

$$\boldsymbol{x}(s) = (s, s^2, 0), \qquad \dot{\boldsymbol{x}}(s) = (1, 2s, 0), \qquad \ddot{\boldsymbol{x}}(s) = (0, 2, 0),$$

a regular point is at $s = 0$. For the second curve

$$\boldsymbol{x}(s) = (s, s^3, 0), \qquad \dot{\boldsymbol{x}}(s) = (1, 3s^2, 0), \qquad \ddot{\boldsymbol{x}}(s) = (0, 6s, 0),$$

a transversal-type singularity appears, while for the third curve

$$\boldsymbol{x}(s) = (s, s^4, 0), \qquad \dot{\boldsymbol{x}}(s) = (1, 4s^3, 0), \qquad \ddot{\boldsymbol{x}}(s) = (0, 12s^2, 0),$$

we have got the reflection type singularity. Notice, that a line $\boldsymbol{x}(s) = \boldsymbol{x}_0 + s\Delta\boldsymbol{x}$ in $\mathbb{R}^3$, being one of the most popular curves to trace by robots, is an example of a singular curve as the versor $\boldsymbol{v}_2$, perpendicular to $\dot{\boldsymbol{x}}(s) = \boldsymbol{v}_1$, is not uniquely determined for any point with $\xi(s) = 1$.

In the case of any type of singularities, placed at isolated points or occupying an interval, it seems natural to interpolate n-SF frames between regular frames and passing through singular ones. To interpolate regular points expressions presented in [6] is used

$$R(s) = R_0 \exp\left(\frac{s - s_a}{s_b - s_a} \cdot \log(R_0^T R_1)\right), \qquad s \in [s_a, s_b] \tag{19}$$

where $\boldsymbol{R}_0, \boldsymbol{R}_1 \in SO(n)$ are regular n-SF frames placed before/after the singular one reached at $s = s_a$ and $s = s_b$, respectively. In Eq. (19) exponent function $\exp : so(n) \rightarrow SO(n)$ was exploited

$$\exp(\boldsymbol{B}) = \boldsymbol{I} + \sum_{i=1}^{\infty} \frac{\boldsymbol{B}^i}{i!},$$

which, for the three dimensional space, takes the Rodriques form

$$\exp(\boldsymbol{B}) = \boldsymbol{I} + \frac{\sin\theta}{\theta}\boldsymbol{B} + \frac{1 - \cos\theta}{\theta^2}\boldsymbol{B}^2, \quad \text{where} \quad \boldsymbol{B} = \begin{bmatrix} 0 & -c & b \\ c & 0 & -a \\ -b & a & 0 \end{bmatrix} \tag{20}$$

and $\theta = \sqrt{a^2 + b^2 + c^2}$. The logarithmic function (the inverse of the exponential function) $\log : SO(n) \rightarrow so(n)$ is not defined uniquely. For $n = 3$ it is given by the equation

$$\log(\boldsymbol{R}) = \frac{\theta}{2 \cdot \sin(\theta)}(\boldsymbol{R} - \boldsymbol{R}^T), \quad \text{where} \quad \theta = \arccos\left(\frac{tr(\boldsymbol{R}) - 1}{2}\right) \tag{21}$$

where $\theta \neq 0$ and tr denotes the trace operator of a given matrix. More complicated expressions to describe $\log(\boldsymbol{R})$ are encountered for $n > 3$. A general method to get the formula for $\exp(\boldsymbol{B})$ is given in [6] while explicit formulas for $n = 4$ and 5 are collected in [7]. It should be noticed that there are alternatives to perform the interpolation. For example Clifford algebras can be used to interpolate matrices from $SO(n)$ [8]. A special case, $SO(3)$, is covered by quaternions [9].

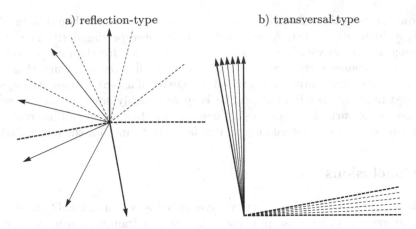

Fig. 1. Evolution of versors v_2 on the YZ plane (dashed line) and v_3 (arrowed) is illustrated while passing through singularity. Initial and final positions of the versors are bolded.

4 Simulations

In this section the interpolation procedure will be illustrated while passing through a singular point. As all characteristics of the passage are clearly visible just for $n = 3$ (and visualization is facilitated in this case), so curves living in $SO(3)$ will be considered. Without loosing generality, $R_0 = I_3$, as the interpolation between R_0 and R_1 is equivalent to the interpolation between I_3 and $R_0^T R_1$, while shifting the results by R_0 (see (19)).

The first example illustrates the reflection-type passage through singularity placed between regular 3-SF frames and described by matrices composed of versors $R = (v_1, v_2, v_3)$:

$$R_0 = \begin{bmatrix} 1 & 0 & 0 \\ 0 & 1 & 0 \\ 0 & 0 & 1 \end{bmatrix} \quad \text{and} \quad R_1 = \begin{bmatrix} 1 & 0 & 0 \\ 0 & 0.985 & -0.174 \\ 0 & 0.174 & 0.985 \end{bmatrix}. \tag{22}$$

It can be checked that $\rho(R_0, R_1)$ is much closer to zero than one, so the reflection-type singularity really appears. Using (19)–(21), the two frames were interpolated and the stroboscopic view of versors v_2, v_3 is presented in Fig. 1a with the variable $s \in [0, 0.01]$ increased by $\Delta s = 0.002$. In Fig. 1 only the YZ plane was presented as the versor v_1 remains constant as s increases. A continuous, small-amplitude change of versors was obtained using the interpolation.

The second example covers the transversal-type singularity passage while planning a motion between the regular 3-SF frames described by matrix R_0 given in (22) and $R_1 = \begin{bmatrix} 1 & 0 & 0 \\ 0 & -0.985 & 0.174 \\ 0 & -0.174 & -0.985 \end{bmatrix}$. Figure 1b, taken for the same range of s variable, visualizes a large-scale reorientation of versors v_2, v_3 as $\rho(R_0, R_1) \simeq 1$.

From a practical point of view, the interpolation procedure should be invoked if only a singularity is met. At an isolated reflection-type singularity met at $s^\star$, the range $s_b - s_a$ of variable $s \in [s_a, s_b]$ $(s_a < s^\star < s_b)$ for the interpolation of regular n-SF frames $(s = s_a$ and $s = s_b)$ can be small. However, when there is a transversal-type singularity, it is advised to take regular n-SF frames with s_a and s_b placed much further from $s^\star$ and to keep reasonably small versors v_i reorientation as the variable s increases. When singularities occupy an interval, it is much simpler to select distant enough regular n-SF frames for the interpolation.

5 Conclusions

In this paper an algorithm to effectively compute the n dimensional Serre-Frenet frame at regular points was presented. Likely, the frames appear in robotics as more complicated robotic systems will be considered. Singular points with the smallest degeneracy were analyzed. At those points the n-SF frame is not determined uniquely. Two types of singularities at isolated singular points were distinguished. It was illustrated that at reflection-type singular points a smooth passage through the singularity can be achieved, just contrary to transversal-type points. An interpolation procedure was proposed to smoothly change orientation of the n-SF frame when pieces composed of regular and singular points should be joined.

References

1. Mazur, A., Plaskonka, J.: The Serret-Frenet parametrization in a control of a mobile manipulator of (nh, h) type. In: the 10th IFAC Symposium on Robot Control, Dubrovnik, pp. 405–410 (2012)
2. Duleba, I, Karcz-Duleba, I.: Algorithmics of Serre-Frenet frame in R^n. In: Moreno-Diaz, R., Pichler, F.R., Quesada-Arencibia, A. (eds.) EUROCAST, Las Palmas, pp. 215–216 (2015). (Extended abstract)
3. Griffiths, P.: On Cartan's method of Lie groups and moving frames as applied to uniqueness and existence questions in differential geometry. Duke Math. J. **41**(4), 775–814 (1974)
4. Gantmacher, F.: Theory of Matrices. AMS Chelsea Publishing, New York (1959)
5. Yilmaz, S., Turgut, M.: A method to calculate Frenet apparatus of the curves in Euclidean-5 space. World Acad. Sci. Eng. Technol. **19**, 771–773 (2008)
6. Gallier, J., Xu, D.: Computing exponentials of skew-symmetric matrices and logarithm of orthogonal matrices. Int. J. Robot. Autom. **17**(4), 2–11 (2002)
7. Andrica, D., Rohan, R.-A.: Computing the Rodrigues coefficients of the exponential map of the Lie groups of matrices. Balkan J. Geom. Appl. **18**(2), 1–10 (2013)
8. Dobrowolski, P.: Evaluation of the usefulness of exact methods to motion planning in configuration space. Ph.D. thesis, Warsaw University of Technology, Faculty of Electronics and Information Technology (2013)
9. LaValle, S.M.: Planning Algorithms. Cambridge University Press, New York (2006)

An Efficient Method for the Dynamical Modeling of Serial Elastic Link/Joint Robots

Hubert Gattringer[1]([✉]), Klemens Springer[1], Andreas Müller[1],
and Matthias Jörgl[2]

[1] Institute of Robotics, Johannes Kepler University Linz,
Altenbergerstr. 69, 4040 Linz, Austria
{hubert.gattringer,klemens.springer,a.mueller}@jku.at
[2] Trotec GmbH, 4614 Machtrenk, Austria
http://www.robotik.jku.at

Abstract. This paper treats the dynamical modeling of elastic robots. A structured way to do this is the usage of the Projection Equation in subsystem representation in combination with the Ritz approximation method for the structural elastic degrees of freedom. Typical subsystems for such robots contain a motor, an elastic gear, an elastic link and a tip mass. Also the effect of dynamical stiffening is treated in the subsystem formulation. A final projection into the minimal space leads to the equations of motion for the whole robot. This model is analyzed in detail regarding the choice of ansatz functions for the elastic degrees of freedom. Therefore, the eigenfrequencies resulting from a linearized model are compared when using different ansatz functions. Finally, the influence of dynamical stiffening w.r.t eigenfrequencies is discussed.

Keywords: Dynamical modeling · Elastic multibody systems · Ritz approximation · Ansatz functions · Eigenfrequencies

1 Introduction

Energy saving is one of the main challenges in this century. Hence, also the automation industry has to contribute its part. Saving energy e.g. in the field of robotics is possible due to the usage of ultra lightweight robots. However, these systems typically suffer from vibration problems. A detailed (analytical) dynamical model provides insights into the dynamic behavior and is the basis for control design, see [7] for a method to control such robots. An overview on the dynamical modeling for elastic robots is presented in [3]. In this contribution, the Projection Equation in subsystem representation as suggested in [2] is used. Such a model depends on the chosen ansatz functions [6] for the elastic degrees of freedom (DoF) and a correct linearization. Details on the correct linearization can be found in [4], while an experimental evaluation of the eigenfrequencies is presented in [5]. In this paper different ansatz functions also called shape functions are compared and their influence on the eigenfrequencies is analyzed. Also the

© Springer International Publishing Switzerland 2015
R. Moreno-Díaz et al. (Eds.): EUROCAST 2015, LNCS 9520, pp. 689–697, 2015.
DOI: 10.1007/978-3-319-27340-2_85

influence of the dynamical stiffening effect is regarded. It is organized as follows. Section 2 presents the calculation of the dynamical model. In this context, mechanical subsystems are introduced taking account of dynamical stiffening. The equations of motion are then linearized about specific positions. This linear system is then analyzed in Sect. 3 regarding eigenfrequencies and eigenmodes.

2   Dynamical Modeling

The dynamical model of a mechanical system is the basis for control design, path optimization, parameter identification and therefore essential for the overall robot performance. The focus in this paper is on articulated flexible link/joint robots as shown in Fig. 1.

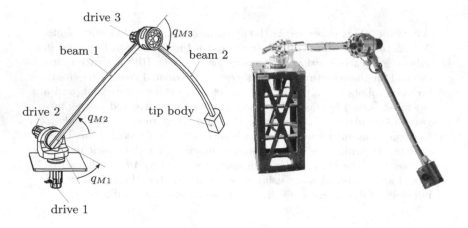

Fig. 1. Left: Coordinate systems and DoF for the considered elastic robot; Right: Photo of the robot

Such robots typically consist of repeated combinations of parts (motor, base body, elastic arm, tip body). Therefore, partitioning them into subsystems simplifies the overall derivations, see also [1]. An efficient method to derive the equations of motion (EoM) is the Projection Equation [2] (here written in subsystem representation)

$$\sum_{n=1}^{N} \left(\frac{\partial \dot{\mathbf{y}}_n}{\partial \dot{\mathbf{q}}} \right)^T (\mathbf{M}_n \ddot{\mathbf{y}}_n + \mathbf{G}_n \dot{\mathbf{y}}_n - \mathbf{Q}_n) = 0, \tag{1}$$

where $\mathbf{M}_n, \mathbf{G}_n, \mathbf{Q}_n$ are mass matrix, gyroscopic matrix and generalized forces of a subsystem, respectively. Each subsystem is associated with describing velocities $\dot{\mathbf{y}}_n$ and $\dot{\mathbf{q}}$ are the minimal velocities of the robot. The Jacobian of the describing velocities w.r.t. the minimal velocities projects the subsystems into the minimal space. An overview about the calculations of the subsystem is presented in the next section.

2.1   Subsystems

Figure 2 shows a possible subsystem for the robot under consideration. Since the elastic link is a distributed parameter system, a Ritz ansatz for the elastic DoF is used

$$
\begin{pmatrix} \vartheta(x,t) \\ v(x,t) \\ w(x,t) \end{pmatrix} = \begin{bmatrix} \boldsymbol{\vartheta}(x)^T & 0 & 0 \\ 0 & \mathbf{v}(x)^T & 0 \\ 0 & 0 & \mathbf{w}(x)^T \end{bmatrix} \begin{pmatrix} \mathbf{q}_\vartheta(t) \\ \mathbf{q}_v(t) \\ \mathbf{q}_w(t) \end{pmatrix} := \boldsymbol{\Phi}^T \mathbf{q}_e. \tag{2}
$$

Variables v, w are the displacements of a mass element dm from the undeformed state, while ϑ is the torsional angle. This distributed coordinates are approximated by a spatial matrix of shape functions $\boldsymbol{\Phi}^T$ multiplied by the time dependent Ritz coefficients $\mathbf{q}_e$.

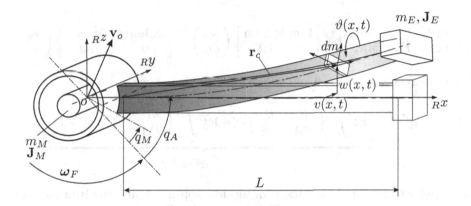

Fig. 2. Subsystem motor, elastic gear, elastic arm, tip body

For a complete description of the subsystem, the describing velocities have to contain the guidance velocities (translational $\mathbf{v}_o$, rotational $\boldsymbol{\omega}_F$) as well as the motor velocity $\dot{q}_M$, link velocity $\dot{q}_A$ and Ritz velocities of the elastic beams $\dot{\mathbf{q}}_e$. The Jacobian $\overline{\mathbf{F}}\boldsymbol{\Psi}^T$ projects the velocities of the mass element dm $(\mathbf{v}_c, \boldsymbol{\omega}_c)$ to the space of describing coordinates $\dot{\mathbf{y}}_n$

$$
\begin{pmatrix} \mathbf{v}_c \\ \boldsymbol{\omega}_c \end{pmatrix} = \overline{\mathbf{F}}\boldsymbol{\Psi}^T \underbrace{(\mathbf{v}_o^T \ \boldsymbol{\omega}_F^T \ \dot{q}_M \ \dot{q}_A \ \dot{\mathbf{q}}_e^T)^T}_{\dot{\mathbf{y}}_n}. \tag{3}
$$

Exemplarily, the mass matrix for the subsystem in Fig. 2, that is composed of N_{rb} rigid bodies and N_{el} elastic bodies, reads

$$
\mathbf{M}_n = \sum_{i=1}^{N_{rb}} (\overline{\mathbf{F}}^T \overline{\mathbf{M}} \mathbf{F})_i + \sum_{i=1}^{N_{el}} \left(\int_o^L ((\overline{\mathbf{F}}\boldsymbol{\Psi}^T)^T \frac{d\overline{\mathbf{M}}}{dx} \overline{\mathbf{F}}\boldsymbol{\Psi}^T) dx \right)_i. \tag{4}
$$

L is the length of the beam. For the calculation of the remaining subsystem matrices we refer to [1] for details.

2.2 Dynamical Stiffening

In the previous section, linearizable small deflections are assumed. This is valid, as long as the forces/torques that act on a mass element are small. For a correct physical linearization also the displacement fields of *second* order

$$\mathbf{r}^{(2)} = \int_o^x \begin{pmatrix} -(v'^2 + w'^2)/2 \\ (x - \xi)\vartheta'w' - \vartheta w' \\ -(x - \xi)\vartheta'v' - \vartheta v' \end{pmatrix} d\xi, \quad \boldsymbol{\varphi}^{(2)} = \int_o^x \begin{pmatrix} (v'w'' - w'v'')/2 \\ \vartheta'v' \\ \vartheta'w' \end{pmatrix} d\xi \quad (5)$$

have to be included. The prime indicates a derivation w.r.t. positions, while φ is the orientation of element dm. If they are combined with the forces/torques of *zero* order (these are equivalent to the forces of the rigid robot - $\mathbf{q}_e = 0$)

$$\begin{pmatrix} d\mathbf{f}^{(o)} \\ d\mathbf{M}^{(o)} \end{pmatrix} = \begin{pmatrix} d\mathbf{f}^e \\ d\mathbf{M}^e \end{pmatrix} - \begin{bmatrix} \mathbf{I}dm & \tilde{\mathbf{e}}_1^T x dm \\ 0 & d\mathbf{J} \end{bmatrix} \begin{pmatrix} \dot{\mathbf{v}}_o \\ \dot{\boldsymbol{\omega}}_o \end{pmatrix} - \begin{bmatrix} \tilde{\boldsymbol{\omega}}_o \mathbf{I}dm & \tilde{\boldsymbol{\omega}}_o \tilde{\mathbf{e}}_1^T x dm \\ 0 & \tilde{\boldsymbol{\omega}}_o d\mathbf{J} \end{bmatrix} \begin{pmatrix} \mathbf{v}_o \\ \boldsymbol{\omega}_o \end{pmatrix}$$

$$(6)$$

it can be seen with the help of the principle of virtual work

$$\delta W_n = \delta \mathbf{q}_e^T \underbrace{\int_o^L \left[\mathbf{F}_1^T \int_x^L \left(\frac{d\mathbf{f}^{(o)}/d\xi}{d\mathbf{M}^{(o)}/d\xi} \right) d\xi + \mathbf{F}_2^T \int_x^L \left(\frac{d\mathbf{f}^{(o)}/d\xi}{d\mathbf{M}^{(o)}/d\xi} \right) (\xi - x) d\xi \right] dx}_{-\frac{d\mathbf{K}_{n,el}}{dx} \mathbf{q}_e},$$

$$(7)$$

that linear terms for the equations of motion appear. Again, the Ritz ansatz is used for the displacement fields. The dynamical stiffness matrix

$$\mathbf{K}_{n,el} =$$

$$\int_o^L \begin{bmatrix} 0 & \int_x^L \left[\frac{df_z^{(o)}}{d\xi}(\xi - x)d\xi \right] d\xi \vartheta'\mathbf{v}'^T & -\int_x^L \left[\frac{df_y^{(o)}}{d\xi}(\xi - x)d\xi \right] d\xi \vartheta'\mathbf{w}'^T \\ & -\int_x^L \frac{df_z^{(o)}}{d\xi}d\xi \vartheta \mathbf{v}'^T & +\int_x^L \frac{df_y^{(o)}}{d\xi}d\xi \vartheta \mathbf{w}'^T \\ \hline & \int_x^L \frac{df_x^{(o)}}{d\xi}d\xi \mathbf{v}'\mathbf{v}'^T & 0 \\ \hline symm. & & \int_x^L \frac{df_x^{(o)}}{d\xi}d\xi \mathbf{w}'\mathbf{w}'^T \end{bmatrix} dx,$$

$$(8)$$

has to be included in the subsystem matrices. Since the *zero* order forces/torques depend on the rigid body accelerations $\dot{\mathbf{v}}_o, \dot{\boldsymbol{\omega}}_o$, velocities $\mathbf{v}_o, \boldsymbol{\omega}_o$ and positions, additional terms for the subsystem mass matrix $\mathbf{M}_{n,add}$, gyro matrix $\mathbf{G}_{n,add}$ and stiffness matrix $\mathbf{K}_{n,add}$, respectively, arise. Details for the derivation of the dynamical stiffness matrix and also the inclusion of the tip mass can be found in [1].

2.3   Equations of Motion - Linearization

Evaluating Eq. (1) delivers the EoM

$$\mathbf{M}(\mathbf{q})\ddot{\mathbf{q}} + \mathbf{g}(\mathbf{q}, \dot{\mathbf{q}}) = \mathbf{Q}_M, \tag{9}$$

with the mass matrix $\mathbf{M}$ the vector of nonlinear terms $\mathbf{g}$ containing centrifugal, Coriolis, friction, gravitational and stiffness terms, while $\mathbf{Q}_M$ are the applied motor torques. The vector of minimal coordinates for our robot (whole model) reads

$$\mathbf{q} = \begin{pmatrix} \mathbf{q}_M \in \mathbb{R}^3 \\ \mathbf{q}_A \in \mathbb{R}^3 \\ \mathbf{q}_e \in \mathbb{R}^n \end{pmatrix}, \tag{10}$$

where n is the number of ansatz functions for the elastic DoF. A statement about the quality of this dynamical model can be given by comparisons with the physical system. This quality depends on the choice and number of shape functions and on the physical effects that are modeled. One possibility is to use different shape functions and compare the calculated eigenfrequencies. Therefore the nonlinear model (9) is linearized at specific stationary points leading to the linear model

$$\mathbf{M}\ddot{\mathbf{y}} + \mathbf{K}\mathbf{y} = 0. \tag{11}$$

$\mathbf{M}$ and $\mathbf{K}$ are the constant mass and stiffness matrix of the linear system and $\mathbf{y}$ are the small deviations from $\mathbf{q}$. The eigenmodes and eigenfrequencies can be calculated by inserting the ansatz $\mathbf{y} = \overline{\mathbf{y}}e^{j2\pi f_{eig}}$ in (11) leading to the characteristic equation for calculating the eigenfrequencies $f_{Eig,i}$

$$\det(-(2\pi f_{Eig,i})^2\mathbf{M} + \mathbf{K}) = 0 \tag{12}$$

and for the eigenmodes $\overline{\mathbf{y}}_i$

$$(-(2\pi f_{Eig,i})^2\mathbf{M} + \mathbf{K})\overline{\mathbf{y}}_i = 0. \tag{13}$$

3   Model Analysis

3.1   Choice of Ansatz Functions

The main demand for the shape functions is, that they are linearly independent and that they have to fulfill the kinematic boundary conditions. In our case this is a clamped/free beam and therefore $\mathbf{v}(0) = 0, \mathbf{v}'(0) = 0, \mathbf{w}(0) = 0, \mathbf{w}'(0) = 0$, $\vartheta(0) = 0$ has to hold. In the following, three different types listed in Table 1 are considered.

The robot under consideration consists of two elastic links. The shape functions in Table 1 are used for each link. Choice 1 is the simplest one, where two functions are used in each bending direction for each beam and one ansatz for the torsion, respectively. For the second choice, only one entry is changed to have an approximation of the exact solution of a single Bernoulli/Euler beam (BEb).

Table 1. Selection of investigated shape functions

Choice 1	Choice 2	Choice 3
$\mathbf{v} = \mathbf{w} = \begin{pmatrix} \frac{x^2}{L^2} \\ \frac{x^3}{L^3} \end{pmatrix}$	$\mathbf{v} = \mathbf{w} = \begin{pmatrix} \frac{x^2}{L^2} \\ \frac{x^3}{L^3} - \frac{4}{5}\frac{x^2}{L^2} \end{pmatrix}$	$\mathbf{v} = \mathbf{w} = \begin{pmatrix} \frac{x^2}{L^2} \\ \frac{x^3}{L^3} - \frac{4}{5}\frac{x^2}{L^2} \\ \frac{x^4}{L^4} - \frac{7}{5}\frac{x^3}{L^3} + \frac{9}{20}\frac{x^2}{L^2} \end{pmatrix}$
$\vartheta = \frac{x}{L}$	$\vartheta = \frac{x}{L}$	$\vartheta = \begin{pmatrix} \frac{x}{L} \\ \frac{x^2}{L^2} \end{pmatrix}$

Table 2. Eigenfrequencies of the elastic robot for different shape functions

	Choice 1	Choice 2	Choice 3
$f_{Eig,1}$ (Hz)	2.8	2.8	2.8
$f_{Eig,2}$ (Hz)	3.0	3.0	3.0
$f_{Eig,3}$ (Hz)	12.0	12.0	12.0
$f_{Eig,4}$ (Hz)	12.8	12.8	12.8
$f_{Eig,5}$ (Hz)	63.3	63.3	63.3
$f_{Eig,6}$ (Hz)	72.7	72.7	66.3
$f_{Eig,7}$ (Hz)	84.3	84.3	75.7
$f_{Eig,8}$ (Hz)	104.7	104.7	99.2
$f_{Eig,9}$ (Hz)	138.6	138.6	121.4
$f_{Eig,10}$ (Hz)	145.7	145.7	123.8

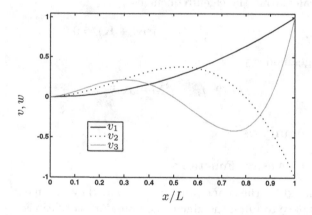

Fig. 3. Shape functions of choice 3

To get a more accurate model, in choice three, the number of shape functions is increased by one and again using an approximation of the BEb, see Fig. 3 for a plot of the used shape functions. In this case, 8 ansatz functions per beam are used leading in total to 16 elastic DoF.

Table 3. Eigenfrequencies for elastic robot for different linearization points

	Linearization Point 1	Linearization Point 2
$f_{Eig,1}$ (Hz)	2.8	5.2
$f_{Eig,2}$ (Hz)	3.0	5.4
$f_{Eig,3}$ (Hz)	12.0	6.9
$f_{Eig,4}$ (Hz)	12.8	7.3
$f_{Eig,5}$ (Hz)	63.3	60.3

An evaluation of the eigenfrequencies in Table 2 shows, that there is nearly no difference between choice 1 and 2 which is obvious since the ansatz functions of choice 2 are linear combinations of choice 1. Increasing the number of shape functions (choice 3) leads to more accurate results. It is well known, that the eigenfrequencies approach from above. As one can see, the first eigenfrequency that is different between choice 2 and 3 is number 6. Therefore convergence for the first 5 frequencies is achieved. Similar results can be observed when again increasing the number of shape functions.

The eigenfrequencies/-modes are the result of the linearized system at a specific point. Obviously, they change with different linearization points. Table 3 presents the frequencies for 2 specific positions that are shown in Fig. 4. It can be seen that the effective inertia for point 2 is much lower since the effective masses are nearer at the center of the robot so that the first eigenfrequency is higher than for point 1.

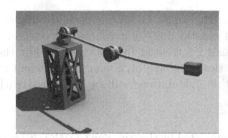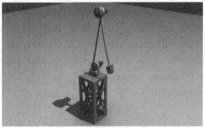

Fig. 4. Left: Linearization Point 1; Right: Linearization Point 2

3.2 Effect of Dynamical Stiffening

An evaluation of the eigenfrequencies of the model with and without dynamical stiffening shows only a very small change of max. 0.2 Hz. A detailed analysis delivers, that only gravitational forces enter the dynamical stiffness matrix in the linearized case that are small in contrast to the elastic stiffness terms, see (6).

However, for a dynamical simulation of the nonlinear model when applying a fast motion, the effect of dynamical stiffening results in a deviation of about 3 cm of the end-effector of the robot during motion. So this effect is important for fast motions.

3.3   Eigenmode Analysis

For a visualization of the approximated eigenmodes, system (11) is transformed to modal form by changing the coordinates $\mathbf{y} = \mathbf{Y}\boldsymbol{\eta}$ to modal coordinates $\boldsymbol{\eta}$ via the modal matrix $\mathbf{Y} = [\overline{\mathbf{y}}_1, ..., \overline{\mathbf{y}}_n]$ containing the eigenvectors of the system. For this, all motor and arm coordinates are locked to evaluate only the elastic behavior. Since our robot consists of two elastic links, the elastic coordinates are

$$\begin{pmatrix} \vartheta_1(x,t) \\ v_1(x,t) \\ w_1(x,t) \\ \vartheta_2(x,t) \\ v_2(x,t) \\ w_2(x,t) \end{pmatrix} = \begin{bmatrix} \boldsymbol{\Phi}_1^T & 0 \\ 0 & \boldsymbol{\Phi}_2^T \end{bmatrix} \begin{pmatrix} \mathbf{y}_{e,1} \\ \mathbf{y}_{e,2} \end{pmatrix} = \mathrm{diag}[\boldsymbol{\Phi}_1^T, \boldsymbol{\Phi}_2^T]\mathbf{Y} \begin{pmatrix} \boldsymbol{\eta}_1 \\ \boldsymbol{\eta}_2 \end{pmatrix} \tag{14}$$

where index 1 indicates beam 1 and index 2 beam 2, respectively. Therefore an approximation of the eigenmodes of the system is found by

$$\boldsymbol{\Phi}_{Eig}^T = \mathrm{diag}[\boldsymbol{\Phi}_1^T, \boldsymbol{\Phi}_2^T]\mathbf{Y}. \tag{15}$$

4   Conclusion

With the Projection Equation and the Ritz approximation method, efficient methods for the dynamical modeling of elastic link/joint robots are on hand. Also the effect of dynamical stiffening can be treated in this context. For the specific robot, a number of 5 ansatz functions e.g. as polynomials is sufficient to get a realistic behavior. In the future, this calculations will be compared with measurements.

Acknowledgments. This work has been supported by the Austrian COMET-K2 program of the Linz Center of Mechatronics (LCM), and was funded by the Austrian federal government and the federal state of Upper Austria.

References

1. Gattringer, H.: Starr-elastische Robotersysteme: Theorie und Anwendungen. Springer, Heidelberg (2011)
2. Bremer, H.: Elastic Multibody Dynamics: A Direct Ritz Approach. Springer, Heidelberg (2008)
3. Dwivedy, S.K., Eberhard, P.: Dynamic analysis of flexible manipulators, a literature review. Mech. Mach. Theorie **41**(7), 749–777 (2006)

4. Höbarth, W., Gattringer, H., Bremer, H.: Modeling and control of an articulated robot with flexible links/joints. In: Proceedings of the 9th International Conference on Motion and Vibration Control (2008)
5. Kleemann, U.: Regelung elastischer Roboter, VDI-Verlag (1989)
6. Pfeiffer, F. (ed.): Mechanical System Dynamic. LNACM, vol. 40. Springer, Heidelberg (2008)
7. Staufer, P., Gattringer, H.: State estimation on flexible robots using accelerometers and angular rate sensors. Mechatronics **22**, 1042–1049 (2012)

On Impact Behavior of Force Controlled Robots in Environments with Varying Contact Stiffness

Herbert Parzer[1]([☒]), Hubert Gattringer[1], Matthias Neubauer[1],
Andreas Müller[1], and Ronald Naderer[2]

[1] Institute of Robotics, Johannes Kepler University Linz,
Altenbergerstr. 69, 4040 Linz, Austria
{herbert.parzer,hubert.gattringer,matthias.neubauer_1,a.mueller}@jku.at
http://www.robotik.jku.at
[2] FerRobotics Compliant Robot Technology GmbH,
Altenbergerstr. 69, 4040 Linz, Austria
ronald.naderer@ferrobotics.at
http://www.ferrobotics.at

Abstract. In this contribution two methods to increase the robustness
of robot force control are discussed and experimental results on a real
system are presented. One way to control end–effector forces of a robot
is to use a force control method which manipulates the desired trajectory of a position controlled robot in a cascaded scheme. The benefit of
this control scheme is that the end–effector is also able to follow position
trajectories in the non–force–controlled directions. For such a direct parallel force/position control the stability depends on the force controller
parameters and the contact stiffness, assuming a stable position control.
Tuning these parameters in environments with varying contact stiffness
is challenging and time consuming. To avoid this, additional feed–back
torques are calculated to increase the dynamic of the force controller. The
first method is based on the classical feed–forward control of a robotic
system which is used in the feed–back loop of the force control. In the
second method the acceleration term of the force control law is used to
calculate a feed–back torque.

Keywords: Robot force control · Varying contact stiffness · Contact
behavior

1 Introduction

In the field of industrial robotics many tasks require predefined contact forces
between the environment and the robot's end–effector. In tasks like cutting,
assembly, grinding or polishing it is also necessary to follow a desired trajectory.
To reach this goal a parallel force/position control of the robot, suggested in [1]
and also implemented in [2,3], is used. With this method the desired trajectory
is modified by the force controller, so that the position controlled robot applies
the desired force in the force–controlled directions and follows the trajectory in

© Springer International Publishing Switzerland 2015
R. Moreno-Díaz et al. (Eds.): EUROCAST 2015, LNCS 9520, pp. 698–705, 2015.
DOI: 10.1007/978-3-319-27340-2_86

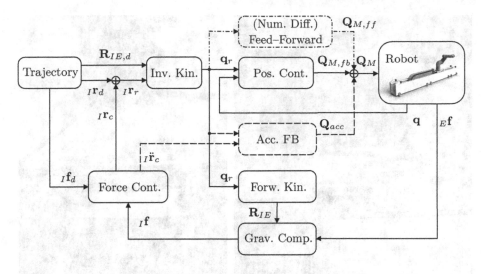

Fig. 1. Robot control scheme

the remaining directions. In an environment with varying contact stiffness, and especially when the robot's end–effector hits the surface, the stability depends on the controller parameters and the contact stiffness. In the case of uncertain system parameters one simple way is to calculate directly a feed–back torque from the force control law, to increase the stability of the force control. Otherwise a precise behavior can be achieved by taking the dynamics of the robot into account.

2   Position and Force Control

The considered robot is a six–axes industrial robot (STÄUBLI TX90L) controlled by decentralized feed–back motor position controllers and by centralized trajectory generation, force control and feed-forward control, see [4]. The mathematical model of the robot is derived with the *Projection Equation* in subsystem representation, see [5]. This leads to the equations of motion

$$\mathbf{M}(\mathbf{q})\,\ddot{\mathbf{q}} + \mathbf{G}(\mathbf{q},\dot{\mathbf{q}})\,\dot{\mathbf{q}} - \mathbf{Q}_r = \mathbf{Q}_M, \tag{1}$$

with the mass matrix $\mathbf{M}(\mathbf{q})$, the matrix of the gyroscopic terms $\mathbf{G}(\mathbf{q},\dot{\mathbf{q}})$, the vector of remainder forces $\mathbf{Q}_r$ (e.g. gravity, friction, ...) and the vector of the motor torques $\mathbf{Q}_M$. The vector of the minimal coordinates of the robot is given with $\mathbf{q}$ and the velocities and accelerations with $\dot{\mathbf{q}}$ and $\ddot{\mathbf{q}}$, respectively. The force control law is described by the differential equation

$$\mathbf{K}_{A,p}\,{}_I\ddot{\mathbf{r}}_c + \mathbf{K}_{V,p}\,{}_I\dot{\mathbf{r}}_c = {}_I\mathbf{f}_d - {}_I\mathbf{f}, \tag{2}$$

where $\mathbf{K}_{A,p}$ and $\mathbf{K}_{V,p}$ denote the positive definite controller parameters which are usually set as diagonal matrices, e.g. $\mathbf{K}_{A,p} = \mathrm{diag}\left(k_{A,px}\ k_{A,py}\ k_{A,pz}\right)$. The vector

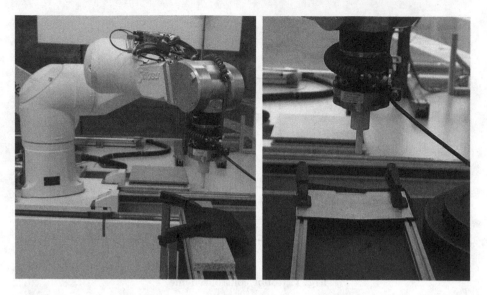

Fig. 2. Experiments: Setup A - contact with a rubber layered wooden board (left), Setup B - contact with a sheet metal (right)

$_I\mathbf{f}_d$ represents the desired and $_I\mathbf{f}$ the measured force in the inertial frame (I). With the parallel composition $_I\mathbf{r}_r = {}_I\mathbf{r}_d + {}_I\mathbf{r}_c$, where $_I\mathbf{r}_c$ is the solution of (2), the desired reference position $_I\mathbf{r}_r$ of the end–effector for the position controlled robot is calculated. In Fig. 1 the control scheme of the parallel force/position controlled robot is shown. The desired orientation of the robot's end–effector is given by a rotation matrix $\mathbf{R}_{IE,d}$ and with the help of forward kinematics the measured force in the end–effector frame (E) is gravity compensated and transformed into the inertial frame. With the inverse kinematics the desired minimal coordinates $\mathbf{q}_r$ are calculated from the desired end–effector position and orientation. Each axis of the robot is controlled with a cascaded position controller in the form $\mathbf{Q}_{M,fb} = \mathbf{K}_D[\mathbf{K}_P\,(\mathbf{q}_r - \mathbf{q}) + (\dot{\mathbf{q}}_r - \dot{\mathbf{q}})]$, with the positive definite controller parameters $\mathbf{K}_P$ and $\mathbf{K}_D$. Through this control scheme (labeled with *FCTRL*) the position controlled robot is able to provide a desired contact force and also follow a given trajectory in the remaining directions. One of the most common cases in robot force control is that the robot starts without contacting a workpiece or the environment and then move towards them to close the contact. This transition from free moving to contact is a critical part for the stability of the system. On the one hand a high dynamic force control is required to follow force trajectories or to simply hold a constant force during a movement along a curved object. On the other hand this high dynamic can cause an instability when the robot hits the surface due to the unilateral contact. Clearly if the exact position of a workpiece or the environment is known, a trajectory close to the object can be planned before activating the force controller. So high impact velocities and thereof high impact forces can be avoided. Further there is also

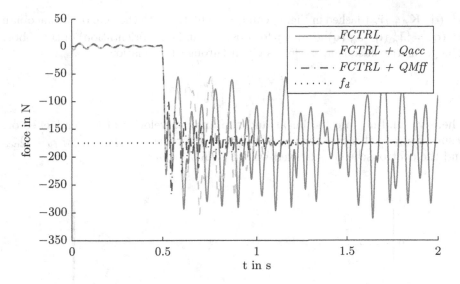

Fig. 3. Measurements 1 Setup A: wooden board, $f_d = -175\,\mathrm{N}$, controller parameters $k_{A,p} = 6.37\,\mathrm{kg}$ and $k_{V,p} = 1000\,\mathrm{Ns\,m^{-1}}$, impact velocity $v_{impact} = -175\,\mathrm{mm\,s^{-1}}$

a problem, if the stiffness of the environment varies strongly along a trajectory. In the following two methods are discussed to increase the robustness of the force control without reducing the dynamic.

2.1 Feed–Forward Control

A common way to increase the positioning accuracy of a robot is to add a feed–forward control based on the mathematical model of the robot. The feed–forward torques $\mathbf{Q}_{M,ff} = \mathbf{M}\,(\mathbf{q}_r)\,\ddot{\mathbf{q}}_r + \mathbf{G}\,(\mathbf{q}_r, \dot{\mathbf{q}}_r)\,\dot{\mathbf{q}}_r - \mathbf{Q}_r\,(\mathbf{q}_r)$ are obtained from (1). In standard robotic applications, the inputs of the feed–forward control are only calculated from the desired trajectory. Since the desired minimal coordinates are part of the outer feed–back loop of the force controller the feed–forward control of the robot (chain–dotted in Fig. 1) is now also part of the force control loop and the motor torques are calculated to $\mathbf{Q}_M = \mathbf{Q}_{M,fb} + \mathbf{Q}_{M,ff}$. This control scheme is labeled with $FCTRL + QMff$ and leads to a more responsive force control, especially when the robot hits the environment. However, if for example the system parameters are uncertain or a numerical differentiation of $\mathbf{q}_r$ is too noisy (since measured end–effector forces are included) such a feed–forward control does not necessarily yield stable behavior.

2.2 Acceleration Feed–Back

Another idea to increase the dynamics of the force control is to use directly the acceleration term, $\mathbf{K}_{A,p}\,_I\ddot{\mathbf{r}}_c$, of (2). This acceleration feed–back torque $\mathbf{Q}_{acc} =$

$\mathbf{J}_p^T\,(\mathbf{q})\,\mathbf{K}_{A,p}\,{}_I\ddot{\mathbf{r}}_c$ (dashed in Fig. 1) can be calculated with the help of the Jacobian $\mathbf{J}^T\,(\mathbf{q}) = [\mathbf{J}_p^T\,(\mathbf{q})\;\mathbf{J}_o^T\,(\mathbf{q})]$ (index p for position and o for orientation) of the robot. The geometric Jacobian, see [6], is given through the relation

$$\begin{pmatrix}\mathbf{v}_E \\ \boldsymbol{\omega}_E\end{pmatrix} = \begin{bmatrix}\mathbf{J}_p \\ \mathbf{J}_o\end{bmatrix}\dot{\mathbf{q}}, \tag{3}$$

where $\mathbf{v}_E$ and $\boldsymbol{\omega}_E$ are the linear and the angular velocity of the end–effector, respectively. In this case the calculated motor torques are $\mathbf{Q}_M = \mathbf{Q}_{M,fb} + \mathbf{Q}_{acc}$ and the control scheme is labeled with $FCTRL + Qacc$.

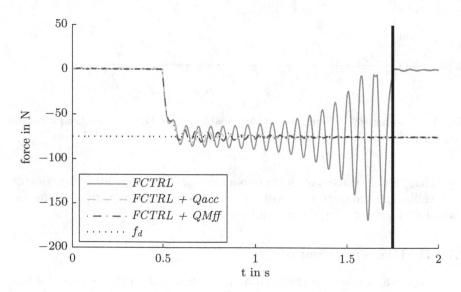

Fig. 4. Measurement 1 Setup B: sheet metal, $f_d = -75\,\mathrm{N}$, controller parameters $k_{A,p} = 6.37\,\mathrm{kg}$ and $k_{V,p} = 1000\,\mathrm{Ns\,m}^{-1}$, impact velocity $v_{impact} = -75\,\mathrm{mm\,s}^{-1}$ (the vertical black line indicates the deactivation of the force control due to safety reasons)

3   Experiment

Based on simulations of the above mentioned methods (*FCTRL*, *FCTRL + QMff*, *FCTRL + Qacc*) an experiment with an industrial robot, described in Sect. 2, was done. For this two different setups, see Fig. 2, were chosen. The first setup, labeled with *Setup A*, consists of a wooden board layered with a thin mat of rubber to build a stiff environment. To analyze the behavior on a more compliant environment a second setup, labeled with *Setup B*, was constructed that consists of a thin sheet metal clamped between two aluminum profiles. In both setups a plastic stick as a tool–dummy was mounted at the end–effector of the robot. The arising forces were measured with a six–axis force/torque sensor mounted between the robot and the tool. Thereby the robot starts in a distance of about

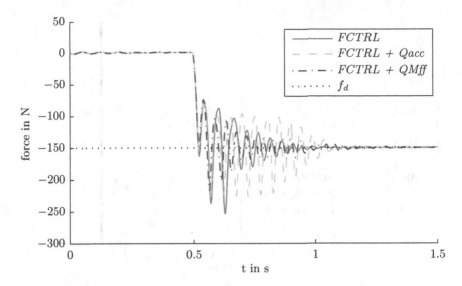

Fig. 5. Measurement 2 Setup A: wooden board, $f_d = -150\,\text{N}$, controller parameters $k_{A,p} = 7.64\,\text{kg}$ and $k_{V,p} = 1200\,\text{Ns}\,\text{m}^{-1}$, impact velocity $v_{impact} = -125\,\text{mm}\,\text{s}^{-1}$

0.1 m above the contact point of the current setup. In the experiments only the force normal to the environment was controlled and the parameters of the force controller were not especially tuned for one of both setups. Starting the force control leads to a steady state movement with a constant velocity of the robot's end–effector, since no contact force is measured. This velocity v_{impact} can be calculated from (2) with $v_{impact} = k_{V,p}^{-1} f_d$. At first the controller parameters were chosen to $k_{A,p} = 6.37\,\text{kg}$ and $k_{V,p} = 1000\,\text{Ns}\,\text{m}^{-1}$. Figures 3 and 4 show the impact behavior of the tool for all three methods. In the setup with the wooden board the pure force control method ($FCTRL$) oscillates very long (about 4 s) before the desired force is reached and becomes even unstable on the sheet metal setup. In the experiment with the sheet metal only a desired force of -75 N was reached and due to safety reasons the force control was deactivated after 1.75 s (indicated with the vertical black line). Additional feed–back torques from the acceleration term ($FCTRL + Qacc$) or using the robot feed–forward control in the control loop of the force control ($FCTRL + QMff$) stabilizes both setups under the same conditions. To compare both setups with the same impact velocity the parameters of the force controller were slightly changed and the measurements were repeated, see Figs. 5 and 6. For both setups the controller parameters were set to $k_{A,p} = 7.64\,\text{kg}$ and $k_{V,p} = 1200\,\text{Ns}\,\text{m}^{-1}$ and a desired force of -150 N was claimed. This results in a impact velocity of 125 mm s^{-1} for both setups. The measurements at the wooden board in Fig. 5 shows a stable behavior of all three methods within 0.5 s after contact. The best result shows the force control with the robot feed–forward control ($FCTRL + QMff$). Adding the acceleration term ($FCTRL + Qacc$) results here in a slightly longer oscillation than the other methods, but with less overshoot than the pure force control

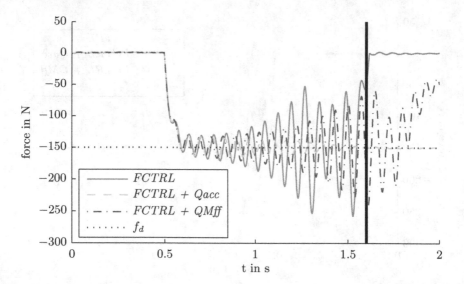

Fig. 6. Measurement 2 Setup B: sheet metal, $f_d = -150\,\text{N}$, controller parameters $k_{A,p} = 7.64\,\text{kg}$ and $k_{V,p} = 1200\,\text{Ns}\,\text{m}^{-1}$, impact velocity $v_{impact} = -125\,\text{mm}\,\text{s}^{-1}$ (the vertical black line indicates the deactivation of the force control due to safety reasons)

method. For the second setup with the sheet metal only the method with the acceleration term ($FCTRL + Qacc$) leads to a stable behavior, while both other experiments had to be aborted due to safety reasons (indicated with vertical black line).

4   Conclusion

In this work two methods to increase the robustness of robot force control in environments with varying or changing contact stiffness are compared. The first method simply uses the feed–forward control of the robot in the feed–back loop of the force controller and the second one uses an additional feed–back torque calculated from the used force control law itself. Both methods are compared to the pure force control method with the result, that non of both methods destabilizes the system, as long as the pure force control method $FCTRL$ is stable. For robot systems where the parameters are well known or identified the method $FCTRL + QMff$ with the robot feed–forward control will improve the stability. If the measured forces are very noisy or the derivatives of the minimal coordinates are calculated with a numerical differentiation this method is not useful. In this case the method $FCTRL + Qacc$, where the acceleration term of the force control law is used, leads to promising results.

Further it has to be said, that for applications which requires very high impact velocities or deals with extreme contact stiffness, force control is still a challenging field. Continuing work has to focus on stability, like in [7], but with the extension of closing the contact between robot and environment. For repetitive tasks also an iterative learning force control, briefly discussed in [8], becomes more and more important.

Acknowledgment. This work has been supported by the Austrian COMET-K2 program of the Linz Center of Mechatronics (LCM), and was funded by the Austrian federal government and the federal state of Upper Austria.

References

1. Siciliano, B., Villani, L.: Robot Force Control. Kluwer Academic Publishers, Dordrecht (1999)
2. Kastner, M., Riepl, R., Gattringer, H.: A novel approach to the robotic automation of industrial contact processes: comparison with classical force control methods. In: The 13th Mechatronics Forum International Conference, Proceedings, vol. 1/3, pp. 21–26. Trauner-Verlag, Linz (2012)
3. Chiaverini, S., Sciavicco, L.: The parallel approach to force/position control of robotic manipulators. IEEE Trans. Robot. Autom. **9**, 9:361–9:373 (1993). (IEEE)
4. Gattringer, H., Riepl, R., Neubauer, M.: Optimizing industrial robots for accurate high-speed applications. J. Ind. Eng. **2013**, 1–12 (2013)
5. Bremer, H.: Elastic Multibody Dynamics: A Direct Ritz Approach. Springer, Heidelberg (2008)
6. Siciliano, B., Sciavicco, L., Villani, L., Oriolo, G.: Robotics: Modelling, Planning and Control. Springer, Heidelberg (2009)
7. Ferretti, G., Magnani, G., Rocco, P.: On the stability of integral force control in case of contact with stiff surfaces. J. Dyn. Syst. Meas. Control **117**, 547–553 (1995). (ASME)
8. Zeng, G., Hemami, A.: An overview of robot force control. J. Robotica **15**, 473–482 (1997). (Cambridge)

A Robotic Platform Prototype
for Telepresence Sessions

A. Martínez-Romero, A. Quesada-Arencibia[✉],
J.C. Rodríguez-Rodríguez, J.D. Hernández-Sosa,
C.R. García, and R. Moreno-Díaz Jr.

Institute for Cybernetic Science and Technology,
University of Las Palmas de Gran Canaria, Las Palmas, Spain
{aaronmartinezromero,jcarlos.ciber}@gmail.com,
{aquesada,dhernandez,rgarcia,rmorenoj}@dis.ulpgc.es

Abstract. In this paper we present a first prototype of a teleoperated telepresence system that uses a range of devices aimed at operating a mobile platform situated in a remote location while offering the user the sensation of being at that remote location. The objective of this first stage of the project is to achieve a sensation of telepresence by simply giving the user the freedom of movement of the platform and the freedom of movement of the camera system.

Keywords: Teleoperation · Telepresence · Robotics · Pioneer 3-AT

1 Introduction

Teleoperation is understood to be an extension of sensorial capacities and human dexterity to a remote location. The term teleactuating is also used to refer to specific aspects of generating orders for actuators and telespeakers to pick up and display sensorial information. The term telepresence refers to a set of technologies and an ideal situation that enable a person to feel that he or she is present in a location other than their present physical location. The use of control mechanisms and visualisation systems that create the illusion of presence for the human operator in a remote location are fundamental to telepresence. The most specific aspect of telepresence is harnessing the interaction between sensorial and motor aspects. This interaction is achieved by integrating effector technologies and sensors.

These two concepts were explored in this project. A study was conducted and a system developed that uses a range of devices aimed at operating a mobile platform situated in a remote location while offering the user the sensation of being at that remote location. The objective of this first stage of the project is to achieve a sensation of telepresence by simply giving the user the freedom of movement of the platform and the freedom of movement of the camera system.

2 Objectives

The main objective of this work has been to develop a low-cost platform that enables a user in another place to connect to the system and conduct a telepresence session.

© Springer International Publishing Switzerland 2015
R. Moreno-Díaz et al. (Eds.): EUROCAST 2015, LNCS 9520, pp. 706–713, 2015.
DOI: 10.1007/978-3-319-27340-2_87

The system should be simple to turn on remotely and easy for users to control remotely [1]. It is designed for users who have no experience in teleoperation and informatics, and should therefore be as intuitive as possible and use common user interfaces that are well known to most users.

3 Critical Design Decisions

The following requirements and restrictions were taken into account in the design and prototype phases as, during the project, we detected new technical requirements for achieving the feel of telepresence. Several prototypes were developed and discarded during the testing phase, mainly because they were not easy to use:

- The system should be wireless and connect to a WiFi router where it is located.
- The system should be turned on with a couple of clicks, allowing inexperienced users to activate the device from another location.
- The user should be able to use immersive devices to achieve the feeling of telepresence, or a PC-based teleoperation station.
- The system should use open-source software.
- The height of the camera should be similar to the eye level of a person of average height.
- The main camera should move intuitively using head movements as input.

4 Architecture Overview

The system has a client-server architecture (see Fig. 1). The server is the mobile platform with cameras and actuators. The client is the controlling software and immersive devices for conducting the telepresence session, operated by the user. The diagram below shows, on the server side, two mobile platforms on which the system has been tested. The land mobile platform is the platform developed for this project and the underwater platform was developed for the SAUC-E underwater robotics competition.

4.1 Hardware Components

The server hardware is listed below:

- Mobile platform Pioneer 3-AT:
  - Odometer: to count wheel rotations
  - Compass: to indicate where north is
  - Sonar: to detect obstacles
  - Bumpers: to detect collisions
  - Embedded computer: handles all system controls and contains the server software

- Camera system:
  - Wide angle camera: the camera that gives the user the main view
  - Pan/tilt system: to move the main camera
  - Rear camera: to see the rear of the robot, for reversing manoeuvres
  - 360° camera: gives a panoramic view and enables steering

The client hardware is listed below:

- User interface
  - HMD 800-26 3D 5DT: virtual reality goggles that immerse the user in the telepresence session.
  - Inertiacube2+: inertial sensor that senses the user's head movements
  - Gamepad: used to teleoperate the robot.
- Control centre
  - PC with Linux system: the operating system used for this project

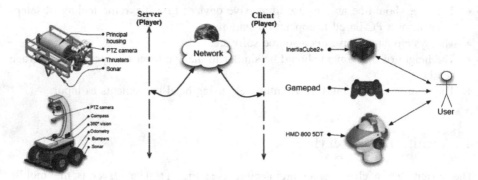

Fig. 1. System structure

4.2   Software System

For this project the Player/Stage programming framework used in the field of robotics was chosen. This software allows us to develop robotic applications fairly quickly, since it has a number of libraries with which to control the Pioneer3-AT platform, send data to another Player/Stage system, etc.

Server Side. We chose to place the project server on the robot platform as this is what the user will connect to. The platform is always listening for requests from users who want to access the system. Once a user begins a session, the server connects the platform and starts reading its sensors. This information is sent via TCP to the user.

A streaming client was also installed for each camera on the platform. When the user activates the cameras from the user interface, the platform begins to send images to the client software. These images are sent via UDP to avoid transmission delays as it is intended to be a real-time system.

There are 3 types of camera mounted on the robotic platform. A motorised pan/tilt camera [5], a rear camera and a 360° camera [2]. Each camera was selected after tests during prototype development and this configuration enables the user to teleoperate the platform while able to visualise its surroundings at all times.

Figure 2 shows 2 of the 3 camera types: 360° and pan/tilt.

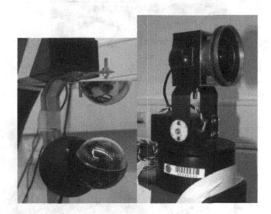

Fig. 2. 360° and pan/tilt cameras

The Player/Stage framework reads the platform sensors and the data are sent to any Player/Stage client that requests them.

Client Side. The Player/Stage client system is located on the user's PC. This client connects to the platform and then sends movement commands generated by the user via the teleoperation devices and also receives the necessary information from the platform to display to the user.

In addition, a streaming server is mounted on the client side to receive the data sent by the platform cameras. The user can enable or disable the images from the platform via the user interface, and can activate or deactivate any of the cameras via a simple button.

The software developed for the client side also shows the camera images to the user. These images are displayed on the HMD-800-26 and the user interface [4]. As mentioned above, there are 3 types of camera, one of which needs processing: the 360° camera. The image that the user receives is a sphere showing everything that is happening around the platform. Figure 3 shows how the image is processed and stitched into a panoramic picture of everything around the platform. This image is also used as the overhead view and is used by the user to steer when there are obstacles close to the platform, such as doors.

The user interface combines these three images in one single view that is displayed to the user through the goggles [3]. Figure 4 shows the basic composition of the user view. The main camera display is the pan/tilt camera and the overhead and rear cameras are displayed as secondary cameras. Also in the user view are a series of indicators that show

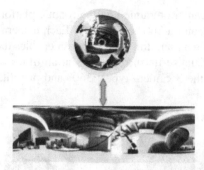

Fig. 3. 360° photo to panoramic image

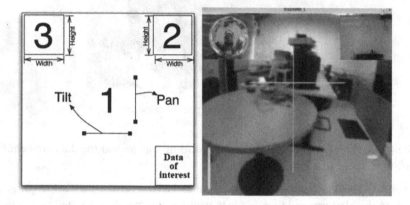

Fig. 4. Vision goggles user interface

the user graphic information that aids handling. The most important indicator is that which shows the user the position of the pan/tilt camera. This is because during testing, the user had no idea of the position of the pan/tilt camera, and therefore ended up looking towards a place that was at the limit of the camera's movement, which made steering uncomfortable and the user unable to figure out what was happening. By incorporating these indicative lines the user now knows at all times the position of the camera.

4.3   Communication Interfaces

The user uses a computer with Linux system and teleoperation software to connect to the robot. The user can use two operating modes: the PC screen or virtual reality goggles for the feeling of immersion. The virtual reality goggles have a tracking system which captures the movements of the user's head to teleoperate the robot's pan/tilt camera. This operating mode enables the user to look anywhere by moving their head as if they were in the robot's location.

The robot's movements are controlled with a PlayStation gamepad (Fig. 5).

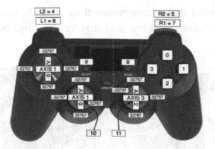

Fig. 5. Gamepad controller

Different types of actions have been assigned to the gamepad buttons. The gamepad has both digital and analog buttons. When the user controls the platform with the digital buttons, it moves at a speed predetermined by the software. When the user operates the analog buttons, he or she can smoothly and precisely alter the speed of the robot. This is necessary when in close proximity to obstacles. The upper gamepad buttons are used to change camera views and configure the speed of the system.

5 Results and Conclusions

During project development we experimented with different telepresence platform prototypes. The final design was arrived at through a series of iterations and tests with real users. Figure 6 shows one of the prototypes.

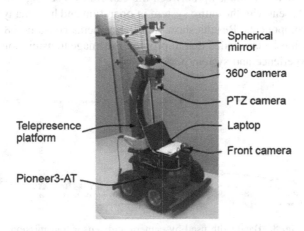

Fig. 6. Components of the second prototype

One of the minimum requirements for the user to be able to feel that they are in another place is having good images of that place. For this reason a study was conducted on the minimum image quality for the user to be able to use the system comfortably. We concluded that a compression ratio of 20 was more than enough for most users to be able to steer the robot and distinguish objects in its vicinity (Fig. 7).

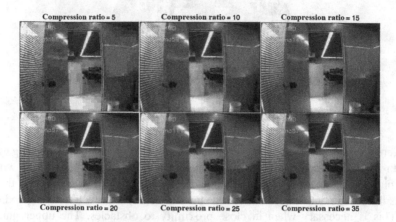

Fig. 7. Tests of image compression acceptable to the user.

By reducing the amount of data sent over the network, the system may be used in networks with low bandwidth, over the internet for example.

As well as studying the minimum image quality acceptable to the user, another study was carried out on the minimum frames per second with which a user could operate the system. We concluded that 15 FPS were more than enough to handle the robot.

Figure 8 shows the relationship between the camera FPS setting and the amount of data sent, the data sent with the entire system in operation and how many data are being sent by which components. Results show that the cameras consume 98 % of the total data sent. It can thus be concluded that improving the image transmission system would improve user experience and system performance.

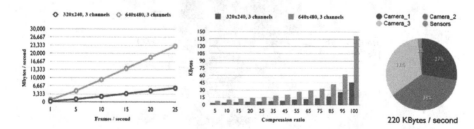

Fig. 8. Bandwidth used by camera and sensor transmission

One of the typical problems of telepresence is signal delay, i.e. the time between data capture and it being displayed to the user. The longer this period, the less useful the system, since the user does not have the feeling of instantaneous teleoperation since he or she has to adapt to signal delays in the system.

We studied the delay in data capture from the camera and calculated that the system needed 0.066 s to capture an image, compress it, send it to the user, decompress it and display it. The time it takes is almost negligible, but the study was necessary because any increase in calculations for one of these steps means that the user will not see an image in real time. This will make operation of the platform inefficient and unstable (Fig. 9).

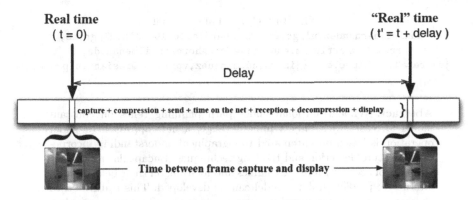

Fig. 9. Process from frame capture to user display.

In conclusion, a low-cost telepresence system has been created using open software (Player/Stage) that has been tested on land and underwater platforms.

Although the project was developed with Player/Stage, it is relatively easy to port it to other frameworks such as ROS (Robot Operative System) because the structure is very similar.

References

1. Babic, J., Budisic, M., Petrovic, I.: Dynamic window based force reflection for safe teleoperation of a mobile robot via internet. In: 2007 IEEE/ASME International Conference on Advanced Intelligent Mechatronics, pp. 1–6 (4–7 September 2007)
2. Fiala, M.: Pano-presence for teleoperation. In: 2005 IEEE/RSJ International Conference on Intelligent Robots and Systems (IROS 2005), pp. 3798–3802 (2–6 August 2005)
3. Stemmer, R., Brockers, R., Drue, S., Thiem, J.: Comprehensive data acquisition for a telepresence application. In: 2004 IEEE International Conference on Systems, Man and Cybernetics, vol. 6, pp. 5344–5349 (10–13 October 2004)
4. Martins, H., Ventura, R.: Immersive 3-D teleoperation of a search and rescue robot using a head-mounted display. In: IEEE Conference on Emerging Technologies and Factory Automation. ETFA 2009, pp. 1–8 (22–25 September 2009)
5. Hayashi, K., Yokokohji, Y., Yoshikawa, T.: Tele-existence vision system with image stabilization for rescue robots. In: Proceedings of the 2005 IEEE International Conference on Robotics and Automation. ICRA 2005, pp. 50–55 (18–22 April 2005)

Ocean Glider Path Planning Based on Automatic Structure Detection and Tracking

Daniel Hernandez$^{(\boxtimes)}$, Leonhard Adler$^{(\boxtimes)}$, Ryan N. Smith, Mike Eichhorn,
Jorge Cabrera, Josep Isern, Antonio C. Dominguez, and Victor Prieto

SIANI, ULPGC, Las Palmas, Spain
daniel.hernandez@ulpgc.es, leonhard.adler101@alu.ulpgc.es,
rnsmith@fortlewis.edu, mike.eichhorn@tu-ilmenau.de,
jcabrera@dis.ulpgc.es, {jisern,adominguez,vprieto}@iusiani.ulpgc.es

Abstract. While traditional glider path planning relies on constant model forecasts with only a limited range, a new approach to glider operation is based on automated topographical understanding incorporating feature detection and tracking techniques. Encapsulating the key elements of ocean structure dynamics and focusing on their behaviour an alternative prediction data model can be developed. This feature-based characterization is then used to improve upon the glider path planning. Additionally a structural comparison of ROMs and global models is conducted as well as a forecast assessment within the model. This approach is applied to the case of mesoscale eddies that form around the canary islands and spin off describing various trajectories depending on origin, type and time of the year.

Keywords: Ocean gliders · Feature detection · Model assessment · Path planning

1   Ocean Features in Path Planning

Ocean currents can be described either by its ocean current functions or by its characteristic features, latter require a procedural understanding of those features. Besides locally static features like upwelling zones, river plumes and tidal currents, mesoscale eddies present an interesting feature that is not yet fully understood but is considerably important in terms of water mass transport but also vehicle navigation.

2   Eddy Detection

2.1   Techniques

In order to be able to track the movement of eddies a new automated eddy detection algorithm is presented based on streamline characteristics on a 2-

Partially funded by Canary Island government - FEDER (proj. 2010/62) and Dep. Informatica y Sistemas ULPGC.

R. Moreno-Díaz et al. (Eds.): EUROCAST 2015, LNCS 9520, pp. 714–719, 2015.
DOI: 10.1007/978-3-319-27340-2_88

dimensional flow field. Streamline examination based on Curvature Center Density to detect centers was introduced by [1], whereas [2] relies on geometric constraints. Eddy detection schemes based on different physical principles can be seen in [3], where the ocean state representation is given by the sea surface height. The detection is based on a logic that looks out for the relative sea surface height change in cold-core or warm-core eddies, with effective threshold control. Another detection scheme can be based on further physical ocean factors like temperature or oxygen values, yet they are not directly captured by satellite.

2.2 Detection Algorithm

The proposed streamline algorithm is a multistep procedure which first focuses on regions with sign changes in u and v component of currents in order to determine the exact location of possible centers. In the following steps the eddies are finally identified on streamline characteristics. The outline of the proposed Eddy Detection can be described as follows:

- Find zero crossing of current components u and v
- Streamlines from grid around crossing points
- Calculate streamline properties based on derived angle
- Get 360 streamline center points, choose lowest velocity
- Recheck complete winding for n-neighborhood
- Detect type and further properties.

2.3 Comparison of Detection

Four different eddy detection algorithms are tested on a current field, with an example seen in Fig. 1, which represents the Aviso data for a specific date. In this case there exist panoptically the sea surface height as well as the derived currents, therefore detection schemes based on 2 different physical principles can be applied at once.

All four detection algorithm detect the same main eddies, whereas detecting smaller ones depends on parametrization of the detection algorithm. An advantage of the streamline algorithm is that the center points are more precise with subgrid resolution in contrast to the Nencioli [2] and adapted Nencioli algorithms. This especially plays an more important data with higher grid spacing like in global ocean models.

3 Feature Tracking

Following the process of features over time permits to further analyze their characteristical behaviour for certain regions and deduce probable outcomes for prediction purposes. In this case as eddies are appearing and constantly moving before they finally dissolve, a characterisation is made regarding is longevity and movement pattern.

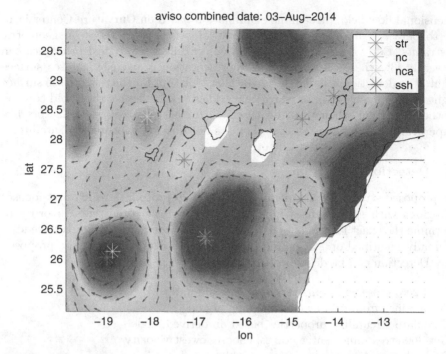

Fig. 1. A typical current grid given as model output, where eddies are discovered by the different detection schemes. Best seen in color (Color figure online).

3.1 Tracking Algorithm

In order to achieve trajectories over time, a robust tracking algorithm was developed, which takes into account short-term detection failures that might occur due to weak current data. In order to achieve robust tracking the algorithm gathers eddies in lists for every available timestep, quite often daily. Results for following timesteps are matched to the previous combination of eddies, with an allowed maximum displacement velocity for eddies per timestep. When an eddy is not detected in the following timestep the object in the list is not yet deleted but rather put into inactive mode, from where it can be reactivated at reappearance of the eddy detection. The maximum inactive mode duration was set up to be a maximum of 3 days, for when it is supposed to have been dissolved.

3.2 Statistical Examination

Eddy development during August and September 2014 in the Canary Islands area is depicted in Fig. 2. The statistical examination shows us a clear channel below the island of Gran Canaria with eddies moving southward as a result of prevalent trade winds in this area during summer time. This was also observed by [4].

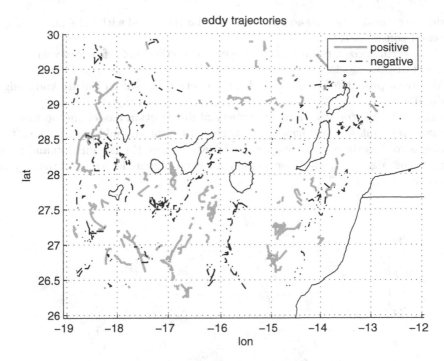

Fig. 2. Appearance of eddies in August/September, 2014, distinguishing between positive (*gray*) and negative (*black*) rotation.

3.3   Multi-model Approach

As there are occasionally multiple models for specific regions available the eddy detection results in incoherent feature positions, the question arises on how to reach model consensus on the exact position? A possible way to resolve such uncertainty is to match model data to in-situ or satellite measurements where available and weight them in. A weighting can be undergone based on simple feature mean positions as well as a more complex weighting scheme applying an Bayes Model Averaging on different ROMS as was outlined in a previous work.

4   Path Planning

The path planning problem can now be approached by a behavioural understanding of ocean dynamics as depicted in. Prevalent synoptic circulation structures [5] can be detected and used for assessment of regional ocean models as a basis for feature-based ensemble forecasts. Identifying and tracking these features can have multiple use cases for path planning purposes, which can be classified by its time horizon as instant, short, mid and long-term:

– Instantly knowing the relative position and the distance to a feature, especially interesting for scenarios with multi-vehicle and multi-feature settings. Higher

degree of automated mission planning can be generated with rules and setting-
based constraints.

- Short-term horizon comprises the movement prediction for features with velocity of displacement.
- Mid-term probable forecast models are generated based on feature knowledge
  database.
- Finally, long-term case analyzes statistical distribution model and occurrence
  maps relevant for deployment strategies. Besides ensemble generation, the
  aim is to directly incorporate detected features into the the mission and path
  planning algorithms in order to gain an even higher degree of autonomy in
  ocean gliders (Fig. 3).

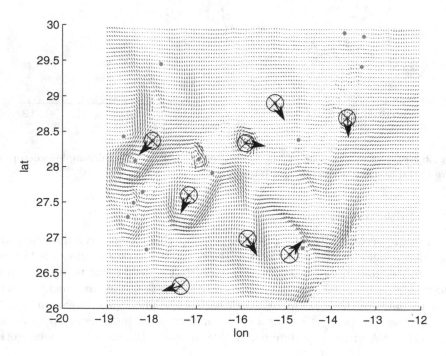

Fig. 3. Example of detected eddies with an estimated proceeding direction and velocity
which can be fed to the planning algorithm

5   Conclusion

Realizing a detection scheme with tracking capabilities aides in targeting scientific research by guiding vehicles into the center of regions of interest (ROI) where
more valuable data can be gathered. For vehicle operation this means there are
dynamic, relative waypoints to which a scientific mission can be planned, which
is highly interesting in terms of exploring the physical and biochemical processes

of those moving ocean features. Without detection it would be rather difficult to make an educated guess of the trajectory in the current field. In the next step the mission objective can be optimized incorporating the needs and restrictions to a planner. This is not part of this investigation but might be a future application.

References

1. Ari Sadarjoen, I., et al.: Detection, quantification, and tracking of vortices using streamline geometry. Comput. Graph. **24**(3), 333–341 (2000)
2. Nencioli, F.: A vector geometry-based eddy detection algorithm. J. Atmos. Oceanic Technol. **27**(3), 564–579 (2010)
3. Faghmous, J.H., Styles, L., Mithal, V., Boriah, S., Liess, S., Kumar, V., Vikebo, F., dos Santos Mesquita, M.: Eddyscan: a physically consistent ocean eddy monitoring application. In: 2012 Conference on Intelligent Data Understanding (CIDU), pp. 96–103, October 2012
4. Sangr, P., Auladell, M., Marrero-Daz, A., Pelegr, J.L., Fraile-Nuez, E., Rodrguez-Santana, A., Martn, J.M., Mason, E., Hernndez-Guerra, A.: On the nature of oceanic eddies shed by the island of gran canaria. Deep Sea Res. Part I: Oceanogr. Res. Pap. **54**(5), 687–709 (2007)
5. Calado, L., et al.: Feature-oriented regional modeling and simulations (forms) for the Western South Atlantic: Southeastern Brazil region. Ocean Model. **25**(1–2), 48–64 (2008)

Mobile Platforms, Autonomous and Computing Traffic Systems

Mobile AgeCI: Potential Challenges in the Development and Evaluation of Mobile Applications for Elderly People

Stefan Diewald[1]([✉]), Barbara Geilhof[2], Monika Siegrist[2], Patrick Lindemann[3],
Marion Koelle[3], Martin Halle[2], and Matthias Kranz[3]

[1] Chair of Media Technology, Distributed Multimodal Information Processing Group,
Technische Universität München, Munich, Germany
stefan.diewald@tum.de
[2] Department for Prevention, Rehabilitation and Sports Medicine,
Technische Universität München, Munich, Germany
{geilhof,siegrist,halle}@sport.med.tum.de
[3] Lehrstuhl für Informatik mit Schwerpunkt Eingebettete Systeme,
Universität Passau, Passau, Germany
{patrick.lindemann,marion.koelle,matthias.kranz}@uni-passau.de

Abstract. Designing mobile applications for elderly users can be very challenging. Their heterogeneous prior knowledge and abilities make user-centered design processes difficult. For that reasons, some measures are necessary to make the applications usable the majority of elderly people and to get useful feedback during the evaluation. In this paper, we summarize central challenges we faced during the user-centered development of a mobile fitness application for seniors. We address differences in interaction, trust issues, fears, functional complexity, and aspects of motivation. Based on these experiences, we present suggestions that can be useful for the future development and evaluation of mobile (fitness) applications for elderly people.

1 Motivation and Setting

With more than 1.3 million mobile applications in Google's Play store[1] and about the same number in Apple's App Store[2], there seems to be apps for everyone and every purpose. The categories reach from communication, news, and business over gaming, entertainment, and education, to physical fitness [7]. However, a 2014 report on app users revealed that there are actually only a few apps for elderly people [8] that cater for impairments many seniors suffer from (such as less acute vision or reduced tactile sense) or for missing prior knowledge (such as special gestures or typing on a soft keyboard). For that reason, many elderly people cannot benefit from the large amount of available mobile apps that could support their activities of daily living or their personal health.

---

[1] http://www.appbrain.com/stats/number-of-android-apps.
[2] http://techcrunch.com/2014/09/09/itunes-app-store-reaches-1-3-million-mobile-applications/.

© Springer International Publishing Switzerland 2015
R. Moreno-Díaz et al. (Eds.): EUROCAST 2015, LNCS 9520, pp. 723–730, 2015.
DOI: 10.1007/978-3-319-27340-2_89

Developing mobile applications for elderly people is especially difficult as their abilities and experiences are quite diverse. With increasing age, there are changes that negatively influence sensory-perceptual processes, motor abilities, response speed, and cognitive processes [1]. The severity of these age-related functional limitations varies widely from person to person, which leads to different requirements on the user interface. Another difficulty is the different amount of prior knowledge on computer technology. Many of the current seniors have never worked with computers and are unaware of possibilities and boundaries of modern technology. Since both factors – the functional limitations and prior knowledge – vary over a broad range, it is necessary to follow worst-case assumptions for the design of digital applications and to adapt the evaluation process to the individual abilities of the subjects [6].

In order to give an overview of central challenges that may occur in the development process of mobile applications for elderly people, we share our insights from the development and evaluation of a mobile physical training app for seniors who use a rollator as mobility aid [2]. In addition, we describe the measures we applied to adapt to the elderly users' abilities. The measures can be seen as recommendations for the development of future mobile (fitness) applications. The physical fitness context was chosen as it is an important topic for most elderly rollator users, which should avoid acceptance problems due to doubts on the usefulness of the application.

The structure of the paper is as follows: We begin with presenting the concept and the prototype of the training application. Subsequently, we describe the evaluation setting of the application and present some results to show the effectiveness of the application. We finally share challenges we faced during the development and evaluation and summarize measures that helped us to counteract the individual challenges.

2   Mobile Training App for Rollator Users

A regular physical training is necessary for rollator users to prevent falls and to improve their ability to walk. The goal of the application is to provide an appropriate training program, which can be performed independently and integrated into daily life [3].

The developed mobile application is an interactive physical training app, where the rollator is used as training equipment (see Fig. 1). The app includes exercises for coordination, strengthening, and flexibility with the aim to increase strength and performance and to reduce the risk of falling. The set of exercises was compiled by sports scientists. Instructional videos and photos of key positions along with written and spoken exercise descriptions were implemented to support a correct exercise execution (see Fig. 1, right). The app reminds the user to exercise regular (recommendation: three times per week) and additionally visualizes the current training progress. A virtual trophy is used to enhance and maintain the motivation if the training session is completed successfully (see Fig. 1, left). The duration of a training session is between 15 and 20 min

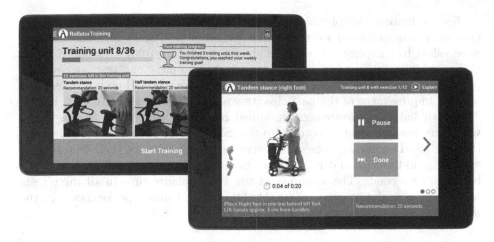

Fig. 1. The main menu of the mobile training app summarizes the current progress and previews next exercises (left). Advanced functions are hidden in the app drawer. The exercise instructions are presented via videos, textual or audio descriptions (right).

and includes initially ten exercises. The number of exercises and their intensity increase with the training progress.

3   Evaluation of the App

The training app has been tested by elderly rollator users with limited walking ability. Ten seniors (1 male, 9 female) aged 75 to 89 years (average: 82 years, standard deviation: 5 years) used the app and trained independently for 12 weeks. During the test period, 7-inch tablet PCs with universal mountings that could be fixed at the rollator were provided to the participants. Since all participants had no experience with smartphones or tablet PCs, three training sessions took place prior to the independent training, where functions of the devices were explained and a correct training technique was taught. For the evaluation, technical data as well as data on physical performance were collected. The technical data consists of application log data (e.g., frequency of use, duration per exercise and activated functions) and subjective assessments of the training sessions. To detect changes on physical performance, tests for strength, balance and walking ability were performed at the beginning and at the end of the exercise period.

The analysis of the log data revealed that only one subject regularly met the recommended exercising repetitions over the 12 weeks. Most other subjects only used the application regularly in the first few weeks. In the after-study interview, many of them stated that they knew many exercises by heart then and performed them without the app. Almost all users exercised at the same time of day. It could also be seen that some subjects regularly skipped exercises. One subject once even skipped 9 out of 11 exercises in one training unit.

For evaluating the physical effects, the functional strength of the lower extremity was measured by the 'Chair Stand Test' (CST) [9]. The patients were asked to complete five rapid chair rise cycles up from a standard chair. Before training, six participants were able to complete the test successfully. After the end of training seven participants were able to stand up five times. The average improvement of the participants was from 29.5 ± 17.1 s to 17.7 ± 6.4 s. The static balance measurement (modified Romberg, *mRomberg* [4]) was tested with three measurements according to the 'Short Physical Performance Battery' (SPPB) [4]. The participants were instructed to stand with their feet side by side, in semi-tandem, and full-tandem position. Each test position had to be held for ten seconds. The summary of the total balance time in all three tests was used for analytics (max. reachable 30 s). The balance performance in the *mRomberg* increased on average from 19.4 ± 9.4 s to 28.8 ± 3.1 s.

4 Challenges and Recommendations

Based on the experiences during the development and evaluation of the mobile training application, the following challenges have been identified. The summary is not limited to usability aspects [5] but also includes factors that may influence the acceptance of the application and the results of the evaluation.

4.1 Deviant Interaction

In order to evaluate whether users recognize the interactive interface elements and whether the elements' size is large enough, the app also recorded the touch positions in the different screens. During the analysis of the recorded touch position data, it was noticed that many users did not press at the center of the elements. In particular, touch events were recorded in the right hand side of the elements, which can be probably explained that most subjects operated the application with their right hand. A temporal analysis of the recorded touch positions revealed also a position shift over time. In Fig. 2, a representative excerpt of recorded touch positions for three buttons is visualized. In contrast to Fig. 1, the labels are in German as the evaluation was performed with the German version of the application. The figure shows touch positions of the first three app uses as well as positions from the tenth to the thirteenth use. When comparing the touch positions, it can be observed that inexperienced users avoided clicking on the text. However, as soon as the users are acquainted with the app the touch positions are shifted towards the center of the element and are no longer around the text. A possible explanation could be that users do not have to read the labels in detail anymore as they know what happens when they click on the color-coded buttons.

This behavior was not expected. A consequence of this observation was that the central elements were enlarged to offer enough space to press next to the text. Since elderly users may have a different mental model of mobile applications, they can show different interaction patterns compared to younger users that are

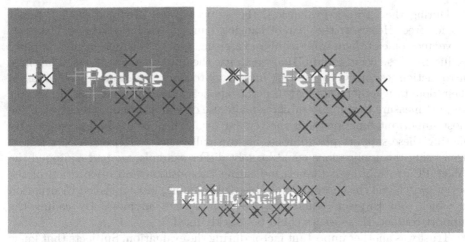

✗ Touch positions from first to third use of application

╶┼╴ Touch positions from tenth to thirteenth use of application

Fig. 2. During the evaluation, the touch positions were recorded in order to check whether interactive elements could be detected. The analysis revealed that experienced users (tenth to thirteenth use of app) more likely press at the center of the elements whereas novice users (first to third use) avoid tapping on the text. In contrast to Fig. 1, the texts are in German as they were during the evaluation.

familiar with modern technology [11]. For that reason, it is advisable to observe or record interactions during the evaluation in detail. The temporal analysis can be useful to reveal changing requirements with the level of experience.

4.2 Fears and Trust

Especially users with little or no previous knowledge on mobile device and PC use had inhibitions to perform experiments without exact instructions. Besides the fear of causing irreparable damage to the system, some subjects were also afraid to embarrass themselves. Even though the experimenter emphasized that only the applications are tested and not the subjects, many participants felt like being in an exam situation.

As part of the iterative development, we performed short laboratory studies with subjects from the target group. In order to create a relaxed situation, we started the evaluation with semi-structured interviews while guiding users through the app, which served at the same time as introduction to the app. When performing task completion experiments, we defined a maximum duration after which we helped to solve the task to keep the subject's motivation. The measures were well accepted by the subjects. However, it was also difficult to perform valid task completion experiments.

During the 12-week evaluation, the subjects were provided with a tablet PC for free. However, the fear of causing damage to the device or losing it, prevented some of them from regular exercising. Only after presenting a liability exclusion, these users could be moved to use the application at home. The three introduction sessions were also very important to many users and helped to dispel their doubts whether they can use the application alone. Another important support measure that many subjects made use of were printed manuals with the most important functions and the regular availability of a contact person. By offering these support possibilities, many small issues that prevented subjects from using the applications could be solved. For example, we had equipped the tablet PCs with adhesive labels indicating the position and orientation of the power switch and the charging plug. In the beginning, lost labels led to situation in which some subjects could not use their devices anymore. By calling the support contact, these issues could be quickly fixed.

Trust was another important factor during the evaluation. Subjects that knew the experimenter before and, thus, had already a certain mutual trust rated the trustworthiness of the app and its exercise content higher than subjects without prior contact did. At the same time, the subjects that had a better bond of trust with the experimenter expressed their opinions more openly. When performing an evaluation, this bias should be considered, but could be also exploited. When choosing the participants, one could distinguish between a more open qualitative and a low-biased quantitative evaluation.

4.3   Reduction of Complexity

An early prototype of the app required input of age and selection of preferred training days. However, initial experiments revealed that the input of data (text, selection of dates and times) was a major problem for many elderly novice users. For that reason, this step was removed and default values were set. As a consequence, the amount of data input should be kept to a minimum. In many cases, default values can be used, which could be changed in the settings if it is desired or necessary. Other supportive measures are auto-completion that is able to compensate for minor typos or the possibility to create favorites to reduce repeated data input.

A good approach to reduce the mobile application's complexity is to analyze which functions are actually used. When a function is only rarely used, the reason for not using it should be examined. Possible results could be that the function is not necessary for the users or that it is currently very difficult to find or use. In general, the main function should be at the center of attention and stand out against auxiliary functions. For example, the main screen of the rollator training app offers only a single visible element for starting or resuming the current training unit. All other functions are accessible via the hidden app drawer menu. The display of single exercises was initially divided into two steps. In the first step, the users should watch the training video and read the instructions. By clicking on the start button, the exercise was started and a stopwatch was displayed. However, observations of training sessions and the analysis of recorded log data have shown that many users started exercising already in the introduction part. This caused situations where the stopwatch had to be started after the exercise execution followed by an immediate click on the finish button to jump to the next exercise. This led to combining the instruction and execution step which then only required a single click to get to the next exercise. The stopwatch function can still be used, but is implemented as an auxiliary function that can be started on demand.

4.4 Fidelity of Prototype

The evaluation of early prototypes was very difficult. Since most of the elderly subjects had no experience with smartphones and tablet PCs, the mock-ups without functionality or even paper prototypes were too abstract for them. Due to the missing experiences, they could not imagine how the functional prototype would work. For that reason, low-fidelity prototypes were then evaluated by experts. However, it is advisable to create a functional digital prototype as early as possible in the process to gather results from the target group. In doing so, it is important to match the prototype's level of detail with the prior knowledge and experiences of the potential users. We also noticed that an incomplete or imperfect prototype could have a negative influence on the future acceptance of an application. Another difficulty was the dissociation of the element under evaluation. Most subjects did not understand the difference of software and hardware during the evaluation. For example, subjects named the slippery surface and the weight of the used tablet PC as negative points of the app. This needs to be considered when questions on stability or similar areas that can refer to hardware as well as software are part of the evaluation.

4.5 Training Motivation

A regular training is necessary to achieve a sustained health benefit. For this reason, it is important that the application promotes long-term training. If the participants themselves determine a success in training, such as improvements in balance or strength, the training motivation will increase. An integration of exercises, which have a fast and positive training effect, is therefore advisable. In addition, the motivation can be reinforced by integrated virtual rewards. In the training app, trophies were displayed when the participants reached the predefined training goals, which was also named as an important motivational factor in the after-study survey. Additionally, variety in training sessions can trigger curiosity and, thus, further boost the participants' motivation [10].

5 Conclusion

By sharing our insights on the development and evaluation of a mobile application for elderly users, we try to contribute to closing the generation gap in mobile app use. The summarized challenges and possible approaches for solving these can be used as basis for the future development of mobile (training) apps for seniors. We are currently optimizing the presented application and its exercising concept and plan to make it available to the public after a second long-term evaluation phase.

Acknowledgments. This research was supported in part by the German Federal Ministry of Education and Research (BMBF, project PASSAge, funding number 16SV5748). Further information on the project can be found on https://www.passage-projekt.de.

References

1. Czaja, S.J., Lee, C.C.: The impact of aging on access to technology. Univ. Access Inf. Soc. **5**(4), 341–349 (2007)
2. Diewald, S., Koelle, M., Stockinger, T., Lindemann, P., Kranz, M.: Mobile AgeCI: insights from the development of a mobile training application for elderly users. In: Proceedings of the 15th International Conference on Computer Aided Systems Theory, Eurocast 2015, pp. 233–234. IUCTC Universidad de Las Palmas de Gran Canaria, February 2015
3. Diewald, S., Möller, A., Roalter, L., Kranz, M.: Today, you walk! - when physical fitness influences trip planning. In: Butz, A., Koch, M., Schlichter, J. (eds.) Mensch and Computer 2014 - Tagungsband, pp. 383–386. De Gruyter Oldenbourg, Berlin (2014)
4. Guralnik, J.M., Simonsick, E.M., Ferrucci, L., Glynn, R.J., Berkman, L.F., Blazer, D.G., Scherr, P.A., Wallace, R.B.: A short physical performance battery assessing lower extremity function. J. Gerontol. **49**(2), 85–94 (1994)
5. Hwangbo, H., Yoon, S.H., Jin, B.S., Han, Y.S., Ji, Y.G.: A study of pointing performance of elderly users on smartphones. Int.J. Hum.-Comput. Interact. **29**(9), 604–618 (2013)
6. Ijsselsteijn, W., Nap, H.H., de Kort, Y., Poels, K.: Digital game design for elderly users. In: Proceedings of the 2007 Conference on Future Play, FuturePlay 2007, pp. 17–22. ACM, New York, NY, USA, November 2007
7. Kranz, M., Möller, A., Hammerla, N., Diewald, S., Plötz, T., Olivier, P., Roalter, L.: The mobile fitness coach: towards individualized skill assessment using personalized mobile devices. Pervasive Mob. Comput. **9**(2), 203–215 (2013)
8. Lee, P., Stewart, D., Barker, J.: The smartphone generation gap: over-55? There's no app for that. In: Technology. Media and Telecommunications Predictions 2014, pp. 42—44. TMT, Deloitte, January 2014
9. Lusardi, M.M., Pellecchia, G.L., Schulman, M.: Functional performance in community living older adults. J. Geriatr. Phys. Ther. **26**(3), 14–22 (2003)
10. Schutzer, K.A., Graves, B.S.: Barriers and motivations to exercise in older adults. Prev. Med. **39**(5), 1056–1061 (2004)
11. Ziefle, M., Bay, S.: Mental models of a cellular phone menu. comparing older and younger novice users. In: Brewster, S., Dunlop, M.D. (eds.) Mobile HCI 2004. LNCS, vol. 3160, pp. 25–37. Springer, Heidelberg (2004)

Cross Pocket Gait Authentication Using Mobile Phone Based Accelerometer Sensor

Muhammad Muaaz[✉] and René Mayrhofer

JRC u'smile and Institute of Networks and Security,
Johannes Kepler University Linz, Altenbergerstr. 69, 4040 Linz, Austria
muhammad.muaaz@fh-hagenberg.at, rene.mayrhofer@jku.at

Abstract. Gait authentication using mobile phone based accelerometer sensors offers an implicit way of authenticating users to their mobile devices. This study explores gait authentication performance under a realistic scenario if gait template and gait test data belongs to left and right side front pocket of the trousers. To simulate this scenario, we used two identical (model, build, and vendor) Android mobile phones to record cross pocket biometric gait data from 35 participants (29 male and 6 female) in two different sessions. Both datasets (left and right pocket) are processed and segmented using the same approach. Our results show that biometric gait performance not only decreases over the time but it is also highly influenced by the placement of the mobile device or the sensor capturing gait data. High number of False Non Matches (FNMR) in cross pocket scenario indicate a significant asymmetry in leg muscle strength.

1 Introduction

Mobile phones have evolved to the stage where they are not only used for calling and texting purposes but also offer a multitude of services such as mobile banking, e-commerce, portable storage, social, and entertainment. Data stored on mobile phones is typically protected with PIN/password based authentication mechanisms. Mobile phones are frequently accessed but for smaller periods of time [3] when compared to desktop/laptop type systems. Therefore, mobile phone users mostly avoid using PIN/password based authentication on their phones as it consumes time and increases cognitive load. Physiological biometrics on the other hand could solve issues related to the PIN/password based authentication mechanism, however they also suffer from some challenges such as; their deployment on mobile phones increases product cost and they consume user time due high Failure to Acquire (FTA) errors (such as user has to swipe his finger over the fingerprint sensor multiple times to authenticate or mobile camera fails to capture face image under improper lightening conditions). Therefore, we need to find a more intuitive way of authenticating individuals to their mobile phones which is not only reliable and robust but also usable.

Gait is a behavioural biometric and has been proposed as an alternative authentication mechanism for mobile phones. Gait is an individual's walking

© Springer International Publishing Switzerland 2015
R. Moreno-Díaz et al. (Eds.): EUROCAST 2015, LNCS 9520, pp. 731–738, 2015.
DOI: 10.1007/978-3-319-27340-2_90

style and the process of identifying and verifying individuals by they way they walk is called gait authentication. Gait authentication using mobile phone based accelerometer sensor is an active research area since 2009. Various studies [1,4,5,7] have reported promising results of gait authentication. However, these studies were conducted on datasets recorded under ideal and controlled scenarios, for example mobile phone was tightly attached to the participants body on a fixed position or participants were asked to wear same clothing and shoes if gait data was recorded on different days. Studies [2,7] have shown that biometric gait alongside offering an implicit way of authenticating individuals also suffers from various challenges such as; it changes over a period of time, it is also sensitive to clothing, shoes, walking speeds, and sensor placement.

When we walk, our limbs exhibit the different pattern of movements for instance our arms movement is different from our legs or hips or feet and so on. Therefore, from gait authentication perspective there exists an interesting question to what degree a realistic scenario can be designed without effecting measurability and user friendliness while maintaining characteristics such as uniqueness and universality. Considering this, most suitable phone placement could be trousers pocket as users often place their mobile phones inside their trousers front pocket. In a previous study [6] we have reported gait authentication performance under this realistic scenario such as placing the mobile phone inside the trousers front pocket and participants walked at their normal pace. However, mobile phone users often do not place their mobile phone in their same pocket, therefore this study focuses on the question how gait authentication would be influenced under cross pocket scenario.

2   Data Collection

For data collection purpose, we developed an Android application which records three-dimensional (X, Y, and Z axis) accelerometer data at a sampling rate of 100 Hz and writes it to a text file with time stamps. This study uses gait data collected from 35 participants (6 female and 29 male) which is also used for [6]. However, for cross pocket analysis as the main focus in the present work, we now use two identical (Samsung Google Nexus) Android phones. Each phone was placed inside the participant's left and right side front pocket as shown in Fig. 1(a) and (b).

Participants were asked to wear a trouser with not-too-loose front pockets. For capturing a distinctive walking style, the phone or sensor must be placed close-to-the-body otherwise it might picks up to much random noise. Participants were asked to walk at their normal pace in a 68 m long straight corridor (with no stairs) as shown in Fig. 1(d). They were told to wait for 1 s at the end of walk, then turn around, and wait for another second before starting their new walk. In one session, every subject walked $4 \times 68 = 272$ m or in other words completed two rounds of the corridor. For every subject, data recording was conducted in two different sessions. An average gap between the sessions is about 25 days. Eight walks were recorded for every subject in two different sessions.

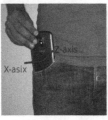
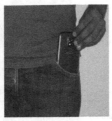
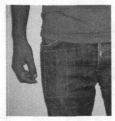
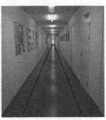

| (a) Left pocket. | (b) Right pocket. | (c) Phone position inside the pocket. | (d) Experimental setup. |

Fig. 1. Phone placement and its orientation at the start of the session for all participants.

3 Data Description and Processing

Figure 2 shows various activities performed in one data recording session. Approximately the first 10–20 s of data is when the phone was being placed inside the pocket, and next 100 s are when person is standing still and listening to the instructions. Then the participant starts walking and reaches the end point. This walking activity lasts around 50 s and varies from person to person as it highly depends upon the walking pace of the person. At the end of the walk participant waits for a second, turns around and waits for another second before the new walk, and so on participant completes the session with four walks. Data processing begins by separating session-wise recorded walks and computing magnitude from tri-axes accelerometer data. This study utilizes similar steps of data processing as mentioned in [6] except the noise removal step. In this study we have used a Savitzky-Golay smoothing filter described in Sect. 3.4, due to its shape preserving property.

3.1 Walk Separation

A simple variance threshold method is used to separate the walks. This is done by monitoring the variance of the y-axis data (any other axis, or the magnitude of accelerometer data can also be used) with a sliding window of one second. If variance within this window rises above a certain threshold, this marks the start of an active walk segment, and when the variance drops below that threshold it marks the stop of that active walk segment. In this study, we use a variance threshold of $0.8 \frac{m}{s^2}$. Once all active walk regions are marked, we pick those segments which are longer than 10 s.

3.2 Zero Normalization

In the steady state (lets say when phone is place on the table), acceleration measured along the axis influenced by gravity must be equal to the earth's gravitational force and acceleration along remaining two axes, which are not influenced

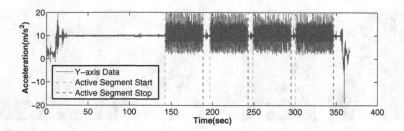

Fig. 2. Acceleration recorded along the y-axis with detected four walk segments.

by the gravity must be zero. However, acceleration recorded by phone-based accelerometer sensors is not stable in the steady state. Therefore, acceleration along all three axes is zero normalized by subtracting their respective mean as shown in Eq. 1, where A is acceleration over time and μ is mean acceleration.

$$\bar{A}_i(t) = A_i(t) - \mu_i, i \in \{x, y, z\} \tag{1}$$

In this step, we simply compute the resultant vector as given in Eq. 2 from individual axis data of each walk which undergoes further data processing steps described in the following subsections. This is done to avoid the influence of continuously changing orientation of the mobile device inside the pocket.

$$R_s = \sqrt{A_x^2 + A_y^2 + A_z^2} \tag{2}$$

3.3 Interpolation

Android phones accelerometer sensor only outputs data when the Android API's (onSensorChange) method is triggered. Therefore an accelerometer sensor does not output acceleration data at equal time intervals. By applying linear interpolation as given in Eq. 3, data can be reshaped in equal intervals in order to mitigate data loss of too many values.

$$a = a_1 + \frac{(a_2 - a_1)(\acute{t} - t_1)}{(t_2 - t_1)} \tag{3}$$

3.4 Noise Removal

A Savitzky-Golay smoothing filter (also called digital smoothing polynomial filter or least-square smoothing filter) is used to remove noise from the data. We preferred a S-G filter over the typical average moving filters because least-square smoothing not only reduces noise but also maintains the shape and hight of waveform peaks. The basic idea behind S-G filter is to find a least-square fit with a polynomial of high degree for each data point, over an odd sized window centred around that data point.

4   Segmentation

We have already reported segmentation process in detailed in [6] and for the sake of completeness we briefly describe it here as well.

4.1   Cycle Length Estimation

Our cycle length estimation as given in [6] begins by extracting a small subset of samples around the centre of the walk called reference-segment and compute its distance with the other sub-segments of the same size extracted from that walk. From this distance vector we find the indices of the minimum distance values and store them to a minimum index vector. Later we compute a difference vector which contains the difference of every two adjacent elements of the minimum index vector. Finally, the cycle length is computed by taking the mode of the difference vector. In case if mode does not exist (which means every step has different length which could happen if an individual is intentionally changing the walking pace) we compute cycle length by averaging the values of difference vector.

4.2   Cycle Detection

Cycle detection as explained in [6] begins by extracting a small segment (2 × estimatedCycleLength) around the center of the walk as it is the most stable section of the walk and we find minimum value in this section of the walk. From this minimum point cycles are detected in forward and backward direction by adding and subtracting the cycle length. From our experiments we found that all minimas in the walk do not occur at equal intervals therefore, we select a small an offset (0.2 × estimatedCycleLength) area around the found end point and find minima in that region. Once all minimas in both direction are found they are called gait cycle starts, which are used to segment walk to gait cycles.

4.3   Omitting Unusual Cycles

Detected cycles are cleaned by removing outlier cycles. This is done by computing the pairwise distance using Dynamic Time Warping (DTW). Cycles which have a distance of at-least half of the other cycles are removed [4]. After removing unusual cycles we are left with remained-cycles as shown in Fig. 3. If less than three cycles are remained threshold is raised and process of deleting unusual cycles starts again until three cycles are remained. These remained cycles are further separated to reference gait cycle and probe cycles. A cycle which has minimum distance to all other cycles is called reference cycle and the rest of the cycles are called probe cycles.

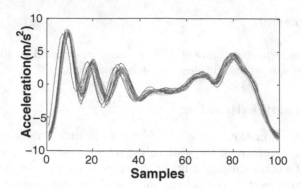

Fig. 3. Remained gait cycles after removing outliers.

5   Results and Discussion

Once reference and probe cycles are generated they are compared against each other to compute the intra-class (genuine) and inter-class (impostor) distances by using the DTW distance metric. Computed distances are passed to a majority voting module to decide if a walk is a genuine or an impostor attempt. If 50 % cycles of a walk have distances lower than the threshold value then the walk is considered a genuine walk.

For this study, we have recorded gait data in two different sessions with an average gap of 25 days between the sessions by placing cell phones inside both (left and right) pocket which gives us four different combinations. Same-Session Same-Pocket (SS-SP) results are achieved when reference and probe cycles are from the same pocket (either left or right side pocket) and same session walks. Same-Session Cross-Pocket (SS-CP) indicates that same session walks are used for reference and probe cycles but reference and probe data is from different pockets. If reference data is from left side pocket then probe data is from right side pocket and vice versa. Cross-Session Same-Pocket (CS-SP) means reference and probe data is from different sessions but belongs to the same pocket. For Cross-Session Cross Pocket (CS-CP), reference and probe data is from different sessions but if reference data is from left pocket then probe data of right pocket is used. Table 1 shows the results of this study under global threshold settings when the single best gait cycle from first walk of first session is used as reference data and Table 2 shows results when thefour best cycles from four walks of first session are used. As False Match Rate (FMR) and False Non Match Rate (FNMR) are highly sensitive to the global threshold value, therefore we have run various tests (such as selecting a range of thresholds and computing FMR and FNMR at every threshold) to find a threshold value which gives good FMR and FNMR for cross day performance. For this study we set a global threshold to 60 DTW distance units for all experiments. If we compare SS-SP and SS-CP results we can see that FMR stays unaffected but on the same time FNMR significantly increases which is also true for CS-SP and CS-CP comparisons.

Table 1. Gait authentication results under same/cross sessions and pockets settings when 1 gait cycle from first walk of first session is used as reference data, and global threshold is set to 60 DTW distance units.

Reference data	Subjects	SS-SP		SS-CP		CS-SP		CS-CP	
		FMR	FNMR	FMR	FNMR	FMR	FNMR	FMR	FNMR
Left pocket	35	0,1064	0,0236	0,0936	0,4753	0,1031	0,3693	0,0985	0,6193
Right pocket	35	0,1168	0,0179	0,1071	0,4668	0,1169	0,3200	0,1041	0,5785

Table 2. Gait authentication results under same/cross sessions and pockets settings when 4 best gait cycles from 4 walks of first session are used as reference data, and global threshold is set to 60 DTW distance units.

Reference data	Subjects	SS-SP		SS-CP		CS-SP		CS-CP	
		FMR	FNMR	FMR	FNMR	FMR	FNMR	FMR	FNMR
Left pocket	35	0,0923	0,0000	0.0862	0.4697	0,0630	0,3561	0.0643	0.6969
Right pocket	35	0.1245	0.0076	0.1084	0.4773	0,0829	0,3106	0.0677	0.5833

Table 3. Gait authentication results under same/cross sessions results after combining 4 gait templates from left pocket and 4 gait templates from right pocket, and increasing global threshold to 70 DTW distance units.

Reference data	Subjects	SS		CS	
		FMR	FNMR	FMR	FNMR
Left and right pocket	35	0.14252	0,04545	0.10464	0.3560

Apparently our legs movement looks similar but our results indicate that both legs movement is different at least from an authentication point of view. To further confirm on this we computed DTW distance between the best gait cycles obtained from left and right leg same session recording, and we found that DTW distance is high enough to mark it as an impostor, given the same global threshold.

From Tables 1 and 2 we can see that increasing numbers of templates do reduce FMR and FNMR for SP results however for CP scenario there is no improvement at all. These results indicate we need to combine left and right side gait templates to achieve better results and rethink global threshold not only from cross day performance perspective but also from cross leg performance point of view as shown in Table 3.

6 Conclusion and Future Outlook

We explore gait authentication using mobile phone based accelerometer sensor under a realistic scenario. Previous work [6] has shown that it is possible to authenticate individuals by placing cell phones inside the trousers front pocket and in this paper we extend that work by posing a question if it is possible to authenticate an individual if we use gait template and test data from two different front (left and right) pockets of the trousers. With our approach we have achieved False Match Rate (FMR = 0.0862) and False Non Match Rate (FNMR = 0.4697) under same session cross pocket scenario at a global threshold. Under cross session cross pocket scenario a FMR is 0.0643 and FNMR is 0.6969. By combining gait templates from left and right pocket cross session FNMR is dropped to 0.3560. Our novel results indicate that under cross pocket scenario, gait is not similar enough to identify an individual. Therefore, we can say that it points out that combining both left and right side templates is necessary. In our future work, we will test run our gait authentication prototype and explore some other features that might help us to improve cross pocket gait authentication performance.

Acknowledgments. We gratefully acknowledge funding and support by the Christian Doppler Gesellschaft, A1 Telekom Austria AG, Drei-Banken-EDV GmbH, LG Nexera Business Solutions AG, and NXP Semiconductors Austria GmbH.

References

1. Derawi, M.O.: Smartphones and biometrics: gait and activity recognition. Ph.D. thesis, Gjøvik University College, November 2012
2. Gafurov, D.: Performance and security analysis of gait-based user authentication. Ph.D. thesis, Universitas Osloensis (2004)
3. Hintze, D., Findling, R.D., Muaaz, M., Scholz, S., Mayrhofer, R.: Diversity in locked and unlocked mobile device usage. In: Proceedings of the 2014 ACM International Joint Conference on Pervasive and Ubiquitous Computing: Adjunct Publication, UbiComp 2014 Adjunct, pp. 379–384. ACM, New York, NY, USA (2014)
4. Muaaz, M., Nickel, C.: Influence of different walking speeds and surfaces on accelerometer-based biometric gait recognition. In: 2012 35th International Conference on Telecommunications and Signal Processing (TSP), pp. 508–512 (2012)
5. Muaaz, M., Mayrhofer, R.: An analysis of different approaches to gait recognition using cell phone based accelerometers. In: Proceedings of International Conference on Advances in Mobile Computing and Multimedia, pp. 293–300. ACM (2013)
6. Muaaz, M., Mayrhofer, R.: Orientation independent cell phone based gait authentication. In: Proceedings of the 12th International Conference on Advances in Mobile Computing and Multimedia, MoMM 2014, pp. 161–164. ACM, New York, NY, USA (2014)
7. Nickel, C.: Accelerometer-based biometric gait recognition for authentication on smartphones. Ph.D. thesis, TU Darmstadt (June 2012)

SIFT and SURF Performance Evaluation and the Effect of FREAK Descriptor in the Context of Visual Odometry for Unmanned Aerial Vehicles

Abdulla Al-Kaff[(⊠)], Arturo de la Escalera, and José María Armingol

Intelligent Systems Laboratory, Universidad Carlos III de Madrid,
Avenida de la Universidad, 30, 28911 Leganés, Madrid, Spain
{akaff,escalera,armingol}@ing.uc3m.es
http://www.uc3m.es/islab

Abstract. Feature points detection and description play very important role in many of computer vision applications. Specifically in robot visual navigation systems (i.e. visual odometry or visual simultaneous localization and mapping), which need reliable high speed processing algorithms with low memory load. This paper presents a performance evaluation of the two robust feature detection/description algorithms (SIFT and SURF) with the effect of combining the FREAK descriptor. The performance of these algorithms was compared for the changes in noise, scale and rotation.

Keywords: Feature points · SIFT · SURF · FREAK · Detectors · Descriptors · Visual odometry

1 Introduction

Features detection, description and matching are considered as important parts in the visual navigation systems, especially for aerial vehicles, such as visual odometry [1,2] or visual simultaneous localization and mapping [3]. During the last decade, a variety of feature detectors (SIFT [4], SURF [5], FAST [6], STAR [7], BRISK [8]) and descriptors (SIFT [4], SURF [5], BRIEF [9], ORB [10], FREAK [11]) are proposed and applied to visual navigation purposes. For real time navigation applications, the performance and the robustness of detection/description process are required; therefore many surveys and comparisons of different feature point detectors and descriptors are presented. In [12], a survey with a comparison of many detectors and descriptors was reported and as a conclusion the SIFT and SURF have the same accuracy and robustness however the SURF is more efficient. Another comparison of affine region detectors was presented in [13], at which the authors concluded that the SIFT has the best results, excluding SURF from the comparison. A comparison of FREAK and SURF descriptors in the context of pedestrian detection was reported in [14],

© Springer International Publishing Switzerland 2015
R. Moreno-Díaz et al. (Eds.): EUROCAST 2015, LNCS 9520, pp. 739–747, 2015.
DOI: 10.1007/978-3-319-27340-2_91

at which the author concluded that SURF is more robust than FREAK for pedestrian detection issued. In [15], an experimental study using indoor mobile robot was reported and the authors concluded that the FAST-BRIEF pair is a good choice when processing speed is a concern, however SIFT was excluded.

The motivation of this work is focusing on SIFT and SURF, due to that both provide an invariant method. In other words, the ability to identify and localize accurately the points, even under different image conditions, such as scale, rotation, illumination or image noise. Additionally, they present results with high level of robustness.

This paper presents a performance evaluation between robust and reliable algorithms of feature point detection/description (SIFT and SURF) using datasets of several images under typical image transformations (noise, scale and rotation). In addition to the effect of pairing FREAK descriptor with SIFT and SURF detectors to be used for real-time visual navigation purposes in aerial vehicles.

2   Methods

In computer vision, the term of feature detection refers to the process of identifying an image point (*keypoint*), which differs from its nearest neighbors in term of texture, color or intensity. Whilst, feature description is the process of extracting a local patch around the detected keypoint to be compared with other features.

This section briefly introduces the three methods of feature detection/ description that are used in the performance evaluation study.

SIFT: Scale Invariant Feature Transform [4] was presented as an algorithm for extracting the feature points from images. These features can be invariant in orientation and scale. SIFT is based on four major steps of computation: Scale-space extrema detection (which uses the Difference of Gaussian (DoG) to identify the Keypoints from a pyramid of scales), Keypoint localization, Orientation assignment and Keypoint descriptor.

SURF: Speed-Up Robust Features [5] is an orientation and scale invariant detector/descriptor inspired by SIFT detector/descriptor. This method takes the advantage of the integral images to gain the speed in the processing. Unlike SIFT, SURF method is based on two major steps: Keypoint detection (which uses a Laplacian of Gaussian (LoG) on the images, then the determinants of the Hessian matrix are used to identify the Keypoints) and Keypoint description.

FREAK: Fast Retina Keypoint [11] descriptor concept is adapted from the biological human visual system (retina), at which the system computes a cascade of binary strings by comparing the intensities of the given image by using a circular retinal sampling grid.

3 Experiments

3.1 Datasets

In the experiments, all detectors and descriptors have been evaluated for image matching using datasets of 27500 high-resolution images. The images are captured by ARDrone 2.0 quadcopter [16] of size 1270×720 in indoor and outdoor environments under various illumination conditions. These datasets are divided into three groups:

- **1st Group:** 8000 images form outdoor flight with total distance of 61.1 m
- **2nd Group:** 8500 images from outdoor flight with total distance of 63.7 m
- **3rd Group:** 11000 images from indoor flight with total distance of 148.6 m.

3.2 Image Transformations

The performance and robustness of each method in this study is evaluated against different image transformations.

Noise Invariance: to test noise invariance, three types of noises are applied on the images: Gaussian white noise with $\sigma^2 = 0.1$, Salt and Pepper with density of 20 % and Multiplicative white (Speckle) noise with zero mean and $\sigma^2 = 0.04$.

Rotation Invariance: to test rotation invariance, the test images are rotated at different angles (15° and 30°) in anti-clockwise direction.

Scale Invariance: scale test images to 50 % of the reference images size

3.3 Evaluation

Using the original images as reference, the performance of the detectors/ descriptors is evaluated by the matching process. The keypoints are detected and the descriptors of each keypoint are extracted in both images (reference and transformed). Applying Brute-Force algorithm to each descriptor in the transformed image, afterwards matching them with all features in the reference image using a distance threshold. If the distance is less than or equal the threshold, the correspondent feature is returned. Generally, the evaluation is focused on three criteria; **Repeatability:** the percentage of the features detected on the scene in both images, **Accuracy:** the localization of the detected features and **Efficiency:** the detection/description should be a time-critical process

To study these criteria, the following points are considered:

- **Speed per frame:** absolute total time required to the feature detection/ description of a single frame
- **Speed per feature:** detection/description time for single feature

$$t_f = \frac{T}{N} \tag{1}$$

where T is the total time divided and N number of features.

- **Percentage of matched features:** ratio of the successfully matched features of the transformed image to the reference
- **Average detection error:** the average distance of the feature position in the reference and transformed image. Large values indicate large number of false positives and less accuracy in the detector
- **Features count deviation:** to estimate how slight exposure changes affect feature detection

$$\tau = \frac{1}{N} \sum_{i=0}^{N} \frac{x_{o_i} - x_{t_i}}{x_{o_i}} \tag{2}$$

where, x_{o_i} and x_{t_i} are the number of features from reference and frame transformed respectively.

On the other hand, the matched features by the four methods are used in a homography-based visual odometry algorithm to estimate the drone position. The four generated trajectories area compared to a predefined ground truth to estimate the accuracy and processing time of each one.

4   Results

To evaluate the performance of the proposed methods, the features are extracted from the reference images and then calculate the time of each method, see Table 1. From the reference image, we found the SIFT detector/ descriptor has the best number of feature points, but it is the slowest in processing time, while SIFT-FREAK can extract large number of feature points as SIFT with significant less computational time, approx. 50 % of SIFT. A comparison of the number of feature points and computational time from the transformed image to the reference image of the second dataset, see (Figs. 1 and 2) respectively.

For the noise/rotation invariance property, Tables 2 and 3 show that both SIFT and SURF have a significant drop in the number of matched features. SIFT has accuracy less than 66 % in rotation and 60 % in noise for SIFT, where SURF has accuracy less than 38 % and 14 % in the rotation and noise effect respectively. Moreover, by studying the effect of FREAK descriptor with SIFT and SURF, the number of matched features extracted by SIFT-FREAK is almost equal as extracted from reference images with accuracy more than 91 % in both noise and rotation. While combining FREAK with SURF reduces the accuracy to less than 11 % because of the detection of a large number of false positives see (Fig. 3).

Table 1. Reference images

		SIFT	SURF	SIFT-FREAK	SURF-FREAK
Number of features	G1	1877	1047	1695	885
	G2	6743	5840	6269	433
	G3	1359	1000	1200	635
Time (ms)	G1	738.4	184.4	392.2	126.8
	G2	3262.1	853.8	1083.9	432.4
	G3	606.6	192.0	440.8	121.6

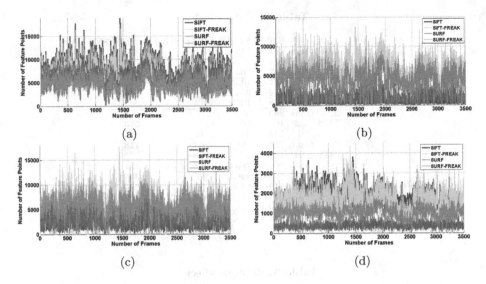

Fig. 1. Number detected feature points from the 2nd dataset; **a:** Reference images, **b:** Gaussian Noise images, **c:** $30°$ Rotated images, **d:** Scaled images

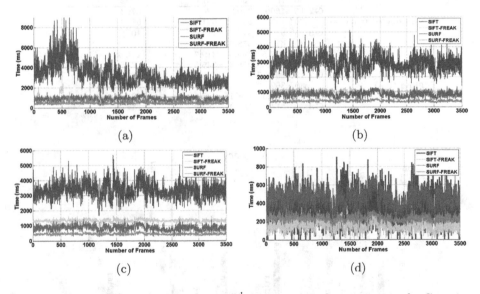

Fig. 2. Processing Time (ms) from the 2nd dataset; **a:** Reference images, **b:** Gaussian Noise images, **c:** $30°$ Rotated images, **d:** Scaled images

Whereas, by comparing the methods in term of time, the SIFT is the slowest in processing time, while SURF-FREAK has the minimum processing time see Tables 2 and 3. However (Fig. 4) shows that the SIFT-FREAK combination has invariance computation time per feature approx. 0.23 ms. For scale invariance

Table 2. Noise effect

			SIFT	SURF	SIFT-FREAK	SURF-FREAK
		Gaus.	251	519	1631	868
	G1	S&P	481	1000	1043	884
		S	247	463	1358	627
		Gaus.	577	1433	6563	1067
Number of featuers	G2	S&P	119	2919	6371	4731
		S	568	1272	6832	4820
		Gaus.	253	551	1276	627
	G3	S&P	103	300	1327	573
		S	243	447	1142	515
		Gaus.	757.5	790.8	319.7	118.4
	G1	S&P	1048.9	278.4	345.5	175.2
		S	766.9	180.5	319.0	121.2
		Gaus.	2908.7	846.6	1067	395.2
Time (ms)	G2	S&P	3626.4	1186.7	1127.8	580.4
		S	2744.8	880.7	1029.7	421.1
		Gaus.	599.3	168.1	280.8	125.3
	G3	S&P	614.5	180.4	282.5	112.7
		S	604.9	171.0	275.9	105.1

Table 3. Rotation effect

			SIFT	SURF	SIFT-FREAK	SURF-FREAK
	G1	15°	735	833	1682	1337
		30°	796	754	1679	1282
	G2	15°	1890	3293	6267	6793
Number of features		30°	1933	3372	6017	5973
	G3	15°	579	645	1128	1041
		30°	619	578	1141	1046
	G1	15°	757.5	790.8	319.7	118.4
		30°	1048.9	278.4	345.5	175.2
	G2	15°	2908.7	846.6	1067	359.2
Time (ms)		30°	3626.3	1186.7	1127.8	580.4
	G3	15°	599.3	168.1	280.8	125.3
		30°	614.5	180.4	282.5	112.7

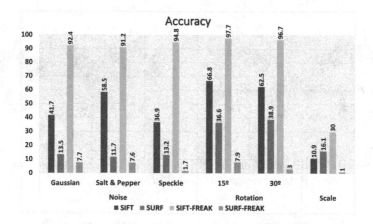

Fig. 3. Accuracy of feature point extraction

Table 4. Scale effect

		SIFT	SURF	SIFT-FREAK	SURF-FREAK
	G1	164	131	484	171
Number of features	G2	1854	375	1662	1033
	G3	165	139	418	133
	G1	447.7	107.5	199.9	83.9
Time (ms)	G2	324.9	455.4	147.1	232.7
	G3	391.9	95.0	177.7	73.7

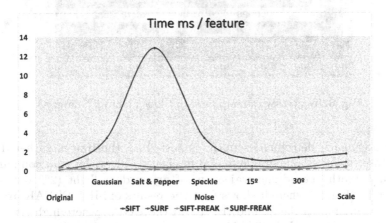

Fig. 4. Time per feature of proposed methods according to image change

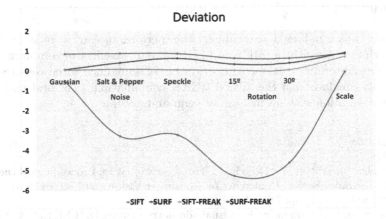

Fig. 5. Deviation of each method against image changes

property, Table 4 and (Fig. 3) show that the four methods have very low accuracy in matching, however SIFT-FREAK combination has the best results.

Finally, (Fig. 5) shows the deviation of each method, at which the SIFT-FREAK has a deviation ratio of 0.0 that means the invariance against image transformation (*Noise, Rotation* and *Scale*), while SURF-FREAK is very sensitive of any small change in the image.

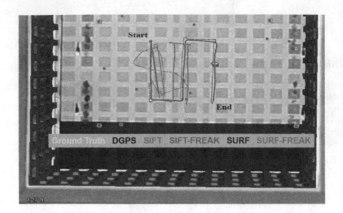

Fig. 6. Trajectory estimation of outdoor flight (2nd dataset)

Moreover, each detector/descriptor is tested on the frames gathered from each dataset using a hompgraphy-based navigation algorithm and compared to the ground truth. The drone trajectory of an outdoor flight (2nd dataset) is presented in (Fig. 6), where it shows that the results of SIFT-FREAK are more accurate compared to the ground truth and the DGPS, where high error rates are generated by the SURF-FREAK.

5   Conclusion

This study was conducted to evaluate the performance of a reliable detection/description algorithms (SIFT and SURF) and the effect of combining with FREAK descriptor for visual navigation system of unmanned aerial vehicles. The experiments conclude that the SIFT-FREAK combination is the best choice for real-time navigation systems in term of time and accuracy.

References

1. Nister, D., Naroditsky, O., Bergen, J.: Visual odometry. In: Proceedings of the 2004 IEEE Computer Society Conference on Computer Vision and Pattern Recognition, CVPR 2004, vol. 1, pp. I-652–I-659 (2004)
2. Scaramuzza, D., Fraundorfer, F.: Visual odometry (Tutorial). IEEE Robot. Autom. Mag. **18**(4), 80–92 (2011)
3. Karlsson, N., Di Bernardo, E., Ostrowski, J., Goncalves, L., Pirjanian, P., Munich, M.E.: The vSLAM algorithm for robust localization and mapping. In: Proceedings of the 2005 IEEE International Conference on Robotics and Automation, ICRA 2005, pp. 24–29 (2005)
4. Lowe, D.G.: Distinctive image features from scale-invariant keypoints. Int. J. Comput. Vis. **60**(2), 91–110 (2004)
5. Bay, H., Tuytelaars, T., Van Gool, L.: SURF: speeded up robust features. In: Leonardis, A., Bischof, H., Pinz, A. (eds.) ECCV 2006, Part I. LNCS, vol. 3951, pp. 404–417. Springer, Heidelberg (2006)

6. Rosten, E., Drummond, T.W.: Machine learning for high-speed corner detection. In: Leonardis, A., Bischof, H., Pinz, A. (eds.) ECCV 2006, Part I. LNCS, vol. 3951, pp. 430–443. Springer, Heidelberg (2006)
7. Agrawal, M., Konolige, K., Blas, M.R.: CenSurE: center surround extremas for realtime feature detection and matching. In: Forsyth, D., Torr, P., Zisserman, A. (eds.) ECCV 2008, Part IV. LNCS, vol. 5305, pp. 102–115. Springer, Heidelberg (2008)
8. Leutenegger, S., Chli, M., Siegwart, R.Y.: BRISK: binary robust invariant scalable keypoints. In: 2011 IEEE International Conference on Computer Vision (ICCV), pp. 2548–2555. IEEE (2011)
9. Calonder, M., Lepetit, V., Strecha, C., Fua, P.: BRIEF: binary robust independent elementary features. In: Daniilidis, K., Maragos, P., Paragios, N. (eds.) ECCV 2010, Part IV. LNCS, vol. 6314, pp. 778–792. Springer, Heidelberg (2010)
10. Rublee, E., Rabaud, V., Konolige, K., Bradski, G.: ORB: an efficient alternative to SIFT or SURF. In: 2011 IEEE International Conference on Computer Vision (ICCV), pp. 2564–2571, November 2011
11. Alahi, A., Ortiz, R., Vandergheynst, P.: FREAK: fast retina keypoint. In: IEEE Conference on Computer Vision and Pattern Recognition (2012)
12. Tuytelaars, T., Mikolajczyk, K.: Local invariant feature detectors: a survey. Found. Trends Comput. Graph. Vis. 3(3), 177–280 (2007)
13. Mikolajczyk, K., Tuytelaars, T., Schmid, C., Zisserman, A., Matas, J., Schaffalitzky, F., Kadir, T., Gool, L.V.: A comparison of affine region detectors. Int. J. Comput. Vis. 65(1–2), 43–72 (2005)
14. Schaeffer, C.: A comparison of keypoint descriptors in the context of pedestrian detection: FREAK vs. SURF vs. BRISK. Citeseer (2013)
15. Schmidt, A., Kraft, M., Fularz, M., Domagala, Z.: The comparison of point feature detectors and descriptors in the context of robot navigation. J. Autom. Mob. Robot. Intell. Syst. 7(1), 11–20 (2013)
16. AR. Drone 2.0. Parrot new wi-fi quadricopter - Civil drone - Parrot. http://ardrone2.parrot.com/. Cited March 2013

Stereo Road Detection Based on Ground Plane

C.H. Rodríguez-Garavito[1,2](✉), J. Carmona-Fernández[1], A. de la Escalera[1],
and J.M. Armingol[1]

[1] Intelligent Systems Laboratory, Universidad Carlos III de Madrid, Madrid, Spain
cesarhernan.rodriguez@alumnos.uc3m.es, jucarmon@ing.ucm3.es,
{escalera,armingol}@ing.ucm3.es
[2] Automation Engineering Department, Universidad de La Salle, Bogotá, Colombia
cerodriguez@unisalle.edu.co

Abstract. This paper presents a robust road perception algorithm
aimed to detect multiple lanes with temporal integration, one of the
most important tasks in Advanced Driver Assistance Systems (*ADAS*).
A new vision-based system is proposed, consisting on three parts: a line
marker detection algorithm, a road line classification and a lane tracking
integration. The goal is to detect the position, type and number of road
lanes. The developed approach is characterized by the use of the bird's
eye view, road marks filtering based on gradient space algorithms, robust
features descriptor for line classification, and road tracking based on time
of life for each detected lane. The road detection is done according to
the Spanish standard IC 8.2. The system was tested on the test platform
IvvI 2.0.

Keywords: Road line detection · Bird eye view

1 Introduction

Since development of computer science and artificial intelligence, one of the most
expected steps to the future has been the autonomous driving. Some of these
researches in this field are the Advanced Driver Assistance Systems, *ADAS*.
Among sensors used in *ADAS*, ones based on computer vision are most spread
given their low cost and due to the fact that all vehicle infrastructure is built
according to human visual perception. The first proposals systems were designed
in 1990s, [1,3], for favourable lighting conditions and simple context scenes such
as highways. They showed similar architecture based on road marks extraction,
normally in Inverse Perspective Mapping or Bird View Perspective, [7], later
a lane detection module is used, which depends on the lane model selected:
linear, parabolic, clothoid, spline or 3D. and tracking lane, [4]. An example of
linear model tracking of road is found in [5], where lanes are detected by Statistic
Hought transform, *SHT* as usually, and a particle filter algorithm is implemented
for tracking process. Nowadays the researches in this field are focus on including concepts such as learning, adaptation and self-tuning algorithms to deal with
challenging conditions in a wide range of traffic scenarios. This paper presents the

© Springer International Publishing Switzerland 2015
R. Moreno-Díaz et al. (Eds.): EUROCAST 2015, LNCS 9520, pp. 748–755, 2015.
DOI: 10.1007/978-3-319-27340-2_92

Road Lane Classification module of the IvvI 2.0 project (Intelligent Vehicle based on Visual Information) inside of the Intelligent System Lab at Carlos III University. [6]. Its goal is to automatically detect the position, type, and number of road lanes with a stereo on-board camera. The article is divided into the following sections: Sect. 2 give the change perspective grounding to *IMP* implementation, Sect. 3 explains how lane and boundary lines are segmented. Section 4 focuses on the algorithms for line description and classification. Section 5 describes the temporal consistency algorithm, and Sect. 6 presents some conclusions for the work.

2   Change Perspective to Bird View

The process begins with the generation of a set of 3D points called point cloud, *PC*, relatively positioned to a reference system on the camera $\{C\}$. The 3D representation is built using a stereo image pair to create a disparity map, then the pixel disparity along the whole image could be associated to a 3D coordinate by triangulation, see Fig. 1, left frame.

2.1   Automatic Extrinsic Extraction from Road Plane

Afterwards, using the *MSAC* [9] algorithm for plane spatial estimation. The parametric plane, $\pi_{(X)} : \overrightarrow{n} \cdot \overrightarrow{p} = h$, is obtained as the most populated in the point cloud scene, this plane is coincident with the road plane, where $\overrightarrow{n}$ is a normal vector to the plane, $\overrightarrow{p}$ is a generic point which belongs to the plane and h is the perpendicular distance from the plane to the camera. Extrinsic camera parameters, pitch (α), roll (σ) and height (h), are extracted from plane representation using the algorithm reported in [8], as shown in Fig. 1, right frame.

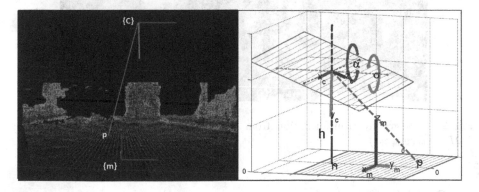

Fig. 1. Left frame: Point Cloud of scene, Right frame: Plane definition.

2.2 Homographic Transform

Now, images could be projected to a more useful perspective, called *"Top view"* or *"Bird view"*, where the lines that define a standard road lane on the highway look parallel. This perpective change is made through an homography transformation.

$$s^cP = {}^cP_s = {}^cH_{bv}{}^{bv}P \tag{1}$$

where, ^{bv}P is the pixel's position in *bird view* perspective image and ^cP_s is the scaled pixel's position in *original camera* perspective image. The homography matrix has three component.

$$^cH_{bv} = K^cT_m{}^mT_{bv}K^{-1} \tag{2}$$

where, K and K^{-1} are the intrinsic matrix and its inverse, ^cT_m is a homogeneous transformation matrix from 3D world to camera pose and $^mT_{bv}$ is a homogeneous transformation matrix from bird view camera pose to world reference system.

$$^cT_m = \left[Rot_x\left(\frac{\pi}{2} - \alpha\right) Rot_{y'}(-\sigma) \mid \begin{bmatrix} 0 \\ 0 \\ h \end{bmatrix} \right], ^mT_{bv} = \left[Rot_x(\pi) \mid \begin{bmatrix} x_{bv} \\ y_{bv} \\ z_{bv} \end{bmatrix} \right] \tag{3}$$

The bird view camera pose's position $[x_{bv}, y_{bv}, z_{bv}]$ allows to change the region of interest where the image in top view is projected in, see Fig. 2.

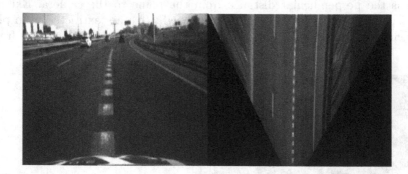

Fig. 2. Homography transformation from road image into bird view, right frame: $ROI_{bv}(x_{bv}, y_{bv}, z_{bv})$.

3 Road Segmentation

Subsequent steps are performed on image in top view. The process continues with road markings detection in accordance with standard *IC 8.2* [2]. In order to avoid distortion induced by wrong transformed points, which do not belong to the road plane, a free space mask is defined, restricting pixels whose 3D position lies within a distance threshold from the road plane.

3.1 Road Markings Mask

The road lines and lanes will be detected over a road marks mask. This mask is the result of applying a filter base on gradient space. Set of points, $p_k(i,j)$, $k = 0, 1, \ldots, n$ whose head and end point gradient match the template approach given in (4), are identified as candidates for belonging to road lines, as shown in Fig. 3.

$$|\|\nabla p_0\| - \|\nabla p_n\|\| < \epsilon_m, |\angle\nabla p_0 + \angle\nabla p_n| < \epsilon_a, |\|p_0 - p_n\| - w_{rm}| < \epsilon_w \qquad (4)$$

where the parameter road mark width, w_{rm}, is set according to the virtual camera height, z_{bv}, previously used in perspective change. ϵ_m, ϵ_a and ϵ_w, are chosen small enough because process noise.

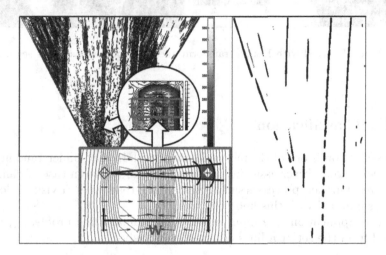

Fig. 3. Left frame: gradient template approach. Right frame: road line mask in bird view perspective, RM.

3.2 Road Lines and Lanes Detection

Once the region of interest, where road marks are, has been defined, line detection based on Hough transformation is performed.

3.3 Identification of Lanes on the Road in Adjacent Fashion

The set of lines extracted does not provide information of the road until it is properly interpreted. To do so, an histogram of line angles is created, where the highest rate identifies the predominant direction of the lanes on the road (ϕ_R). In order to build a road structure, all pairs of lines, l (hereinafter lane), are constrained to be parallel, have an orientation equal to ϕ_R and have a normal distance in the range of tolerance, w_l. The set of fitting lanes is then stored according to an adjacency and no redundancy rule. See Fig. 4.

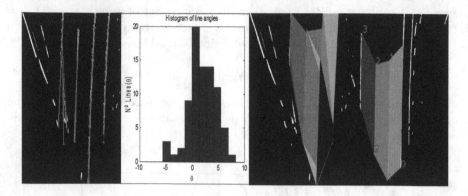

Fig. 4. Lines detected with Hough transform and non-consecutive lanes segmented.

4   Line Classification

Line classification is one of the most important task in road understanding. This information allows driver assistant system detect and warn in case of dangerous manoeuvres. Further, processes such as tracking of road lanes or visual odometry could be simplified with this knowledge.

For this application, the input classifier is a binary line profile, $\mathcal{P}_i$, that is extracted from the set of n lines detected previously.

$$\mathcal{P}_i(t) = RM(l_i(t)) \tag{5}$$

$$l_i(t) = (lenght(line_i) - t)P0_i + tP1_i \tag{6}$$

where $i = 1, 2, \ldots, \#$ detected lines, and $t \in \mathbb{R}$, $t = 1, 2, \ldots, lenght(line_i)$, $P0_i$ and $P1_i$ are the head and end points of line i^{th}.

4.1   Descriptor

The descriptor chosen in this case is based on a mix of features in both spatial and frequency domain. The two first features are the mean value, $\overline{\mathcal{P}_i}$, of the ith line profile, and its length measured in meters, $\|\mathcal{P}_i\|$. The other features correspond to the frequencies of the three first power peaks, in descendent order $Peaks_j(\mathcal{F}(\mathcal{P}_i))$, $j = 1, 2, 3$. See Fig. 5.

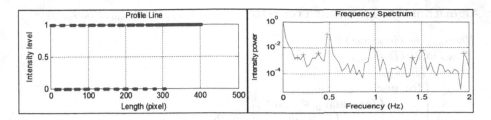

Fig. 5. Space and frequency descriptor line.

4.2 Classifier

The decision rules are obtained by analysing a collection of eight thousand of sample lines, manually labelled as Solid, dashed, merge and unknown lines, along with their corresponding space and frequency spectrum.

$$\omega_1 : \sum_{j=1}^{3} Peaks_j(\mathcal{F}(\mathcal{P}_i)) - 0.5 < 0.05$$
$$\omega_2 : \overline{\mathcal{P}_i} > 0.4 \wedge \overline{\mathcal{P}_i} < 0.8$$
$$\omega_3 : \|\mathcal{P}_i\| > 3\|dls\|$$
$$\omega_4 : \overline{\mathcal{P}_i} > 0.52$$
$$\omega_5 : \|\mathcal{P}_i\| > \|dls\|$$
$$\omega_6 : \overline{\mathcal{P}_i} > 0.2 \wedge \overline{\mathcal{P}_i} < 0.52$$
$$\omega_7 : \|\mathcal{P}_i\| > 2\|dls\| \wedge \|\mathcal{P}_i\| < 3.3\|dls\|$$

$$C_1 : \omega_1 \wedge \omega_2 \wedge \omega_3 \Rightarrow \text{ then merge line}$$
$$C_2 : \neg C_1 \wedge \omega_4 \Rightarrow \text{ then solid line}$$
$$C_3 : \neg C_2 \wedge (\omega_5 \wedge \omega_6) \vee (\omega_7 \wedge \neg \omega_5) \Rightarrow \text{ then dashed line}$$

Where $\sum$ mean OR logic operator, and *dls* is the lenght of dashed line segment.

5 Temporal Consistency

Finally, a temporary lane filtering is done based on updating two lane road structures: $Road_{mem}$, $Road_{new}$. The current structure road detection, $Road_{now}$, allows the lanes to be added or deleted according to the detections history, thus, the algorithm increase its reliability against occlusions and spurious noise generated by other vehicle's movement on the field of view and deformation induced by objects that do not belong to the road plane, upon which the algorithm is based.

Algorithm 5.1. TEMPORAL CONSISTENCY($Road_{now}$, $Road_{mem}$, $Road_{new}$)

$Road_{now} \leftarrow Capture()$
if $Is\_empty\,(Road_{mem})$
   then $\{Road_{mem} \leftarrow Road_{now}$
      for each $i \in Road_{mem}$
         for each $j \in Road_{now}$
            do $\begin{cases} \textbf{if } Road_{mem}\,(i) \approx Road_{now}\,(j) \\ \textbf{then} \begin{cases} Road_{mem}\,(i) \leftarrow Road_{now}\,(j) \\ Inc\,(Road_{mem}(i).LifeTime) \\ Set\_true\,(Road_{mem}(i).change) \\ Inc\,(cnt\_match\_mem(j)) \end{cases} \end{cases}$

      do $\begin{cases} \textbf{if } Is\_true(Road_{mem}\,(i)\,.change) \\ \textbf{then} \begin{cases} Set\_false(Road_{mem}\,(i)\,.change) \\ Inc\,(Road_{mem}\,(i)\,.LifeTime) \end{cases} \\ \textbf{else } Predict\,(Road_{mem}\,(i)) \\ Dec(Road_{mem}(i).LifeTime) \end{cases}$

      if $Is\_zero\,(First\,(Road_{mem})\,.LifeTime)$
         then $Remove\,(First\,(Road_{mem})\,.LifeTime)$
      if $Is\_zero\,(Last\,(Road_{mem})\,.LifeTime)$
         then $Remove\,(Last\,(Road_{mem})\,.LifeTime)$
      for each $i \in Road_{now}$
         for each $j \in Road_{new}$
            do $\begin{cases} \textbf{if} \begin{cases} Road_{now}\,(i) \approx Road_{new}\,(j) \wedge \\ Is\_zero\,(cnt\_match\_mem(i)) \end{cases} \\ \textbf{then} \begin{cases} Set\_true(Road_{now}(i).change) \\ Road_{new}(j) \leftarrow Road_{now}(i) \\ Inc(Road_{new}(j).LifeTime) \\ Inc\,(cnt\_match\_new(i)) \end{cases} \end{cases}$

else $\begin{cases}$

      do $\begin{cases} \textbf{if} \begin{cases} Is\_zero\,(cnt\_match\_new(i)) \wedge \\ Is\_zero\,(cnt\_match\_mem(i)) \end{cases} \\ \textbf{then} \begin{cases} Set\_true(Road_{now}(i).change) \\ Insert(Road_{new}, Road\_now(i)) \end{cases} \end{cases}$

      $Empty(cnt\_match\_new)$
      $Empty(cnt\_match\_mem)$
      for each $i \in Road_{new}$
         do $\begin{cases} \textbf{if } Is\_true(Road_{new}(i).change) \\ \textbf{then } Set\_false(Road_{new}(i).change) \\ \textbf{else } Dec(Road_{new}(i).LifeTime) \\ \textbf{if} \begin{cases} Is\_max(Road_{new}(i).LifeTime) \wedge \\ (Is\_join(Road_{new}(i), First(Road_{mem})) \vee \\ Is\_join(Road_{new}(i), Last(Road_{mem}))) \end{cases} \\ \textbf{then} \begin{cases} Flood(Road_{new}(i).LifeTime) \\ Insert(Road_{mem}, Road_{new}(i)) \end{cases} \\ \textbf{else } Remove(Road_{new}(i)) \end{cases}$

Acknowledgments. This work was supported by automation engineering department from de La Salle University, Bogotá-Colombia; Administrative Department of Science, Technology and Innovation (COLCIENCIAS), Bogotá-Colombia and the Spanish Government through the CICYT projects (TRA2013-48314-C3-1-R) and (TRA2011-29454-C03-02) and Comunidad de Madrid through SEGVAUTO_TRIES ($S2013/MIT - 2713$).

References

1. Bertozzi, M., Broggi, A.: Gold: a parallel real-time stereo vision system for generic obstacle and lane detection. IEEE Trans. Image Process. **7**(1), 62–81 (1998)
2. de Carreteras, I.: 8.2 ic marcas viales. (1987)
3. Crisman, J.D., Thorpe, C.E.: Scarf: a color vision system that tracks roads and intersections. IEEE Trans. Robot. Autom. **9**(1), 49–58 (1993)
4. Felisa, M., Zani, P.: Robust monocular lane detection in urban environments. In: 2010 IEEE Intelligent Vehicles Symposium (IV), pp. 591–596. IEEE (2010)
5. Liu, G., Worgotter, F., Markelic, I.: Combining statistical hough transform and particle filter for robust lane detection and tracking. In: 2010 IEEE Intelligent Vehicles Symposium (IV), pp. 993–997. IEEE (2010)
6. Martín, D., García, F., Musleh, B., Olmeda, D., Peláez, G., Marín, P., Ponz, A., Rodríguez, C., Al-Kaff, A., De La Escalera, A., et al.: Ivvi 2.0: an intelligent vehicle based on computational perception. Expert Syst. Appl. **41**(17), 7927–7944 (2014)
7. Muad, A.M., Hussain, A., Samad, S.A., Mustaffa, M.M., Majlis, B.Y.: Implementation of inverse perspective mapping algorithm for the development of an automatic lane tracking system. In: 2004 IEEE Region 10 Conference TENCON 2004, pp. 207–210. IEEE (2004)
8. Rodríguez-Garavito, C., Ponz, A., García, F., Martín, D., de la Escalera, A., Armingol, J.: Automatic laser and camera extrinsic calibration for data fusion using road plane. In: 2014 17th International Conference on Information Fusion (FUSION), pp. 1–6. IEEE (2014)
9. Torr, P.H., Zisserman, A.: Mlesac: a new robust estimator with application to estimating image geometry. Comput. Vis. Image Underst. **78**(1), 138–156 (2000)

Clustering Traffic Flow Patterns by Fuzzy C-Means Method: Some Preliminary Findings

Mehmet Ali Silgu[✉] and Hilmi Berk Celikoglu

Department of Civil Engineering,
Technical University of Istanbul (ITU), Istanbul, Turkey
{msilgu, celikoglu}@itu.edu.tr

Abstract. In this paper, performance of fuzzy c-means clustering method in specifying flow patterns, which are reconstructed by a macroscopic flow model, is sought using microwave radar data on fundamental variables of traffic flow. Traffic flow is simulated by the cell transmission model adopting a two-phase triangular fundamental diagram. Flow dynamics specific to the selected freeway test stretch are used to determine prevailing traffic conditions. The performance of fuzzy c-means clustering is evaluated in two cases, with two assumptions. The procedure fuzzy clustering method follows is systematically dynamic that enables the clustering, and hence partitions, over the fundamental diagram specific to selected temporal resolution. It is seen that clustering simulation with dynamic pattern boundary assumption performs better for almost all the steps of data expansion when considered to simulation with the corresponding static case.

Keywords: Vehicular traffic flow · Flow pattern · Clustering · Fuzzy C-Means

1 Introduction

In this paper, performance of fuzzy c-means (FCM) clustering method in specifying flow patterns, which are reconstructed by a macroscopic flow model, is sought using microwave radar data on fundamental variables of traffic flow.

The literature on the effort to quantify flow conditions, as either a service level or by a macroscopic fundamental diagram, and input to local and/or global traffic network-wide management implementations (see for example [1–4]) has been our motivation to classify dynamically the flow patterns in the form of a fundamental diagram scatter and to signify the consequent temporal changes on flow in order to capture flow pattern variations, especially in cases of non-recurrent effects on traffic.

Pattern, or alternatively state, specification is generally described as to estimate flow variables along a road stretch with an adequate spatial resolution at each time instant based on a limited amount of available measurements, for example by detectors, where pattern variables are the flows, space-mean speeds and densities [5]. Volume or flow as a single variable is insufficient to exactly specify any pattern since a certain value of volume or flow corresponds to two distinct density and speed pairs in two completely different flow conditions, i.e., congested and un-congested, when the existence of a linear dependency between speed and flow is assumed. In the present study, we have utilized

© Springer International Publishing Switzerland 2015
R. Moreno-Díaz et al. (Eds.): EUROCAST 2015, LNCS 9520, pp. 756–764, 2015.
DOI: 10.1007/978-3-319-27340-2_93

the variables of traffic flow in order to obtain the fundamental diagrams and considered density as the pattern indicator. These variables are reconstructed as the resultants from a macroscopic traffic simulation that adopts the cell transmission theory [6] for flow modeling. Though the ultimate aim in our research is to capture the time to time considerable changes on flow states within an overall frame composed of flow modeling, pattern classifying and pattern variation analysis as in [7, 8], the present study concentrates on the classification performance of fuzzy c-means clustering method applied directly to simulated data.

In the following, the traffic pattern classification problem and the relevant literature are summarized. The fuzzy c-means method employed to obtain clustering is explained in the third section. The fourth section presents results of the analyses conducted and consequent discussions. The final section concludes the paper with possible future research directions.

2   Relevant Literature

The terms classification and clustering are used disconcertedly in the relevant literature. By definition, clustering analysis is the organization of a collection of patterns, usually represented as a vector of measurements, or a point in a multidimensional space, into clusters based on similarity [9]. Clustering has been employed within a wide range of analysis including pattern analysis, grouping, decision-making, data mining, image segmentation, and pattern classification. In case there is little prior information available on data and there has to be made a number of assumptions about the data, a clustering method is appropriate in part for the exploration of relationships among the data points to figure out their structure. A typical pattern clustering involves: i- pattern representation (optionally including feature extraction and/or selection); ii- definition of a pattern proximity measure appropriate to the data domain; and iii- clustering or grouping [10].

Since a careful investigation of the available features and any available transformations can yield significantly improved clustering results, we've analyzed flow patterns by coupling variables of traffic as in the representation of the fundamental diagrams of traffic flow in a number of our previous works [7, 8, 11]. Previously, we've proposed a dynamic flow pattern classification procedure [7] for the traffic simulated by the original cell transmission model (CTM) adopting a two-phase fundamental diagram that is further extended to analyze in details the wave propagation employing a discrete approximation to the CTM for making use of the multiple mode of flow conditions and transitions within them [8]. We've further employed a non-hierarchical multivariate clustering method to classify traffic flow patterns simulated in [7]. Considering both the dynamic approach proposed [7, 8] and the multivariate clustering [11] that is dynamic due to its structure, we've comparatively evaluated the relative performance of these methods by re-simulating the overall modeling and classification process with transferring the level of service measures in [12].

3 Flow Pattern Specification Process

The flow pattern classification procedure is adopted by simplifying the approach in [7]. The overall procedure involves two sub-processes succeeding the pre-process of noisy traffic flow measurements. The flow modeling follows the noise removal and incorporates a discrete approximation to a simple continuum model of macroscopic approach that adopts a two-phase triangular fundamental diagram under stationary and spatially homogeneous equilibrium conditions.

Since the ultimate aim of the present study is to evaluate the classification performance of fuzzy clustering method on flow patterns in a dynamic fashion, the time-dependent densities of freeway test stretch are matched on the partitioned fundamental diagram. Filtered and simulated flow data is clustered alternating the temporal resolution through 2 min to 24 h. In order to comparatively evaluate the performance of fuzzy clustering approach, an example by re-simulating the overall process with transferring the level of service measures [12] is provided.

3.1 Traffic Flow Simulation Process

For modeling, we follow the fluid dynamics approach to theory of continuous vehicular traffic flow, defined upon the variables of flow-rate, q, density, ρ, and speed, u, and referred to as the LWR theory [13, 14]. This theory assumes that flow is strictly a function of density, $q = Q(\rho)$, and consequently speed is strictly a function of density, $u = U(\rho)$. The LWR model can be described by a single partial differential equation in conservation form as given by Eq. 1 or alternatively as given by Eq. 2,

$$\frac{\partial \rho}{\partial t} + \frac{\partial (\rho \cdot U\rho)}{\partial x} = 0 \tag{1}$$

$$\frac{\partial \rho}{\partial t} + \left(C(\rho) \cdot \frac{\partial \rho}{\partial x} \right) = 0 \tag{2}$$

where; $C(\rho) = (\partial Q(\rho))/\partial \rho$. The LWR theory expresses that slight fluctuations in flow are propagated upstream along kinematic waves, where the speed is given by $c = C(\rho)$, such as the slope of flow-density curve. Given the appropriate boundary conditions, solution to this model can be obtained by determining the function $\rho(x, t)$, where x and t represent space and time respectively. Different variations of the macroscopic model given by Eq. 2 can be characterized by the speed-density relationship $u = U(\rho)$ and, consequently, by the adopted fundamental diagram.

In order to obtain a convergent approximation to the continuous LWR model, we utilize the discrete cell transmission approach of Daganzo [11] that adopts a two-phase simplified fundamental diagram, in which u_{ff} is the free-flow speed, u_{cong} is the backward wave propagation speed in congestion, ρ_{jam} is the jamming density, ρ_{opt} is the optimum density and q_{max} is the capacity. The CTM divides the freeway into sections called 'cells' where traffic flow entering a cell bounded by points s and s + 1, is considered to be constant between two successive times t and t + Δt and is determined by Eq. 3 [11].

$$q^{s,s+1}(t) = \min\left\{\left(u_{ff}^{s-1,s} \cdot \rho^{s-1,s}(t)\right), \left(u_{cong}^{s,s+1} \cdot \left(\rho_{jam}^{s,s+1} - \rho^{s,s+1}(t)\right)\right), \left(q_{max}^{s,s+1}\right)\right\}$$

(3)

Here; $\rho^{s,s+1}(t)$ is the average density of cell s, s + 1 between times t and t + Δt, $\rho_{jam}^{s,s+1}$ is the jamming density of cell s, s + 1, $u_{ff}^{s-1,s}$ is the free flow speed in cell s − 1, s, $u_{cong}^{s,s+1}$ is the congestion wave speed in cell s, s + 1, and $q_{max}^{s,s+1}$ is the capacity of cell s, s + 1. Considering the prevailing phase speeds and densities, Eq. 3 determines the flow on each section for each time interval Δt.

The flow modeling component uses the procedure explained above for the real-time simulation of actual traffic dynamics and the consequent reconstruction of section performances. The real-time reconstruction of flow variables are sequentially used to update and partition the fundamental diagrams of speed-flow and flow-density at each computation time interval, as explained in the following.

3.2 Flow Pattern Classification by Fuzzy C-Means Clustering

The dynamic classification approach in [7] is analogous to the level of service concept with a pre-defined pattern class number but differing in terms of bounding density measures all of which change temporally throughout the simulation. In order to obtain a consistent comparative evaluation with the static case, transferring level of service boundaries in [12], we set the user-defined class number to six, as presented in the comparative evaluations in [7, 8]. In each time step, dynamic segmentation on the fundamental diagram is updated by the fuzzy clustering considering the critical values of flow and density and partitioning the current density range into classes upon user-defined rules.

3.2.1 Fuzzy C-Means Clustering Method
A large family of fuzzy clustering algorithms is based on minimization of the fuzzy c-means functional that is formulated as given by Eq. (4) [13–15]:

$$J(\mathbf{Z}; \mathbf{U}, \mathbf{V}) = \sum_{i=1}^{c} \sum_{k=1}^{N} (\mu_{ik})^m \| \mathbf{z}_k - \mathbf{v}_i \|_A^2$$

(4)

where;

$$U = [\mu_{ik}] \in M_{fc}$$

(5)

is a fuzzy partition matrix of Z,

$$\mathbf{V} = [\mathbf{v}_1, \mathbf{v}_2, \ldots, \mathbf{v}_c], \mathbf{v}_i \in \mathbb{R}^n \tag{6}$$

is a vector of cluster prototypes, which have to be determined,

$$D_{ik\mathbf{A}}^2 = \| \mathbf{z}_k - \mathbf{v}_i \|_\mathbf{A}^2 = (\mathbf{z}_k - \mathbf{v}_i)^T A (\mathbf{z}_k - \mathbf{v}_i) \tag{7}$$

is a squared inner-product distance norm, and

$$m \in [1, \infty) \tag{8}$$

is a parameter which determines the fuzziness of the resulting clusters.

3.2.2   Fuzzy C-Means Algorithm

The basic version of fuzzy c-means clustering can be arranged in four steps following [15]. Given the data set Z, choose the number of clusters $1 < c < N$, the weighting exponent $m > 1$, the termination tolerance $\varepsilon > 0$ and the norm-inducing matrix A. Initialize the partition matrix randomly, such that $U^{(0)} \in M_{\mathrm{fc}}$.

(1) Compute the cluster prototypes (means):

$$\mathbf{v}_i^{(l)} = \frac{\sum_{k=1}^{N} (\mu_{ik}^{(l-1)})^m \mathbf{z}_k}{\sum_{k=1}^{N} (\mu_{ik}^{(l-1)})^m}, 1 \leq i \leq c. \tag{9}$$

(2) Compute the distances:

$$D_{ik\mathbf{A}}^2 = \left(\mathbf{z}_k - \mathbf{v}_i^{(l)} \right)^T A \left(\mathbf{z}_k - \mathbf{v}_i^{(l)} \right), \tag{10}$$

$$1 \leq i \leq c, 1 \leq k \leq N.$$

(3) Update the partition matrix:

$$\text{For } 1 \leq k \leq N;$$
$$\text{if } D_{ik\mathbf{A}} > 0 \text{ for all } i = 1, 2, \ldots, c$$
$$\mu_{ik}^{(l)} = \frac{1}{\sum_{j=1}^{c} (D_{ik\mathbf{A}}/D_{jk\mathbf{A}})^{2/(m-1)}} \tag{11}$$

Otherwise;

$$\mu_{ik}^{(l)} = 0 \text{ if } D_{ik\mathbf{A}} > 0, \text{ and } \mu_{ik}^{(l)} \in [0, 1] \text{ with } \sum_{i=1}^{c} \mu_{ik}^{(l)} = 1 \tag{12}$$

(4) Repeat until

$$\| \mathbf{U}^{(l)} - \mathbf{U}^{(l-1)} \| < \varepsilon \tag{13}$$

The parameters, i.e., the number of clusters, "c", the 'fuzziness' exponent, "m", the termination tolerance "ε", and the norm-inducing matrix "A", the fuzzy partition matrix "U" have to be initialized prior to employing the FCM algorithm [15]. The FCM algorithm stops iterating when the norm of the difference between U in two successive iterations is smaller than the termination parameter ε and the shape of a cluster is determined by the choice of the matrix A in the distance measure, given by Eq. (7) [15]. A common choice is A = I, that is the standard Euclidean norms given by Eq. (14) [15];

$$D_{ik\mathbf{A}}^2 = (\mathbf{z}_k - \mathbf{v}_i)^T (\mathbf{z}_k - \mathbf{v}_i) \tag{14}$$

4 Numerical Implementations Using Fuzzy C-Means Clustering

In order to obtain a consistent comparative evaluation with the static case, the user-defined class number is set to six. Fuzziness parameter, termination tolerance and norm- induce matrix are relatively selected as 2, 0.00001 and A = I considering [16].

In order to comparatively evaluate the clustering performances of fuzzy method on lane-based densities relative to deterministic clustering, a number of statistical criteria, including the root mean squared error (RMSE), the mean square error (MSE), the mean absolute error (MAE), and the mean absolute percentage error (MAPE), [17] is calculated using the fuzzy centroid displacement information with the corresponding static centroid figures.

The performances of fuzzy c- means clustering are evaluated in two cases, with two assumptions. First is the case that static centroids for deterministic HCM method is assumed, and referred to SHCM, where: i- Each level of service is accepted as a cluster; ii- Centroids are calculated by subtracting the boundary values of the LOS; and iii- the result is divided into two [18]. Second case assumes dynamic centroids for deterministic HCM method and, is referred to DHCM, where: i- Each level of service is accepted as a cluster; ii- Mean for each level of service is calculated; and iii- the previous step is repeated for each loading [18]. In the light of the information given on computing centroids for level of service, the boundaries are defined in Highway Capacity Manual – 2010 [12].

The RMSE measure is provided figure out the difference between values obtained by the FCM and the values actually resulted from the clustering that is being modelled. Figure 1 shows the variation of RMSE measure for fuzzy c-means clustering with the corresponding DHMC and SHMC respectively.

Figure 2 shows the variations of MAE and MSE measures for fuzzy c-means clustering with the corresponding DHMC and SHMC respectively.

Figure 3 shows the variation of MAPE measure for fuzzy c-means clustering with the corresponding DHMC and SHMC respectively.

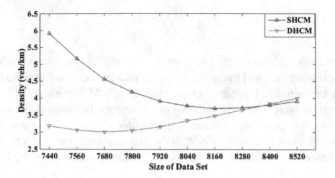

Fig. 1. Variations of RMSE on Fuzzy C- Means clustering

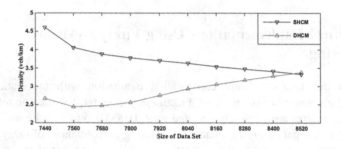

Fig. 2. Variations of MAE on Fuzzy C- Means clustering

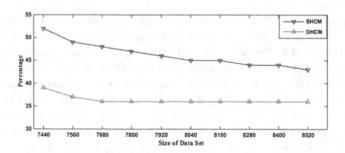

Fig. 3. Variations of MAPE on Fuzzy C- Means clustering

5 Conclusions

The aim of the current study has been to employ and comparatively evaluate the
performance of fuzzy c-means clustering in helping to capture flow state variations over
the fundamental diagram of traffic flow. On this purpose the dynamic classification

performance of fuzzy clustering method is investigated using outputs of a traffic simulation model run with the point measurement data over a freeway segment.

Fuzzy c-means clustering which is dynamic due to its processing nature, is separately applied to cluster flow conditions that are simulated by a macroscopic traffic flow model. The comparative evaluation is presented considering the static level of service classification approach in Highway Capacity Manual.

It is straight to conclude from the comparative evaluations provided that the FCM clustering when compared to DHCM performs better than when compared to SHCM throughout the simulation where each clustering simulation step stands as a step of data set's expansion. Investigating the classification performance of FCM on traffic flow patterns reproduced by an elaborated CTM extension, as in [8], and in comparison to existing multivariate clustering techniques are the possible future research directions that the present preliminary study motivates.

Acknowledgments. The authors would like to thank Onur Deniz for contributions in coding.

References

1. Daganzo, C.F.: Urban gridlock: macroscopic modeling and mitigation approaches. Transp. Res. Part B: Methodol. **41**(1), 49–62 (2007)
2. Geroliminis, N., Daganzo, C.F.: Existence of urban-scale macroscopic fundamental diagrams: some experimental findings. Transp. Res. Part B: Methodol. **42**(9), 759–770 (2008)
3. Lu, X.-Y., Varaiya, P., Horowitz, R., Skabardonis, A.: Fundamental diagram modeling and analysis based NGSIM data. In: 12th IFAC Symposium on Control in Transportation Systems, Redondo Beach California (2009)
4. Dervisoglu, D., Gomes, G., Kwon, J., Horowitz, R., Varaiya, P.: Automatic calibration of the fundamental diagram and empirical observations on capacity. In: 88th Annual Meeting of the Transportation Research Board, Washington, D.C. (2009)
5. Wang, Y., Papageorgiou, M., Messmer, A.: Real-time freeway traffic state estimation based on extended kalman filter: a case study. Transp. Sci. **41**(2), 167–181 (2007)
6. Daganzo, C.F.: The cell transmission model: a dynamic representation of highway traffic consistent with the hydrodynamic theory. Transp. Res. Part B: Methodol. **28**(4), 269–287 (1994)
7. Celikoglu, H.B.: An approach to dynamic classification of traffic flow patterns. Comput. Aided Civ. Infrastruct. Eng. **28**(4), 273–288 (2013)
8. Celikoglu, H.B.: Dynamic classification of traffic flow patterns simulated by a multi-mode discrete cell transmission model. IEEE Trans. Intell. Transp. Syst. **15**(6), 2539–2550 (2014)
9. Jain, A.K., Murty, M.N., Flynn, P.J.: Data clustering: a review. ACM Comput. Surv. **31**(3), 264–323 (1999)
10. Jain, A.K., Dubes, R.C.: Algorithms for Clustering Data. Prentice Hall, College Div. (1988)
11. Silgu, M.A., Celikoglu, H.B.: K-means clustering method to classify freeway traffic flow patterns. Pamukkale J. Eng. Sci. **20**(6), 232–239 (2014)
12. Highway Capacity Manual 2010, Transportation Research Board of the National Academies (2010)

13. Dunn, J.C.: A fuzzy relative of the ISODATA process and its use in detecting compact well-separated clusters. J. Cybern. **3**(3), 32–57 (1974)
14. Bezdek, J.C.: Pattern Recognition with Fuzzy Objective Function Algorithms. Kluwer Academic Press, New York (1981)
15. Babuska, R.: Fuzzy clustering algorithms with applications to rule extraction. In: Sczepaniak, P.S., et al. (eds.) Fuzzy Systems in Medicine, pp. 139–173. Springer, Heidelberg (2000)
16. Pal, N.R., Bezdek, J.: On cluster validity for the fuzzy c-means model. IEEE Trans. Fuzzy Syst. **3**(3), 370–379 (1995)
17. Spiegel, M.R., Stephens, L.J.: Schaum's Outline of Statistics, 4th edn. McGraw Hill, New York (2011)
18. Silgu, M.A.: Multivariate and fuzzy clustering approaches to dynamic classification of traffic flow states. M.Sc. thesis submitted to Istanbul Technical University Graduate School of Science Engineering and Technology (2015)

Platoon Driving Intelligence. A Survey

Samuel Romero Santana[✉], Javier J. Sanchez-Medina,
and Enrique Rubio-Royo

CICEI – ULPGC, Las Palmas, Spain
sam_r_s@hotmail.com, javier.sanchez@ulpgc.es, rubio@cicei.com

1 Introduction

Mobility is a crucial element for this century's societies. We are at a crossroad where the two most important and challenging goals are:

- Safety
- Sustainability:

According to the European Commission, in 2011, more than 30000 people died on the roads. Even worse, "For every death on Europe's roads there are an estimated 4 permanently disabling injuries such as damage to the brain or spinal cord, 8 serious injuries and 50 minor injuries".

These are terrible numbers that we must fight as researchers.

Regarding Sustainability, we must rush to drastically cut down the environmental impact of mobility, probably through brave investments in Clean Energies. This may be also linked to a progressive but firm global move towards transportation electrification.

The United Nations includes *"Ensure environmental sustainability"* in the Eight Goals for 2015, within the Millenium Development Goals ([1]). Back in 1992 the European Commission in its "Green Paper on the impact of transport on the environment - A Community strategy for sustainable mobility" ([2]) recommends:

> *"Traffic management schemes in areas most vulnerable congestion and the introduction of advanced telematics to improve efficiency of transport operations"*

In a tight relationship to these two goals, in the last 20 years many research groups all around the world have carried out extensive research on platoon driving or Platooning. To many, that will be an essential part of future driving, where automated driving will play a central role.

In a few words, automated vehicles will hooked in raws to circulate at high speeds through highways. Their occupants will delegate the driving tasks to a fully automated system that will use Vehicle to Vehicle (V2V) and Vehicle to Infrastructure (V2I) systems to keep a small distance between cars and a high speed in a very efficient way.

This approach to high-speed driving will bring lots of benefits. The energy consumption and the consequent environmental impact will be lower, mainly

© Springer International Publishing Switzerland 2015
R. Moreno-Díaz et al. (Eds.): EUROCAST 2015, LNCS 9520, pp. 765–772, 2015.
DOI: 10.1007/978-3-319-27340-2_94

because of a highly efficient management of the platoon speed and the reduction of air drag that circulating close behind another vehicle yields.

Human factors will not play any role regarding safety because human will not need to operate any controls during the platooning stage.

Finally, while circulating in a so tight platoon, with a very reduced distance between cars, a huge saving of space is obtained. In other words, it will mean a much more efficient use of the current highways, probably alleviating traffic jams and congestion. Plus, the resulting contention on construction pace of new traffic infrastructures will be also beneficial.

The general philosophy of such systems can be summarized as follows: The leader car, the first car in the platoon, will be driven by a professional driver, at least until this task can be done automatically. Each vehicle will be equipped with sensors and intelligence to measure the distance with its predecessor, speed, and heading. There will be safe procedures for vehicles to join or leave the platoon. The platoon leader will manage speed, and it will be able to take decisions that will affect to the rest of vehicles.

To ensure a very small vehicle to vehicle gap it is necessary a good communication between the vehicles in the platoon. So the information flow efficiency is of utmost importance, sharing data as position, speed, acceleration, and heading. We can read about the importance of this variables at [3,4].

Another important factor that must be taken into account is the braking, acceleration and stirring control systems. They must be extremely fast, precise and safe. They must be specially regarding collision avoidance intelligence. We can read a good research about it at ([5]). Any failure in this sense may be disastrous. between vehicles of the platoon, or with other external vehicles trying to control the formation like a set.

Thus, extremely sophisticated algorithms, that take into account a wide range of scenarios, number of lanes, weather, intersections, etc., has to be employed (We can read more about this sophisticated methods in [6]).

In the rest of this paper we will discuss the intelligence of such algorithms, classifying a number of works regarding how research groups deal with Intersections, Communications, Platooning Control and Safety, to end with some comments on Future Directions of this research area.

This paper has been divided in these four sections because they are four basic areas in platoon driving researches, where the improvement of one of them makes better to the others. A fluid Communication is fundamental to keep a good formation, sharing information while the section Platooning Control try to keep the formation and apply math algorithms to face up to Special Situations like overtaking or intersections where the platoon has to take a crucial decision in a few time, putting the formation at risk. Finally, in these situations must exist Safety Systems that should act whether things don't occur how they had been planned.

2 Intersections

Intersections are one of the most complex driving scenarios for autonomous vehicles. Nowadays, many of the black points in our streets are our intersections. When a platoon of autonomous vehicles follow a leader approaches the intersection, the convoy has to take a decision quickly to cross the intersection safely. Some of these decisions could be to stop at the intersection, to cross the intersection keeping the convoy or to split the convoy to avoid a collision (Fig. 1).

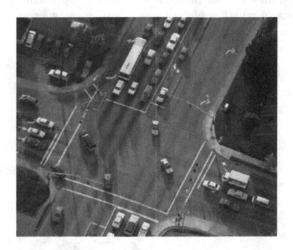

Fig. 1. Intersection

There are two kinds of intersections; Signalized and unsignalized intersections.

A signalized intersection is controlled by traffic lights. Whereas the second type does not include signalizing lights and is called unsignalized Intersection.

At unsignalized intersection, the safety demands a system which alert to convoy about, positions, speed, accelerations of other vehicles or convoys that come to the same place, to take a good decision in real time. It is possible to find information about communications in real time at [7]. On the other hand if a convoy try to cross a signalized intersection, the convoy should have some information to know if it can pass in time, stop, or split the convoy in two sets.

Today, there are some solutions to these problems. One of them is to implement a system at the intersection which gives information to the convoy leader. Reducing queues at intersections are being researched through math algorithms (we can find some of them at [6]) that help platoon crossing these intersections reducing the waiting time at the stop.

The gradient of a line (it is quoted in this paper [8]) is another problem to resolve, where researchers try to investigate how to keep the formation in these situations because vehicles could separate each other whether they don't have similar characteristics like the engine, weight or even the size.

To implement algorithms that can resolve the problem of the intersections it is necessary to have a good infrastructure at intersections which help to share relevance data between the different platoons or vehicles that approach to the intersection.

For it, each vehicle should have hardware (ultrasonic sensors, cameras, and microcontrollers) to measure the position, velocity, heading, and acceleration of each vehicle and mainly of the leader, which indicates the face of the platoon. That information will be sending to hardware of the intersection which will have other information about other platoons or vehicles approaching to the intersection and will control whether platoons can pass, must wait at stop line or can split in sets to cross safely the intersection.

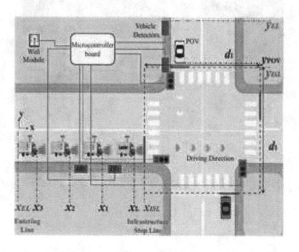

Fig. 2. Platoon at intersection

For example, in the Fig. 2 it is shown have a platoon formed by trucks, and other vehicle which try to cross the intersection. We can see the intersection has special hardware like Wi-Fi module (share information between microcontrollers of the intersection and trucks), vehicle detectors and semaphores that help us to control the traffic at intersection. Each truck is able to measure interconexion distance using sensors and cameras, the speed and the acceleration. The variable x indicates the position of each truck (i is the position of each truck in the platoon, and l means that is the position of the leader.) With these data it is possible to implement an array where the dynamics of whole platoon is given by (it is possible to find a research about it at [4]):

$$\dot{x} = A_p + X_p + B_p A_L$$

$$X_p$$

is the array of truck's positions, AL is the leading vehicle's acceleration, (A, B are the system matrices.)

In the image, Pov means position of other vehicle.

With these data it is possible to take a decision, calculating whether the platoon or the other vehicle can cross without causing an accident.

The most important information for algorithms is the position of platoons and other vehicles. Other proposal considers a infrastructure at intersection composed by four vehicles detectors(satellites) with known positions.

Given the distances of at least three satellites, the position of the vehicle can be calculated by a trilateration algorithm which computes the intersection points of three circles around the satellites (it is possible to find a research about it at [3]). Using it we will get the position of platoon to able to take a good decision about to cross or not the intersection.

3   Communications

Keeping close the vehicles of the platoon is one of the most important objectives in platoon driving. If we get to reduce the distance between a vehicle and its preceding vehicle we will get to reduce fuel (it is quoted at [9]), CO2 and to increase the traffic fluidity.

On the other hand, in applications like cooperative driving it is crucial that a vehicle has exact knowledge of the location of its neighbors. Today it's being researched about communications using LAN, WIFFI, GPS, laser and other spread spectrum techniques.

Communications between vehicles is called V2V (we can find more about it at [10,11]). Communications between a vehicle and the infrastructure is known as V2I (see [10]).

We could say that platoon driving must have a good communication because everything; reaction time, special situations, security and control depend of information about the vehicles to apply the best solution to the real problem.

To share information between vehicles is possible to use a dedicated short-range communication DSRC (A good research can be found in [7]). Many researchers have concluded that DSRC cover a good range and it is cheaper than other infrastructures because it is much extended around the world. But this technology has a disadvantage. This technology has been implemented for local area networks with no or low mobility. However, in IVC systems the mobility can be very high. Other disadvantage can be that not exist access point and all features available in infrastructure mode are unavailable in an IVC context.

Other alternative is the Bluetooth (A good research can be found in [7] because is inexpensive and easy to use, but this technology has a drawback that imposes a piconet structure difficult to maintain in IVC systems, and has delays that make difficult the platoon communication. Other solution when vehicles are outside major cities is cellular networks (it is possible to find more about it at [7]) which have a large cover. The main arguments for using a mobile telephony standard for IVR systems is that the infrastructure is already there, and in the future vehicles will have access to these networks. Cellular system were not designed and provided for simultaneous utilization by a large numbers of users for long periods of time.

4 Formations (Platooning Control)

Keeping the convoy is the principal idea to get all benefits we read before. But keeping the platoon requires algorithms to control the speed between vehicles, split and join of vehicle formations doing obstacle avoidance (we can read more about these algorithms at [12]) where vehicles join and leave formations, cooperative autonomous platoon maneuvers on highways, performance limitations in vehicle platoon control, etc.

Many algorithms to keep a good formation need information to have a longitudinal and latitudinal control (for further explanation [11,13,14]). The Latitudinal control governs the vehicle steering and impairs the ability for a vehicle to stay in a lane and follow a specified path. On the other hand the longitudinal control governs the speed of the vehicle and impairs the ability for a vehicle to maintain the correct velocity or spacing from a preceding vehicle.

The desired speed and acceleration for a specific vehicle can vary based on enforce highway speed limits and the temporal gap to the preceding vehicle. The efforts in this kind of research are to try that each vehicle has the same behavior than the leader and just in the same place. For example in a bidimensional model street if the leader heading five degrees to left at (x,y) position, the others vehicles should have the same behavior at the same position to able in this case that the platoon turn left . It results very difficult because the leader's' behavior change constantly (accelerating, turning and braking).

5 Security

The convoys vehicles have to go to a little distance each other to ensure the environmental impacts reducing, fuel consumption, and traffic fluid [14,15]. But if we reduce the distance between vehicles, we should have a security system to avoid conflicts and collisions between the vehicles of the convoy. Many researches are based on brake systems which allow decelerating the convoy or avoiding collisions in the face of unusual situations.

The behavior of the convoy depend of traffic, highways, weather, and others vehicles that interact with the convoy. There are other systems that control the security like algorithms, and manual braking systems(there is a good research about it at [5]). The driver could break the vehicle if he detects that the brakes fail. The experimental results indicated that emergency braking is an effective method for avoiding a rear-end collision when there is a system failure in the automatic platooning, resulting in the mean maximum deceleration for the following vehicle being higher than that for the preceding vehicle.

6 Future Directions

It is very possible that we will see platoon driving in Highways very soon. It will probably be platoons of trucks the first application of platoon driving to be put in service.

Considering the huge benefits that may be obtained from such systems, including a considerable impact on safety and sustainability of transportation, more and more transportation modes are expected to be joining in.

In our group we are working on possible new coordination intelligent algorithms to make this possible. For example, in [16] we published the first results of a brand new coordination system, based on the detection, transmission and mimicing of the leader's acceleration signal by the rest of the cars in the platoon. Results were promising. We believe that approach to be full of potential mainly because most of the current platoon driving coordination systems are based on the car following paradigm, where each car try to keep a distance just the front car, and that is system where small errors accumulate as we go back in the platoon.

We also propose and are working on a new idea to facilitate long trips without overusing the distracting and error proning GPS based navigators. We are exploring algorithms to use platoon driving to help people driving to unknown places, in a way resembling a subway system. When you travel by subway, there are a number of lines and you switch from one to another until you reach your desired station. We propose the implementation of a system where a user inputs his/her destination and then he/she gets information on what platoon he must join in, when he must leave it to transfer to another one, and so on until he/she reaches a virtual destination station to finally drive manually to his actual destination.

Finally, there is also a very open and wide front on platoon overtakings. It may happen that two different platoons are circulating in the same lane but with different speeds. Therefore, a safe and robust automatic overtaking system must be designed to cope to that situations. We are also laborating on that and will be producing some results soon.

References

1. U.G. Assembly, "United nations millennium declaration," resolution adopted, vol. 18 (2000)
2. CEC, A community strategy for sustainable mobility; green paper on the impact of transport on the environment. In: COM (92) 46 Final, Commission of the European Communities (1992)
3. Diab, H., Makhlouf, I.B., Kowalewski, S.: A platoon of vehicles approaching an intersection: a testing platform for safe intersections, pp. 1918–1923. IEEE (2012)
4. Ben Makhlouf, I., Diab, H., Kowalewski, S.: Reachability analysis for managing platoons at intersections, pp. pp. 1141–1147. IEEE (2013)
5. Zheng, R., Nakano, K., Yamabe, S., Aki, M., Nakamura, H., Suda, Y.: Study on emergency-avoidance braking for the automatic platooning of trucks. IEEE Intell. Transp. Syst. Mag. 15(4), 1748–1757 (2014)
6. Wu, J., Yan, F., Abbas-Turki, A.: Mathematical proof of effectiveness of platoon-based traffic control at intersections, pp. 720–725. IEEE (2013)

7. Sichitiu, M.L., Kihl, M., I. vid LTH, L. University, E. och informationsteknik, L. Lunds tekniska hgskola, Electrical, information technology, L. universitet, D. at LTH, and L. a. L. U. Faculty of Engineering: Inter-vehicle communication systems: a survey. IEEE Commun. Surv. Tutorials **10**(2), 88–105 (2008)

8. Ros, B.G., Knoop, V.L., van Arem, B., Hoogendoorn, S.P.: Reducing congestion at uphill freeway sections by means of a gradient compensation system, pp. 191–198. IEEE (2012)

9. Xu, L., Wang, L., Yin, G., Zhang, H.: Communication information structures and contents for enhanced safety of highway vehicle platoons

10. Abualhoul, M.Y., Marouf, M., Shagdar, O., Nashashibi, F.: Platooning control using visible light communications: a feasibility study, pp. 1535–1540. IEEE (2013)

11. Hashimoto, N., Kato, S., Saito, Y., Tsugawa, S.: Preliminary experiments about following distance for obtaining benefit under some conditions, pp. 128–133. IEEE (2012)

12. Gren, P.: Split and join of vehicle formations doing obstacle avoidance, In: Proceedings of the IEEE International Conference on Robotics and Automation, vol. 2004, no. 2, pp. 1951–1955 (2004)

13. Lam, S., Katupitiya, J.: Cooperative autonomous platoon maneuvers on highways, pp. 1152–1157. IEEE (2013)

14. Solyom, S., Coelingh, E., tekniska hgskola, C., I. fr signaler och system, D. of Signals, Systems, C. U. of Technology, and S. of Electrical Engineering, Performance limitations in vehicle platoon control, pp. 1–6. IEEE (2012)

15. Suzuki, M., Harada, R., Kanda, S., Shigeno, H.: Overtaking priority management method between platoons and surrounding vehicles considering carbon dioxide emissions (poster), pp. 260–267. IEEE (2011)

16. Sánchez-Medina, J.J., Broggi, A., Galan-Moreno, M.J., Rubio-Royo, E.: Acceleration signal based linear formation driving model: algorithmic description and simulation results. In: Moreno-Díaz, R., Pichler, F., Quesada-Arencibia, A. (eds.) EUROCAST. LNCS, vol. 8112, pp. 47–54. Springer, Heidelberg (2013)

How to Simulate Traffic with SUMO

Samuel Romero Santana, Javier J. Sanchez-Medina[✉],
and Enrique Rubio-Royo

CICEI – ULPGC, Las Palmas, Spain
sam_r_s@hotmail.com, javier.sanchez@ulpgc.es, rubio@cicei.com

In this paper we want to give a quick introduction about how to install and use SUMO to build a first simulation in a few steps. SUMO, (Simulation of Urban Mobility") ([1–4]) is a free an open traffic simulation suite which is available since 2001 allows modeling of intermodal traffic.

SUMO is very important to researchers who work in modeling traffic because allows to watch the behavior of the vehicles, the traffic in general and our infrastructures, and being able to correct mistakes or improve behaviors before implementing them in real life. For example in platoon driving we can model behaviors, distances between vehicles or improve algorithms solutions for special situations like intersections before seeing it in the real life where a mistake can cost very expensive.

The first step to run SUMO is choosing which platform we want to install it. For a quick install in Windows, you only have to extract the zip file you have downloaded in a simple path and execute the executable file sumo-gui.

If your platform is Linux or MacOS, you have to follow four steps to be able to run SUMO; Install all of the required tools and libraries, get the source code, build the SUMO binaries and install the SUMO binaries to another path (optional).

Once executed SUMO we will open a simulation file with the extension cfg which is formed by a link of at least other two files (Fig. 1).

```
<configuration>
    <input>
        <net-file value="highwaynet.xml"/>
        <route-files value="ruta.rou.xml"/>
    </input>
</configuration>
```

Fig. 1. Configuration file

In our paper the file highwaynet.xml (Fig. 1) determines the map of street over we want to do the simulation. This file has a special structure. We can get a map from several ways; Google, Openstreetmap, Mapbox, or even a map drawn by ourselves. For that we must know that a street, via, motorway or highway is formed by a set of nodes. The union of a set of nodes form the via. JOSM can be

R. Moreno-Díaz et al. (Eds.): EUROCAST 2015, LNCS 9520, pp. 773–778, 2015.
DOI: 10.1007/978-3-319-27340-2_95

a tool to draw or get a real map from a determined place. This map will be saved with the extension osm and achieve with the requisites written before. So, we have to convert the osm file in a xml file [1,4]. For that, SUMO has a tool called netconvert which does this work. We must write in our console an instruction like this: netconvert highway.osm -o highwaynet.xml. This instruction converts the input file highway.osm (map from Josm) in an output file called highwaynet.xml.

Now, the map is a net of edges, where an edge has the following characteristics. Each description of an edge ([3] should include information about the name of the edge, the number of lanes, the maximum speed allowed (m/s) on this edge, etc. An edge starts in a node and finishes in other one. We can define it with the properties "from" and "to". To define the vehicles ([1,3] and the route that our vehicles have to take in the map it is necessary to built other file. In our case, this file is called ruta.rou.xml (Fig. 1).This file defines the type of vehicles we want to have in our simulation. So, we have to declare the special word vtype followed of a set of properties like id (indicates the name of the vehicle type), accel (the acceleration ability of vehicle of this type in m/s), decel (the deceleration ability of vehicle of this type in m/s too), sigma (the driver imperfection in a range from 0 to 1), length (the length of the vehicle), color (the color of the vehicle defined in RGB), depart (the time step at which the vehicle shall enter the network), departlane (the lane on which the vehicle shall be inserted), and much more like vclass (an abstract vehicle class that SUMO has defined with several properties to simulate busses, public transport, public emergency etc.). Not it is necessary to write all the properties. We only have to declare the properties we need. On the other hand, we need to define the route ([1,3] of this class of vehicle using the special word "route". Routes must have an edges (indicates which edges form the route. These edges must be connected.).

```
<routes>
   <vType id="type1"  accel="0.8" decel="4.5" sigma="0.5" length="7"
        maxSpeed="60" vClass="emergency"/>
     <vehicle id="0" type="type1" depart="0" color="1,0,0" departLane="2">
       <route  edges="180171905#0 180171905#1 180171905#2" color="0,0,1"/>
   </vehicle>
</routes>
```

Fig. 2. "ruta.rou.xml". Definition of vehicles and their routes

In our file we have declared a red ambulance which departs in lane 2 (our highway has three lanes). This ambulance [Fig. 3] is seven meters width, has an acceleration of 8 m/s, a deceleration of 4,5 m/s and the maximum speed it can take is 60 m/s.The driver of the ambulance will have an imperfection in his decisions of 0, 5 (Fig. 2).

Now we have the map, vehicles and the route that these vehicles must take on the map. We have to open the cfg file and watch our simulation pressing the

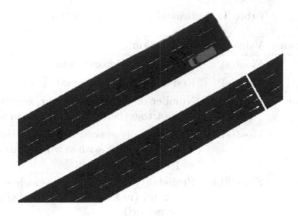

Fig. 3. Special vehicle in SUMO (Color figure online)

button play situated in the main menu. If we want to decelerate the simulation to watch better what happen we must write a value in the box delay. Otherwise we can stop the simulation pressing the button stop in the main menu.

On the other hand, one of the most important ideas in SUMO is to simulate traffic jams or to see how a set of vehicles can take different behaviors in several situations. For that, researchers have two options to introduce vehicles. The first one is to declare each vehicle, one by one in the file which declares the route. (In our case ruta.rou.xml). It isn't very efficient because if we need a busy highway to simulate a traffic jam, we will have to copy a declaration for each vehicle (vehicles and their routes) we want in our highway.

The second one is to build an automatic file which declares a set of vehicles and their routes automatically. So, we can build a battery of vehicles in a few steps. For that, It is possible to define repeated vehicle emissions ("flows"), which have the same parameters except for the departure time. The following additional parameters are known:

To build a battery of vehicles in an automatic way, we need two files.

– car.flow.xml
– highwaynet.xml

The first one indicates the characteristics and routes for our set of vehicles, and the second one is the map we have used before.

In this new file, we have declared five hundred vehicles, which will be distributed uniformity, where the first one will depart in 0 s and the last one in 10 s (Table 1).

To build our new route-file, where will have our battery of vehicles and their routes, we will have to use a tool called duarouter (Fig. 4). Duarouter mixes the flow file and our net file to get our final route file (output-file). For that, we have to write in our console the following commands:

```
duarouter-flows=cars.flow.xml-net=highwaynet.xml-output-file=newrou.rou.xml.
```

Table 1. Additional parameters for flows

Atrtibute name	Value type	Description
Begin	Float(s)	First vehicle departure time
End	Float(s)	End of departure interval
VehsPerHour	Float(n/h)	Number of vehicles per hour, equally spaced (not together with period or probability)
Period	Float(s)	Insert equally spaced vehicles at that period (not together with vehsPerHour or probability)
Probability	Float([0,1])	Probability for emitting a vehicle each second (not together with vehsPerHour or period)
Number	Int(n)	Total number of vehicles, equally spaced

```
<routes>
  <vType id="0" type="type1" />
  <flows>
    <flow id="type1" from="180171905#0" to="180171905#2" begin="0" end="10" number="500" />
  </flows>
</routes>
```

Fig. 4. Flow file

Now, we have to change our configuration file to replace our old file route for the new one. We will get something like [Fig. 5].

Finally, researchers usually want to take the control of his simulation, (for example to take the control of an specific car, or to try to extract interesting data like the speed of a particular vehicle, the fuel consumption, the position of a vehicle in the highway or the position of a particular car in a platoon) (Fig. 6). For that, SUMO allows us to interact with it through TraCI. In a few words we can define TraCI like the short term for "Traffic Control Interface" which gives the access to a running road traffic simulation, it allows to retrieve values of simulated objects and to manipulate their behaviour "on-line". TraCI allows to connect SUMO with an script (preferably written in Python) and do what we want in a real time inside of our simulation. To carry out this process, we have to do some changes in our cfg file. We have to put the port where we are going to link our SUMO with the script. This port will be the number 8813 [Fig. 7].

Tutorials of SUMO say about to use python like language script to take the total control of our simulation online, although we can use the script we want. We have to be sure we have installed our script (for example Python in our computer). If you choose Linux like your Operating System, you will have to:

- (a) Install the python devel package files.
- (b) Call configure using the –with-python option.
- (c) Make and make install as usual.

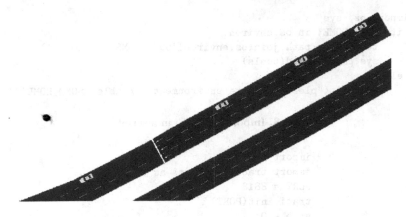

Fig. 5. Flow: "Set of vehicles put into the simulator in a range of tim"

```
<configuration>
  <input>
     <net-file value="highwaynet.xml"/>
     <route-files value="newrou.rou.xml"/>
  </input>
</configuration>
```

Fig. 6. New configuration file with flows

```
<configuration>
  <input>
     <net-file value="highwaynet.xml"/>
     <route-files value="ruta.rou.xml"/>
     <remote-port value="8813"/>
  </input>
</configuration>
```

Fig. 7. Configuration file with TraCi

If your Operating System is Windows:

- (a) Make sure python is installed and is in your PATH.
- (b) Call tools/build/pythonPropsMSVC.py to generate a python.props file.
- (c) Enable the inclusion of python.props by uncommenting the relevant line in build/msvc10/Win32.props.
- d) Build the Win32 Release version as usual.

Once, you have installed Python in your operating System, you have to write some lines in your script to connect your script with Sumo. The first step is to import TraCi in your script. It s very easy. To use the library, the SUMO HOME/tools directory must be on the python load path [Fig. 8].

```
import os, sys
if 'SUMO_HOME' in os.environ:
    tools = os.path.join(os.environ['SUMO_HOME'], 'tools')
    sys.path.append(tools)
else:
    sys.exit("please declare environment variable 'SUMO_HOME'")
```

Fig. 8. Importing TraCi in a script

```
import traci
import traci.constants as tc
PORT = 8813
traci.init(PORT)
step = 0
while step < 1000:
            "Here we take the control"
        step += 1
traci.close()
```

Fig. 9. Interfacing TraCi with SUMO

The second step is to interface with SUMO from Python. You have to insert some lines in your script [Fig. 9]. After opening the connection to the port which was given to SUMO as the remote port Option in your configuration file, you can emit various commands and execute simulation steps until you close your connection. The commands you can emit are based in variables which can be found (them and their descriptions) in the file "traci/constants.py". There are variables which allow us to move a car, get all data we want about it, for example its speed, acceleration, CO_2 emission, fuel consumption, give a heading, a direction, etc. Definitely, to do what we want in our simulation in a real time.

References

1. Behrisch, M., Bieker, L., Erdmann, J., Krajzewicz, D.: Sumo-simulation of urban mobility-an overview. In: The Third International Conference on Advances in System Simulation, SIMUL 2011, pp. 55–60 (2011)
2. Krajzewicz, D., Brockfeld, E., Mikat, J., Ringel, J., Rössel, C., Tuchscheerer, W., Wagner, P., Wösler, R.: Simulation of modern traffic lights control systems using the open source traffic simulation sumo. In: Proceedings of the 3rd Industrial Simulation Conference, vol. 2205 (2005)
3. Krajzewicz, D., Erdmann, J., Behrisch, M., Bieker, L.: Recent development and applications of sumo-simulation of urban mobility. Int. J. Adv. Syst. Meas. **5**(3–4), 128–138 (2012)
4. Krajzewicz, D., Hertkorn, G., Rössel, C., Wagner, P.: Sumo (simulation of urban mobility). In: Proceedings of the 4th Middle East Symposium on Simulation and Modelling, pp. 183–187 (2002)

Cloud and Other Computation Systems

Using Data Mining to Improve the Public Transport in Gran Canaria Island

Teresa Cristóbal[1], José J. Lorenzo[2], and Carmelo R. García[1(✉)]

[1] Institute for Cybernetic Science and Technology,
University of Las Palmas de Gran Canaria, Las Palmas, Spain
teresa.cristobalb@gmail.com, rgarcia@dis.ulpgc.es
[2] Institute of Intelligent Systems and Numerical Applications in Engineering,
University of Las Palmas de Gran Canaria, Campus Universitario de Tafira,
35017 Las Palmas, Spain
jlorenzo@dis.ulpgc.es

Abstract. In this work Business Intelligence and Data Mining techniques have been used to extract useful knowledge for the main corporation of intercity public transportation on Gran Canaria island. The aim has been to find a pattern to predict the number of passengers who want to travel from one point to another. To achieve it, events files generated in the vehicles of the company and additional data have been used as information source: temporal (time of the trip, type of the day, month and season) and geographic and demographic (departure and destination bus stop, type of bus stop and zip codes of the origin and destination bus stop.

Keywords: Data mining · Intelligent transport systems · Public transport management

1 Introduction

Data mining can be defined as the non-trivial extraction of implicit, previously unknown, yet potentially useful information from data [1], this field is an important research frontier for machine learning, database technology and many other related areas. Fundamentally, Data Mining is an applied science: it studies a problem, how to find useful knowledge in data, interested in all the relevant methods that can be used. The process consists of several steps: data cleaning, feature construction/extraction, algorithm and parameter selection, and interpretation and validation.

This paper describes the use of Data Mining process in order to provide a tool for the Global Salcai-Utinsa, the main corporation of intercity public transportation of Gran Canaria. The main goal was to predict passengers demand to adjust its resources and its use planning, using records generated in its vehicles fleet during one year.

This document is organized as follows: first we introduce related works, the third section describes the methods and tools used, the fourth describes the data mining project made and, the last one, presents the conclusions.

© Springer International Publishing Switzerland 2015
R. Moreno-Díaz et al. (Eds.): EUROCAST 2015, LNCS 9520, pp. 781–788, 2015.
DOI: 10.1007/978-3-319-27340-2_96

2   Related Works

In the bibliography there are multiple related works with a common goal: to promote the use of public transport over private transport. Some of these, such as Arentze [2], Levner [3], Lathia y Capra [4–6], use the data provided by the automatic payment systems and tracking systems installed in the vehicles of the fleet, developing algorithms that produce rules used for modeling travel demand in transportation networks.

We note the work of Du [7] using data from payment systems and location of urban buildings to anticipate demand in areas of sprawl. This work explains a new framework to use the data through Automated Fare Collection Systems (AFCS) to discovering regions with high passenger gathering intensity and it also classifies points in these regions with similar passenger gathering feature varying with time in dynamic way, which is called spark region. Furthermore, the novel definition group mobility pattern (GMP) is proposed to mine the regular group behavior among these spark regions. A series of analysis is employed by using large-scale and real-world data, which consists of nearly 17 million people daily public transit records, bus intervals generated by over 14,854 buses organizations in Beijing at 20 s interval. The application indicates that group mobility pattern is helpful for diagnosis and understanding residence of each region with their demand for public transportation in a significant way.

3   Methodology and Tools

The standard and more frequently data mining methodology, named CRISP-DM (Cross-Industry Stan- dard Process for Data Mining) [8], has been applied in this work. The tool used for preprocessing and analysis of data has been Pentaho Community Edition [9], and Weka framework [10] for data modeling. A brief description of each tool is outlined below.

3.1   CRISP-DM

This is an industry-proven way to guide the data mining efforts [11]. This methodology includes descriptions of the typical phases of a data mining project, the tasks involved with each phase, and the explanation of the relationships between these tasks. From the point of view of the process model, CRISP-DM provides an overview of the data mining life cycle. The particular phases of the CRISP-DM methodology are:

- Business understanding and process planning: Gather information about the company, assess your situation and know their priorities.
- Data understanding. Collect, describe and explore the available data using tables and graphics and determine its quality.
- Data preparation. Merge and classify data, deriving new attributes and define training and test sets.

- Modeling. Use data modeling tools and determine the checking and evaluation methods of the patterns.
- Evaluation. Verify that the results meet the needs presented.
- Deployment. Implement new knowledge into the organization to participate in the planning and decision making.

3.2 Pentaho Community Edition

This is the open source version of *Pentaho Data Integration* and *Pentaho Business Analytics Platform*, two of the main applications of the *Pentaho Business Intelligence* platform, designed for decision making [12]. Data Integration (DI or Kettle) delivers powerful Extraction, Transformation, and Loading (ETL) capabilities, using a groundbreaking, metadata-driven approach, with an intuitive, graphical, drag and drop design environment and a proven, scalable, standard-based architecture. Pentaho Business Analytics Platform (BA) provided ad-hoc tools to analyze and visualize data, using pre-created contents with different types for analyzing, reporting, dashboarding and data mining. Plugins created by users community can be seamlessly connected.

3.3 Weka

Weka (Waikato Environment for Knowledge Analysis) is a popular suite of machine learning software written in Java, developed at the University of Waikato, New Zealand [13]. Weka contains a collection of visualization tools and algorithms for data analysis and predictive modeling together with graphical user interfaces for easy access to this functionality.

4 The Data Mining Project

The development of the project was carried out using the methodology CRISP-DM previously explained. So the application of the different phases to the project is presented in this section.

4.1 Business Understanding

Global Salcai-Utinsa Company installed in 2005 in each vehicle of its fleet an intelligent system to control the transport operations. This system records all the relevant events produced in the vehicles that can affect the operations planning. Examples of this events are:

- The beginning and end of a service from a driver.
- The beginning and end of an expedition vehicle.
- Each change of fare stop.
- Each cash payment made in the vehicles.
- Each card payment made.

From the events generated by these systems, we decided to find a pattern to predict the number of passengers who want to travel from one point to another in a given moment of the day, in this way the company can streamline its resources and benefit their users. We consider the following types of information:

- Temporal.
  - Time of the trip.
  - Type of the day (working day or holiday day).
  - Month.
  - Season.
- Geographic and demographic.
  - Departure and destination bus stops.
  - Type of bus stop: urban, residential, rural, high school or campus area.
  - Zip code origin and destination bus stop.

4.2 Data Understanding

In this phase the Pentaho tools were used to explore the data, obtaining the following information:

- The data of all network lines during one year are available.
- The most frequent errors arise in the date, number of passengers and destination bus stop. Because of the number of these errors is low, then the disposal of the erroneous registers is decided.
- The 30 % of travelers are concentrated in just five lines.

4.3 Data Preparation

With the conclusions reached in the previous phase several decisions are taken that will determine the data to be modeled finally:

- Lines studied. Three of the five lines with more travelers correspond to a very limited area of the island close to the capital, Las Palmas de Gran Canaria. These lines and their bus stops constituting a corridor who was called "Capital-Centre Corridor".
- Zero traveller register. During the first attempts at modeling it became apparent the lack of an important fact: "no one at the bus stop". To include this data in the original file we included an additional control process over the stop sequence, increasing the robustness of data.
- Temporal grain. Since in intercity routes the fare stops are formed by several physical stops, after analyzing the data it is observed that the temporal grain of 5 min is significant.

We decide to use classification algorithms to predict demand, then at this stage, we build new fields to discretize those involved in modeling:

- for the number of passengers going to the same stop from the same stop at the same interval of five minutes in an hour, three new fields were created:
- for time intervals:

And depending on the location of the stop we define various types that also incorporated in the file data:

Field	Meaning
np1_class	0 = no passenger, 1 = 1 or more
np2_class	0 = no passenger, 1 = 1, 2 = 2 or more
np3_class	0 = no passenger, 1 = 1 or 2, 2 = 3 or more

Field	Meaning
timetable_1	0 = 21 h-7 h, 1 = 7 h-21 h
timetable_2	0 = 21 h-7 h, 1 = 07 h-12 h, 2 = 12 h-16 h, 3 = 16 h-21 h

Type	Description
1	Urban stop (Las Palmas de G.C.)
2	Residential stop
3	Village stop
4	Rural stop
9	High school/Campus stop

4.4 Modeling

In data preprocessing phase, fields were incorporated with some redundancy (for example on the number of passengers), for this reason the first step done in this phase was to eliminate the less significant attributes in order to improve the effectiveness of the methods.

The dataset to which the modeling algorithms were applied consists of the following fields:

- From the original file:
  - Month
  - Origin bus stop.
  - Destination bus stop.
- Created or incorporated into the preprocessing phase:
  - Season.
  - *np1_class*
  - *np2_class*
  - Weekday indicator.
  - *timetable_2*
  - For the departure stop: type and zip code.
  - For the destination stop: type and zip code.

As discussed above, we decided to use classifier algorithms because they are the most common methods and generate good results, specifically:

- Naive Bayes [14], probabilistic classifier based on applying Bayes theorem with strong (naive) independence assumptions between the features.

- C4.5 [15], an algorithm used to generate a decision tree which is usually inter-
pretable.
- Random Forest [16], one of the most accurate algorithms, it is an ensemble
learning method for classification that operate by constructing a multitude of
decision trees at training time.

To model two of the fields created with the number of passengers, np1_class
and np2_class, each of these algorithms were executed twice with each lines in
the corridor and with the complete set of lines. The complete set of lines also
was modeled in two ways: based on departure and destination stop (designated
as P in figures) and based on departure and destination stop type (designated as
Tp in figures). In total 80 models were created. In all cases was used as training
set 66 % of the instances and the remaining as test set.

4.5   Evaluation

The results have been evaluated using three measures: the accuracy, the precision
and the recall values. Means of precision and recall values obtained for each line
studied and for the complete sets of lines are shown in the Table 1.

Table 1. Means of precision and recall values.

Lines	J48		Random Forest	
	Precision	Recall	Precision	Recall
214	0,98	1,00	0,88	1,00
301	0,99	1,00	0,99	1,00
302	1,00	1,00	1,00	1,00
303	1,00	1,00	1,00	1,00
305	0,81	0,90	0,81	0,90
306	0,90	0,99	0,93	0,95
307	0,90	0,97	0,90	0,97
311	1,00	1,00	1,00	1,00
318	0,84	0,66	0,85	0,65
326	1,00	1,00	1,00	1,00
327	1,00	1,00	1,00	1,00
328	0,90	0,81	0,90	0,81
330	0,98	1,00	0,98	1,00
331	1,00	1,00	1,00	1,00
P	1,00	1,00	1,00	1,00
Tp	0,88	1,00	0,88	1,00

From the obtained results the following conclusions arise:

- Of the three methods chosen, Naive Bayes is the one that yields worst result with np1_class, so it was not used to estimate the np2_class.
- When the field is np1_class, it is "take the bus any passenger on the stop or none", close to 100 % correct clasified instances in the lines with more passengers is achieved with the other methods.
- When the field is np2_class, it is "take the bus one passenger, more than one or none", the average percentage of well classified instances is around 75 % and the values of precision and recall of both methods are also very high in lines with more number of passengers.
- In lines with more passengers, modeling algorithms have used the variables considered the start of work: month, origin and destination bus stop, weekday indicator and times.
- If bus stop type is used in the prediction a simple decision tree is generated, therefore it is understandable, as show in Table 2 with the results with the complete set of lines for np2_class.

Table 2. Decision matrix obtained by J48 for bus stop's types (Tp).

		Destination				
		1	2	3	4	9
	1	0	1	1/2*	1	1
	2	1	0	1	1	1
Departure	3	1/2**	1	0	1	1
	4	1	1	1	0	1
	9	1/2**	1	1	1	0

* depending on day and season
** depending on day

5   Conclusions

This paper is a practical application of how to use Data Mining techniques with a basic set of travel data, consisting of journeys made by anonymous users in a fleet of vehicles equipped with an onboard computer, regardless of the payment method used (cash or card). It is also an example of using free software tools that allow you to apply statistical techniques, analysis and data cleaning, modeling algorithms in an immediate way, allowing to develop projects at low cost and in a short time.

The results obtained have been limited by the nature of the Data Mining data: it corresponds to transport services realized, stops recorded in the file are fare stops (no physical stops), and like public service some lines has few passengers, but nevertheless has been able to model the trunk lines and get some knowledge and, as demand is modeled using data directly related to the offer, this knowledge can be applied to adjust the planning of routes and schedules.

References

1. Frawley, W., Piatetsky-Shapiro, G.Y., Matheus, C.: Knowledge discovery in databases: an overview. AI Mag. **13**(3), 213–228 (1992)
2. Arentze, T.A., Timmermans, H.: ALBATROSS - A Learning-Based Transportaion Oriented Simulation System. Urban Planning Group/EIRASS, Eindhoven University of Technology, Netherlands (2007)
3. Levner, E., Ceder, A., Elalouf, A., Hadas, Y., Shabtay, D.: Detection and improvement of deficiencies and failures in public-transportation networks using agent-enhanced distribution data mining. In: IEEE International Conference on Industrial Engineering and Engineering Management, art. no. 6118006, pp. 694–698 (2011)
4. Lathia, N., Froehlich, J., Capral, L.: Mining public transport usage for personalised intelligent transport systems. In: IEEE International Conference on Data Mining, pp. 887–892 (2010)
5. Lathia, N., Capra, L.: Mining mobility data to minimise travellers'spending on public transport. In: Proceedings of the ACM SIGKDD International Conference on Knowledge Discovery and Data Mining, pp. 1181–1189 (2011)
6. Lathia, N., Smith, C., Froehlich, J., Capra, L.: Individuals among commuters: building personalised transport information services from fare collection systems. Pervasive Mob. Comput. **9**(5), 643–664 (2013)
7. Du, B., Yang, Y., Lv, W.: Understand group travel behaviors in an urban area using mobility pattern mining. In: Proceedings of the IEEE 10th International Conference on Ubiquitous Intelligence and Computing, UIC 2013 and IEEE 10th International Conference on Autonomic and Trusted Computing, ATC 2013, art. no. 06726200, pp. 127–133 (2013)
8. Shearer, C.: The CRISP-DM model: the new blueprint for data mining. J. Data Warehouse. **5**(4), 13–23 (2000)
9. Pentaho. http://community.pentaho.com/. visited on 04 February 2014
10. Weka. The University of Waikato. http://www.cs.waikato.ac.nz/ml/weka. visited on 15 June 2014
11. Manual CRISP_DM de IBM SPSS Modeler. Copyright IBM Corporation 1994 (2012)
12. Roldán, M.C.: Pentaho Data Integration Beginner's Guide. Packt Publishing (2003)
13. Hall, M., Frank, E., Holmes, G., Pfahringer, B., Reutemann, P., Witten, H.: The WEKA Data Mining Software: An Update. SIKDD Explor. **11**(1), 10–18 (2009)
14. Duda, R.O., Hart, P.E., Stork, D.G.: Pattern Classification. Wiley, New York (2001)
15. Quinlan, J.R.: C4.5: Programs for Machine Learning. Morgan Kaufmann, San Mateo (1993)
16. Pavlov, Y.L.: Random Forest. VSP, Utrecht (2000)

A New Large Neighborhood Search Based Matheuristic Framework for Rich Vehicle Routing Problems

Simona Mancini[✉]

Politecnico di Torino, Corso Duca degli Abruzzi 24, 10129 Torino, Italy
simona.mancini@polito.it

Abstract. In this paper a New Large Neighborhood Search Based Matheuristic Framework for Rich Vehicle Routing Problems is presented. The innovative aspect of the proposed approach concern the possibility to address large neighborhoods in reasonably small computational time exploiting the search directly by the mathematical model. In this way it is possible to obtain the local minimum respect to the addressed neighborhood, which make the intensification phase of the algorithm more powerful and precise. The method is extremely flexible and can be adapted to many rich vehicle routing problems. This procedure can be used as a stand alone heuristic or can be embedded in a more complex metaheuristic framework such as Variable Neighborhood Search (VNS) and Adaptive Large Neighborhood Search (ALNS). The proposed algorithm has been tested on a new rich Vehicle Routing Problem arising in real life context, the Multi Depot Multi Period Vehicle Routing Problem with Heterogeneous Fleet. Computational results on realistic instances, showing the effectiveness of the proposed method, are provided.

1 Introduction

The Large Neighborhood search heuristic, (LNS), belongs to the class of heuristics known as Very Large Scale Neighborhood search (VLSN) algorithms as stated in [1]. All VLSN algorithms are based on the observation that searching a large neighborhood results in finding local optima of high quality, and hence overall a VLSN algorithm may return better solutions. However, searching a large neighborhood is strongly time consuming, hence various filtering techniques are used to limit the search. In VLSN algorithms, the search is typically restricted to a subset of the solutions belonging to the neighborhood which can be searched efficiently. Differently from what happens in other VLSN, in LNS the neighborhood is implicitly defined by the moves used to destroy and repair an incumbent solution. For a detailed survey on LNS applications to routing problems the reader may refer to [2]. The destroy operators may be defined in different ways. For routing problems, for instance, a destroy operator could consist into break k routes letting the others unvaried, or to remove a fixed percentage of the arcs in the current solution. A random (or randomized) component is used to select

© Springer International Publishing Switzerland 2015
R. Moreno-Díaz et al. (Eds.): EUROCAST 2015, LNCS 9520, pp. 789–796, 2015.
DOI: 10.1007/978-3-319-27340-2_97

the arcs to be removed. The repair method rebuild a feasible solution starting from the partially destroyed one. Generally a greedy construction heuristic is used to rebuild the solution, which is very fast but not always very accurate, since only a sample solution is analyzed in the neighborhood. The innovative aspect of the LNS proposed in this paper concern the possibility of address the whole neighborhood in reasonably small computational time. In fact, the large neighborhood search is exploited directly by the model. In this way it is possible to obtain the local minimum respect to the addressed neighborhood, which make the intensification phase of the algorithm more powerful and precise.

2   The Multi Depot Multi Period Vehicle Routing Problem with Heterogeneous Fleet

This problem deal with the weekly planning of delivery operations for a company which dispose of several depots where the good is stored and/or produced, a known fleet of vehicles, located at the depots. Each customer must be served in one of the time slots in which he/she is available. Differently from what happens in classical Multi-Depot vehicle routing problems (MDVRP), [3] in which routes must end at the same depot from which it started, we allow routes ending on a different depot. This version of MDVRP, which did not receive a greatest interest by the academic community, is very common in practical applications. In fact, it could be more convenient to end a route in a different depot with respect to the starting one, avoiding long trip back to the depot. An heterogeneous fleet is considered, composed by vehicles characterized by capacity and cost per Km, as occurs in most of the VRPs with heterogeneous fleet in literature ([4–6]) in which a fixed usage cost, different for each vehicles classes, is considered. Furthermore, vehicles may have different characteristics (for instance, refrigerated vehicles) which can be required by some customers and must be avoided for other ones. The location of each vehicle at the beginning of the time-horizon analyzed is supposed to be known in advance. Not every customer may be served by all the vehicles and from all the depots. Restrictions on the maximum route duration coming out from drivers working hours limitations are considered too. The goal is to minimize the global travel time.

2.1   Problem Definition

In this subsection we formally define the MDMPVRPHF. The problem consist of serving a set of customers, I, at the minimum cost. Each customer i requires a quantity of goods q_i which can be delivered from one of more depots d belonging to the set of depots D, depending on the availability of the requested products at the depots. Delivery may be carried out by vehicles which are compatible with customers request, during a time-slot (day) in which the customer is available. Further temporal constraint may be given by strictly deadlines imposing that customer i must receive his order before day s or by goods availability (in some cases goods may be available only after day s'). For each couple of nodes is known the distance r_{ij}. The average speed is fixed equal to a constant ν known in advance. A set of vehicles V is located at the depots. For each vehicle v is known the capacity C_v, the cost per min of usage μ_v, and the depot d where the vehicle is located. We define as α the maximum duration of a route. A set of possible routes K is given, where for each route k is known the vehicle v to which it is associated and the day s in which it is scheduled. A customer may be assigned to a route only if it is performed. A vehicle v is supposed to be located at depot d on day s (for $s > 1$) if d is the arrival depot of the routes performed by v on day $s - 1$ or v. If v has not been used in day $s - 1$ he is supposed to be located at the arrival depot of its last performed route, or if it has not been used yet, at the depot where it was located at the beginning of the time-horizon. To help the reader, the definitions of variables and constants are summarized in the following:

2.2   Definitions and Notations

To help the reader, the definitions of variables and constants are summarized in the following:

Input data:
$I = \{1 \ldots Imax\}$: set of customers
$D = \{Imax + 1 \ldots Dmax\}$: set of depots
$N = \{1 \ldots Imax + Dmax\}$: set of nodes ($N = I \cup D$)
$K = \{1 \ldots Kmax\}$: set of routes
$V = \{1 \ldots Vmax\}$: set of vehicles
$S = \{1 \ldots Smax\}$: set of days
M: very large constant
ϵ: very small constant
α: maximum route duration
ν: average speed (expressed in Km/h)
q_i: demand of customer i
r_{ij}: distance between node i and node j
v_k: vehicle associated to route k
t_k: day on which route k is scheduled
C_k: capacity of route k (i.e. capacity of vehicle v performing route k)
F_{id}: equal to 1 if customer i can be served by depot d
E_{iv}: equal to 1 if customer i can be served by vehicle v
G_{is}: equal to 1 if customer i can be served on day s
l_{kd}: equal to 1 if vehicle v associated to route k is initially located at the depot d
μ_v: cost per minute of usage for vehicle v

Variables:
X_{ijk}: boolean variable equal to 1 if arc ij is used by route k
Y_{ik}: boolean variable equal to 1 if customer i is served by route k
Z_k: boolean variable equal to 1 if route k belongs to the solution
T_i: time at which node i is visited

L_{kd}: boolean variable equal to 1 if route k can start from the depot d
W_k: duration of route k

3   A Mixed Integer Programming Model for the MDMPVRPHF

Using the notation above introduced a MIP model to minimize the total cost for delivery operations over a fixed time-horizon, can be formulated as follows:

$$\min \sum_{i \in N} \sum_{j \in N} \sum_{k \in N} \frac{\nu}{60} r_{ij} \mu_{v_k} X_{ijk} \tag{1}$$

s.t.

$$\sum_{j \in N | j \neq i} X_{ijk} = Y_{ik} \quad \forall i \in I, \forall k \in K \tag{2}$$

$$\sum_{j \in N | j \neq i} X_{jik} = Y_{ik} \quad \forall i \in I, \forall k \in K \tag{3}$$

$$\sum_{k \in K} Y_{ik} = 1 \quad \forall i \in I \tag{4}$$

$$\sum_{j \in N | j \neq i} X_{djk} \leq L_{kd} \quad \forall k \in K, \forall d \in D \tag{5}$$

$$\sum_{j \in N | j \neq i} \sum_{d \in D} X_{djk} = Z_k \quad \forall k \in K \tag{6}$$

$$\sum_{j \in N | j \neq i} \sum_{d \in D} X_{jdk} = Z_k \quad \forall k \in K \tag{7}$$

$$\sum_{i \in I} Y_{ik} \leq M \cdot Z_k \quad \forall k \in K \tag{8}$$

$$X_{iik} = 0 \quad \forall i \in I \forall k \in K \tag{9}$$

$$T_i \geq T_j + \frac{\nu}{60} r_{ij} X_{jik} - M(1 - X_{jik}) \quad \forall i \in I, \forall j \in N, \forall k \in K \tag{10}$$

$$T_d = 0 \quad \forall d \in D \tag{11}$$

$$\sum_{i \in I} q_i Y_{ik} \leq C_k \quad \forall k \in K \tag{12}$$

$$W_k \leq \alpha \quad \forall k \in K \tag{13}$$

$$W_k = \sum_{i \in N} \sum_{j \in N} \frac{\nu}{60} r_{ij} X_{ijk} \quad \forall k \in K \tag{14}$$

$$L_{kd} = l_{kd} \quad \forall k \in K | t_k = 1 \; \forall d \in D \tag{15}$$

$$\sum_{d \in D} L_{kd} \leq 1 \quad \forall k \in K \tag{16}$$

$$L_{kd} = l_{kd}(1 - Z_{k - Vmax}) + \sum_{j \in N} \sum_{\substack{w \in K| \\ v_w = v_k \\ t_w = t_k - 1}} X_{jdw} \quad \forall k \in K | t(k) \geq 1, \forall d \in D \tag{17}$$

$$L_{kd} \leq \sum_{j \in N} \sum_{\substack{w \subset K| \\ v_w = v_k \\ t_w = t_k - 1}} X_{jdw} + l_{kd} \quad \forall k \in K | t(k) \geq 1, \forall d \in D \tag{18}$$

$$L_{kd} \geq \sum_{j \in N} \sum_{\substack{w \in K| \\ v_w = v_k \\ t_w = t_k - 1}} X_{jdw} \quad \forall k \in K | t(k) \geq 1, \forall d \in D \tag{19}$$

$$Y_{ik} \leq \sum_{d \in D} F_{id} L_{kd} \quad \forall i \in I, \forall k \in K \tag{20}$$

$$Y_{ik} \leq E_{iv_k} \quad \forall i \in I, \forall k \in K \tag{21}$$

$$Y_{ik} \leq G_{it_k} \quad \forall i \in I, \forall k \in K \tag{22}$$

The objective function which minimize the total cost is reported in (1). Constraints (2) and (3) ensure that a customer is visited by a route only if it has been assigned to it, while constraint (4) implies that each customer must be assigned to one and only one route. A customer i can be served by a route k only if he can be served by the depot d from which k starts, as stated in constraint (5). Constraints (6) and (7) imply that if a route k is performed, it must start from and end to a depot, and, on the other hand, if it is not performed, it can not exit or enter any depot. Constraint (8) state that a customer can be assigned to a route only if that route is performed. Subtours elimination is guaranteed by constraints (9)–(11). Limits on the duration of the routes are imposed by (13) and (14), while vehicle capacity satisfaction is ensured by constraint (12). Constraints (15)–(19) allow to determine the starting depot for each routes, depending on the initial location of the vehicle and the routes performed by it on the previous days. Constraints (20)–(22) check customer-route compatibility. Variables related to arrival time at nodes, T_i may take real non-negative values, while all the other variables are binary.

4   Algorithm Description

The proposed matheuristic, from now on called MH, works on the customers-to-route assignment variables Y_{ik}. More precisely at each iteration of the algorithm, p customers are randomly selected; all the others $|I| - p$ customers are assigned to the same route to which they are assigned in the current solution, while the p selected ones are let free to be assigned to any route. More in details, being P the set of selected customers, and being $Y*_i k$ the value of the assignment variables in the current solution, we impose the following additional constraints:

$$Y_{ik} = Y_{ik}^* \quad \forall i \in I - P \tag{23}$$

The parameter p can be arbitrary chosen keeping in mind that small values of p allow a limited perturbation with the risk to remain trapped into local minima, while very big values generate such a large neighborhood search which cannot be easily exhaustively explored in a short computational time. Preliminary tests indicate that $p = 10$ represent a good compromise between diversification and neighborhood evaluation speed. The new obtained solution, which is the local minimum in the neighborhood, is chosen as current solution for the next iteration. The procedure terminates after a maximum number of iteration, $MAXITER$, or after a maximum number of iterations without any improvement, $MAXNOIMPROVE$, which are given parameters of the algorithm. This procedure need an initial feasible solution form which to start, that could be computed in different ways, both with a simple greedy constructive heuristic and with more complex meta-heuristic or directly with the model. The initial solution quality is not a crucial issue, because, due to the strong diversification inserted in the algorithm, the matheuristic is capable to explore regions potentially far, in the solutions space, from the starting point and to converge to a very good solution even starting from a poor quality one. This is a strong good point of the method. In this case it has been chosen to take as initial solution the best feasible solution obtained by the model within a given short time limit, TIMELIMIT. The value of this parameter should be short but, at the same time must allow to find at least one feasible solution.

5   Computational Results

In this section computational results obtained on instances with different characteristics are reported. Three depots and six vehicles are available. Thirty customers must be served within a time-horizon of five days. The maximum route duration is imposed to be equal to eleven hours.

Three different levels of customers-vehicles compatibility and of customer availability have been defined (high, medium and low). One instance for each combination of these two parameters have been generated.

These levels have been constructed in order to represent realistic cases which may arise in practical applications. In fact, availability and compatibility level may sensibly very depending on the analyzed context. For instance, in food delivery to the supermarkets, vehicles compatibility is generally low; in fact, frozen or perishable items require specific vehicles, like freezer or refrigerated ones, which generally are a very small subset of the global fleet. Customers availability, instead, is very high because supermarket do not have strictly deadlines, and may be served each day of the week. In other contexts, like electronic products home delivery (carried out by amazon or other online shopping website), strictly delivery deadline are imposed, but vehicles compatibility is around 100 %, because products do not have any specific requirement. Since the goal of this project was to create a tool which can be applied on several contexts, we decided to test the model on instances having different characteristics, in order to recreate realistic situations.

The perturbation size p has been taken equal to 10, the time limit for the initial solution search is imposed equal to 10 seconds. While the maximum number of iterations, MAXITER, is equal to 100, while the maximum number of iterations without any improvements, MAXNOIMPROVE, is equal to 10.

Matheuristic results are compared with the results obtained running the model on XPRESS 7.3. with a time limit of 3600 seconds. Detailed results are reported in Table 1, which is organized as follows. First column contains the name of the instance, while customer-vehicle compatibility and customers availability are reported in columns 2 and 3, respectively. In columns 4 and 5 we show the best solution obtained by the model within the time limit (UB) and the initial solution (IS). Column 6 reports the averaged objective function obtained by MH over 10 runs, while in columns 7 and 8 are reported the averaged percentage improvement with respect to the model solution and to the initial solution, respectively. Column 9 reports the best objective function obtained over 10 runs and columns 10 and 11 the related percentage improvements. Averaged computational time for the MH is around 200 seconds.

Table 1. Computational results

ISTANZA	V-COMP	DAY-AV	MODEL-LB	MODEL-UB	INIT-SOL	MH (AVG)	IMPROVE (UB)	IMPROVE(IS)	MH (BEST)	IMPROVE (UB)	IMPROVE(IS)
I1	HIGH	HIGH	1292.79	1902.85	2290.65	1673.05	-12.08%	-26.96%	1626.89	-14.50%	-28.98%
I2	HIGH	MEDIUM	1346.74	1848.79	1981.54	1577.43	-14.68%	-20.39%	1544.50	-16.46%	-22.06%
I3	HIGH	LOW	1359	1715	2466.64	1713.15	-0.11%	-30.55%	1649.92	-3.79%	-33.11%
I4	MEDIUM	HIGH	1341.11	1913.14	1975.44	1594.07	-16.68%	-19.31%	1574.42	-17.70%	-20.30%
I5	MEDIUM	MEDIUM	1364.49	1779.92	2529.48	1753.41	-1.49%	-30.68%	1720.08	-3.36%	-32.00%
I6	MEDIUM	LOW	1384.01	1673.03	2377.26	1612.40	-3.62%	-32.17%	1582.56	-5.41%	-33.43%
I7	LOW	HIGH	1422.71	1743.33	2408.86	1661.39	-4.70%	-31.03%	1646.54	-5.55%	-31.65%
I8	LOW	MEDIUM	1650.32	1811.37	2257.23	1863.60	2.88%	-17.44%	1809.75	-0.09%	-19.82%
I9	LOW	LOW	1700.01	1796.14	2236.9	1848.05	2.89%	-17.38%	1791.71	-0.25%	-19.90%
AVG			1429.02	1798.174	2280.444	1699.62	-5.29%	-25.10%	1660.71	-7.46%	-26.80%

As shown in Table 1, MH provide a remarkable percentage improvement with respect to the model within much quicker computational time. The improvement with respect to the initial solution is above 25 % on average, which means that the algorithm is capable to converge to a good solution even starting from a poor one. Improvements are smaller on highly constrained instances (I8 and I9), which are the less common in practice. This behavior can be explained by the fact that the model perform better on more constrained problem, and therefore, solutions obtained by the model on I8 and I9 are already high quality ones. Averaged results on 10 runs are quite similar to best results which is another good point of the algorithm because shows its robustness respect to the random component.

6   Conclusions

In this paper a new A New Large Neighborhood Search Based Matheuristic Framework for Rich Vehicle Routing Problems is proposed and tested on the Multi Depot Multi Period Vehicle Routing Problem with Heterogeneous Fleet, a complex routing problem arising in real contexts. The most innovative aspect of the proposed approach is the capability of exhaustively exploring a large (or very-large) neighborhood in very small computational time, which make the LNS framework much more effective than to traditional implementation of LNS in which only a subset of the solutions in the considered neighborhood are analyzed. Another good point of this approach is that it is extremely portable, i.e. it can be easily adapted to other vehicle routing problems dealing with assignment variables, such as the 2E-VRP in which customers are assigned to intermediate facilities, or as standard Multi-Depot and Location-Routing problems. Furthermore, this neighborhood search technique may be used in the local search phase in more complex metaheuristics such as Variable Neighborhood Search (VNS), Adaptive Large Neighborhood Search (ALNS) and others.

References

1. Ahuja, R., Ergun, Ö., Orlin, J., Punnen, A.: A survey of very largescale neighborhood search techniques. Discrete Appl. Math. **123**, 75–102 (2002)
2. Pisinger, D., Ropke, S.: Large Neighborhood Search. In: Gendreau, M., Potvin, J.-Y. (eds.) Handbook of Metaheuristics. International Series in Operations Research & Management Science, vol. 146, pp. 399–419. Springer, Berlin (2010)
3. Toth, P., Vigo, D.: The Vehicle Routing Problem. SIAM, Philadelpia (2002)
4. Salhi, S., Imran, A., Wassan, N.: The multi-depot vehicle routing problem with heterogeneous vehicle fleet: Formulation and a variable neighborhood search implementation. Comput. Oper. Res. (to appear)
5. Brandao, J.: A tabu search algorithm for the heterogeneous fixed fleet vehicle routing problem. Comput. Oper. Res. **38**, 140–151 (2011)
6. Choi, E., Tcha, D.: A column generation approach to the heterogeneous fleet vehicle routing problem. Comput. Oper. Res. **34**, 2080–2095 (2007)

A Cloud Architecture Approximation to Collaborative Environments for Image Analysis Applications

Francisca Quintana-Domínguez[1](✉), Carmelo Cuenca-Hernández[2],
and Abraham Rodríguez-Rodríguez[1]

[1] Instituto Universitario de Ciencias Y Tecnologías Cibernéticas,
Universidad de Las Palmas de Gran Canaria, Campus de Tafira,
35017 Las Palmas de Gran Canaria, Spain
{francisca.quintana,abraham.rodriguez}@ulpgc.es
[2] Departamento de Informática y Sistemas,
Universidad de Las Palmas de Gran Canaria, Campus de Tafira,
35017 Las Palmas de Gran Canaria, Spain
carmelo.cuenca@ulpgc.es

Abstract. This work describes a flexible cloud computing architecture intended to be used in collaborative groups where each group member develops image analysis processes that are made available to the rest of the group in a flexible, robust and easy-to-use way. The cloud computing approximation makes the whole system elastically scalable and reliable to failures. Computing resources are provisioned when needed, used for a specific task and finally relinquished after the job is done. In the proposed architecture each individual process takes its input data from a queue, carries out the task and leaves the output in another queue. Building a complex task starting from individual ones is performed by chaining processes, just matching output and input queues of subsequent processes.

Keywords: Cloud computing architectures · Collaborative environments · Image analysis · Amazon web services

1 Collaborative Environments and Cloud Architectures

In a collaborative environment, like for example a scientific laboratory of image analysis, group members develop different software processes for a common pool. The aim is that these different processes are available for the whole group, to be easily used and integrated in any general task. Traditionally, these individual pieces of code are packed up in software libraries that are included whenever needed. However, this scenario entails several sources of problems. First of all, compiling the whole code can become a challenge. Group members must deal with compiling considerations of other's code which makes it a burden to get a running version of the whole application. Second, a good planning and coordination must be done so that each funcionality is only developed once (applying the

© Springer International Publishing Switzerland 2015
R. Moreno-Díaz et al. (Eds.): EUROCAST 2015, LNCS 9520, pp. 797–804, 2015.
DOI: 10.1007/978-3-319-27340-2_98

"Don't Repeat Yourself" principle). Third, each group member must know in every moment what is the version of the different pieces of code that he is using where are located. All these considerations make sharing, reusing and integrating code a challenging situation that can be difficult to successfully solve [1].

These drawbacks can be overcome by using a cloud computing architecture design for the whole application and for each individual process. In that case we could see other's routines as a service, running somewhere in the cloud. To use them we just connect to them, send parameters and receive results. This scenario abstracts us from developing details of other's code, we could have a running version serving to many users, while assuring a reasonable response time.

1.1   Cloud Architectures

Cloud computing architectures are design patterns of software applications that use Internet-accesible on-demand services [2,3]. Applications developed based on cloud architectures run on a service model so that they are used only when needed, and can scale up and down according to the instant workload [4]. Moreover, cloud applications run in the cloud (in our case Amazon Web Services, AWS [5]), using a provider's infrastructure whose location is transparent to the user. They provide reliable, scalable resources in a pay-per-use service model. Following these patterns means provisioning resources only when needed, using them to carry out a task, and releasing them as soon as they are not needed any more. Moreover, resources are elastically provisioned, which means dinamically increasing or decreasing the ammount of provisioned resources to meet the applications demands in every moment. On the other hand, using the cloud services of public providers allows a quick resources provision with a simple API-based connection through the Internet. It also allows deploying applications without any initial investment, as the cloud economic model is pay-per-use based. In this way, cloud developments can be done with a modest budget, as we only pay for what we really use, during the amount of time that we have provisioned the resources.

All in all, developing and deploying applications using the cloud architecture patterns allows a considerable cost reduction and a better service to users, even in high workload situations.

1.2   Background

We have identified several public solutions that deal with similar problems, although none of them solve exactly the same situation. Among the different options we have found Cloudinary [6], 6px [7], Blitline [8], Imgix [9] and the IPOL journal [10]. Some of them provide with a Graphical User Interface, others allow interaction through an API, and a few of them allow both. Except for the IPOL journal, none of these services permit including your own new image transformations, so they are not suitable for a collaborative environment where members develop new code. In the case of the IPOL journal, although you can upload new transformations, it is restricted to those that implement new methods that have been previously publised in the journal. And even in this case, the execution time is limited to one minute. Therefore, we haven't found an implementation of a collaborative environment based on cloud architecture patterns like the one that we describe in this work.

2 Our Proposal: A Collaborative Cloud Computing Architecture

Our proposal is based on hiding the implementation details and the integration procedures. In this way, only the developer of the process knows how a process works internally, how is implemented, the environment for running the process, which libraries are needed, the dependencies with other processed, etc. The rest of the group members just uses it. This is acomplished by executing the process in the cloud, as a service. The process accepts requests of use that are carried out, and the resulting outputs are sent back to the users.

2.1 Architecture of a Basic Process

In our architecture each single process executes in the cloud (in our case EC2 of AWS) following a service model. It takes its input data from an input queue and leaves the results in an output queue, as seen in Fig. 1(a), and it is not conscious about the complex task it is working for in every moment. In fact, parameters and results are really stored in the cloud (Simple Storage Service, or S3, of AWS [5]), so the messages only have the information of where data are located in the S3. The use of queues allow decoupling one process from the others, isolating processes from each other and buffering requests (which means that the difference of speeds between processes is balanced). It also provides with an asynchronous execution of processes, sharing processes between different users, and it is a fault tolerant solution because if the process fails it can be automatically launched again and it continues processing the pending incoming messages.

Moreover, the architecture is also scalable so that if a process has too many pending requests in its input queue, more processes of the same type are launched

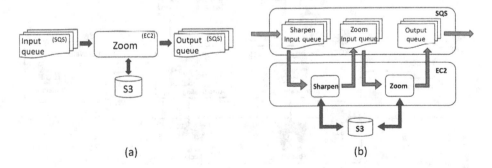

(a)   (b)

Fig. 1. Cloud architecture of (a) a single Zoom process and (b) a complex task made up of two single processes (Sharpen and Zoom).

to deal with this workload. Similarly, as the input queue empties, the extra processes are disposed. When the input queue is completely empty, all the processes are removed, so the computational resources are relinquished.

Cloud Implementation in AWS. We have chosen AWS as the public cloud provider for the implementation due to several reasons: it's a leader among the cloud providers, it's mature and consolidated, it includes all the services that we need in just one provider, and it has a free layer (and a grant program). Among the more then thirty different services provided by AWS we have used Elastic Compute Cloud (EC2), AutoScaling, Simple Storage Service (S3), Simple Queue Service (SQS), CloudWatch, Simple Notification Service (SNS) and Identity and Access Management (IAM).

In Fig. 2 we can see the basic implementation. On the right there is a Sharpen process that is being used by only one user, and on the left there is a Zoom process that is being used by two different users. In the later case, both users send their requests to the same input queue. To execute a process the user logges in AWS with its secure credentials through the IAM. It builds the input message and sends it to the in_queue of the process in SQS. The structure of the input message includes the process identification, the params that the process need to execute (e.g. input image, specific params for the image process and output image), and some optional information like the destination for the output image (the S3 bucket name) and whether we want a notification upon termination of the process. Then, the running EC2 instance reads the message from the input queue, does its job and stores the result in S3. After that, it builds the

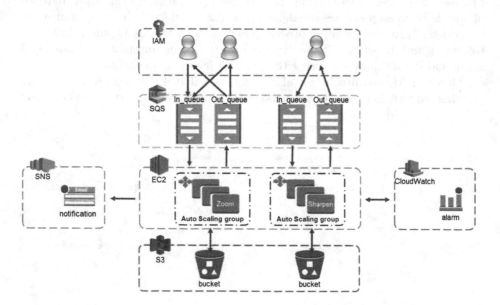

Fig. 2. Cloud architecture implementation for single processes Zoom and Sharpen.

```
InitCloud (Input_image, in_queue, S3_bucket)
    Sqs new
    S3 new
    Read in_queue until valid_message
    Analyze message
    Download Input_image from S3_bucket
```

```
EndCloud (Output_image, out_queue, S3_bucket)
    Upload Output_image to S3_bucket
    Build output_message
    Send message to out_queue
```

Fig. 3. The steps that the `InitCloud()` and `EndCloud()` utilities execute.

output message and sends it to the output queue. The output message structure includes the idenfication of the process, a status code of the finished process and the place in the S3 where the output image has been stored. Optionally, the EC2 instance sends a notification through SNS (if needed). In the mean time, the CloudWatch service provides the measures for the alarms. If the alarm triggers, the AutoScaling service increases or decreases the number of running instances for that process.

Adapting to the Cloud: Adding and Using a New Process. From the programmer's point of view the adoption of the new architecture is quite simple. He has to include the appropriate libraries to work with the cloud services and start the new process code with a reading of the input queue. Once the queue has a message to be delivered, the process downloads the input image from the cloud storage and it does exactly the same as in the non-cloud programming model. Finally, at the end of the process a new step to be done is to build the output message and send it to the ouput queue. All this process can be automated, which is the key for the sucess of the implementation. A new process just makes a call to an `InitCloud()` function at the beginning, and `EndCloud()` at the end. These functions execute the steps in Fig. 3. Once the process is developed it must be launched to the cloud. A new EC2 instance must be created, which includes the code with its execution environment. This can also be automated with a call to a `Register()` utility, with the information about the proccess, that is, its name and params. This `Register()` utility doesn't launch the instance to prevent having idle instances running (which would unnecesarily increase costs). The instance will automatically be launched when some process needs to use it. At that time the process asks for a running instance, and if there isn't any, it will be launched.

From the user's point of view, instead of doing a traditional function call, now the user must build the message with the params for the process and send

```
CloudExec (Zoom, Input, HorizontalZoom, VerticalZoom,
Output)
    Sqs new
    S3 new
    SetUpCloud (EC2, SQS,  CloudWatch, AutoScaling)
    Upload Input image to S3_bucket
    Build message (Zoom, Input, HorizontalZoom, VerticalZoom,
    Output)
    Send message to in_queue
    Read out_queue until valid_message
    Analyze message
    Download Output image from S3_bucket


                    SetUpCloud (EC2, SQS,  CloudWatch, AutoScaling)
                        Launch EC2 instance
                        Create in_queue and out_queue
                        Create a set of alarms in CloudWatch
                        Create AutoScaling group with appropiate rules
```

Fig. 4. The steps that the CloudExec() and SetUpCloud() utilities execute.

it to the input queue. However, before sending the message it must ask for the existence of a running instance for that process. If there isn't any, it must launch the EC2 instance, create the input and output queues, create a set of alarms in CloudWatch and create the AutoScaling group with the appropriate rules that allow launching more instances if needed. All these steps can be automated in a SetUpCloud() utility. After building the message and send it to the input queue, it must wait for a valid message in the output queue, analyze the message to check if the status is successfull and download the output image from the S3 bucket. Again, all these steps can be automated with a CloudExec() utility with the definition of the process and the needed parameters. All these execution steps are shown in Fig. 4.

2.2 Complex Tasks: Chaining Processes

Going one step further, we define a complex task by chaining simple processes. In that case we match the output queue of a process with the input queue of the following one, so the output queue of every single process will be no longer needed as the result will be directly sent to the input queue of the next process, as shown in Fig. 1(b).

Now, the structure of the initial message is more complex as it must define the full task. It must include the different processes involved and their params, as well as the destination of the resulting images, whether we want the intermediate images to be stored or not, and whether a notification must be sent after

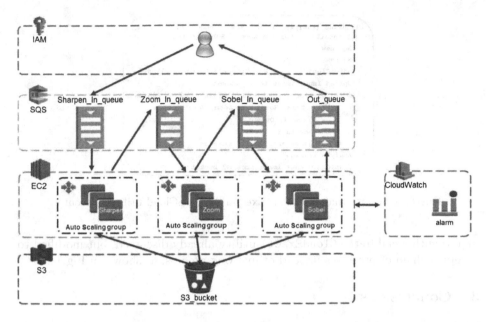

Fig. 5. Cloud architecture implementation for a complex task out of chained processes.

the complex task is finished. As the message moves from one process queue to another, it also includes the different processes that have been finished, their status code, and their output images.

Cloud Implementation in AWS. In Fig. 5 we can see the implementation of a complex task with three simple processes: Sharpen, Zoom and Sobel. The user sends the initial message to the Sharpen_In_queue. Sharpen reads from that queue and before finishing it sends a message to the Zoom_In_queue. In the same way, Zoom and Sobel read from their input queues and before finishing they send output messages to the appropriate queues. The last process sends the final output message to the Out_queue. As in the previous case, CloudWatch alarms are set for the different AutoScaling groups of the instances so that if there are many pending requests in the input queues, additional instances are launched.

Complex Tasks: Adding and Using a New Process. The only difference with the previous case is that at the end of every single process it must be checked if there is a running instance for the following process. If that is the case, the output message must be sent to its input queue. But if there isn't, then an instance for the following process must be launched. This can be achieved with a call to the `SetUpCloud()` utility already described.

Regarding the use of a new process, all we have to do is to build a complex initial message that includes the definition of the whole task. This can be auto-

```
CloudExec (Sharpen, Input, Sharpeness, Radius, Zoom,
HorizontalZoom, VerticalZoom,  Sobel, Output)
    Sqs new
    S3 new
    SetUpCloud (EC2, SQS,  CloudWatch, AutoScaling)
    Upload Input image to S3_bucket
    Build message (Sharpen, Input, Sharpeness, Radius,
                Zoom, HorizontalZoom, VerticalZoom,
                Sobel, Output)
    Send message to in_queue
    Read out_queue until valid_message
    Analyze message
    Download Output image from S3_bucket
```

Fig. 6. The steps that the CloudExec and SetUpCloud utilities execute.

mated with a call to the `CloudExec()` utility already discussed, but modified to accept a chain of processes instead of just one process, as shown in Fig. 6.

3   Conclusions

We have proposed a cloud architecture for collaborative environments in the field of image analysis applications. It provides with characteristics that improve the efficiency of collaboration: isolation of the processes, decoupling of the different tasks and buffering of the requests. These characteristics rely on the fact that every process takes its input data from an input queue and leaves the results in an output queue. Building a complex task starting from individual ones is performed by chaining processes, matching output and input queues of subsequent processes. Our proposed architecture is easy to use and elastically scalable. Furthermore, the architecture is robust, reliable to failures and flexible. This is acomplished by provisioning resources only when needed, carrying out the process and relinquishing them when they are no longer needed.

References

1. Highsmith, J.: Adaptive Software Development. A Collaborative Approach to Managing Complex Systems. Dorset House, New York (2000)
2. Varia, J.: Building GrepTheWeb in the Cloud, Part1: Cloud Architectures. Amazon Web Services (2008). http://aws.amazon.com/articles/1632
3. Reese, G.: Cloud Applications Architectures: Building Applications and Infrastructure in the Cloud. O'Reilly, USA (2009)
4. Wilder, B.: Cloud Architecture Patterns. Building Cloud-Native Applications. O'Reilly, USA (2012)
5. Amazon Web Services. http://aws.amazon.com
6. Cloudinary. http://www.cloudinary.com
7. 6px. http://www.6px.io
8. Blitline. http://www.blitline.com
9. Imgix. http://www.imgix.com
10. IPOL Journal. http://www.ipol.im

Deployment Models and Optimization Procedures in Cloud Computing

Jerzy Kotowski[1,2]([✉]), Jacek Oko[1,2], and Mariusz Ochla[1,2]

[1] Wroclaw University of Technology, Wroclaw, Poland
[2] IBM Polska Sp. z o.o, Warsaw, Poland
{jerzy.kotowski,jacek.oko}@pwr.edu.pl, mariusz_ochla@pl.ibm.com

Abstract. Cloud computing is a category of computing solutions in which a technology and service lets users access computing resources on demand, as needed, whether the resources are physical or virtual, dedicated, or shared, and no matter how they are accessed. In any case a Virtual Machine (VM) is putted into the motion. The mathematical model of the deployment process varies of the detailed properties of the particular hosts putted into the work in the considered cloud. We will present these properties in the full paper and show the road that leads to appropriate optimization model.

Keywords: Cloud computing · Deployment process · Optimization · Mathematical model

1 Cloud Computing

Cloud computing's importance rests in the cloud's potential to save investment costs in infrastructure, to save time in application development and deployment, and to save resource allocation overhead. Typical benefits of managing in the cloud are: reduced cost, increased storage and flexibility. Cloud platform facilitates deployment of applications without the cost and complexity of buying and managing the underlying hardware and software layers.

2 Virtual Machine

A virtual machine is a software implementation of a machine (i.e. a computer) that executes programs like a physical machine. An essential characteristic of a virtual machine is that the software running inside is limited to the resources and abstractions provided by the virtual machine - it cannot break out of its virtual environment. At the moment, there exists hundreds of application that support cooperation between server and user PC, which are being installed by user. Among them, we can distinguish such as: VMware, VM from IBM, etc. A virtual machine is a "completely isolated guest operating system installation within a normal host operating system". Modern virtual machines are implemented with either software emulation or hardware virtualization. In most cases, both are implemented together [1].

© Springer International Publishing Switzerland 2015
R. Moreno-Díaz et al. (Eds.): EUROCAST 2015, LNCS 9520, pp. 805–812, 2015.
DOI: 10.1007/978-3-319-27340-2_99

3 Deployment Model – Problem Description

Cloud platform services often consuming cloud infrastructure and sustaining cloud applications. It facilitates deployment of applications without the cost and complexity of buying and managing the underlying hardware and software layers [3,4]. The problem itself may be, in general, formulated as follows:

Given: The number of virtual machines. Each of them is described by needed resources (CPU performance, memory). Required working hours are also known. These requirements may be different for each machine. There is a cloud computing system consisting of multiprocessor computers (host machines) with defined parameters.

Assumptions: Each virtual machine must be deployed on a single host. The hardware resources of at least one host machines are larger than those required by the virtual machine. Working hours for each VM are known. The most important parameter for the VM is its performance. The minimal feasible performance is known as like as its advisable value.

Task: Deploy virtual machines on the particular host.

4 Optimization Problem

Problem presented above may be transformed to the Strip Packing (Cutting) Problem. This problem is formulated as follows: to pack (or cut) a set of small rectangles (pieces) into a bin (strip) of fixed width but unlimited length. The aim is to minimize the length to which the bin is filled.

In this paper the most imported idea is to put into the motion properties of the host memory operating system. The most popular systems now are FAT and NTFS. FAT (File Allocation Table) is a table that the operating system uses to allocate files on the disk. The FAT system allows for defragmentation of files into the small pieces. NTFS (New Technology File System) has features to improve reliability, such as transaction logs to help recover from disk failures. To control access to files, you can set permissions for directories and/or individual files. For large applications, NTFS supports spanning volumes, which means files and directories can be spread out across several physical disks. The memory operating system has a crucial influence on the shape of the optimization problem [3,5,6].

5 Orchestrator

Orchestrator is a workflow management solution for the data center. Orchestrator lets to automate the creation, monitoring, and deployment of resources. Cloud orchestration solutions from IBM are designed to reduce the IT management complexities introduced by virtual and cloud environments and accelerate cloud service delivery, allowing enterprises to quickly respond to changing business needs. IT administrators perform many tasks and procedures to keep the health of their computing environment up-to-date and their business running. Tasks might include the diverse activities. Individual tasks and subtasks are automated, but typically, not for the whole process [2].

By using Orchestrator, we can carry out the following tasks:

- Automate processes in the data center,
- regardless of hardware or platform,
- automate IT operations and standardize best practices to improve operational efficiency and
- connect different systems from different vendors without having to know how to use scripting and programming languages.

Orchestrator provides tools to build, test, debug, deploy, and manage automation in environment. The standard activities defined in every installation of Orchestrator provide a variety of monitors and tasks with which it is possible to integrate a wide range of system processes.

Any IT organization can use Orchestrator to improve efficiency and reduce operational costs to support cross-departmental objectives. Orchestrator provides an environment with shared access to common data. By using Orchestrator, an enterprise can evolve and automate key processes between groups and consolidate repetitive manual tasks. It can automate cross-functional team processes and enforce best practices for incident, change, and service management.

5.1 Smarter Cloud Orchestrator at Wroclaw University of Technology

Future education will be not only widely available, but also much smarter than today. Due to a rapid growth of technologies, among which cloud computing plays a key role, the education supporting systems will use all available information in order to personalize the process of teaching. It is already happening and predicts a fast development of such technologies within 5 years. The revolution of process of teaching will affect all levels of education, not only academia. The adoption of new mentality as well as the development of necessary systems will obviously take some time, however it is particularly academia's role to lead the process.

All the changes in education will not be possible without a flexible system that would support cooperation between all types of schools and interactions with businesses. Smarter Cloud Orchestrator (SCO) at Wroclaw University of Technology (WrUT) is a base on which such systems for the entire region of Lower Silesia will be built. The first phase of the project consists of implementation of an IT Cloud for education at the University with the architecture and technology already prepared to support future extension.

5.2 Lower Silesia Educational Cloud

Following chapter presents the concept developed by Wroclaw University of Technology on the execution and implementation of pilot of the services called "Lower

Silesia Educational Cloud" – hereon called . The proposed concept assumes to adapt processing solutions in the cloud computing to the specifications and requirements of the educational sector. On the basis of the infrastructure virtualization layer (software layer) we will build, both hardware resources, to ensure access to computing power, and resources to ensure access to space.

Workstations operating in schools are affected by hypertrophy, inconsistencies, bad management and maintenance of IT infrastructure. Most schools build their teaching facilities based on incremental purchases that are not correlated with any unified concept. The life cycle of a workstation is a disadvantage economically, and affects any justification of the continued functioning of schools in the currently adopted model. Another problem is the lack of interoperability between different schools. Lack of this interoperability leads to the creation of specific barriers preventing the free transfer of knowledge and good practice between schools/learning centers - schools.

5.3   Target LSEC Model

Model realization of Lower Silesia Educational Cloud should be considered at three levels:

– Infrastructure; Content and services; Maintenance and operation.

When considering an appriate model of LSEC one may recognise the seven characteristics of cloud computing:

– Scalability; Accessibility; Measurability; Ease of deployment; Performance; Security; Savings.

5.4   Functional Assumptions of LSEC

For the purposes of the organization of Lower Silesia Educational Cloud the following functional assumptions were adopted:

– Educational Portal providing science subjects materials; Team work;
– Virtual computer labs; The ability to use resources outside the timetable;
– Elements of "personalized education" for each student;
– The possibility of introducing an examination platform;
– Possibility to use the Cloud for the scientific research tasks;
– Availability of materials usage statistics;
– Creating a single repository of information about participants of the educational system; Remote administration of IT resources; Opening the portal in several languages.

The proposed solution involves the use of blade environment, external storage, backup system, and an extensive section of proactive monitoring of all areas at many levels. The use of blade solutions will enable a dramatic reduction in the requirements for the space (physical space in server racks, server rooms).

The concept involves the construction of Lower Silesia Educational Cloud in the following phases:

- Phase 1 - Needs Analysis;
- Phase 2A - Implementation of a pilot;
- Phase 2B - Implementation of basic services (selected geographical area subjective);
- Phase 3 - Implementation of basic services (the rollout of basic services in the area of the Lower Silesia Province);
- Phase 4 - Implementation of the target model for multiservice (along with the model of self-provisioning);

6 Reflections Concerning Cloud Computing

Seven years ago, we saw the emergence of a Smarter Planet —a world becoming instrumented, interconnected and intelligent.

Big Data is the planet's new natural resource. Hundreds of billions of connected sensors and devices have created massive, invisible flow of digital "1s" and "0s" - a global gusher of information.

Advanced analytics enable us to mine it. Enterprises and institutions are analyzing this flow of streaming, unstructured data and acting upon those insights in real time.

Cloud computing is coming of age. The model of computing known as "the cloud" delivers on-demand computing over the internet. It brings new scale and efficiency to service delivery and enables more agile ways of doing business.

Social and mobile create a new platform for work. With devices in hand, individuals now expect to interact with the world around them - as consumers, as students, as citizens.

The concepts of building a Smarter Planet, through Smarter Education and Research, are enabled by a business infrastructure that is instrumented, interconnected, and intelligent.

- Access to learning resources from a variety of mobile devices
- Sensors that allow to manage the campus and buildings facilities (e.g. Energy Grids, Digital video surveillance to protect students)
- Sensors to collect data for large scale research projects

Anywhere anytime learning access for students and teachers Access to leading reference databases anywhere in the world Collaborative cross-institution research on major projects.

- Effective measurement and analysis of individual student and overall school system performance.

- Assessment of individual student needs and predictive interventions to prevent failures.
- Extensive data analysis to support large research projects.

In a rapidly changing world, education and government leaders have the opportunity to ensure successful outcomes for students, the economy and society.

Smarter Classroom. Bring together deep analytics with advanced technology, learning resources and research to create new insights and guide decisions.

Smarter Research. Collaborate with researchers and industry to create knowledge, innovation, intellectual assets to contribute to education and the economy.

Smarter Administration. Create an intelligent infrastructure with open applications and flexible processes that drive down cost, dynamically respond to new requirements and provides security and safety.

Students are at the center with a focus on enhancing academic success and career/college readiness. Smarter Education ensures the student is on the right track for success:

- Mobility plays a key role in Smarter Education. Student centered personalized approach to learning and teaching.
- Digital instructional resources uses the data and analytics.
- Tools to enhance learning by increasing learner engagement delivering an exceptional student experience and outstanding outcomes.

Delivering smarter education means:

- Quality education is delivered effectively, efficiently and at lower costs.
- The future needs of students are anticipated and planned.
- Programs and resources are matched to the learning styles of students.
- Technology builds compelling engagement across the student life-cycle.
- Curriculum is built for the needs of students and the requirements of employers. More, Services and learning opportunities are delivered to students flexibly and easily.

Data and Analytics - Enabling personalized education at scale

- Identifying students at risk; Predicting best interventions per student;
- Integrating outcomes across an institution or geography;
- Management reporting and dash boarding; Better recruitment and retention.

Mobile and Social - Enabling any where, any time, any device learning

- Personalized information and experience; Rationalizing challenging application estate.

Learning is a social enterprise

- Student engagement across full life-cycle; Expertise location, mentoring and coaching.

Cloud - Flexible, scalable IT infrastructure across operational, aadministrative and teaching realms

- Faster to deploy; Simpler to operate and alter;
- Reliable, Secure, Privacy protecting;
- Improving Back Office Operations is key to sustainability, and to enable investment in Front Office Transformation.

Managing resources effectively and efficiently means:

- Budgets are prepared and executed against program goals;
- Tuition and other revenue is collected;
- Institutional advancement strategies are long-term versus short-term;
- Top performers are retained and salaries and benefits competitive and aligned;
- Outages in key services are prevented; Operational costs are lowered;
- Physical assets are maintained and aligned to teaching goals.

Data and Analytics

- Enrollment systems; Alumni information systems; Budget & finance systems;
- Program data systems; HR systems; Operational data of physical systems.

Business Process Improvement

- ERP modernization; Facilities and asset management;
- Energy, traffic, water management; Compliance and risk management;
- Score carding & Dash boarding; Predictive Analytics.

Infrastructure and Operations

- IT operations; Campus and IT security; Converged networks;
- Shared services within and across institutions;
- Accelerate research discovery and innovation capabilities.

6.1   Roadmap for Education Transformation and Sustainability

Create a personalized learning environment built on a 21st century digital curriculum and tools, and individualized intervention plans for student achievement. Enable mobility and pervasive access via an agile infrastructure that supports institutionally and personally owned devices.

Provide secure, authenticated access to collaboration and productivity tools for learners, teaching faculty, researchers and administrators. Leverage data and analytics as a cornerstone of decision-making and insights for teaching faculty and administrators Support students and employers succeed with workforce skills and post-secondary readiness that align with economic development goals.

6.2   Personalized Education Through Analytics on Learning Systems

Teacher uses a dashboard to identify students at risk. Predictive analytics capability identifies at-risk students and their skill gaps. Prescriptive and content analytics capabilities recommend behavior and curriculum interventions for the student.

Teacher selects appropriate interventions and creates an intervention plan for the student. Student consumes the recommended content from the intervention plan using web-based or mobile app. Teacher monitors the progress of the student and adjusts the plan.

7   Summary

As we stated at the beginning in any case at cloud computing a Virtual Machine (VM) is putted into the motion. The mathematical model of the deployment process varies of the detailed properties of the particular hosts putted into the work in the considered cloud. We presented these properties in the paper and showed the road that leads to appropriate optimization model.

References

1. Brzozowska, A., Greblicki, J., Kotowski, J.: Cloud computing in educational applications methods of virtual desktops deployment. In: Moreno-Díaz, R., Pichler, F., Quesada-Arencibia, A. (eds.) EUROCAST 2011, Part I. LNCS, vol. 6927, pp. 568–575. Springer, Heidelberg (2012)
2. Kotowski, J., Oko, J., Ochla, M.: SmartCloud Orchestrator - the first implementation in the world at WrUT for supporting design processes in education at universities. In: 2nd Asia-Pacific Computer-Aided System Engineering Conference, APCASE 2014, Bali, Indonesia, 10–12 February 2014
3. Greblicki, J., Kotowski, J.: Analysis of the properties of the harmony search algorithm carried out on the one dimensional binary Knapsack problem. In: Moreno-Díaz, R., Pichler, F., Quesada-Arencibia, A. (eds.) EUROCAST 2009. LNCS, vol. 5717, pp. 697–704. Springer, Heidelberg (2009)
4. Kotowski, J.: Internships as an application of cloud computing solutions for education at universities. In: Moreno-Díaz, R., Pichler, F., Quesada-Arencibia, A. (eds.) EUROCAST. LNCS, vol. 8112, pp. 156–165. Springer, Heidelberg (2013)
5. Brzozowska, A., Greblicki, J., Kotowski, J.: State encoding and minimization methodology for self-checking sequential machines. In: Moreno-Díaz, R., Pichler, F., Quesada-Arencibia, A. (eds.) EUROCAST 2011, Part I. LNCS, vol. 6927, pp. 551–558. Springer, Heidelberg (2012)
6. Kotowski, J., Wilkocki, M.: Dynamic Tivoli Data Warehause. Komputerowe wspomaganie badań naukowych XIX / red. Jan Zarzycki. Wrocławskie Towarzystwo Naukowe, Wrocław (2012) (in Polish)

A Model for Intelligent Treatment
of Floodwaters

Walter Zajicek[✉]

HTL-Leonding, Technical High School, Limesstraße 12-14,
4060 Leonding, Austria
w.zajicek@htl-leonding.ac.at

Abstract. This model reflects the situation of floodwaters of the river Danube in Upper Austria. The main idea is to use statistical data in this model, so that it will come very close to the real behavior of an inundating Danube in this area. Important input parameters are the water throughput at some crucial locations along the river and the amount of precipitation in the influencing region. This model shows how significant damages on areas nearby the river can be avoided after the installation of flood preventing constructions (e.g. flood polder). It will be adaptable for other territories by changing parameter values.

1 Introduction

In the years 2002 and 2013, during the period of summer, the nearby region of the river Danube was flooded. In Linz on June 4th, 2013 the maximum water level was at 9.3 meters, whereas the normal gauge height is about 3.5 m.

The two pictures below give an impression of this situation: Fig. 1.

The most important goal of this work is to be able to take efficient measures to minimize the damage of an inundating Danube that could go up to millions of Euros in particular when enterprises like *voestalpine* in Linz are affected. See also the documentation of the above mentioned floodwater: *Hochwasser Juni 2013, Donau, Ereignisdokumentation, Verbund AG* [3].

2 Brief Description of the Model

The most important input data are the values of the amount of the flowing water at the power stations. Some important parameters enable the computation of the amount of water of an inundated area depending on the actual water throughputs in that area. The output is a measure of the damage in a given situation.

With the help of this model I make suggestions for an intelligent control of the water power stations in such situations. Some more flood preventing actions like eliminating sediments in the river and their impact will be investigated.

Here is a map of the affected area: Fig. 2.

© Springer International Publishing Switzerland 2015
R. Moreno-Díaz et al. (Eds.): EUROCAST 2015, LNCS 9520, pp. 813–821, 2015.
DOI: 10.1007/978-3-319-27340-2_100

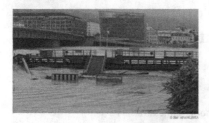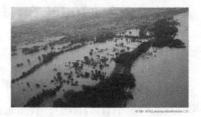

Fig. 1. Left: right riverbank, Ars Electronica Center and Nibelungen Bridge of Linz [1]. Right: deliberately flooded municipality area of Ottensheim [2].

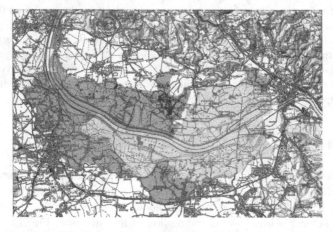

Fig. 2. The area of the Eferdinger Becken. The yellow depicted part was seriously affected, whereas the lila zone was less afflicted [5] (Colour figure online).

3   Mathematical Notation of the Model

This notation is made up of a DEVS (Discrete EVent System) and its functions. The most important one is the state transition function that transforms a given state s of the inundation model at some elapsed discrete time e to the next state s' that will be valid at the time **e + 1**. The time slot will be one hour. This system will start at time **e = 1** and stop after a given number **n** of hours. So we consider a certain interesting time interval within a few days.

Here is the DEVS formalism of the flooding model:

$$DEVS = <X, Y, S, \delta, \lambda >$$

with

X is the input set: a table (e, q) where e is a number between **1** and **n** and **q** is the amount of outflowing water in **m³** at time **e**. This amount of water depends on the throughputs of water from the above power station and the one beneath after the saturation delay **d**.

Y is the output set: it represents the caused **damage** in **euros**.

S is the set of all possible states including the elapsed time: formed by a table (**e, s**) where s is the sum of already outflowed water at time **e**.

δ: S → S is the state transition function: it simply sums up the **q** values:

(**e', s'**): = (**e + 1, s + q**) for (**e, q**) of X and (**e, s**) of S.

For (**e <= d**) the value of **q** is **0**. For **e = 1** the value of **s** starts with 0.

λ: S → Y is the output function: it takes the maximum value **s**, compares it with values in the damage table and takes the corresponding cost value from that table.

More details are stated in the next paragraph. The specific input table in this model mainly depends on the actual flowing water at the small village of Brandstatt (river km 2157). And this water flow depends on the operation mode and throughput of the power stations in Aschach and Ottensheim.

The difference $Q_{Aschach} - Q_{Ottensheim}$ (Q is measured in m^3 per second) is the approximate amount of outflowing water to the region called "Eferdinger Becken" which is about 50 km^2 large. About half of this region is severely affected. The input function table takes values on the basis of the real situation of **June 2013**. It reflects the observed amount of outflowed water and with the help of the damage table one can estimate the damage that adds up to about **100 million euros**.

4   The Computational Model

All the data and parameter values are stored in tables. The input table is generated by a PLSQL stored procedure. Here is a description of the most important parts:

4.1   The Tables and Their Values

There is a table that holds the data of the two power stations of interest. The next figure is a graphical representation of the input table during 27 h. At both power stations the peak of water throughput was reached about 20 h after the model starting time which is Monday 3rd of June 2013 at 5:15 am Fig. 3.

This diagram describes the outflowing water **q** in m^3 per hour at time e: Fig. 4.

The next figure shows the actual amount of outflowed water at the elapsed hour **e**: Fig. 5.

The following diagram shows that the overall damage is about **100 million euros** Fig. 6.

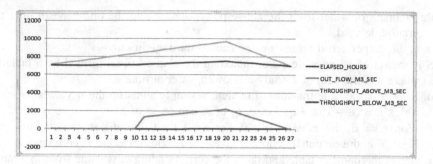

Fig. 3. The throughput data of Aschach and Ottensheim and the outflow.

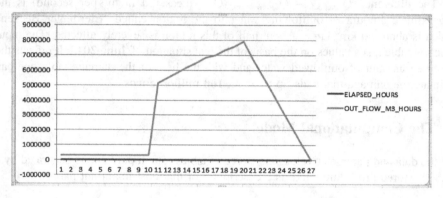

Fig. 4. The amount of outflowing water during 27 h in m³ per hour.

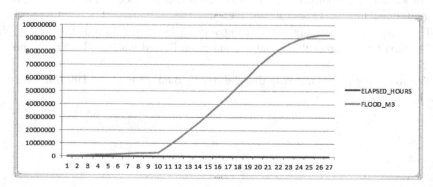

Fig. 5. The accumulated amount of outflowing water in m³.

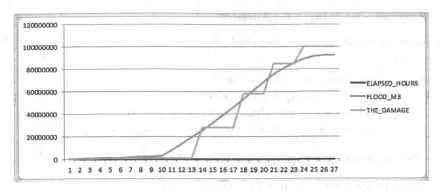

Fig. 6. The growth of the damage in euros relative to the increase of outflowing water.

4.2 The Parameters, Variables and Their Values

The following table lists the relevant characteristics with their names and values.

Characteristic	Variable names	Value
Name of the area	region_name	"Eferdinger Becken"
Size of this area	total_size	$\sim 50\,000\,000$ m^2
Size of the most affected area (yellow)	size_yellow	$\sim 25\,000\,000$ m^2
Size of the less affected area (lila)	size_lila	$\sim 25\,000\,000$ m^2
Stowage space of power station Aschach	stowage_A	$\sim 114\,000\,000$ m^3
Sediments increase during one year	sed_incr	$\sim 2\,000\,000$ m^3
Size of future flood polder	polder_size	$\sim 12\,500\,000$ m^2
Stowage space of future flood polder	stowage_P	$\sim 30\,000\,000$ m^3
Peak water throughput KW Aschach	max_Q_A	$\sim 9\,700$ m^3/sec
Peak water throughput KW Ottensheim	max_Q_O	$\sim 7\,500$ m^3/sec
Maximum water outflow June 2013	max_out	$\sim 2\,200$ m^3/sec
Monitoring starting time	start_time	3rd June 2013, 5:15 am.
Time to fill stowage space KW Ottensheim	saturation_delay	10 h
Monitoring period from start time	duration	27 h
Tailback water amount	tailback_water	$\sim 5\,000\,000$ m^3
Sum of water outflow + tailback water	sum_out	$\sim 92\,500\,000$ m^3
Percentage of ground water	percent_gw	~ 50 %
Sum of water above ground	sum_over	$\sim 46\,250\,000$ m^3
Average water hight in yellow area	avg_yellow	1,6 m
Average water hight in lila area	avg_lila	0,25 m

4.3   Dependencies Between the Variables

The following equations must be satisfied:

total_size = size_yellow + size_lila
max_out = max_Q_A - max_Q_O
sum_out = sum_over + sum_out * percent_gw/100
sum_over = size_yellow * avg_yellow + size_lila * avg_lila

4.4   The Definition of a Typical View Written in SQL

Here is one typical view, used to get the results above:

```
CREATE VIEW actual_damage AS
SELECT elapsed_hours, flood_m3, MAX(extent_of_damage_euros) as the_damage
    FROM actual_flood, flooding_damage
    WHERE flooding_m3 <= flood_m3
    GROUP BY elapsed_hours, flood_m3
    ORDER BY elapsed_hours;
```

4.5   The Input Data Generator

For this purpose I wrote a PLSQL procedure to generate a plausible curve of throughputs at the power stations Aschach and Ottensheim. If available, this code can be replaced with statistical input data to store into the table "flow_rates_m3_sec".

5   Case Studies

Now it is possible to consider some typical flood water situations. The first one describes an inundation of type "June 2013", the second one assumes the elimination of sediments before this event and the third one includes a yet not existing flood polder of a plausible size.

5.1   The June 2013 Inundation

Taking the results of the model described above, this inundation caused an amount of outflowed water of approximately **92.5 million m^3** in this region and a damage that rounds up to **100 million euros**. It is a fact that the sediments above the power station of Aschach were constantly increasing and no flood preventing constructions were installed.

5.2   Same Inundation After Eliminating Sediments

Let us consider the constant elimination of the sediments. According to the above parameter of sediments increase, after 30 years about half of the stowage space of the power station Aschach was filled with **stones, gravel and sludge**. So it is not surprising that the company **Via Donau**, that manages the power stations, wanted to increase the water level upstream of (not only) this hydropower station. Because of the increase of the sediments the water amount in the stowage space decreases and therefore the performance of this power station also reduces to a certain extent.

After the elimination of the sediments we would have had **60 million m^3** more stowage space upstream this power station, and then the amount of outflowed water could obviously have been 60 million m^3 less which would have reduced the amount of the inundation to approximately **32.5 million m^3** in this region. So the damage could have been reduced from about **100 million** euros to only about **28 million** euros according to the damage table.

5.3   Same Inundation Having Flood Preventing Constructions

Additionally after the construction of a **flood polder** almost all the remaining **32.5 million m^3** of water can be hold in it and the flow off can be controlled so that the downriver areas are protected to that dimension. As a result, there is no need to deliberately flood the Eferdinger Becken and there will be **no damage at all**.

All the assumed parameter values are realistic and based on official documents and a discussion on this subject in a conference of the Landtag Oö held by Landesrat Rudolf Anschober [3, 4].

6   Recommendations

So far I have not mentioned the possibility of reducing the water amount in all stowage spaces before an obvious flooding event. This will also help a lot to minimize the devastating consequences of a natural catastrophe of this kind. The below stated recommendations are a summary of what I have learned by studying this subject.

6.1   Define Appropriate Rules of Operation

The reduction of the amount of water in all stowage spaces should begin more than 2 days before a critical rainy weather situation in the affecting areas. In such a situation rain probably will continue and therefore the flowing speed of the river is to accelerate to make sure that a maximum amount of water flows downstream, still without causing serious damage. A weather forecast with high quality prediction will facilitate decisions of this kind. These rules should operate in two modes:

(A) **pre-emptying** all stowage spaces upriver at least **54 h before** and
(B) **holding back as much water** as possible when the wave arrives.

Last time the prediction was based on a 24 h time window, but during 30 h it is possible to transport approximately **1 000 000 000 m³ (one cubic kilometer)** of water downriver, so it is recommendable to extend this period to about 54 h.

6.2 Eliminate Sediments

The elimination of sediments along the whole river Danube in Bavaria and Austria and its tributary streams will contribute a lot to prevent floodwaters. There will be more space to temporarily store water and the throughput of water will be significantly higher as in the actual situation. There is one disadvantage, namely, during the period of pre-emptying the stowage spaces the power stations are almost out of service. In his speech on the 12th of June 2014, Landesrat Rudolf Anschober [4] made clear that flood prevention had a much higher priority than electricity generation.

6.3 Build Flood Polders

The existence of appropriate flood polders allows that a high amount of water can be stored temporarily and after a certain time it can be released without causing any damage. These constructions will make it possible to cope with extreme floodwaters caused by heavy precipitations.

6.4 Develop an App for Smart Phones

This **"Flood Warner"** application should alert the users and display important data such as water throughputs and water levels at all power stations and important places of residences. Moreover, it should also give a **prognosis** of the **expected maximum water level** and when it will be reached at a given user location.

7 Conclusion

Applying the above written recommendations will result in an intelligent treatment of floodwaters. I hope that in the near future we always will be able to say: *"We have been lucky, not even that heavy rainfall has caused any serious damage!"*

References

1. NewsAT: Hochwasser bedroht Museen. http://www.news.at/a/hochwasser-linz-museen. Accessed 4 June 2013
2. NewsAT: Absichtlich geflutet. http://www.news.at/a/hochwasser-verbund-absichtlich-oberoesterreich-geflutet. Accessed 4 June 2013
3. Verbund, A.G.: Hochwasser Juni 2013. http://www.bmlfuw.gv.at/dms/lmat/wasser/nutzung-wasser/Hochwasserbericht/Beilage_2_Bericht_Verbund.pdf. Accessed 27 July 2013

4. Speech of LR R. Anschober. 44. Sitzung des Oö Landtages, Fragestunde: 1. Mündliche Anfrage von LAbg. Eidenberger. Video: ~37 minutes. http://www2.land-oberoesterreich.gv. at/internetlandtag/Start.jsp. Accessed 12 June 2014

5. Map of the Eferdinger Becken. 138 households affected to move house, http://www.nachrichten. at/oberoesterreich/Absiedelung-im-Eferdinger-Becken-138-Haushalte-betroffen;art4,1221623 and http://www.nachrichten.at/storage/med/download/219762_absiedlungskarte1.pdf. Accessed 22 October 2013

Hybrid Method for Forecasting Next Values of Time Series for Intelligent Building Control

Andrzej Stachno and Andrzej Jablonski[(⊠)]

Faculty of Electronics, Wroclaw University of Technology, Wroclaw, Poland
{andrzej.stachno,andrzej.jablonski}@pwr.edu.pl

Abstract. The method for forecasting successive values of time series with the application of Artificial Neural Networks and Moving Window Fourier takes into account additional parameters. Such parameters are determined by an external observer based on an analysis of the accuracy of forecasts obtained. For the purpose of automating the above method, a parameter selection module based on decision trees has been proposed. In this way the Hybrid Method for Forecasting (HMF) successive values of time series has been created.

Keywords: Artificial neuron networks · FFT · Forecasting · Successive values of a time series · Moving Window Fourier · Environmental measurements in an intelligent building

1 The Need for Forecasting Measurement Data in an Intelligent Building

The field of intelligent building management, combined with optimized control of comfort and energy, is an important part of automation and information technology. Measurements of environmental parameters in particular, are an important part of data acquisition systems in the intelligent building. Outdoor temperature, external light intensity, wind speed, solar radiation, etc. are specific examples of the parameters that influence control algorithms in building automation [1]. Their values are independent of operation of these algorithms, and at the same time have a significant impact on the functioning of the entire building automation system. For example, the taking into account of outside temperature is essential for controlling room temperature.

Owing to the impossibility of impacting on objective environmental (weather) parameters, it is necessary to take into account the current values of parameters in a control process. These values vary with time very often, and their dynamics cannot be determined by an explicit algebraic equation. For this reason, a prediction of the very measurement values of environmental parameters based on historical data [2] is a good and effective solution. Owing to that, the control parameters that determine a final result can be taken into consideration well in advance.

© Springer International Publishing Switzerland 2015
R. Moreno-Díaz et al. (Eds.): EUROCAST 2015, LNCS 9520, pp. 822–829, 2015.
DOI: 10.1007/978-3-319-27340-2_101

2 The Neural Model and Forecast Behavior of an Object

The methodology for ensuring a satisfactory accuracy of forecasts consists in the use of artificial neural networks (ANNs) [2]. The unavailability of a mathematical model of an object is the rationale for the construction of a neural model. This is typical of objects that generate independent measurement data, such as outdoor temperature, CO2 concentration, wind speed and other environmental parameters. These are important quantities and parameters, which must be considered while algorithms for building automation are created. Moreover, objects of this type prevent the application of conventional methods for determining mathematical models due to the impossibility of influencing model inputs. Only the states at outputs can be observed (Fig. 1).

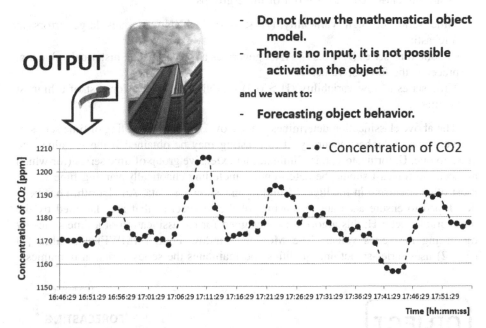

Fig. 1. Example of an object that generates independent measurement data - CO2 concentration. A premise for the construction of the neural model.

The neural model reflecting the behavior of the object over time is constructed based on an analysis of the data generated at its output. This data is presented as a sequence of values at regular time intervals – and it forms a time series. The time series creates a vector of data that is present at the inputs and at the output of a neural network during training. Historical data is presented at the inputs, whereas forecast data is presented at the output. This adopts the internal structure of artificial neural networks to changes that occur over time in the object that generates measurement data. An initial classification of time series takes into account the dynamics of each of the values (the classification by Hurst exponent value [3]). Therefore it can be assumed that a time series of a given type subjected to classification varies in a stable way. Owing to that, the adaptation of the internal structure of a neural network, based on historical data coming from a time series, reflects the same dynamics at moments to come in the future with a high accuracy. This means that successive values of a time series can be forecast based on historical data through the application of the neural model constructed in that way.

3 Time Series Smoothing and Forecast Accuracy

The research conducted [4] showed a significant impact of the initial classification of time series on forecast accuracies. The classification helps determine time series variability. The variability is expressed by means of the Hurst exponent (H). Time series are pre-classified into one out of three groups:

- Time series of high variability (H < 0.5) – ANN generates large errors in forecasting,
- Chaotic time series (H = 0.5) – ANN generates a forecast as the historical value that precedes the forecast value,
- Time series of low variability (H > 0.5) – ANN generates a forecast of a highest accuracy.

The above classification determines the use of ANN for forecasting of time series of a given type. A highest accuracy of forecasting may be obtained if the H values are close to one. Unfortunately, this eliminates an extensive group of time series (for which an accurate forecast should be determined), including chaotically varying time series, most often occurring in Intelligent Building measurement data. An algorithm has been developed to ensure accurate forecasting of the time series that are classified by the unfavorable factor H; this algorithm is designed for reclassification of a time series by modifying the series values. The Moving Window Fourier (MWF) algorithm [4] (Fig. 2) uses series-smoothing qualities and maintains the series variation dynamics.

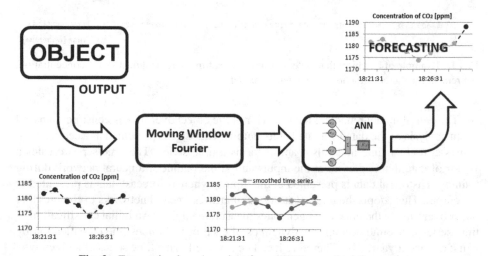

Fig. 2. Forecasting based on data from MWF-smoothed time series.

The following three parameters need determining:

k – the width of a Fast Fourier Transform window,
e – a number of eliminated harmonics,
se – the number of a selected item to be assigned to the smoothed time series.

The parameters are selected experimentally.

4   Classification of Training Vectors by Means of Decision Trees

Automated operation of the algorithm for generating forecasts with the application of ANN and for smoothing time series with the MWF method requires that k, e, se be determined. These parameters are selected experimentally for a specific period of a given time series. The selection of a specific parameter value determines the accuracy of the forecast obtained for a given series value (Table 1).

Table 1. Parameters of MWF transformation and their impact on the forecast.

Parameter	The impact on forecast
k – the width of the window Fast Fourier Transform,	Determines the number of points taken into account time series during its smoothing.
e – number of eliminated harmonics,	Determines the quality of smoothing time series. The elimination of a large number of harmonics resulting in a significant delay resulting time series,
se - the desired item number, which is assigned to the smoothed time series.	Determines the what part of the dynamics of change is transferred from the original time series to a series of smoothed. This parameter is very irregular and should be modified in short intervals for each time series.

An analysis of the accuracy of forecasts in the MWF method shows a significant influence of the selection of the item number (se) from the resulting time window because the number is transferred to the target, smoothed time series.

The se parameter is very irregular. It is selected for a given time series based on observations of the forecast accuracy. A change in se values significantly affects the accuracy of the forecast. For a given time series, the se parameter also needs modifying at short intervals. The objective of this modification is to adjust the algorithm to the nature of changes of individual values of the time series. Moreover, the se parameter significantly affects the delays generated by the MWF-based smoothing method. Owing to the above issues, se values need adjusting while a forecast is being calculated.

In order to make the time series smoothing algorithm independent of the observer, we have proposed a method for linking the MWF method with the decision tree-based classification algorithm [5]. The automatic decisiveness of the selection of the best *se* value in a given period, automates a forecast calculation process. The *se* factor is selected by creating as many time series (based on an original time series) as is the number of potential *se* parameters (Fig. 3). Thereby a feature vector V consisting of all possible time series is created. Every time series corresponds to the position of a consecutively selected *se* item (Fig. 4).

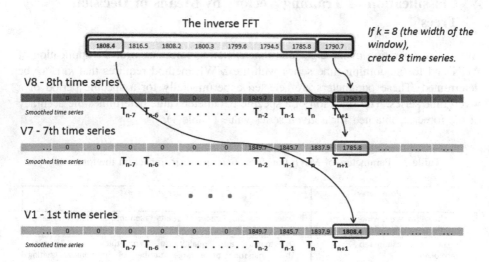

Fig. 3. The idea of creating an *se*-based time series vector.

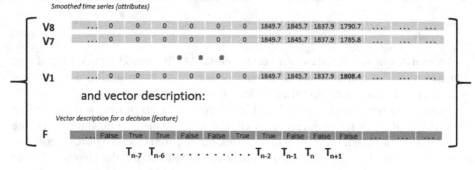

where:

F - Vector description for a decision (feature) is forecast
   to increase or decrease the value in step n + 1:
   - *True - if the value increases*
   - *False - if the value decreases*

Fig. 4. Constructions a feature vector transferred to the decision-tree module.

The vectors created in this way reflect a time series. Then, these vectors are collated with the vector that defines an increase (True) or a decrease (False) of the following time series value relative to the previous value. This collation creates a global data vector whose elements are composed of time series based on various MWF location items (various *se* values) in combination with an incremental forecast vector (Fig. 4).

The collation made in this way, *i.e.* a time series vector - attributes and incremental forecasts as a feature - are subject to classification to create a decision tree. This decision tree defines the extent of links between each of the time series with the incremental forecast. This procedure results in the decision tree whose trunk defines the time series mostly associated with the incremental forecast. This series was originally constructed from a given *se* factor, which was therefore considered the best in a given period. In order to ensure possibly good matching between the resulting time series and the original series - by selecting the right *se* factor - it is necessary to cyclically repeat the classification/selection of the time series that is mostly associated with the incremental forecast. A combination of MWF supported by decision tree algorithms allowed us to develop and test a new forecasting approach described as the Hybrid Method for Forecasting (HMF).

5 Forecast Generation Algorithm - Hybrid Method for Forecasting

The combination of the MWF-based method for smoothing a time series and the classification with the application of a decision tree resulted in the development of an HMF algorithm that is the tool for forecasting successive values of a time series (Fig. 5). This algorithm consists in the following:

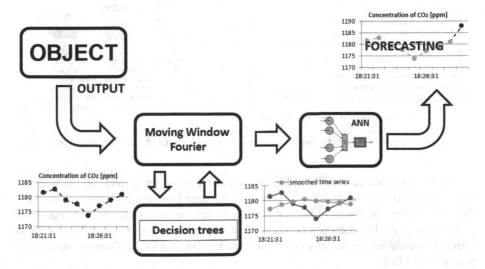

Fig. 5. Block diagram of the HMF algorithm for the hybrid (MWF and decision tree) method.

(a) Preparation of input data.
(b) Determination of the window width for FFT.
(c) Calculation of Fast Fourier Transform.
(d) Determination of a quantity of MWF components eliminated.
(e) Elimination of high harmonics.
(f) The inverse FFT.
(g) Using the MWF to create a set of time series.
(h) Selection of time series by means of decision trees.
(i) Selection of the time series of highest importance to the selection.
(j) Construction of input vectors for artificial neural networks.
(k) Determination of original time series forecasts.

6   Example of Forecasts

In order to illustrate the differences in the accuracies of the forecasts obtained, please consider an example of time series forecasting for CO_2 concentration that may occur in a laboratory (Fig. 6).

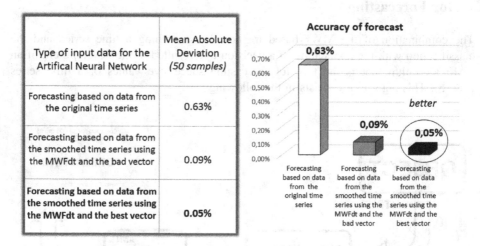

Fig. 6. The accuracy of forecasting of successive values of a CO_2 concentration time series.

All the forecasts used ANN as the primary mechanism for generating the forecast. The accuracy of the forecast that is based on the data from the original time series is shown in white. The forecast obtained with an *se* time series rejected by a decision tree is shown in gray. The accuracy of the forecast determined on the basis of the *se* factor selected by the decision tree as most adjusted to incremental vector forecast (best value) is shown in black.

7 Summary

The decision tree method has been proposed for implementing a k, e and se parameter selection process in the Moving Window Fourier (MWF) algorithm. The implementation of this method and the selection of best results of a forecast results in prediction of the parameters for which the forecast gives best results. A classification with the application of the decision tree method is an auto adaptation of the general forecasting algorithm. Such a procedure adjusts the basic parameters of the MWF algorithm to forecasting needs. The combination of the selection (decision tree) and forecasting (neural networks) methods makes it possible to adopt the prediction algorithm to a given time series. For this reason the term (concept) Hybrid Method for Forecasting (HMF) has been introduced. The research conducted shows that predicting by means of a neural network, complemented by the decision trees-based selection method gives comparable results for the entire time series that is analyzed based on historical measurement data. Potential changes (tuning) of the k, e and se parameters shall be made in time intervals significantly distant one from another, in the series under analysis [4]. For time series diversely classified by the Hurst exponent [2], it is necessary to select new MWF parameters. Summing up, it should be confirmed that the original forecasting method called the Hybrid Method for Forecasting, brings a new and better quality to comfort (environment) control in intelligent buildings.

References

1. Jabłoński, A.: Intelligent buildings as distributed information systems. Int. J. Comput. Anticip. Syst. **21**, 385–394 (2008). (Liege)
2. Stachno, A., Suproniuk, M.: Environmental performance measurement system designed for forecasting in intelligent buildings, Przegląd Elektrotechniczny, R89, 9, pp. 152–155 (2013). ISSN 0033-2097
3. Peitgen, H.O., Jurgens, H., Saupe, D.: Introduction to Fractals and Chaos. PWN (2002)
4. Stachno, A., Jablonski, A.: Application of artificial neuron networks and hurst exponent to forecasting of successive values of a time series representing environmental measurements in an intelligent building. In: Moreno-Díaz, R., Pichler, F., Quesada-Arencibia, A. (eds.) EUROCAST. LNCS, vol. 8111, pp. 483–490. Springer, Heidelberg (2013)
5. Mitchell, T.M.: Machine Learning. McGraw-Hill, New York (1997)

Marine Sensors and Manipulators

Low-Cost Plug-and-Play Optical Sensing Technology for USVs' Collision Avoidance

Andrea Sorbara[✉], Marco Bibuli, Enrica Zereik, Gabriele Bruzzone, and Massimo Caccia

National Research Council of Italy, Institute of Intelligent Systems for Automation, Via De Marini 6, 16149 Genova, Italy
andrea.sorbara@ge.issia.cnr.it
http://www.issia.cnr.it

Abstract. In the field of marine robotics it is particularly important to endow the robot with a safe and highly reliable Navigation Guidance and Control (NGC) system which enables the Unmanned Surface Vehicles (USVs) to safely navigate even in presence of human activities such as commercial and recreational traffic, swimmers, rowers, etc... A key aspect to achieve a safe autonomous navigation is the ability of the robot to recognize well in advance the presence of an unexpected, potentially moving, obstacle. This function represents the base brick for the development of a collision avoidance systems smart enough to reactively detect unexpected obstacles and perform the necessary avoidance maneuvers to prevent collisions. The present article describes the design of an a innovative obstacle detection sensor, combining both passive and active optical devices and based on a new concept of optronic system. It is specifically conceived for collision avoidance tasks in marine environments and it is designed to be easily mounted on small-medium sized USVs.

Keywords: Marine robotics · Obstacle detection · Optronic system

1 Introduction and Related Works

The employment of highly autonomous Unmanned Surface Vehicles (USVs) and, following the trend on the recent years, the exploitation of cooperative multi-vehicle teams requires to face and find a very reliable solution to the problem of collision detection and avoidance.

Safe and autonomous navigation of USVs in restricted and controlled area, free of obstacles and obstructions, is already a reality (as reported in [1–3]), however the utilization of autonomous robotic technologies in complex scenarios where the interaction with human activities is a needed (i.e. recreational and commercial traffic, swimmers, buoys and other fixed installations) still represents an open issue for safety reasons.

The patrolling of a harbor or the sampling of an area subject to commercial traffic are common scenarios that highlight the need for robust sensing capabilities in order to ensure the execution of safe autonomous operations. Thus, robots

© Springer International Publishing Switzerland 2015
R. Moreno-Díaz et al. (Eds.): EUROCAST 2015, LNCS 9520, pp. 833–840, 2015.
DOI: 10.1007/978-3-319-27340-2_102

have to be endowed with very robust NGC (Navigation Guidance and Control) systems in order to be able to navigate autonomously and safely in such kind of environments. One of the main aspects of the safe navigation consists in the capability to reactively detect unexpected obstacles with suitable advance in terms of time and distance, in such a way to perform the necessary avoidance maneuvers to safely prevent collisions.

For this reason, the obstacle detection sensor should have a field of view of at least 180 degrees and, in order to give time to the vehicle to safely perform the necessary avoidance maneuvers, a field of action of about 100 m. In this way the vehicle will be able to identify and avoid moving objects that are found not only in front of it, but also laterally and that can potentially cross its path.

To achieve this performance, in general, unmanned surface vehicles have a large sensoristic endowment such as a high number of fixed cameras (to cover the 180 degrees), X-band radar and multi-beam laser like in [4]. However, this approach often results in a poorly integrated solution and in a rather expensive and bulky system which is not suitable for a small-medium sized vehicle. Another interesting approach exploits radar imagery techniques for small vessels as for instance in [5] where the employment of commercial radar systems on USVs is discussed, drawing the conclusion that such systems are designed for manned operation and need interpretation by the human pilot.

Beside being reliable and effective, a collision avoidance system for USVs should be also 'low-cost' and 'plug-and-play' (meaning highly integrated and compact). Since efficient and robust sensing is still an open issue, the robotic community would greatly benefit from the availability of such a reliable low-cost and compact sensor.

2   Functional Architecture

The present work aims to design and develop an integrated active and passive optical sensor, based on a new concept of optronics system, specifically conceived for collision avoidance tasks in marine environments. The system has been designed in such a way to be able to detect small surfacing obstacles in a range of 100 m and 180° ahead the vehicle in order to effectively early detect mobile traversing obstacles. It employs low-cost off-the-shelf devices and consists of two subsystems: the first one equipped with a LWIR (Long Wave Infra-Red) uncooled camera and a DLTV (Day Light Television) camera, and the second endowed with a LRF (Laser Range Finder) with its related scanning system. The two cameras (representing the passive subsystem) are devoted to determine two of the coordinates that characterize the position of the obstacles (azimuth and elevation), while the LRF (representing the active subsystem) is in charge of computing the distance component of the obstacle position.

The innovation of the proposed architecture, with respect to commercial optronic systems, consists in the way the different sensors work together. The basic idea consists in acquiring, as quickly as possible, a panoramic view of the 180 degree ahead the vehicle with the passive sensors and, in a second phase, using the LRF to inspect the possible obstacles identified in such a view. To minimize the recognition time, it is convenient to run the two phases in parallel as described below:

- the passive subsystem, with the two cameras, is posed in permanent alternative motion spanning the 180 degree and creating a panoramic view. For each acquired frame, a list of candidate obstacles is built through appropriate vision and data fusion algorithms. Any identified obstacle is now localized only by the azimuth and elevation coordinates;
- the list built by the passive subsystem is continuously reviewed by the active subsystem which directs the laser beam towards each obstacle in the list. The laser creates a point cloud in the neighborhood of each obstacle thus determining the third coordinate of the position.

To implement the above described strategy it is clear that the passive and active subsystems must be mechanically decoupled and free to independently move from one another: while the panoramic view acquired by the two cameras is continuously built in order to be able to detect traversing obstacles, the laser can momentarily stop on each obstacle just for the time needed to build the point cloud. The proposed sensor is thus composed by two independent actuated heads that are integrated in a single pedestal in order to maintain a good level of compactness. The pedestal will be in turn installed on a gyro-stabilized platform in order to compensate for the sea motion. The design of such a platform does not represent a key aspect of the proposed system hence it will not be discussed in this paper. The overall architecture concept is represented in Fig. 1.

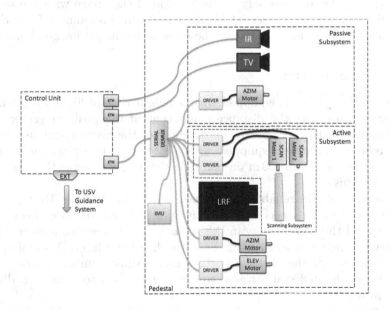

Fig. 1. Architecture concept

2.1   Passive Subsystem

The time employed by the Passive Subsystem to capture a full view is a key parameter to determine the performance of the whole collision avoidance system. The subsystem is actuated by a single motor performing a sinusoidal azimuthal motion. It was estimated that, to obtain a good situation awareness, the scan time of the surrounding 180 degrees must not exceed 1.5 s. In this way, considering the average speed of the obstacles on the image plane, it is still possible to spatially correlate the obstacle positions in two successive scans with a good level of confidence. Moreover, a low scan time considerably increases the ability to distinguish a real obstacle footprint, which lasts between successive scans, from the background noise mainly given by the sea glitter, which instead will change significantly from scan to scan.

However, with a high rotation speed, the images captured by the cameras suffer from a noticeable motion blur. This phenomenon is even more pronounced using low cost cameras not allowing high frame rates and requiring relatively high exposure times. In addition, it has to be considered that the blurring phenomenon on a microbolometer detector, which is often employed in uncooled thermal cameras, is even more evident than in CCD- or CMOS-based cameras. To prevent this problem the azimuthal motion of the passive subsystem is not executed in a smooth continuous way but rather in an intermittent fashion, following a "train of trapezoids" speed profile. The frame acquisition is synchronized with the pedestal motion so that each frame is captured while the cameras are standing still. The acquired frames are then processed in order to identify the obstacles circumscribing the analysis only on the portion of the image with the sea; this can be done thanks to an Inertial Measurement Unit providing information on the vehicle attitude, useful to detect the horizon line in the image plane.

2.2   Active Subsystem

The Active Subsystem is equipped with a pulsed time-of-flight LRF which is in charge of providing the distance component of the position vector of the obstacles identified by the passive part. Many of the lasers commonly used in mobile robotics, although equipped with a system of linear scanning, have a maximum range of about 30 m on non reflective targets; hence they cannot be employed in this case.

In order to obtain reliable measurements even beyond the 100 m, without using high power, it is necessary to employ a very narrow laser beam which doesn't spread the pulse energy in the air. However, a beam so narrow requires an extremely high precision in the line of sight of the laser. A small error in the identification of the obstacle by the passive subsystem or an error in the positioning of the pedestal can lead to a wrong, or even to a missing, distance measurement.

To overcome this problem a laser scanning mechanism has been introduced with the task of creating a point cloud in the neighborhood of each potential obstacle identified. In this way the space region covered by the laser is increased, together with the detection probability. It has been decided to employ Risley-prism scanner, a mechanism for optical beam steering based on a couple of rotating wedge-shaped prisms. This kind of device is very compact if compared with the largely diffused Palmer scanners which are based on mirrors.

The Active Subsystem head is endowed with an elevation degree of freedom, in addition to the azimuthal one, in order to be able to point the laser toward any point framed by the cameras of the passive subsystem.

3   Mechanical Design

In this section the mechanical design of the obstacle detection sensor will be described. The first prototype is currently under construction. As stated before, the sensor is composed by two mechanically decoupled actuated heads and the resulting conceptual device is shown in Fig. 2. The design is very compact (450 mm (H) × 250 mm (W) × 250 mm (L) × 6 Kg) in order to be easily employed on medium-small USV. The used materials are low-cost yet resistant in marine environment (marine aluminum, Derlin, Nylon, Inox Steel) and all the standard elements come from mechanics market. The machined elements can be easily realized with a lathe and a milling machine in few hours. Also the employed main sensors (DLTV, LWIR, LRF) are low-cost components commercial-off-the-shelf that can be found for a total amount of less than 8 K€.

3.1   Passive Subsystem

This subsystem (lower head in Fig. 2) is characterized by 1 degree of freedom (azimuthal rotation) necessary for the TV and IR to build the panoramic view. The selected motor (Maxon EC 90 flat) permits the realization of a trapezoidal intermittent movement in an angular range of 180° in about 1.1 s. The azimuth

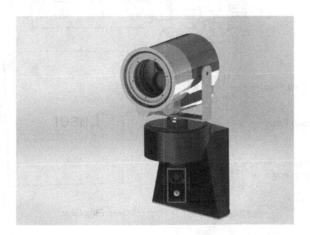

Fig. 2. Object detection sensor

mechanism is quite simple: it is constituted by a watertight box containing the two cameras. The box is mounted on a shaft rotating on two angular contact ball bearings that guarantee a good stability and angular precision. The movement of the box is directly driven by the brushless motor, hence since there are no gears the mechanical backlash is zeroed, lowering significantly the position error.

3.2 Active Subsystem

The Active Subsystem (higher head in Fig. 2) is a 2 degrees of freedom mechanism (azimuth and elevation).

The azimuth mechanism is very similar to the one used for the Passive Subsystem: brushless motor, shaft without gearbox and angular contact ball bearings. In this case the shaft is connected to a fork on which the tilt mechanism is mounted. This last employs a second brushless motor for realizing the $-15°$ to $15°$ movement from the horizontal position. Also in this case, no gearboxes have been employed in order to increase the precision of the LRF line of sight. The motor is enclosed in a weathertight box that contains the LRF device and an ad-hoc developed the Risley-prism scanner.

The design has been aimed to develop a new, light and ultra-compact scanner that can be used with most of the commercial LRF. The solution adopted (shown in Fig. 3) consists in two twin mechanisms driven by two brushless motors. Each mechanism is realized by enclosing a prism between the two extremities of a double flanged bush. The flange is indeed inserted inside the inner ring of a thin ball bearing. One of the flanges of the bush is connected to a ring gear driven by a cogwheel directly connected to a small diameter brushless motor.

The two elements are closed inside a watertight cylinder comprising the two scanner motors, the laser and the elevation motor. A small counterweight placed

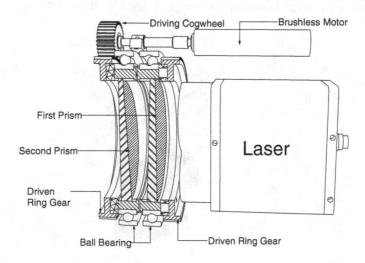

Fig. 3. Section of laser scanner (only one motor visible)

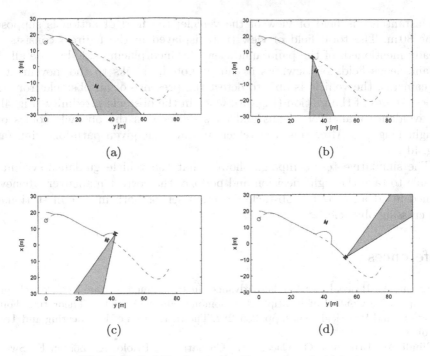

Fig. 4. Path following task with crossing obstacle

on the back of the cylinder is used in order to reduce the torque required to the elevation motor.

4   Simulative Results

In order to verify the effectiveness of the proposed methodology, a simulation campaign for a path-following task has been conducted. The simulations use a geometric and statistic approach rather than replicate the characteristics of the actual physical detectors employed in the design (not yet available at the time of the campaign). The obstacle detection sensor has been simulated associating a detection probability to the obstacles that are inside the field of view of the passive sensors. Such probability increases as the estimated distance decreases and increases with the number of times the obstacle is seen by the sensor. The estimated distance measurement accuracy increases as the obstacle become closer to the vehicle and with the time the obstacle remains in sight. The position of each recognized obstacle is forwarded to the guidance system of the vehicle which is in charge to perform the proper avoidance maneuvers. The Charlie USV (refer to [6] for details) guidance algorithm and dynamic model has been used for the test. In Fig. 4, as representative of the most challenging situation, the reaction of the vehicle in the case of a mobile obstacle crossing its path is reported. The dashed line represents the path to be followed while the triangle represents the instantaneous field of view of the vehicle; the field of action is supposed to be 80 m. The total field of view (not displayed in the figures) consists, as already mentioned, of the panoramic view obtained placing side by side all the instantaneous fields of view. As it can be noted, thanks to the movement of the cameras, the vehicle is able to detect the presence of an obstacle from the earliest stages of the motion (Fig. 4a). Once in the obstacle proximity (Fig. 4b), the avoidance maneuver begins and ends as soon as the obstacle comes out of sight (Fig. 4c). After this, the vehicle resumes the given path-following task (Fig. 4d).

The simulative test campaign showed that the vehicle guidance system is capable to take the right decision and perform the correct maneuver whenever warned in advance by the obstacle detection sensor both in case of stationary and crossing obstacle.

References

1. Aguiar, A., Pascoal, A.: Further Advances in Unmanned Marine Vehicles, chapter Cooperative Control of Multiple Autonomous Marine Vehicles: Theoretical Foundations and Practical Issues, pp, 255–282. The Institution of Engineering and Technology (2012)
2. Bibuli, M., Bruzzone, G., Caccia, M., Gasparri, A., Priolo, A., Zereik, E.: Swarm based path-following for cooperative unmanned surface vehicles. Proc. Inst. Mech. Eng. Part M: J. Eng. Marit. Environ. **228**(2), 192–207 (2014)
3. Bibuli, M., Bruzzone, G., Caccia, M., Fumagalli, E., Saggini, E., Zereik, E., Buttaro, E., Caporale, C., Ivaldi, R.: Unmanned surface vehicles for automatic bathymetry mapping and shores' maintenance. In: Proceedings of the MTS/IEEE OCEANS 2014 Conference, Taipei (Taiwan), April 2014
4. Fioravanti, S., Grati, A., Stipanov, M.: Icarus project: sensor suite integration and implementation of autonomous behaviors on USVs for SAR operations. In: Breaking the Surface 2014 - Invited Talk (2014)
5. Almeida, C., Franco, T., Ferreira, H., Martins, A., Santos, R., Almeida, J.M., Carvalho, J., Silva, E.: Radar based collision detection developments on USV ROAZ II. In: Oceans 2009-Europe, pp. 1–6. IEEE (2009)
6. Caccia, M., Bibuli, M., Bono, R., Bruzzone, Ga, Bruzzone, Gi, Spirandelli, E.: Unmanned surface vehicle for coastal and protected waters applications: the charlie project. Mar. Technol. Soc. J. **41**(2), 62–71 (2007)

Experimental Evaluation of Sealing Materials in 6-Axis Force/Torque Sensors for Underwater Applications

G. Palli[✉], L. Moriello, and C. Melchiorri

DEI - University of Bologna, Viale Risorgimento 2, 40136 Bologna, Italy
{gianluca.palli,lorenzo.moriello,claudio.melchiorri}@unibo.it

Abstract. In this paper, the effects of sealing materials on the performance of an optoelectronic Force/Torque (F/T) sensor designed for underwater robotic applications are investigated. The design of the sensor has been conceived to exhibit a considerable compliance if compared to commercial F/T sensors, such as the ones for industrial applications. Moreover, optoelectronic components have been used as sensible elements for the sensor development, allowing a relatively simple and quite reliable implementation. In particular, these properties are introduced to deal with uncertain environments and to ease the sensor integration in complex robotic systems, such as in the fingers of robotic a gripper for underwater applications.

After a brief introduction of the robotic gripper this sensor is designed for, the paper presents the basic working principle and the design of the proposed F/T sensor, and its main features are illustrate and discussed by means of experimental data. Finally, the evaluation of the sensor as an intrinsic tactile sensor is investigated and experimentally validated, and the sensor performance are compared considering different materials for the sealing, with particular attention on dynamic application like slip detection.

1 Introduction

The autonomous interaction with dynamic environments and the cooperation with humans is actually one of the most challenging goal in robotics. In order to achieve a suitable level of flexibility and to operate in a safe and autonomous way, a robot must be able to sense and recognize what surrounds it, no matter if it is operating in a domestic, industrial, underwater or space environment. In this scenario, Force/Torque (F/T) sensors play a fundamental role since they allow to perceive the interaction with the environment, paving the way toward the implementation of robotic systems designed for manipulating and, more in general, modifying the environment in an autonomous manner, eventually collaborating with humans. In particular, F/T sensors are also useful for the manipulation of uncertain objects, allowing the online adaptability of the robot to the real object characteristics and to different working conditions.

© Springer International Publishing Switzerland 2015
R. Moreno-Díaz et al. (Eds.): EUROCAST 2015, LNCS 9520, pp. 841–852, 2015.
DOI: 10.1007/978-3-319-27340-2_103

In most of the cases, commercial F/T sensors are based on strain-gauges. The reliability of this solution, the wide literature about the optimization of this sensing principle [4,13], the relatively simple numerical methods for the estimation of strain in multi-axis F/T sensors [16] and the large stiffness of the sensor that does not introduce destabilizing effects when applied on conventional industrial manipulators are among the main motivations behind this fact. This type of sensors has been used in a wide number of different robotic applications, e.g. a 6-axis F/T sensor has been embedded in an intelligent robotic foot in [14] or a 4-axis strain-gauge sensor has been developed for measuring interaction forces in haptic devices in [25].

Taking into account grasping and manipulation tasks, the sense of touch plays an essential role for manipulating objects properly. A complete review on tactile sensor technologies and features can be found in [6]. Due, on one hand, to the high manufacturing complexity and cost and, on the other hand, to the lack of knowledge about the interpretation and the exploitation of tactile sensors data and despite the relevance of the application, a limited number of commercial tactile sensors are available on the market. In spite of the many different design solutions that have been proposed in literature and the several physical transduction principles that have been exploited for their design, reliable and accurate tactile sensors are still very complex and expensive devices, then the use of simpler F/T sensors as intrinsic tactile sensors has been proposed in literature [3].

Conventional strain-gauge based F/T sensors measure the strain induced on the mechanical structure by the an external force/torque. On the other hand, an alternative solution based on optoelectronic components may introduce several advantages, as already shown by many different implementations of F/T sensors based on this concept that have been proposed in literature. This kind of sensors exploit the scattering or the reflection of a light beam emitted by a source and received by suitable detectors to directly measure the deformation of a compliant structure or the relative displacement between elastically coupled elements caused by the external force/torque. Optoelectronic F/T sensors range from conventional mono-axial sensors, like the one described in [20] where discrete optoelectronic components are used to measure the forces in a tendon based transmission system, to 6-axis F/T sensors, like the one reported in [15] where the authors adopt optoelectronic devices mounted on a compliant structure to measure human-robot interaction forces, or the one reported in [11] where Hirose and Yoneda implemented an optical 6-axis F/T sensor adopting a 2-axis photosensor for measuring the deformation caused by the external load on a compliant structure. In the field of tactile sensors, a quite common optoelectronic technology makes use of Fibre Bragg Gratings (FBG), exploiting the relationship between the variations of the FBG wavelength and the external force applied to the FBG [10]. Alternative implementations of optoelectronic tactile sensors are based on CCD or CMOS camera to acquire the deformation of a surface caused by external force [12]. In [8,9,26] the light beam of a Light Emitting Diode (LED) scattered by a silicon dome and a urethane foam cavity is exploited. An optical tactile sensor based on a matrix of LED/PD couples covered by a deformable elastic layer is described in [7].

    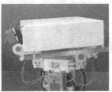

(a) Power grasp.   (b) Parallel grasp on a thin object.   (c) Pen tripod grasp.   (d) Parallel grasp on a plastic bottle.   (e) The gripper grasping a 340 mm width box.

Fig. 1. The gripper executing grasps on various objects.

The development activity reported in this paper has been started during the TRIDENT FP7 project (www.irs.uji.es/trident/) [23] where we were in charge of developing the gripper of an autonomous robot for search and rescue operations [1,2]. According to the project requirements, the gripper should be equipped with force or tactile sensors for the online regulation of the grasping force and the adaptation to objects of unknown shape and dimension. In Fig. 1 several grasps executed by the gripper are shown. The gripper is able to perform power grasps, see Fig. 1(a), to grasp different objects both in tripod configuration, as shown in Fig. 1(c), and in parallel configuration, see Fig. 1(b) and (d). In particular, Fig. 1(e) shows the ability of the gripper of grasping objects up to 340 mm width, whereas Fig. 1(b) shows the ability of grasping very thin objects. The whole integrated system composed by the gripper, the arm and the Girona 500 AUV [21, 22] has been then tested in real undersea operations in the harbor at Port de Soller, Spain, operating at a working depth of about 25 m, according to the goals of the TRIDENT project. Autonomous operations of the overall system have been successfully executed, as shown in Fig. 2. A video showing the final experiments of the TRIDENT project is also available at http://www.irs.uji.es/2nd-i-auv/ videos/E3-Autonomous-Intervention/TRIDENT-Final-Exp.mp4. In particular, after getting the seafloor mosaic (generated on the survey phase), the AUV performed autonomous detection of the dummy black box to be recovered, and the grasp was specified by the human operator using a purposely designed user interface. Then, with the aid of the AUV vision system, the black box recovery stage was autonomously initiated by the system, as detailed in Fig. 2(d). For that purpose, a robust vision system has been implemented on the AUV by using both a 2D camera and a 3D vision system. Once the black box has been autonomously grasped by the gripper, the AUV brought it to the surface. The success of the experiment was observed thanks to the images provided by the onboard cameras of the AUV, and with the help of divers that recorded the experiment from outside, as shown in Fig. 2(b) and (c).

In this paper, the attention is focused on the development of the 6-axis F/T sensor that equips the above described gripper. The sensor is based on optoelectronic components and its working principle is based on the reflection of the

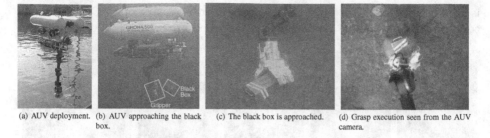

(a) AUV deployment. (b) AUV approaching the black   (c) The black box is approached.   (d) Grasp execution seen from the AUV
                          box.   camera.

Fig. 2. The AUV with integrated arm and gripper during the experimental tests at Port de Soller, Spain.

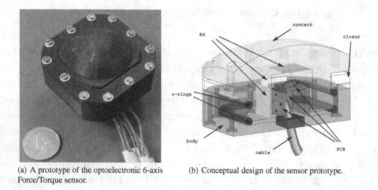

(a) A prototype of the optoelectronic 6-axis   (b) Conceptual design of the sensor prototype.
Force/Torque sensor.

Fig. 3. A prototype of the optoelectronic 6-axis Force/Torque sensor and internal design of the sensor.

light emitted by a Light Emitting Diode (LED) over a moving Reflecting Surface (RS) and the consequent change in the intensity of the light received by an array of 4 PhotoDetectors (PDs). The work here reported is based on a previous investigation of the basic concepts and implementation tests for an optical 6-axis F/T sensor [18,19]. Due to the advantages of optoelectronic-based solutions, an easily scalable and low-cost F/T sensor is obtained, suitable to be used as an intrinsic tactile sensor. Moreover, the proposed sensor requires an extremely simple conditioning electronics. Additionally, since the proposed sensor is designed to work in the underwater environment, this paper takes into account the problem of sealing of the internal components. Finally, the sensor design has been conceived in such a way that all the electronic components are allocated in a single Printed Circuit Board (PCB), making it easier the sensor integration into complex mechanical structures such as grippers for underwater robots.

2   Sensor Prototype

The basic element for building up the proposed 6-axis F/T sensor is a PCB with a LED and four PDs symmetrically arranged around it on a circle of radius 3 mm.

The PCB is a 10×10 mm electronic board (1 cm^2). According to what described in [19], this basic element allows to detect the distance of the RS from the PCB together with its orientation with respect to two rotational axes parallel to the PCB plane. Therefore, with the aim of measuring forces and torques along the three axes with a proper redundancy, 3 of these basic elements have been placed on three faces of a cube. Even thought different arrangements can be also used for the same purpose, this configuration allows an easy manufacturing and assembly of the sensor. In Fig. 3(a) a prototype of the sensor is shown. It is worth noticing that the geometry of the sensor and the arrangement of the PCB may change according to the specific application the sensor is designed for. The internal frame of the sensor (where the PCBs are fixed) is connected to the external contact surface, i.e. the cover (where the RSs are attached), by means of a compliant frame that allows the relative motion of the RS with respect to the PCBs. By a suitable design of the compliant frame, the sensor working range can be freely adjusted according to the application requirements. The simple electronics adopted for the proposed sensor signal conditioning is shown in Fig. 4. Due to its simplicity, the whole circuit in Fig. 4 can be implemented in the same PCB where the LED and the PDs are hosted, and the three PCB shown in Fig. 3 can be then connected to a microcontroller board located into the sensor base through the SPI digital bus. The microcontroller is in charge of elaborating the PDs output signals to perform noise filtering and providing the force estimation on the base of the calibration data, see Sect. 3. The microcontroller is also used to transmit the estimated forces and torques via digital bus using different protocol and bus types: in the specific case of the application described in this paper, the CAN bus and CanOpen protocol have been adopted for compatibility reasons with the other components of the robots. Since the sensor is placed on the fingertips of a underwater three-fingered robot gripper [1], the external surface of the sensor prototype is a spherical cap with radius $R = 44$ mm.

3   Calibration and Characterization

As a reference sensor for the calibration of the sensor prototype, a commercial sensor, the ATI Gamma SI-130-10 F/T sensor, has been adopted. The proposed sensors prototype is connected to the reference sensor in such a way that, by means of a suitable changes of the coordinate reference frame, the measurement of the two sensors can be directly compared. The calibration procedure consists in applying a variable load in terms of both forces and torques to the two sensors, while and the data from both sensors are collected. Assuming that the compliant frame is working within the elastic regime, a linear relationship between the applied force/torque vector $w = [f^T, \, m^T]^T$ and RS displacement can be assumed. Then, a polynomial mapping between the PD output voltages and the applied force/torque can be established

$$w = \mathbf{C} \, v \tag{1}$$

where

$$v = \begin{bmatrix} v_1^n \cdots v_{12}^n \cdots v_1 \cdots v_{12} \, 1 \cdots 1 \end{bmatrix}^T$$

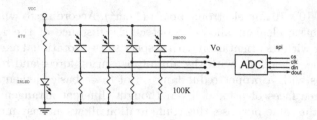

Fig. 4. Simplified measuring circuit of the PCB with one LED and four PDs.

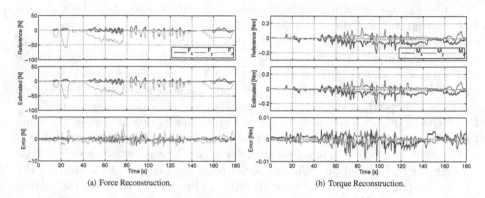

(a) Force Reconstruction.   (b) Torque Reconstruction.

Fig. 5. Performance of the optoelectronic F/T sensor: Force and Torque reconstruction.

is the vector of the 12 sensor output voltages, and the corresponding powers up to the order n. Note that the 12 ones at the end of the vector are used to remove the output voltage offset. The calibration matrix $\mathbf{C}$ can be derived from experiments as

$$\mathbf{C} = \Omega \, \Sigma^+ \tag{2}$$

where Σ^+ denotes the pseudoinverse of the matrix Σ and

$$\Omega = \begin{bmatrix} w_1 \; w_2 \cdots w_i \cdots w_m \end{bmatrix}$$
$$\Sigma = \begin{bmatrix} v_1 \; v_2 \cdots v_i \cdots v_m \end{bmatrix}$$

are the matrices of the m experimental measures of the external forces/torques applied to the optoelectronic sensor and of the PD output voltages respectively. A 3rd-order interpolation polynomial has been adopted for deriving the external force/torque vector from the sensor output signals since this represents a good trade-off between precision in the force/torque reconstruction and computational complexity.

According to the project requirements, the operating range of the sensor prototype has been selected as $[-50 \div 50]$ N along the linear axes, while torques are limited to $[-1 \div 1]$ Nm. In Fig. 5 the comparison between the force and torque measured by the reference sensor and by the proposed optoelectronic sensor as well as the estimation errors are reported. From the plots, it can be

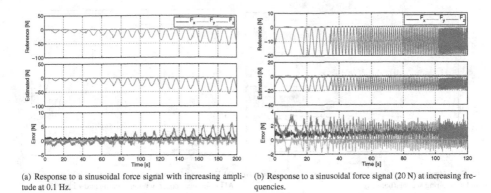

(a) Response to a sinusoidal force signal with increasing amplitude at 0.1 Hz.

(b) Response to a sinusoidal force signal (20 N) at increasing frequencies.

Fig. 6. Response of the sensor to a sinusoidal force signal with increasing amplitude and frequency.

noted that, while the sensor allows a good estimation is quasi-static condition (i.e. if the force/torque is constant), the estimation error increases during the force and torque variations. In order to fully characterize the sensor not only in static conditions but also to evaluate its dynamic behavior, the response of the sensor to a sinusoidal force with increasing amplitude and frequency along the z-axis as been verified. Figure 6(a) shows a test in which a sinusoidal force with constant frequency (0.1 Hz) and increasing amplitude is applied to the sensor. From these plots it is possible to see that the estimation error increases as the force gradient becomes larger and larger. As a matter of fact, because of the visco-elastic properties of the rubber used to seal the optical sensor, this is 'slower' than the reference sensor in recovering the unloaded position. This effect is more evident in Fig. 6(b) where a 20 N sinusoidal force is applied at increasing frequencies, from 0.01 to 3 Hz. In this experiment, the error increases with the frequency of the input signal.

It is important to remark that this effect is not due to some intrinsic limitations of the sensor, and in particular of its working principle, but rather to its mechanical design and, more specifically, to the need of employing rubber sealing for the isolation of the electronic parts from water. As a verification of this fact, the force/displacement response of the sensor without and with o-ring sealing has been experimentally measured, and the results reported in Fig. 7(a) show that a significant frequency dependent hysteresis is introduced in the sensor response by the o-rings. Additional experiments have been also executed to measure the frequency response of the sensor. Figure 7(b) shows how the introduction of the sealing elements reduce the frequency range of the sensor, limiting in this way also the possibility of the using the sensor information for dynamic applications, such as slip detection, as further investigated in the following. Then, the effect of the sealing material needs to be considered during the calibration of the system for a proper identification of the slip events, in particular in case frequency based detection techniques are used. As a first tentative toward the limitation of this

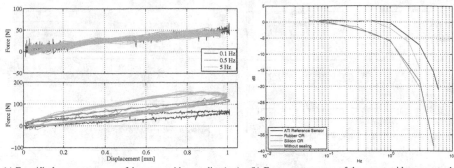

(a) Force/displacement response of the sensor without sealing (top) and with o-ring sealing (bottom).

(b) Frequency response of the sensor with respect to the ATI reference sensor, without sealing and with sealing.

Fig. 7. Force/displacement and frequency response of the sensor with and without o-ring sealing.

problem, a couple of different materials, silicon and rubber o-rings, have been also evaluated for the sensor sealing: as can be seen in Fig. 7(b), no significant difference exists in the sensor response in case of rubber or silicon sealing.

4   Characterization as Intrinsic Tactile Sensor

The use F/T sensors as intrinsic tactile sensors, i.e. for the computation of the contact point between e.g. the fingers of a robot hand and the grasped object, has been reported in literature by several authors, see [3,5,17,24]. With the aim of providing additional information about the contact between the gripper and the grasped object, the use of the proposed device as an intrinsic tactile sensor has been investigated considering the hard finger contact hypothesis, i.e. only forces and not torques can be applied at the contact point. In case of a sensor with spherical surface (with radius r) the position p_c of the contact point can be obtained from the force f and torque m measured by the F/T sensor as [3]

$$\lambda = -\frac{1}{\|f\|}\sqrt{r^2 - \frac{\|f \times m\|^2}{\|f\|^4}}, \quad r_0 = \frac{f \times m}{\|f\|^2}, \quad p_c = r_0 + \lambda f \tag{3}$$

Due to the geometry of the system, these equations admit up to two solutions representing the intersection of a line with a spherical surface. The solution representing the effective contact point can be selected assuming that the contact force acts on the sensor external surface, while the other solution will be out of the fingertip surface. The experimental tests reported in Fig. 8 show the measured forces and the corresponding contact point position on the sensor surface represented by blue lines and red dots respectively. For the sake of comparison, in Fig. 8 also the forces measured by the ATI reference sensor and the corresponding contact point positions are reported with green lines and black dots respectively. The comparison of these results allow to state that the proposed optoelectronic device can be successfully used as intrinsic tactile sensor.

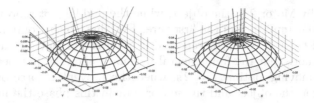

Fig. 8. Comparison of the contact point reconstruction tests: force directions (blue lines) and contact point positions (red dots) measured by the optoelectronics F/T sensor, force directions (green lines) and contact point positions (black dots) measured by the reference ATI sensor (Colour figure online).

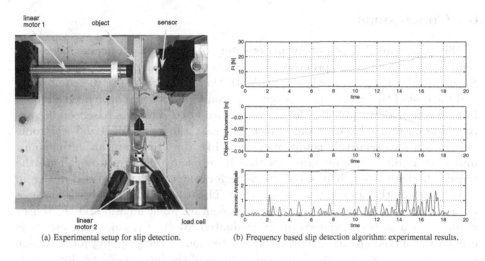

(a) Experimental setup for slip detection.   (b) Frequency based slip detection algorithm: experimental results.

Fig. 9. Experimental setup for the evaluation of the slip detection algorithms.

5   Slip Detection

As a possible dynamic application, the use of the sensor information for the implementation of a slip detection algorithm has been investigated by means of the experimental setup shown in Fig. 9(a). The setup is composed by two linear motors LinMot-37x160: the first motor (Motor 1) is mounted with its motion axis aligned with the sensor z-axis and is used to hold an object against the optoelectronic sensor by means of a rounded tip (to simulate the contact between the object and a second fingertip); the second motor (Motor 2) is positioned perpendicularly to Motor 1 in order to apply a tangential force to the object and is equipped with a precision load cell. Motor 2 is used both to apply to the object a tangential force and to measure the object displacement during slip by means of the integrated encoder. Motor 2 is controlled using the force signal of the load cell mounted on its slider.

The typical response of the sensor with sealing o-rings obtained during the slipping of the object is reported in Fig. 9(b): the top plot reports the increasing force applied by Motor 2 to the object, while the middle plot reports the object position and the amplitude of the first three FFT harmonics computed from the force signal of the F/T sensor is reported in the bottom plot. From these plots, it possible to note that the fundamental harmonic shows a first peak when the object starts moving at time $t = 2$ s, when the tangential force overcome the friction between the object and the sensor, but in this phase the motion is not still continuous but is characterized by a stick-slip behavior. Later, an higher peak can be seen at time $t = 14$ s when the continuous motion of the object is achieved due to the high level of the tangential force. This experiment allows to see how it is also possible to discriminate between this two slipping regimes.

6   Conclusions

In this paper, an F/T sensor for underwater robotic applications has been presented. In particular, the proposed device has been developed for equipping the fingertips of a three-fingered gripper. With the aim of reducing the complexity and the cost of the device, discrete optoelectronic components have been adopted for the sensor development. Moreover, the proposed sensor is based on a compact and customizable electronics, fact that easy the mechanical and electronic integration into relatively complex systems like the gripper of an autonomous underwater robot. The experiments that have been performed to evaluate the sensor characteristics show satisfactory performance of the proposed device in the estimation the applied force and torque. The usage of the proposed sensor as an intrinsic tactile sensor for detecting the contact point location on the sensor surface has also been experimentally evaluated. Moreover, since this aspect is crucial for all the application where the detection of the gripping force change rate is more important than the absolute value of the force itself, i.e. for detecting the object slipping, particular attention has been given to the verification of the o-ring sealing effects on the frequency response of the sensor. To this end, the sensor information has been exploited for the implementation of a frequency based slip detection algorithm, enabling the detection of incipient object slip from the sensor signals. Further activities are in progress for the experimental validation of the sensor in grasping and manipulation task on a robotic gripper, to develop more compact sensors and to customize the design for different applications.

References

1. Bemfica, J., Melchiorri, C., Moriello, L., Palli, G., Scarcia, U., Vassura, G.: Mechatronic design of a three-fingered gripper for underwater applications. In: 6th IFAC Symposium on Mechatronic Systems, pp. 307–312, Hangzhou, China (2013)
2. Bemfica, J., Melchiorri, C., Moriello, L., Palli, G., Scarcia, U.: A three-fingered cable-driven gripper for underwater applications. In: Proceedings of the IEEE International Conference on Robotics and Automation, pp. 2469–2474, May 2014
3. Bicchi, A., Salisbury, J., Brock, D.: Contact sensing from force measurements. Int. J. Robot. Res. **12**, 249–262 (1990)

4. Bicchi, A.: A criterion for optimal design of multi-axis force sensors. Robot. Auton. Syst. **10**(4), 269–286 (1992)
5. Cicchetti, A., Eusebi, A., Melchiorri, C., Vassura, G.: An intrinsic tactile force sensor for robotic manipulation. In: Proceedings of the 7th International Conference on Advanced Robotics, ICAR 1995, pp. 889–894, Sant Feliu de Guixols, Spain (1995)
6. Dahiya, R., Metta, G., Valle, M., Sandini, G.: Tactile sensing - from humans to humanoids. IEEE Trans. Robot. **26**(1), 1–20 (2010)
7. De Maria, G., Natale, C., Pirozzi, S.: Force/tactile sensor for robotic applications. Sens. Actuators A: Phys. **175**, 60–72 (2012)
8. Torres-Jara, E., Vasilescu, I., Coral, R.: A soft touch: compliant tactile sensors for sensitive manipulation. In: CSAIL Technical Report MIT-CSAIL-TR-2006-014 (2006)
9. Hellard, G., Russell, A.R.: A robust, sensitive and economical tactile sensor for a robotic manipulator. In: Proceedings of Australasian Conference on Robotics and Automation, pp. 100–104 (2002)
10. Heo, J., Chung, J., Lee, J.: Tactile sensor arrays using fiber bragg grating sensors. Sens. Actuators A: Phys. **126**(2), 312–327 (2006)
11. Hirose, S., Yoneda, K.: Development of optical 6-axial force sensor and its signal calibration considering non linear calibration. In: Proceedings of the IEEE International Conference on Robotics and Automation, vol. 1, pp. 46–53, Tsukuba, Japan (1990)
12. Kamiyama, K., Vlack, K., Mizota, T., Kajimoto, H., Kawakami, N., Tachi, S.: Vision-based sensor for real-time measuring of surface traction fields. IEEE Comput. Graph. Appl. **25**(1), 68–75 (2005)
13. Kang, M.K., Lee, S., Kim, J.H.: Optimal design of a mechanically decoupled six-axis force/torque sensor based on the principal cross coupling minimization (2014)
14. Kim, G.S., Shin, H.J., Yoon, J.: Development of 6-axis force/moment sensor for a humanoid robot's intelligent foot. Sens. Actuators A: Phys. **141**(2), 276–281 (2008)
15. Lorenz, W., Peshkin, M., Colgate, J.: New sensors for new applications: force sensors for human/robot interaction. In: Proceedings IEEE International Conference on Robotics and Automation, vol. 4, pp. 2855–2860 (1999)
16. Ma, J., Song, A.: Fast estimation of strains for cross-beams six-axis force/torque sensors by mechanical modeling. Sensors **13**(5), 6669–6686 (2013)
17. Melchiorri, C.: Tactile sensing for robotic manipulation. In: Nicosia, P.S., Siciliano, P.B., Bicchi, P.A., Valigi, P.P. (eds.) Ramsete: Articulated and Mobile Robotics for Services and Technologies. LNCIS, pp. 75–102. Springer, Heidelberg (2001)
18. Melchiorri, C., Moriello, L., Palli, G., Scarcia, U.: A new force/torque sensor for robotic applications based on optoelectronic components. In: Proceedings of the IEEE International Conference Robotics and Automation, pp. 6408–6413, May 2014
19. Palli, G., Moriello, L., Scarcia, U., Melchiorri, C.: Development of an optoelectronic 6-axis force/torque sensor for robotic applications. Sens. Actuators A: Phys. **220**, 333–346 (2014)
20. Palli, G., Pirozzi, S.: Force sensor based on discrete optoelectronic components and compliant frames. Sens. Actuators A: Phys. **165**, 239–249 (2011)
21. Prats, M., Ribas, D., Palomeras, N., García, J.C., Nannen, V., Wirth, S., Fernández, J.J., Beltrán, J.P., Campos, R., Ridao, P., Sanz, P.J., Oliver, G., Carreras, M., Gracias, N., Marín, R., Ortiz, A.: Reconfigurable AUV for intervention missions: a case study on underwater object recovery. J. Intell. Serv. Robot. **5**(1), 19–31 (2012)

22. Ribas, D., Palomeras, N., Ridao, P., Carreras, M., Mallios, A.: Girona 500 auv: from survey to intervention. IEEE/ASME Trans. Mechatron. **17**(1), 46–53 (2012)
23. Ribas, D., Ridao, P., Turetta, A., Melchiorri, C., Palli, G., Fernandez, J., Sanz, P.: I-AUV mechatronics integration for the TRIDENT FP7 project. IEEE/ASME Trans. Mechatron. **20**(5), 2583–2592 (2015)
24. Salisbury, J.: Interpretation of contact geometries from force measurements. In: Proceedings 1984 IEEE International Conference on Robotics and Automation, pp. 240–247 (1984)
25. Song, A., Wu, J., Qin, G., Huang, W.: A novel self-decoupled four degree-of-freedom wrist force/torque sensor. Measurement **40**(9–10), 883–891 (2007)
26. Tar, A., Cserey, G.: Development of a low cost 3d optical compliant tactile force sensor. In: Proceedings of the IEEE/ASME International Conference Advanced Intelligent Mechatronics, pp. 236–240 (2011)

Underwater Glider Path Planning and Population Size Reduction in Differential Evolution

Aleš Zamuda[1][✉] and José Daniel Hernández-Sosa[2]

[1] Faculty of Electrical Engineering and Computer Science,
University of Maribor, Smetanova ul. 17, 2000 Maribor, Slovenia
ales.zamuda@um.si
[2] Institute of Intelligent Systems and Numerical Applications in Engineering,
University of Las Palmas de Gran Canaria, Campus de Tafira,
35017 Las Palmas de Gran Canaria, Spain
dhernandez@iusiani.ulpgc.es

Abstract. This paper presents an approach to underwater glider path planning (UGPP), where the population size reduction mechanism is introduced into the differential evolution (DE) meta-heuristic and two types of DE strategies (DE/best and DE/rand) are applied interchangeably. The newly proposed DE instance algorithms using population size reduction on the best and rand DE strategies are assessed and compared on 12 test scenarios using the proposed approach. A Bonferroni-Dunns statistical hypothesis testing is conducted to confirm out-performance of the favoured DE/best strategy over the DE/rand strategy for the 12 UGGP scenarios utilized. The analysis suggests that the approach can benefit from gradually reducing the population size and also tuning the DE parameters. Thereby, this contributes to extend the operational capabilities of the glider vehicle and to improve its value as a marine sensor, facilitating the implementation of flexible sampling schemes.

Keywords: Differential evolution · Population size reduction · Glider path planning · Underwater robotics · Autonomous underwater vehicle

1 Introduction

This paper fosters the meta-heuristics research on Underwater Glider Path Planning (UGPP) [13] and Differential Evolution (DE) [24], as initially proposed in the first study on DE and UGPP [26]. Compared to this first study [26], two additional mechanism are included now into the DE metaheuristic and used for the UGPP, (1) the population size reduction from [5,24] and (2) interchangeable use of two types of DE strategies (DE/best and DE/rand) from [24]. The extended abstract of this paper was published in [25]. The proposed improvement aims in contributing to extend the operational capabilities of the glider vehicle and to improve its value as a marine sensor, facilitating the implementation of flexible sampling schemes.

© Springer International Publishing Switzerland 2015
R. Moreno-Díaz et al. (Eds.): EUROCAST 2015, LNCS 9520, pp. 853–860, 2015.
DOI: 10.1007/978-3-319-27340-2_104

2   Related Work

In this section, related work on optimization with differential evolution and the underwater glider path planning challenge are presented, defined in [5,26].

2.1   Differential Evolution and Optimization

Differential Evolution (DE) was introduced by Storn and Price [22] with a floating-point encoding evolutionary algorithm [10] for global optimization over continuous spaces. Its main performance advantages over other evolutionary algorithms [3,4] lie in floating-point encoding and a good combination of evolutionary operators, the mutation step size adaptation, and elitist selection. The DE has a main evolution loop in which a population of vectors is computed for each generation of the evolution loop. During one generation g, for each vector $\mathbf{x}_i$, $\forall i \in \{1, 2, ..., NP\}$ in the current population, DE employs evolutionary operators, namely mutation, crossover, and selection, to produce a trial vector (offspring) and to select one of the vectors with the best fitness value. NP denotes population size and $g \in \{1, 2, ..., G\}$, the current generation number [26].

Mutation creates a mutant vector $\mathbf{v}_{i,g+1}$ for each corresponding population vector. Among many proposed, one of the most popular DE mutation strategies [19,22] are the 'rand/1':

$$\mathbf{v}_{i,g+1} = \mathbf{x}_{r_1,g} + F(\mathbf{x}_{r_2,g} - \mathbf{x}_{r_3,g})$$

and the 'best/1':

$$\mathbf{v}_{i,g+1} = \mathbf{x}_{best,g} + F(\mathbf{x}_{r_1,g} - \mathbf{x}_{r_2,g}),$$

where the indexes r_1, r_2, and r_3 represent the random and mutually different integers generated within the range $\{1, 2, ..., NP\}$ and also different from index i. The $\mathbf{x}_{best,g}$ denotes the currently best vector. F is an amplification factor of the difference vector within the range $[0, 2]$, but usually less than 1. The first term in the mutation operators defined above is a base vector. Following, the difference of two chosen vectors denotes a difference vector which after multiplication with F, is known as amplified difference vector. The simple DE mutation 'rand/1' is by far most widely used [8], however, a form of 'best/1' mutation has also been signified beneficial, especially in more restrictive evaluation scenarios [2,15,24,26].

After mutation the mutant vector $\mathbf{v}_{i,g+1}$ is taken into recombination process with the target vector $\mathbf{x}_{i,g}$ to create a trial vector $\mathbf{u}_{i,g+1} = \{u_{i,1,g+1}, u_{i,2,g+1}, ..., u_{i,D,g+1}\}$. The binary crossover operates as follows:

$$u_{i,j,g+1} = \begin{cases} v_{i,j,g+1} & \text{if } rand(0, 1) \leq CR \text{ or } j = j_{rand} \\ x_{i,j,g} & \text{otherwise} \end{cases},$$

where $j \in \{1, 2, ..., D\}$ denotes the j-th search parameter of D-dimensional search space, $rand(0, 1) \in [0, 1]$ denotes a uniformly distributed random number, and j_{rand} denotes a uniform randomly chosen index of the search parameter, which is always exchanged to prevent cloning of target vectors. CR denotes the crossover rate [23].

Finally, the selection operator propagates the fittest individual [7] in the new generation (for minimization problem):

$$\mathbf{x}_{i,g+1} = \begin{cases} \mathbf{u}_{i,g+1} & \text{if } f(\mathbf{u}_{i,g+1}) < f(\mathbf{x}_{i,g}) \\ \mathbf{x}_{i,g} & \text{otherwise} \end{cases}.$$

In [5], population size reduction was introduced, where population size is reduced by half, when number of generations exceeds ratio between the number of function evaluations allowed and the population size:

$$G_p > \frac{N_{max\_Feval}}{p_{max} NP_p}.$$

2.2   Underwater Glider Path Planning

An ocean glider is an autonomous vehicle that propels itself changing its buoyancy. The resultant vertical velocity is transformed into an effective horizontal displacement by means of the active modification of the pitch angle and the effect of the control surfaces. The glider motion pattern is constituted by a series of "v" descending/ascending profiles between two target maximum and minimum depths, after which the vehicle returns to surface to transmit data and update its target way-points [26].

Ocean gliders constitute an important advance in the highly demanding ocean monitoring scenario. Their efficiency, endurance, and increasing robustness make these vehicles an ideal observing platform for many long-term oceanographic applications [20]. Nevertheless, they have proved to be useful as well in the opportunistic short-term characterization of dynamic structures. Among these, mesoscale eddies are of particular interest due to the relevance they have in many oceanographic processes [13]. The characterization of pollution and harmful algal bloom episodes have been also included as part of recent glider missions. Having the potential of fully autonomous operation, usual control scheme of ocean gliders does not exploit this capacities too much and relies mainly in a human-in-the-loop approach.

Path planning plays a main role in glider navigation [9] as a consequence of the special motion characteristics these vehicles present. Indeed, ocean current velocities are comparable to or even exceed low speed of a glider, typically around 1 km/h (0.28 m/s). In such situations a feasible path must be prescribed to make the glider reach the desired destination. This can be accomplished by analyzing the evolution of the ocean currents predicted by a numerical model. The problem is not trivial, as the planner must take into account a 4D, spatio-temporally varying field over which to optimize. Also, since increasing the number of function evaluations (FES) degrades the optimization execution time and jeopardizes mission planning time (limiting the optimization time to minutes), it is inevitable to put a restriction on FES, e.g. limit to roughly 2000 FES which may compute in a few minutes.

Different solutions to the glider path planning problem can be found in the literature. Inanc et al. [14] propose a method that applies Nonlinear Trajectory Generation (NTG) on a Lagrangian Coherent Structures (LCS) model to generate near-optimal routes for gliders on dynamic environments. Alvarez et al. [1] use Genetic Algorithms (GA) to produce suitable paths in presence of strong currents while trying to minimize energy consumption. Other authors have put the focus on the coordination of glider fleets to define optimal sampling strategies [17]. A multi-objective GA was also applied to autonomous underwater vehicles for sewage outfall plume dispersion observations [18], which considered two objectives, i.e. the maximum number of water samples besides total travel distance minimization.

In the particular case of eddies, the complexity of the path planning scenario is aggravated by the high spatio-temporal variability of these structures and their specific sampling requirements [12]. Garau et al. [11] use an A* search algorithm to find optimal paths over a set of eddies with variable scale and dynamics. Smith et al. [21] propose an iterative optimization method based on the Regional Ocean Modeling System (ROMS) predictions to generate optimal tracking and sampling trajectories for evolving ocean processes. Their scheme includes near real-time data assimilation and has been tested both in simulation and real field experiments. The current state-of-the-art for glider path planning uses optimization based on a Nelder-Mead algorithm [6] (the `fmisearch` Matlab implementation [16]) or genetic algorithms (GA) [13]. In [26], UGPP was addressed using DE and other evolutionary algorithms, where it was suggested that the use of DE is beneficial on the 12 test scenarios, and a real mission was carried out to confirm the viability of the approach.

3 Approach Extension

The population size reduction [5] is used inside DE in this study. Two mechanism are included now into the DE metaheuristic and used for the UGPP, extending the initial approach [26]:

1. the population size reduction from [5,24]
2. interchangeable use of two types of DE strategies (`DE/best` and `DE/rand`) from [24].

All other parameter are kept same as in [26]. In the following section, we present the performance differing with the parameterization of the population size reduction mechanism for different NP, $pmax$, and NP_{min} parameter values. Also, the difference among using `DE/best` and `DE/rand` with different parameter sets, is studied.

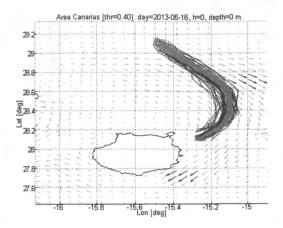

Fig. 1. Phenotype paths obtained using DE/best (Color figure online).

4 Results

In Fig. 1, phenotype paths obtained using DE/best are shown. Trajectory simulations for the 12 bearings computed with best taking population size (NP) as the study factor. For DE/best and NP values are 8 (blue), 32 (purple), 128 (yellow), and 512 (green). Shown are the 120 runs subsampled with step 10 (one run drawn per NP, resulting in 12 trajectories shown).

In Fig. 2, different population sizing settings impact on mean final fitness value for different minimal NP (NP_{min}) and number of reductions ($pmax$) are shown for DE/best, aggregated on 10 independent runs. Also, standard deviation values of the means values are drawn.

In Fig. 3, Bonferroni-Dunn's statistical test of DE/best and DE/rand with some selected different parameter sets are presented. The control algorithm is DE/best setting #47, i.e. DE/best with NP=64, $pmax$=5, NP_{min}=20), this is a setting #47 out of 84. The control algorithm (we propose this one as favorable) outperforms some DE/best and all DE/rand variants. The sample index identifiers are denoted using the Sample number, listing NP_{min} values and then repeating these for different values of $pmax$ (as indicated in Fig. 2). The value Sample No equals the zero-based index number in the $NP_{min} = \{40, 20, 10\}$ array, added the zero-based index in the $pmax = \{20, 15, 10, 5\}$ array multiplied by 3 and added the zero-based index in the initial $NP = \{512, 256, 128, 64\}$ array multiplied by 12, e.g. for the setting #47 this is $47 = 1 + 0 * 3 + 3 * 12$: these indices are 1, 0, and 3, respectively, i.e. $NP_{min} = 20$, $pmax = 20$, and $NP = 64$.

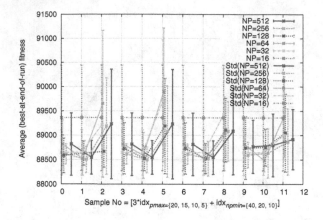

Fig. 2. Different population sizing settings impact on mean final fitness value for DE/best.

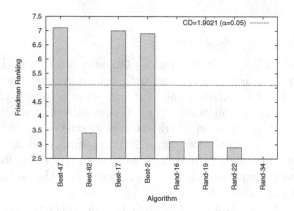

Fig. 3. Bonferroni-Dunn's statistical test of DE/best and DE/rand with different parameter sets.

5   Conclusion

In this paper, we presented an extension of our meta-heuristics research on Underwater Glider Path Planning (UGPP) [13] and Differential Evolution (DE) [24], as initially proposed in the first study on DE and UGPP [26]. Compared to this first study [26], two additional mechanism are included now into the DE metaheuristic and used for the UGPP, (1) the population size reduction from [5,24] and (2) interchangeable use of two types of DE strategies (DE/best and DE/rand) from [24]. The extended abstract of this paper was published in [25].

All other parameter are kept same as in [26]. We presented experimental results for the performance differing with the parameterization of the population size reduction mechanism for different NP, $pmax$, and $NP_{\min}$ parameter values.

Also, the difference among using DE/best and DE/rand with different parameter sets, was presented and the DE/best proposed as a better candidate in the test framework. Thereby, the proposed confirmed improvement contributes to extend the operational capabilities of the glider vehicle and to improve its value as a marine sensor, facilitating the implementation of flexible sampling schemes.

In the future work, the approach could be extended using even more aspects of evolutionary algorithm features, including multi-objective optimization and constraint handling.

Acknowledgments. This work was partially funded by the Slovenian Research Agency under project P2-0041 and the Canary Island government and FEDER funds under project 2010/62. The codes in Matlab for extending the optimization algorithms utilized are provided by Qingfu Zhang at http://dces.essex.ac.uk/staff/qzhang/code/.

References

1. Alvarez, A., Caiti, A., Onken, R.: Evolutionary path planning for autonomous underwater vehicles in a variable ocean. IEEE J. Oceanic Eng. **29**(2), 418–429 (2004)
2. Bošković, B., Brest, J., Zamuda, A., Greiner, S., Žumer, V.: History mechanism supported differential evolution for chess evaluation function tuning. Soft Comput. Fusion Found. Method. Appl. **15**(4), 667–682 (2011)
3. Brest, J., Greiner, S., Bošković, B., Mernik, M., Žumer, V.: Self-adapting control parameters in differential evolution: a comparative study on numerical benchmark problems. IEEE Trans. Evol. Comput. **10**(6), 646–657 (2006)
4. Brest, J., Korošec, P., Šilc, J., Zamuda, A., Bošković, B., Maučec, M.S.: Differential evolution and differential ant-stigmergy on dynamic optimisation problems. Int. J. Syst. Sci. **44**(4), 663–679 (2013)
5. Brest, J., Maučec, M.S.: Population size reduction for the differential evolution algorithm. Appl. Intell. **29**(3), 228–247 (2008)
6. Cabrera-Gámez, J., Isern-González, J., Hernández-Sosa, D., Domínguez-Brito, A.C., Fernández-Perdomo, E.: Optimization-Based Weather Routing for Sailboats. In: Sauze, C., Finnis, J. (eds.) Robotic Sailing 2012, pp. 23–34. Springer, Heidelberg (2013)
7. Darwin, C.: On the Origin of Species by Means of Natural Selection, or the Preservation of Favoured Races in the Struggle for Life. John Murray, London (1859)
8. Das, S., Suganthan, P.N.: Differential evolution: a survey of the state-of-the-art. IEEE Trans. Evol. Comput. **15**(1), 4–31 (2011)
9. Davis, R.E., Leonard, N.E., Fratantoni, D.M.: Routing strategies for underwater gliders. Deep Sea Res. Part II **56**(3), 173–187 (2009)
10. Eiben, A.E., Smith, J.E.: Introduction to Evolutionary Computing. Natural Computing Series. Springer, Heidelberg (2003)
11. Garau, B., Alvarez, A., Oliver, G.: Path planning of autonomous underwater vehicles in current fields with complex spatial variability: an A* approach. In: Proceedings of the 2005 IEEE International Conference on Robotics and Automation, ICRA 2005, pp. 194–198. IEEE (2005)
12. Hátún, H., Eriksen, C.C., Rhines, P.B.: Buoyant eddies entering the Labrador Sea observed with gliders and altimetry. J. Phys. Oceanogr. **37**(12), 2838–2854 (2007)

13. Hernández Sosa, D.J., Smith, R., Fernández-Perdomo, E., Isern-González, J., Cabrera, J., Domínguez-Brito, A.C., Prieto-Marañón, V.: Glider path-planning for optimal sampling of mesoscale eddies. In: Moreno-Díaz, R., Pichler, F., Quesada-Arencibia, A. (eds.) EUROCAST 2013, Part II. LNCS, vol. 8112, pp. 321–325. Springer, Heidelberg (2013)

14. Inanc, T., Shadden, S.C., Marsden, J.E.: Optimal trajectory generation in ocean flows. In: Proceedings of the American Control Conference, Portland, OR, USA, pp. 674–679 (2004)

15. Joshi, R., Sanderson, A.: Minimal representation multisensor fusion using differential evolution. IEEE Trans. Syst. Man Cybern. Part A Syst. Hum. 29(1), 1083–4427 (1999)

16. Lagarias, J.C., Reeds, J.A., Wright, M.H., Wright, P.E.: Convergence properties of the Nelder-Mead simplex method in low dimensions. SIAM J. Optim. 9(1), 112–147 (1998)

17. Leonard, N.E., Paley, D.A., Davis, R.E., Fratantoni, D.M., Lekien, F., Zhang, F.: Coordinated control of an underwater glider fleet in an adaptive ocean sampling field experiment in Monterey Bay. J. Field Rob. 27(6), 718–740 (2010)

18. Moura, A., Rijo, R., Silva, P., Crespo, S.: A multi-objective genetic algorithm applied to autonomous underwater vehicles for sewage outfall plume dispersion observations. Appl. Soft Comput. 10(4), 1119–1126 (2010)

19. Price, K.V., Storn, R.M., Lampinen, J.A.: Differential Evolution: A Practical Approach to Global Optimization. Natural Computing Series. Springer, Heidelberg (2005)

20. Rudnick, D.L., Davis, R.E., Eriksen, C.C., Fratantoni, D.M., Perry, M.J.: Underwater gliders for ocean research. Marine Tech. Soc. J. 38(2), 73–84 (2004)

21. Smith, R.N., Chao, Y., Li, P.P., Caron, D.A., Jones, B.H., Sukhatme, G.S.: Planning and implementing trajectories for autonomous underwater vehicles to track evolving ocean processes based on predictions from a regional ocean model. Int. J. Rob. Res. 29(12), 1475–1497 (2010)

22. Storn, R., Price, K.: Differential evolution - a simple and efficient heuristic for global optimization over continuous spaces. J. Global Optim. 11, 341–359 (1997)

23. Zaharie, D.: Influence of crossover on the behavior of differential evolution algorithms. Appl. Soft Comput. 9(3), 1126–1138 (2009)

24. Zamuda, A., Brest, J., Mezura-Montes, E.: Structured population size reduction differential evolution with multiple mutation strategies on CEC 2013 real parameter optimization. In: 2013 IEEE Conference on Evolutionary Computation, vol. 1, pp. 1925–1931, 20–23 June 2013

25. Zamuda, A., Sosa, J.D.H.: Underwater glider path planning and population reduction in differential evolution. In: Fifteenth International Conference on Computer Aided Systems Theory, Museo Elder de la Ciencia y la Tecnologa, Las Palmas de Gran Canaria, Canary Islands, Spain, 8–13 February 2015, pp. 274–275 (2015)

26. Zamuda, A., Sosa, J.D.H.: Differential evolution and underwater glider path planning applied to the short-term opportunistic sampling of dynamic mesoscale ocean structures. Appl. Soft Comput. 24, 95–108 (2014)

On Underwater Vehicle Routing Problem

Wojciech Bożejko$^{(\boxtimes)}$, Szymon Jagiełło, Michał Lower, and Czesław Smutnicki

Faculty of Electronics, Wrocław University of Technology,
Janiszewskiego 11-17, 50-372 Wrocław, Poland
{wojciech.bozejko,szymon.jagiello,michal.lower,
czeslaw.smutnicki}@pwr.edu.pl

Abstract. In the paper we consider a problem of underwater vehicle routing (also called path planning) which can be described as follows: Given positions under water have to be inspected by the mobile robot taking under consideration water currents, minimizing the total time of the inspection. Two elements of such an approach are described here: vehicle positioning method and routing algorithm. We proposed to apply tabu search and dynasearch metaheuristics as routing alogrithms. As efficient metaheuristics, proposed algorithms allows us to determine good solutions (paths) in a very short time.

1 Introduction

Underwater mobile robot which is considered in this paper is small and its dimensions are in the range of the cube $50 \times 50 \times 70$ cm. The device has a low positive buoyancy close to zero and it is equipped with three electric drive motors with the rotors. The two drive motors are used to change the direction of movement of the robot in the horizontal plane, whereas the third motor is used to immerse the robot and to change its vertical position. A permanent connection via a power cable is used to supply energy to electric motors. This means that the maximum range of the robot is associated with the position of the floating base station and the length of the connecting cable. Hence it is assumed that the maximum range of the robot is about 300 m from the base station. The base station is located on the surface of the water. Therefore, determination of its position is not a big problem using e.g. measurements by GPS (Global Positioning System) or GNSS (Global Navigation Satellite Systems). However, the satellite navigation is impossible under water.

Recognizing the problem as a vehicle routing one can observe, that mostly metaheuristics are used for its solving nowadays. Tabu Search (TS) metaheuritics was introduced by Glover [6] as an extension of classical local search methods. It explores the solution space by local search procedure with the use of neighborhoods. Most of TS efficient implementations are based on the multi-start model, a neighborhood decomposition [3] or move acceleration [4]. Congram et al. proposed so-called dynasearch neighborhood [5] based on the idea of exploration of the exponential-size neighborhood in the polynomial time. In the paper we propose to applyt the tabu search metaheuristics and tabu search with backtracking-jump as well as dynasearch to determine underwater vehicle routing path.

© Springer International Publishing Switzerland 2015
R. Moreno-Díaz et al. (Eds.): EUROCAST 2015, LNCS 9520, pp. 861–868, 2015.
DOI: 10.1007/978-3-319-27340-2_105

2   Positioning System

Due to the limited technical capabilities to determine the position of the object underwater a dead reckoning navigation, assisted with the inertial navigation system (INS) and the inertial measurement units (IMU), are often used [8]. Due to the fact that our task refers to an object moving in a short distance and in regular contact with the base station the most preferred method is the short baseline acoustic positioning system (SBL) [7,10]. The measurement of the position of the mobile robot is performed with respect to the position of the base station which position is determined from satellite navigation. It is assumed that the mobile robot moves under water at a speed up to 1 m/s. The measurement of the position of the object in the real aquatic environment must take the characteristics of the environment into account. It turns out that the most effective measuring medium in these conditions are ultrasounds. With the use of ultrasound one can determine the distance in the water, which is proportional to the distance travelled, what is more, one can also determine the speed of the object moving away, which is possible with the use of Doppler effect. The sound propagates in the water at a speed of 1490 m/s which is four times faster than in the air. Thus, the distance measurement by means of ultrasounds at the section of 300 m can be performed in 0.2 s. Assuming a maximum speed of movement of the robot at 1 m/s, it is possible to obtain the position update every 20 cm.

When making distance measurement on the basis of the average of the ultrasonic wave movement in two directions (both: from object to the reference point and from the reference point to the object) it is possible to eliminate data errors resulting from the water movement in which the measurements are taken.

2.1   Underwater Position Determination

Determination of underwater location of object in 3D space by measuring the distance from the points of reference requires designation of appropriate location of the points [2,7,10]. In determination of the robot location under water only by distance measuring, at least three such sensors are necessary. Distribution of reference points has a significant impact on the accuracy of the designated position of the underwater object. The line connecting two basis points is called the baseline (BL). Most preferred is an arrangement in which the lines from the reference points to the position of the underwater object intersect at a right angle. This means that the spacing between the reference points (BL length) should be close to twice the distance between the positioned object and the BL line. On one hand, a practical relationship can be observed here: the greater the immersion of the positioned object or the robot's work area, the greater the BL spacing between reference points. On the other hand, the specificity of the activities carried out by underwater robot determines the required measurement accuracy. Thus, the measurement system used is a compromise between technical capabilities and required expectations regarding the accuracy of the measurement. For large depths exceeding 100 m and for objects working in a large measure space there are such systems as (LBL) Long BaseLine type. In such systems BL has a length of more than 100 m, sometimes reaching several kilometres. For distances of up to several kilometres there is a problem with the enlargement of absolute error of ultrasonic distance measurement. To increase the absolute accuracy of position measuring of the entire work space in LBL system there are often more than three points of reference fixed. In some publications, e.g. [2], LBL system is further narrowed as a measurement system based on the reference points located on the bottom of the tank. If the reference points are located on the surface of the water and their position is corrected with GPS bearing, then this type of system is called GPS intelligent buoys (GIB) system. If the required BL length does not exceed 100 m, measuring systems of this type are called Short baseline (SBL) acoustic positioning systems. The measurement principle is the same as in LBL systems. In SBL systems reference points are often placed on the hull of a ship (vessel) leading or supervising underwater research. Such placement of reference points provides a stable measurement results relative to the vessel. Rigid arrangement between the reference points is preserved, while the position of the vessel can be determined on the basis of GPS data.

Due to the fact that the measurements of the position of the underwater object are often monitored involving small vessels with limited technical possibilities related to the spacing of reference points there are (USBL) Ultra Short BaseLine type measuring systems used. In such solutions BL is small, no more than several meters and, at the same time, many times smaller than the measured distance. In such systems, there is a problem with accurate position measure based only on the distance to the reference points. Such a situation can be seen for instance when working depth of underwater robot is several times greater than the possibility of BL spacing. Therefore, the type of USBL solution is combined with other measurement systems. Location coordinates are combined with dead reckoning navigation, e.g. on the basis of determining the speed and direction of the robot movement from IMU module, based on water pressure there is the depth of immersion defined. By setting the propagation direction of the sound wave it is possible to reduce such system to one reference point located on the vessel which supervisors measurements.

2.2 Design of Measurement System

The task refers to an object that is in constant contact with the base station with the use of a cable connection. The measured object moves approximately 150 m from the vessel which supervises measurements. In the large water area such as in the sea the supervising vessel may have a length of a several dozen meters, which means that in this case the system can be classified as SBL. When using data collected from small vessels - measuring system can be categorized as USBL [2,7,10].

On the object, that is on the underwater robot there is placed a transponder emitting ultrasonic signal, while in reference points there are receivers of this signal. The underwater mobile robot will be equipped with sensors of INS and IMU type, e.g. namely in a magnetometer and a pressure sensor. On the basis of pressure measurement the depth of immersion can be determined. If the object and reference points are in motion, direction of the object movement is known and we have an influence on the position of basis points, then, not only on the basis of the depth of immersion but also two measurements of the distance from the base station the location of an underwater object can be determined. If the base station is a vessel of a length of several meters, then ultrasonic signal receivers (reference points for measuring distances) can be placed on the bow and stern of the ship. Ultrasonic transponder is placed on the mobile robot. If on a small object reference points are located on the stern and on the bow of the vessel, a satisfactory accuracy of the measurements can be obtained when the work distance of the object is not more than twice the length of the vessel.

3   Routing Algorithm

The problem considered can be modelled as a variation of Traveling Salesman Problem (TSP) in which topology positions are modelled as a graph with weighted arcs. Weights of arcs are connected with times of travel between positions (vertexes of the graph), which are combinations of distances and influences of water currents. For the considered problem a tabu search and dynasearch metaheuristics are proposed.

Table 1. Percentage relative deviation for time of calculations 0.01 [s].

problem	%diff TS	TSAB	DS	problem	%diff TS	TSAB	DS	problem	%diff TS	TSAB	DS
gr202	16.7	16.2	12.9	berlin52	14.9	14.9	11.1	gr137	39.3	39.3	30.8
a280	22.4	22.4	21.2	eil101	16.1	16.4	15.7	pr124	15.1	14.2	13.2
pr299	24.3	24.3	21.8	eil51	12.0	12.0	10.6	att48	13.5	13.5	5.7
bier127	6.5	6.5	5.7	pr136	23.8	24.3	23.8	ali535	29.4	29.4	25.0
pr1002	27.8	27.8	26.9	burma14	8.3	3.9	9.4	gr229	25.4	25.4	21.0
pr107	4.6	3.8	1.7	ch130	21.3	21.3	21.1	pr439	22.4	22.4	19.7
eil76	13.8	13.8	13.8	lin105	37.5	37.5	36.5	pr264	17.8	17.8	14.4
att532	28.3	28.3	26.4	ch150	24.6	24.6	24.2	gr431	29.2	29.2	24.8
gil262	30.6	30.6	19.5	gr96	12.0	16.4	10.7	gr666	23.6	23.6	21.8

problem	%diff TS	TSAB	DS
Average	20.8	20.7	18.1

3.1   Tabu Search

Tabu search algorithm was proposed by Fred Glover in 1986 [6]. The idea lies in metaheuristics designed in a way so as to take local optimization methods beyond local optima. Initially, there is a move defined, which is an operation that transforms the solution S into the new solution S'. The set of all elements

Table 2. Percentage relative deviation for time of calculations 0.1 [s].

	%diff				%diff				%diff		
problem	TS	TSAB	DS	problem	TS	TSAB	DS	problem	TS	TSAB	DS
gr202	13.0	12.9	12.9	berlin52	14.9	13.5	6.6	gr137	38.8	38.8	20.4
a280	21.2	21.2	21.2	eil101	14.6	14.3	10.0	pr124	13.2	13.2	9.8
pr299	22.6	22.5	21.8	eil51	12.0	11.7	3.8	att48	13.5	13.5	3.5
bier127	5.6	5.6	5.7	pr136	20.8	20.8	23.8	ali535	27.2	27.2	23.7
pr1002	27.8	27.8	24.8	burma14	8.3	3.9	9.4	gr229	22.1	21.8	21.0
pr107	1.7	1.7	1.7	ch130	21.1	21.1	21.1	pr439	22.1	21.8	19.7
eil76	13.8	13.8	11.0	lin105	35.9	35.9	26.0	pr264	15.1	15.5	14.4
att532	28.1	28.1	25.0	ch150	24.2	24.2	24.2	gr431	28.2	28.2	24.3
gil262	23.5	23.2	19.5	gr96	10.7	10.3	10.7	gr666	23.6	23.6	21.2

	%diff		
problem	TS	TSAB	DS
Average	19.4	19.1	16.2

that can be generated from a given solution S by means of a defined move is called the neighborhood $N(S)$ of the given solution.

The primary TS mechanism consists of iterative search of neighborhood $N(S)$. The element from neighbourhood $S' \in N(S)$, for which the value of the cost function $\Theta[S']$ is the best (usually the smallest) becomes the new solution. In order to avoid getting stuck in a local optima there is an additional structure called tabu list T introduced in the algorithm, which in its simplest form contains prohibited solutions or moves. Elements from the list cannot be selected by a static (pre-set) or dynamic (variable during operations) number of iterations. The length of the list directly affects the speed of the method and its ability to exit local minima. Too short list will quickly cause 'getting stuck', whereas too long will adversely affect the speed of the algorithm. In addition, the use of too long list does not guarantee a route out of the current minimum [1].

Typically, the algorithm stops after having executed a preset number of iterations, exceeded maximum runtime, finding a solution that is sufficiently close to the lower estimate or failure to improve after the specified number of iterations or specific time. It should be noted that each TS algorithm implementation is dependent on a given problem.

3.2 Swap-Type Neighborhood

Checking the neighborhood $N(S)$ of *swap*-type consists of generating of all solutions S', which can be obtained by changing the values of the two positions p_1 and p_2 of solution S and designating for them values of the function $\Theta[S']$. The size of the neighborhood without repetitions (a number of possible generated solutions is)

$$|N| = \frac{|S|^2 - |S|}{2}, \tag{1}$$

Table 3. Percentage relative deviation for time of calculations 1 [s].

	%diff				%diff				%diff		
problem	TS	TSAB	DS	problem	TS	TSAB	DS	problem	TS	TSAB	DS
gr202	12.9	12.9	12.9	berlin52	14.9	13.5	4.9	gr137	38.8	35.3	20.9
a280	20.8	20.8	21.2	eil101	14.6	14.3	14.6	pr124	13.2	13.2	13.2
pr299	21.8	21.8	21.8	eil51	12.0	11.7	1.4	att48	13.5	13.5	1.6
bier127	5.6	5.6	5.7	pr136	20.8	16.1	21.1	ali535	25.3	25.3	23.7
pr1002	27.5	27.5	23.9	burma14	8.3	3.9	9.4	gr229	21.0	20.6	21.0
pr107	1.7	1.7	1.7	ch130	21.1	21.1	20.5	pr439	19.8	19.8	19.7
eil76	13.8	13.8	9.7	lin105	35.9	34.8	17.9	pr264	13.7	13.7	14.4
att532	26.8	26.8	25.0	ch150	24.2	24.2	24.2	gr431	25.1	25.1	24.3
gil262	18.4	18.4	19.5	gr96	10.7	9.2	10.7	gr666	22.3	22.3	21.2

	%diff		
problem	TS	TSAB	DS
Average	18.7	18.0	15.8

thus, the computational complexity of generating of all the solutions S' without designation the values of given functions is $O(n^2)$.

3.3 Tabu Search Algorithm with Back Jump Tacking

Use of the best solutions from the given neighbourhood as the start solutions results in the loss of history of previous searches. In case of 'being stuck' in the local minimum, the only thing left is to choose a new solution starting with an empty tabu list. In 1996, E. Nowicki and C. Smutnicki proposed a modification to the basic version, which enables the multiple use of neighborhoods of the selected solutions [9].

During its operation, the proposed method uses an additional tabu list L. Each time when the algorithm encounters a solution better than the previous one, it saves the current solution and T list on L list. The solution chosen in the next iteration is added to the saved T list. The elements on L list are sorted by cost function value $\Theta[S]$ [12].

In case of 'being stuck' in the local minimum, the algorithm returns to the best solution from L list. The return concerns also T list [9]. This approach ensures that the next chosen solution will be different than previously selected. In addition, in such an implementation the new solution is added to the stored T list, what allows for multiple returns, whereas the number of possible returns is equal to the length of T list minus one. After having used this limit, the solution is removed from L list. It is possible to compare the basic TS algorithm to exploration of the segment of the solution space, whereas TSAB - to the procedure of its exploration.

3.4 Dynasearch

Descent and iterative improvement algorithms are a simple and fast optimization method. The algorithm searches a better solution in the neighbourhood $N(S)$ of a given solution S. If it exists it becomes the current solution and the procedure is repeated. If there is no better solution then the algorithm terminates. An effective approach is to create a new starting solution by performing a permutation procedure on the final one and restarting the algorithm.

The quality of the obtained result depends heavily on the neighbourhood. A small one will be checked faster but will cause to terminate quickly. A big one will give better results but the computational effort will be higher. The main idea of the DS algorithm is to provide an efficient way of checking neighbourhoods which are obtained by performing series of moves instead a single one and which size is exponential [5]. The neighbourhood is explored in polynomial time by using dynamic programming techniques.

The dynasearch algorithm finds the best solution which can be obtained by using a combination of independent moves. The size of such neighbourhood for the swap move is $2^{n-1} - 1$ but the result can be obtained in $O(n^2)$ time.

4 Computational Experiments

In order to verify the proposed algorithms there were tests carried out on selected instances taken from TSPLIB [11]. The study was performed on a machine equipped with Inter i7 X980 processor, the operating system with the kernel 3.2.0.70-generic or gcc 4.6.3 compiler. During its work, the device may encounter unforeseen obstacles that prevent it to visit all the required points on the pre-planned route. Such situation will require designation of a new route, which takes into account the above problem. All the computations will have to be made in very limited time, so the emphasis is placed on the quality of the solutions obtained in specific units of time: 0.01[s], 0.1[s], 1[s]. Percentage deviation between the obtained result and the best known result for each problem and average percentage deviation was calculated. The obtained results are shown in Tables 1, 2, 3.

The environment in which the device is working is diverse and vulnerable to unpredicted changes. In this situation we can not use an algorithm which gives even the optimal solution for a single problem but fails at other instances. Therefore the current research stage was focused on selecting the most universal method. The proposed procedures were tested by using 27 problem instances. The results confirmed the superiority of the TSAB method over the TS method. A very fast exploration of a large neighbourhood caused that the DS algorithm turned out to be the best choice. In this situation it will be used in further development of the project.

5 Conclusions

The paper presents tabu search and dynasearch algorithms for the underwater vehicle routing problem. Tests were carried out on literature test data taken from the TSPLIB [11]. Computational experiments shows, that dynasearch algorithm outperforms other approaches in the matter of solutions quality as well as running time, in all time ranges (0.01, 0.1, 1 s) which makes it a very good algorithmic solution for vehicle route determination.

References

1. Abdullah, S., Ahmadi, S., Burke, E.K., Dror, M., McCollum, B.: A tabu based large neighbourhood search methodology for the capacitated examination timetabling problem. J. Oper. Res. **58**(11), 1494–1502 (2006)
2. Alcocer A., Oliveira P., Pascoal, A.: Underwater acoustic positioning systems based on buoys with GPS. In: Proceedings of the Eighth European Conference on Underwater Acoustics, 8th ECUA, Carvoeiro, 12–15 June 2006
3. Bożejko, W., Pempera, J., Smutnicki, C.: Parallel tabu search algorithm for the hybrid flow shop problem. Comput. Ind. Engi. **65**, 466–474 (2013)
4. Bożejko, W., Uchroński, M., Wodecki, M.: Parallel hybrid metaheuristics for the flexible job shop problem. Comput. Ind. Engi. **59**, 323–333 (2010)
5. Congram, R.K., Potts, C.N., Van de Velde, S.L.: An iterated dynasearch algorithm for the single maschine total weighted tardiness scheduling problem. INFORMS J. Comput. **14**(1), 52–67 (2002)
6. Glover, F.: Future paths for integer programming and links to artificial intelligence. Comput. Oper. Res. **1**(3), 533–549 (1986)
7. Hegrenaes, O., Berglund, E., Hallingstad, O.: Model-aided inertial navigation for underwater vehicles. In: IEEE International Conference on Robotics and Automation, pp. 1069–1076 (2008)
8. Kaniewski, P.: Integrated positioning system for Auv. Mol. Quantum Acoust. **26**, 115–128 (2005)
9. Nowicki, E., Smutnicki, C.: A fast taboo search algorithm for the job shop problem. Manage. Sci. **42**(6), 797–813 (1996)
10. Stutters, L., et al.: Navigation technologies for autonomous underwater vehicles. IEEE Trans. Syst. Man Cybern. Part C: Appl. Rev. **38**(4), 581–589 (2008)
11. TSPLIB: http://www.iwr.uni-heidelberg.de/groups/comopt/software/TSPLIB95/
12. Watson, J.P., Howe, A.E., Whitley, L.D.: Deconstructing Nowicki and Smutnicki's i-TSAB tabu search algorithm for the job-shop scheduling problem. Comput. Oper. Res. **33**, 2623–2644 (2005)

Belief Space Planning for an Underwater Floating Manipulator

Enrica Zereik[1]([✉]), Francesco Gagliardi[1], Marco Bibuli[1], Andrea Sorbara[1],
Gabriele Bruzzone[1], Massimo Caccia[1], and Fabio Bonsignorio[2,3]

[1] Institute of Intelligent Systems for Automation -
National Research Council, Genova, Italy
enrica.zereik@ge.issia.cnr.it
[2] The BioRobotics Institute - Scuola Superiore Sant'Anna, Pisa, Italy
[3] Heron Robots s.r.l., Genova, Italy

Abstract. Control of robots for underwater intervention and manipulation in real world applications is very challenging due high environmental uncertainties. Techniques based on Belief Space Planning (BSP) are very promising in order to achieve robust robot behaviors in the presence of uncertainties within complex and unstructured scenarios. Here a BSP strategy is developed to control an underwater robotic manipulator. Experiments proved the method effectiveness and reliability.

Keywords: Belief space planning · Stochastic control · Underwater manipulation

1 Introduction

The control of manipulators within real-world applications poses great challenges: non-linear dynamics, quickly changing environmental factors and limited information gathering strongly affect its effectiveness. More specifically, in subsea scenarios, robotic researchers have to cope with huge uncertainties, affecting the state estimation and the measurement accuracy. Additional noise is further introduced on underwater measurements by the usually employed video/acoustic systems and by the sea condition that can cause low predictability.

The present work deals with stochastic mobile manipulation problems, focusing on the control of a robotic arm mounted on-board a (possibly unmanned) stochastic floating platform (i.e. an AUV - Autonomous Unmmanned Vehicle or a ROV - Remotely Operated Vehicle). The desired task consists in grasping an object whose absolute position is unknown; its relative position (with respect to the end-effector) can be measured by a proper sensor (e.g. a simple camera or a sonar), providing inaccurate measurements due to dirty water and turbolences.

The selected strategy is the Belief Space Planning (BSP) approach, which is able to plan a finite horizon trajectory in the belief state, i.e. the set of all possible distributions of the system states. Thus, two concurrent control goals can be fulfilled: (i) reduction of the distance between the end-effector and the

© Springer International Publishing Switzerland 2015
R. Moreno-Díaz et al. (Eds.): EUROCAST 2015, LNCS 9520, pp. 869–876, 2015.
DOI: 10.1007/978-3-319-27340-2_106

target object; (ii) decrease of the uncertainty on the system state. Manipulation planning via the BSP approach (based on the assumption of maximum likelihood observation) has already been proposed in [9], where only simulative results have been reported in a highly simplified scenario. The main contributions of the present work with respect to [9] are:

- the integration of the BSP to drive the arm inverse kinematics
- the generalization from 2D to 3D
- the discussion of the role of the LQR optimization in the overall control loop
- the application on a real world arm

As already suggested, the great benefit of such BSP technique is the ability to explicitly take into account and handle measurement uncertainties that often impair task execution. At the same time, there are also many open issues such as the required computational effort and time constraint to be satisfied in order to plan a trajectory in a real-time fashion.

The remainder of this paper is organized as follows: Sect. 2 provides a brief state-of-the-art, while Sect. 3 describes the employed methodology. Finally, Sect. 4 depicts the robotic setup and reports the experimental results. Final remarks, future work and conclusion are drawn in Sect. 5.

2   Related Works

The problem of manipulating in an underwater environment can be modeled as a POMDP (Partially Observable Markov Decision Process); since work in [8] showed the impossibility to find an exact solution, several approaches have been developed to find an approximate solution to the problem. In [6] non spherical robots are handled by exploiting the 'sigma hulls' associated to their geometry through the Unscented Kalman Filters. In [1,2] the viability of BSP methods is shown for real time application in mobile robotics by using a multi-query POMDP method.

Many works can be found in literature, simulating algorithms for motion planning able to take into account robot uncertainties. Simulation of a new point-based POMDP algorithm that improves computational efficiency is reported in [5]. Other solutions to the robot path planning problem are detailed in [7,11]. The computational cost of such approaches is discussed in [10], which show that planning in belief space can be performed efficiently for linear Gaussian systems.

3   Proposed Methodology

In the present work, the BSP method has been extended and applied to a real ECA ARM 5E MICRO manipulator, refer to [4], that has to be mounted on a AUV. The developed system integrates a belief space planning on top of a classical inverse kinematics-control. The arm kinematics is assumed to be deterministic, with high repeatabilty and accuracy. Up to now, the vehicle and arm

control systems are assumed to be separate; note that the motion of the floating platform is stochastically independent from the motion of the object to be
grasped. In the considered problem, the measures are affected by significant
errors but can anyhow be modeled as linear Gaussian (the platform controller
ensures that this assumpion holds); the reduction of uncertainty (optimized by
BSP) together with the probability of reaching the goal position is very desirable. Assuming maximum likelihood observations, as demonstrated by [9], it is
possible to effectively use techniques of non linear optimization, such as Direct
Transcription and Linear Quadratic Programming, see [3], in the belief space.
A belief space trajectory for the end-effector of the robot moves it from its current
position to a goal (with mean value in the desired position and lower variance),
both expressed as Gaussian PDFs (Probability Density Functions). For example
the belief space for a material point moving along a single dimension is given
by the cartesian product of all the possible real values of the mean and variance
that can represent, by a Gaussian, its position. In general this trajectory will be
non linear for a manipulation system like the employed one.

First, the trajectory is approximated by a series of segments in the belief
space, optimized by Direct Transcription. Then a Linear Quadratic Regulator
is applied to move from a segment to the following one. An iteration on the
segments of the linearized trajectory is performed until the desired end point
is reached in the belief space. The actions in the belief space actually weigh
the objectives to move the end-effector in the desired position and to reduce
the variance of the observations. As a consequence, they can be regarded as
information gathering actions. In general, even in the case of a coarse-grained
approximation of the belief space, the planning has to be performed in an higher
dimensional state than the state space; moreover the belief state dynamics is
non linear, stochastic and inherently and significantly under actuated (as the
number of control input is lower than the dimensions of the belief space). With
the assumption of maximum likelihood observations, the problem is simplified.
In other terms, it is assumed that the state of the system is the most likely
state according to the past observations and the performed action, i.e. that the
actions achieve their intended purpose. In [9] it is demonstrated that this kind of
linearization is optimal under linear Gaussian process assumptions and generates
reasonable behaviors in a neighbourhood of the linearization points. Experiments
so far seem to confirm this, although more extensive test campaigns are needed
and will be performed in the near future.

The controller moves the end-effector on the basis of the information gathered
by the sensors and the estimation of the state of the system. A deterministic
function f links the new state to the old one under the control action u_t and the
observations z performed by the system are a stochastic function g of the state
of the system and of a zero mean Gaussian noise ω as in:

$$x_{t+1} = f(x_t, u_t) \tag{1}$$
$$z_t = g(x_t) + \omega$$

The controller is assumed to know the state through a probabilistic density function $P(x)$. The parameters of this distribution are the "belief state". Assuming linear Gaussian belief state dynamics, the belief state can be updated by the following rules:

$$x_{t+1} = A_t (x_t - m_t) + f (m_t, u_t) \tag{2}$$
$$z_t = C_t (x_t - m_t) + g (f (m_t, u_t)) + \omega$$

where m_t is the mean of the belief state and A_t and C_t are the Jacobian matrices $A_t = \frac{\delta f}{\delta x} (m_t, u_t)$, $C_t = \frac{\delta g}{\delta x} (m_t)$. The Gaussian distribution is given by:

$$\Sigma_t : P(x) = \mathcal{N}(x/m_t, \Sigma_t) \tag{3}$$

In these hypotheses, by assuming maximum likelihood of the observations, it is possible to derive by iteration a series of segments with an associated set of control actions by minimizing the cost function J,

$$J(b_{\tau:T}, u_{\tau:T}) = \sum_{i=1}^{k} w_i \left(\hat{n}_i^T \Sigma_T \hat{n}_i \right)^2 + \sum_{t=\tau}^{T-1} \tilde{m}_t^T Q \hat{m}_t + \tilde{u}_t^T R \tilde{u}_t \tag{4}$$

where $b_{\tau:T}$ is the subset the state space, $u_{\tau:T}$ are the corresponding actions, for a given state space trajectory, Q and R are weight matrices, n_i, are the belief space versors along which the optimization is performed; Σ_T is the covariance matrix at the end of the segment, m_t^T the value of the mean of the Gaussian of the measures. The cost function J is minimized by a standard SQP (Sequential Quadratic Programming) algorithm. The interested reader can refer to [3,9] for details.

4   Experiments

The previously defined strategy, based on a trajectory planning in the belief space, has been simulated and then implemented on the ECA robotic arm described below. Results are here reported.

4.1   Robotic Setup

The 5E MICRO ARM by ECA Robotics is designed to work in an underwater environment at a maximum depth of 3000 m. It has 5 Degrees of Freedom (DoFs) with 5 brushless 24 VDC electric motors, that control four rotational links plus a simple gripper at the end-effector. It can be modelled as a planar arm constituted by a shoulder (θ_2) and an elbow (θ_3); the work plane can be modified through the elevator joint (θ_1). The wrist joint (θ_4) is responsible only for the orientation of the end-effector and will be not considered in the following discussion. The electronics of the robotic arm is constituted by a surface control unit and a subsea housing. These two units communicate with

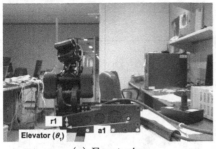

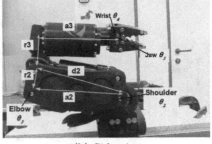

(a) Front view   (b) Side view

Fig. 1. Scheme of ECA arm 5E Micro: geometrical parameters and joint rotation axes are illustrated.

the manipulator through serial port (RS232) and CAN (Controlled Area Network) bus. The manipulator has been geometrically characterized by evaluating its direct and inverse kinematics functions; it is depicted in Fig. 1(a) and (b), highlighting all its geometric parameters. Controls on geometrical constraints and joint velocities of the manipulator are applied to prevent any damage to the structure.

4.2 Results

Many experiments were conducted, up to now on the arm in air, demonstrating the effectiveness of the approach. In fact, the trajectory planner was able to find a path for the manipulator that allowed it to reach the object detected by the sensor. During the test campaign, without loss of validity for the control strategy, such sensor has been simulated. Because of the complexity of the underwater environment, the simulation scenario was modeled to be as more realistic as possible. Therefore, the target is modeled as a sphere of given radius: outside this radius the measurement function gradient is defined to be zero, hence the sensor is not able to detect the target. Furthermore, state-dependent noise is defined to be directly proportional to the distance between the end-effector and the target: the measurements become more precise while the end-effector approaches the target. The dynamics of the system and the observations are modeled as $f(x_t, u_t) = x_t + u_t$ and $z_t = x_t + \omega$, respectively.

The object was placed in $x_{goal} = [4.3\ 23.7\ -0.05]\ m$ and the end-effector started from $x_0 = [2.2\ 8.8\ 6.85]\ m$. The covariance matrix was initialized as $V = diag(1, 1, 1)$ while the acceptance threshold for the final position was set to $\xi = 0.5\ m$. Note that this threshold assesses the accepted error on the final end-effector position and represents a trade-off between the final grasping precision and the time required to execute the task (the more accuracy required, the more time needed). In Fig. 2(a) the 3D end-effector trajectory found by BSP algorithm is shown. The arm end-effector converges to the object location, indicated by the red circle, in a defined number of steps (in this case $n = 20$) reaching the final

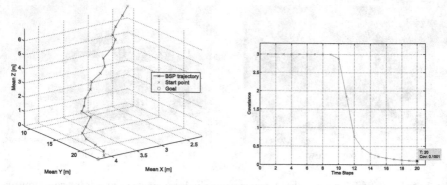

(a) 3D end-effector trajectory found by BSP (b) Covariance time evolution along the
algorithm   trajectory depicted in Fig. 2(a)

Fig. 2. Planned trajectory and related covariance (Color figure online)

belief mean $[m_x, m_y, m_z] = [4.16\ 23.7\ 0.13]\ m$, which correctly falls within the
imposed threshold. The evolution of the 3×3 covariance matrix is reported in
Fig. 2(b) where the quadratic sum of the covariance matrix elements is reported
as a function of the time steps. Covariance begins to decrease when the system
detects the object, i.e. when the end-effector enters the region of space where
the measurement function gradient is not zero; before that, the covariance of the
system does not change.

The efficiency of BSP planning is improved by the adoption of LQR (Linear
Quadratic Regulation) standard control: the evaluation of the optimal control
action for the system leads to the stabilization of the trajectory in spite of
the non linear dynamics. LQR control, allowing to handle small divergences
from the planned motion, minimizes the number of needed replanning steps,
improving the algorithm computational efficiency. Figure 3 shows a comparison
between trajectories evaluated by using the LQR optimal control technique or
not. In the reported example the necessary replanning steps are 12 and 80,
respectively; it has been observed that the statistical LQR calculation produces
a decrease of computing time of about 70 %, leading also to smoother and more
efficient motion of the end-effector. The planned trajectory had to be scaled
before being sent and executed by the real robot, in order to comply with the
manipulator workspace limitations. In particular, the object was placed in $\hat{x}_f =$
$[0.11\ 0.75\ -0.04]\ m$ and the end-effector started from $x_0 = [0.04\ 0.26\ 0.195]\ m$,
reaching the final position $x_f = [0.1041\ 0.7415\ -0.0288]\ m$. Note that the
workspace is really very limited. However, this neither affects the correctness of
the experiment, nor represents a problem: in the planned perspective of applying
the algorithm to an arm mounted on-board an AUV, the vehicle can support
the manipulation system with its own motion, bringing the robot close to the
object to be grasped. Figure 4 shows the time evolution of both the manipulator
cartesian position $[x\ y\ z]$ and the end-effector cartesian error. Note that, apart

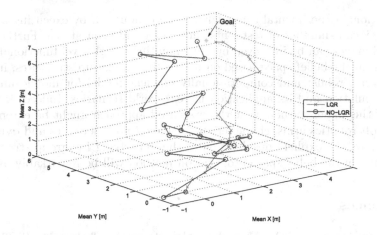

Fig. 3. BSP trajectories evaluated with and without LQR stabilization.

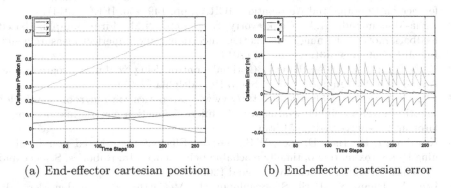

(a) End-effector cartesian position   (b) End-effector cartesian error

Fig. 4. Time evolution of the end-effector cartesian postion and error during the execution of BSP algorithm applied on ECA manipulator (number of steps $n = 10$). A classical Jacobian-based control system is used to drive the robot in each step of the trajectory

from the gripper, only 3 of the 4 arm DoFs are involved in the motion (the end-effector orientation is up to now disregarded).

5 Conclusion and Future Work

One of the main challenges of underwater robotic manipulation and grasping consists in facing and managing the uncertainty introduced by both the harshness of the working environment by and the employed sensors. BSP techniques are a powerful tool in order to obtain motion planning and control, as well as to increase the manipulator grasping effectiveness.

Further development steps are foreseen. First of all, the experimental setup will be refined by substituting the simulated distance sensor with a real sensor.

An additional experimental campaign will be conducted, by executing a statistical significant number of tests, first in a pool and then at sea. Furthermore, BSP techniques can be improved by implementing a high level functional representation of the belief space based on underlying Lie group structures, in order to develop a robust and computationally efficient model for mobile underwater manipulation and its application in real world scenarios. Indeed, it is firm belief of this paper authors that the presented approach might be extended to lighter soft robotics arms, characterized by uncertain kinematics and dynamics. In that case, the explict consideration of the underlying Lie group structure of the motion in the belief space propagation method will be remarkably useful.

References

1. Agha-mohammadi, A.A., Agarwal, S., Mahadevan, A., Chakravorty, S., Tomkins, D., Denny, J., Amato, N.M.: Robust online belief space planning in changing environments: Application to physical mobile robots. In: 2014 IEEE International Conference on Robotics and Automation (ICRA), pp. 149–156. IEEE (2014)
2. Agha-Mohammadi, A.A., Chakravorty, S., Amato, N.M.: Firm: sampling-based feedback motion planning under motion uncertainty and imperfect measurements. Int. J. Robot. Res. **33**(2), 268–304 (2014)
3. Betts, J.T.: Practical Methods for Optimal Control Using Nonlinear Programming. Advances in Design and Control. Siam, Philadelphia (2001)
4. ECA Robotics Arm 5E Micro. http://www.eca-robotics.com/en/robotic-vehicle/robotics-naval-manipulator-arms-arm-5e-micro-5-function-electric-micro-manipulator-arm-of-only-2.7-kg/551.htm
5. Kurniawati, H., Hsu, D., Lee, W.S.: Sarsop: Efficient point-based pomdp planning by approximating optimally reachable belief spaces. In: Robotics: Science and Systems, vol. 2008, Zurich, Switzerland (2008)
6. Lee, A., Duan, Y., Patil, S., Schulman, J., McCarthy, Z., van den Berg, J., Goldberg, K., Abbeel, P.: Sigma hulls for gaussian belief space planning for imprecise articulated robots amid obstacles. In: 2013 IEEE/RSJ International Conference on Intelligent Robots and Systems (IROS), pp. 5660–5667. IEEE (2013)
7. Ong, S.C., Png, S.W., Hsu, D., Lee, W.S.: Planning under uncertainty for robotic tasks with mixed observability. Int. J. Robot. Res. **29**(8), 1053–1068 (2010)
8. Papadimitriou, C.H., Tsitsiklis, J.N.: The complexity of markov decision processes. Math. Oper. Res. **12**(3), 441–450 (1987)
9. Platt Jr., R., Tedrake, R., Kaelbling, L., Lozano-Perez, T.: Belief space planning assuming maximum likelihood observations. In: Proceedings of Robotics: Science and Systems (2010)
10. Prentice, S., Roy, N.: The belief roadmap: efficient planning in belief space by factoring the covariance. Int. J. Robot. Res. **28**(11–12), 1448–1465 (2009)
11. Spaan, M.T.: A point-based pomdp algorithm for robot planning. In: Proceedings of IEEE International Conference on Robotics and Automation, ICRA 2004, vol. 3, pp. 2399–2404. IEEE (2004)

Intervention Payload for Valve Turning with an AUV

Marc Carreras[✉], Arnau Carrera, Narcís Palomeras, David Ribas,
Natàlia Hurtós, Quim Salvi, and Pere Ridao

Computer Vision and Robotics Institute, University of Girona, 17071 Girona, Spain
marc.carreras@udg.edu
http://cirs.udg.edu

Abstract. This paper presents an intervention payload for an AUV
working in a valve turning operation in free-floating control mode. The
payload consists of a stereo camera for panel detection, a 4 degrees of
freedom electrical manipulator and a specifically designed end-effector,
which contains a force and torque sensor, an in-hand camera and a passive effector for valve operation. This payload was designed to be integrated in Girona 500 AUV in the context of an oil application, in which
a valve panel must be operated by turning some of the T-bar handles.
The paper describes the design of the payload and its interaction with
AUV. It also describes the perception systems that have been developed
to detect and operate the valves. Experiments in a water tank show the
performance of the AUV and the suitability of the payload.

Keywords: Autonomous underwater vehicle · Intervention AUV

1 Introduction

Intervention-AUVs (I-AUVs) will substitute in the future some of the repetitive
tasks that nowadays are being done by ROVs in Oil & Gas infrastructures and
other domains. Simple touching applications, such as galvanic measurement at
different junction points of long pipes, will be automated by using I-AUVs. Also,
intervention applications such as valve turning in a ROV panel, will be done by
I-AUVs, which will be in charge of operating underwater infrastructures.

In order to achieve these extended capabilities, several research projects have
already done the first steps towards this future technology. ALIVE project [2]
developed an I-AUV which was able to dock using an hydraulic gripper to an
underwater panel and perform a simple manipulation. The SAUVIM project [5]
performed the manipulation of an underwater object using an I-AUV in free-
floating mode. TRIDENT project [7] developed a system to search and recover
known objects from the seabed using an I-AUV. TRITON project [6] demonstrated the manipulation of valves and connectors while being docked in a sub-sea
station. Finally, Pandora [4] project worked in the operation of valves in free-
floating control mode. This paper presents the intervention payload that was

© Springer International Publishing Switzerland 2015
R. Moreno-Díaz et al. (Eds.): EUROCAST 2015, LNCS 9520, pp. 877–884, 2015.
DOI: 10.1007/978-3-319-27340-2_107

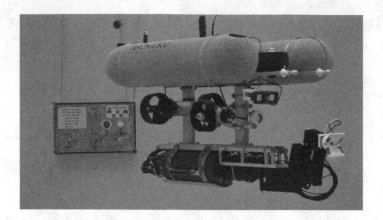

Fig. 1. Girona 500 AUV in the water tank, equipped with a stereo camera, a manipulator and a customized end-effector. At the background there is a mock-up of a valve panel.

developed in the Pandora project [4] for valve turning (see Fig. 1). The payload consist of: (1) a stereo camera with lighting for accurate panel detection and positioning with respect to it; (2) a 4 Degrees Of Freedom (DOF) electrical manipulator with position feedback from each joint; and (3) a specifically designed end-effector mounted at the end of the manipulator, which also contains a passive V-shape for T-bar handle turning, a video camera in the middle of the V-shape for handle detection and a Force/Torque (F/T) sensor for detecting the contact between the end-effector and the panel.

The paper describes how the payload was designed and integrated in Girona 500 AUV. It describes the video processing system done for panel and valve detection, and the F/T sensor processing for contact estimation. The paper is structured as follows. After the introduction in Sect. 1, Sect. 2 will present the design of the payload and the integration of all systems: manipulator, end-effector and stereo camera. Section 3 will detail all perception systems required for the valve turning application: manipulator-AUV calibration, panel and valve detection and F/T contact detection. Section 4 will show some results, pointing out the suitability of the intervention payload for I-AUV applications, and it will also conclude the paper.

2   Payload Design

2.1   Manipulator

Girona 500 can operate as an I-AUV when a manipulator is integrated in the payload area. For the panel intervention task, a 4 rotational DOFs commercial manipulator (ECA ARM 5E Micro) has been used, shown in Fig. 2a. The manipulator can control the Cartesian position (X,Y,Z) and the *roll* (Φ) of the end-effector. Since the manipulator is under-actuated, *pitch* and *yaw* depend on

(a) (b)

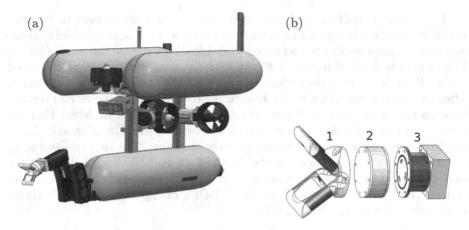

Fig. 2. (a) Girona 500 AUV with the 4 DOFs ECA manipulator equipped with a custom end-effector. (b) 3D model of the disassembled customized end-effector, in which three blocks can be distinguished: (1) passive gripper, (2) camera in-hand and (3) F/T sensor.

the reached Cartesian position. The manipulator is rated for 300 meters and is one of the few commercial electrical manipulators available today. It maintains the typical mechanical configuration of ROV manipulators, which is useful when tele-operating with visual feedback. However, for autonomous intervention, the manipulator has a reduced workspace and low speed, which requires the control of the AUV in combination with the manipulator to compensate previous drawbacks. Also, internal joint sensors do not provide absolute orientation, and forward kinematics must be done with an accurate calibration. Improved manipulators in the future will allow more advanced underwater intervention applications.

2.2 Custom End-Effector

In order to correctly detect and operate T-bar handles of panel valves with the 4 DOFs manipulator, a custom end-effector was designed and built, as shown in Fig. 2b. The main goal of the end-effector is to compensate the small misalignments in *pitch* and *yaw* that cannot be compensated from the manipulator side, due to the reduced DOFs commented in the previous section. These misalignments depend on the position and orientation of the AUV, which sustains the manipulator, and cannot be corrected at a centimeter scale, unlike the manipulator. Also, there are always some detection and calibration errors which generate some inherent error in the position of the end-effector. Therefore, the external part of the end-effector is a flexible V-shape part which passively corrects the end-effector position and orientation errors, driving the handle of the T-bar valve to its center. The shape of this passive gripper allows the connection of the end-effector and the T-bar handle for rotating the valve, when the manipulator *roll* DOF is actuated.

The second goal of the end-effector is to integrate some sensors to perceive at the intervention point. A first module contains a small analog camera, in the center of the passive gripper, to provide visual feedback during the manipulation. The camera is fixed with respect to the V-shape part and, therefore, it is used to directly measure the orientation error between the end-effector and the valve. After the camera module, a F/T sensor measures the contact forces and torques between the manipulator and the valve. This sensor is used to detect that the contact with the valve handle has been established, by measuring an axial force, and to measure the torque done when rotating the valve. The forces measured by the sensor must take into account the depth of the end-effector, to discount the force generated by the water pressure in the F/T housing. Finally, the complete custom end-effector is mounted in the 4 DOFs manipulator, and will rotate according to the manipulator *roll* DOF.

2.3 Stereo Camera

In order to detect the panel and valve handles, a stereo camera (Point Grey Bumblebee 2) was integrated in the front top side of the vehicle (see Fig. 2a), with a specifically designed underwater aluminium housing for a maximum depth of 500 meters (see Fig. 3a).

3 Perception Systems

3.1 Manipulator-AUV Calibration

The manipulator needs an accurate calibration procedure, since it has no absolute encoders to determine an exact position. The authors have proposed a complete procedure to find the state of all joints.

A visual and mechanical calibration method has been designed. To do so, a visual landmark has been integrated at the last joint (wrist), which connects the end-effector with the manipulator. Then, the manipulator is moved to a predefined position where, if the manipulator is approximately calibrated, the marker will be visible by the stereo camera of the vehicle. The wrist will start rotating slowly the end-effector, first 180° and then −360°. During this process, if the marker is detected in a suitable position and orientation (to avoid false positive detections), the inverse kinematic is computed and the arm is calibrated with the values obtained by the visual feedback. Otherwise, the manipulator is moved to the limit of all joints and calibrated using these known positions. The visual landmark provides a more accurate calibration, and it can be regularly applied whenever the user wants a precise calibration.

The algorithm used to compute the position of the landmark with respect the AUV camera relies on the ARToolkit software library [3] to identify, detect and track marks using a monocular camera (see Fig. 3b).

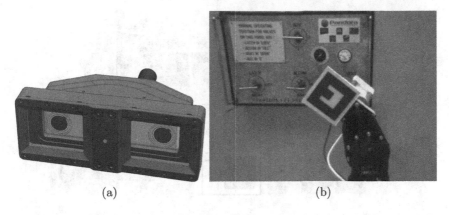

(a)   (b)

Fig. 3. (a) Stereo camera with housing. (b) ARToolkit algorithm detecting landmark mounted on the wrist of the manipulator.

3.2 Panel and Valve Detection

To compute the position of a known landmark, without having to add extra markers, the images gathered by the on-board camera can be compared against an *a priori* known template. In order to extract key-points in the current camera image we use the oriented FAST and rotated BRIEF (ORB) feature extractor that relies on features from accelerated segment test (FAST) corner detection and a binary descriptor vector based on binary robust independent elementary features (BRIEF). These kind of features are present on man-made structures like a valve panel and can be quickly detected.

With these markers, differences between descriptors can be calculated rapidly, allowing real-time matching of key-points at high image frame-rates when compared to other commonly used feature extractors such as scale invariant feature transform (SIFT) and speeded-up robust features (SURF).

Figure 4 illustrates the matching procedure between the *a priori* known template and an image received by the camera. A minimum number of key-points (i.e., 25–40) must be matched between the template and the camera image to satisfy the landmark detection requirement. The detected correspondences are used to compute the transform that relates the template image to the detected landmark. Then, using the camera parameters and the known dimensions of the landmark (i.e., the panel), the landmark's pose can be determined in the camera frame and therefore also in the vehicle frame.

Additionally, since the geometry of the panel is known, the centres of valves on the panel is known in relation to the panel centre. Taking advantage of this, we search a small bounded region of the image for the orientation of the valve. The Hough line transform provides a straightforward method for detecting the orientation of the valves. Outliers are limited by constraining the length of lines and permissible orientations. For more information, please refer to [6].

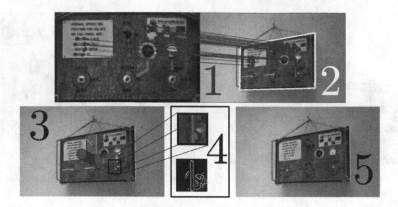

Fig. 4. Steps of the landmark detection: (1) Matching of keypoints between the template and camera image. (2) Estimation of the panel corners in the camera image. (3) Estimation of the template's position and rotation in the image by using the camera parameters and the known geometry of the landmark. (4) Extraction of regions of interest and edges. (5) Estimation of valve orientation using Hough transform to detect lines from the edges.

3.3   F/T Contact Detection

The F/T sensor is used to detect the contact between the end-effector and the valve handle. In order to correctly use this sensor, several corrections must be done:

Depth compensation: The F/T sensor measures the forces and torques that pass through the underwater housing containing the sensor, which resists the water pressure. Therefore, the sensor must discount the force that the water pressure is exerting. In order to do this, the vehicle depth and arm kinematics are used to compute the depth of the end-effector. The pressure of the water generates a force according to the housing area that is compressed, and this force is sustained by the F/T sensor. This force is computed and subtracted from the axial F/T reading.

Drift compensation: F/T sensors use strain gauges to determine applied forces and torques. The output signal of strain gauges drift over time even if there is no applied stimulus. Drift compensation is commonly used in industrial and academic applications of strain gauge based sensors. We use the force/torque data just before a contact to calculate a bias point. The bias point is subtracted from the force/torque output.

Filtering: F/T data are sampled at 250 Hz. The signals are oversampled to avoid aliasing. The F/T data is filtered using a digital filter with a 3 dB point of 2 Hz. After application of the digital filters, the data is down sampled by a factor of 25.

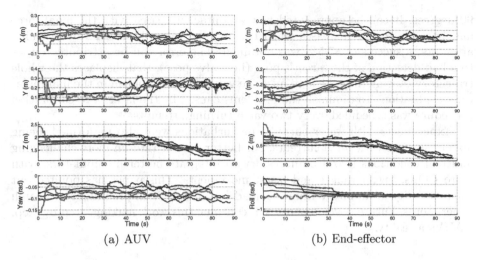

(a) AUV   (b) End-effector

Fig. 5. Tele-operated trajectories (black) for the valve turning task, the upper and lower limit is depicted in dashed-blue and an autonomous trajectory is depicted in red. All trajectories are represented in the frame of the target valve. Each plot shows a single DoF for the AUV and the end-effector (Color figure online).

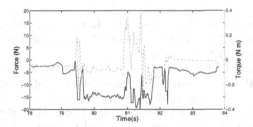

Fig. 6. Force and torque in Z axis measured in the end-effector during grasping and turning. It can be appreciated how a negative force was detected when touching the valve, and how the torque increased when operating the roll DOF (at second 81).

4   Results and Conclusions

The intervention payload has been extensively used in the context of the Pandora EU project, in a valve turning scenario, in which Girona 500 AUV performs autonomous valve turning operations. Figure 5 shows several trajectories in which the 4 DOFs from the AUV and the 4 DOFs from the manipulator were controlled to approach the valve panel and move the end-effector to the valve handle. The coordinates of the trajectories are relative to the valve handle, so it can be appreciated how the trajectories converged to the correct distance for performing the intervention. From these trajectories, 4 of them (in black) were done in teleoperation mode, and one of them (in red) was done in autonomous mode after a learning process, based on Learning by Demontration [1]. Figure 6 shows the force and the torque applied during the action of turning the valve

90 degrees. It can be appreciated how a contact is sensed with the axial force and how the torque increases when turning the valve. From 24 valve turning attempts, a success of 87.5 % was obtained. The error can be attributed either to a bad detection of the target's pose (i.e. valve pose), that displaces the whole trajectory causing the vehicle to miss the valve, or to a problem in the manipulator's calibration. To diminish the problems caused by the later, a re-calibration procedure was scheduled every two valve turning attempts.

Experiments with water currents perturbations were also performed, being able to succeed with small currents. For better success rates in more challenging and real conditions it will be necessary to integrate better manipulators, with more DOFs, bigger ranges and faster movements. This paper has pointed out the suitability of an intervention payload for an I-AUV in preliminary research experiments. Future developments will continue this work making, step by step, I-AUVs a reality.

Acknowledgments. This research was sponsored by PANDORA EU FP7-Project under the Grant agreement FP7-ICT-2011-7-288273. We are grateful for this support.

References

1. Carrera, A., Palomeras, N., Ribas, D., Kormushev, P., Carreras, M.: An intervention-auv learns how to perform an underwater valve turning. In: OCEANS - Taipei, 2014 MTS/IEEE, pp. 1–7 (2014)
2. Evans, J., Redmond, P., Plakas, C., Hamilton, K., Lane, D.: Autonomous docking for intervention-AUVs using sonar and video-based real-time 3D pose estimation. In: OCEANS 2003, vol. 4, pp. 2201–2210 (2003)
3. Kato, H., Billinghurst, M.: Marker tracking and HMD calibration for a video-based augmented reality conferencing system. In: 2nd International Workshop on Augmented Reality (IWAR 1999), San Francisco, USA, October 1999
4. Lane, D., Maurelli, F., Kormushev, P., Carreras, M., Fox, M., Kyriakopoulos, K.: Persistent autonomy: the challenges of the PANDORA project. In: 9th IFAC Conference on Manoeuvring and Control of Marine Craft (MCMC 2012), Arenzano, Italy, September 2012
5. Marani, G., Yuh, S.: Underwater autonomous manipulation for intervention missions AUVs. Oceans Eng. **36**(1), 15–23 (2009)
6. Palomeras, N., Peñalver, A., Massot-Campos, M., Vallicrosa, G., Negre Carrasco, P.L., Fernández, J.J., Ridao, P., Sanz, P.J., Oliver, G.A., Palomer, A.: I-AUV docking and intervention in a subsea panel. In: Intelligent Robots and Systems (IROS 2014). IEEE (2014)
7. Prats, M., Garcia, J., Wirth, S., Ribas, D., Sanz, P., Ridao, P., Gracias, N., Oliver, G.: Multipurpose autonomous underwater intervention: a systems integration perspective. In: 2012 20th Mediterranean Conference on Control Automation (MED), pp. 1379–1384, July 2012

Author Index

Printed in the United States
By Bookmasters